AF898264

# THE SCIENTIFIC BASIS OF CHINESE INTEGRATIVE CANCER THERAPY

Including

# A COLOR ATLAS OF CHINESE ANTICANCER PLANTS

# THE SCIENTIFIC BASIS OF CHINESE INTEGRATIVE CANCER THERAPY

by

Bruce W. Halstead, M.D.

and

Terri Lee Holcomb-Halstead

North Atlantic Books
Berkeley, California

Copyright © 2002 by Bruce W. Halstead, M.D. and Terri Lee Holcomb-Halstead. All rights reserved. No portion of this book, except for brief review, may be reproduced, stored in a retrieval system, or transmitted in any form or by any means—electronic, mechanical, photocopying, recording, or otherwise—without the written permission of the publisher. For information contact North Atlantic Books.

All photographs by Jeffrey McConnell reproduced with permission of Terri Lee Holcomb-Halstead.

All scientific and historical illustrations and drawings reproduced with permission of the World Life Research Institute.

All botanical illustrations reproduced with permission of Terri Lee Holcomb-Halstead and the World Life Research Institute.

Published by
North Atlantic Books
P.O. Box 12327
Berkeley, California 94712

Distributed to the book trade by Publishers Group West

Printed in Hong Kong

*The Scientific Basis of Chinese Integrative Cancer Therapy* is sponsored by the Society for the Study of Native Arts and Sciences, a nonprofit educational corporation whose goals are to develop an educational and cross cultural perspective linking various scientific, social, and artistic fields; to nurture a holistic view of arts, sciences, humanities, and healing; and to publish and distribute literature on the relationship of mind, body, and nature.

**Disclaimer**

This book does not endorse any commercial product. It was written for the express purpose of providing scientific and clinical information on a wide variety of immune enhancing medicinal plants that have shown to have positive therapeutic results in a number of patients suffering from cancer. No cancer cure claims are made. Any person desiring to use any of the medicinal herbs discussed, does so at their own risk and should seek the advice of a physician.

- Bruce W. Halstead
- Terri Lee Holcomb-Halstead

Library of Congress Cataloging-in-Publication Data

Halstead, Bruce W.
The Scientific Basis of Chinese Integrative Cancer Therapy / by Bruce W. Halstead MD and Terri Lee Holcomb-Halstead.
p. ; cm.
Includes bibliographical references and index.
ISBN 1-55643-585-1 (hardcover)
1. Cancer--Treatment. 2. Medicine, Chinese. 3. Cance--Alternative treatment.
I. Holcomb-Halstead, Terri Lee, 1952- . II. Title.
[DNLM: 1. Neoplasms--drug therapy--China. 2. Drugs, Chinese Herbal--China. 3. Medicine, Chinese Traditional--China. 4. Phyto-therapy--methods--China.
QZ 267 H196s 2005]
RC261.H225 2005
616.99'4--dc22

2005022882

1 2 3 4 5 6 7 8 9 Golden Cup Printing, Hong Kong, PRC 10 09 08 07 06 05

# Dedication

**Shen Nung**
The Father of Chinese Herbal Medicine (3494 B.C.)

**Huang Ti**
The brilliant Yellow Empire who first provided and wrote the foundational concepts and structure of Chinese Medicine (2600 B.C.)

**Li Shih-chen**
First to compile a comprehensive written text on these herbs in the *Pen Tsao Kang Mu*

**Professor Zhenguo Wang**
Changbai Mountain Research Institute
Our friend and colleague who has dedicated his entire life to furthering the potential of Chinese Herbal Medicine

**William Harry Moore Jr.**
(June 4, 1928 - August 15, 2002)
Scholar, Lawyer, Warrior, M.D., Mentor, and Beloved Friend. May your work continue forever!

**Marjorie W. Moore**
Thank you for being the wind beneath your husbands wings. May your mission be blessed as you carry on the "great work"!

**John ("Jay") Stewart Holcomb**
(1948-1979)
You gave the world so much compassion and love. Thank you for being a mentor to so many. You inspired us all to look to nature and natural medicine for remedies. You set an example of living in harmony with your own body, mind, and soul. You live on as a part of the wholistic, integrative, and complimentary movement.

**Jack Troop**
Friend, mentor, and colleague. Dedicated to bringing safer and more effective cancer therapies into public awareness.

And to:

**All cancer victims and their families the world over**

# Acknowledgements

This publication was made possible by the China-Japan Feida Union Corporation whose headquarters are in the Kowloon District of Hong Kong, China. Thank you Mr. Lu, Mr. Lee, and all of the CJFU family. May your mission be blessed!

To the cooperation of Professor Zhengou Wang and his entire staff at the Changbai Mountain Research Institute.

Thanks to Mr. Michael Ng and Mr. Frank Cousineau and everyone at Innovative Marketing Group (Modesto, California).

The authors are indebted to Leonette C. Medrano for her monumental contribution in researching, all aspects of editing, design layout, and the preparations necessary for this manuscript for publication. We are also thankful to her for preparing the numerous amounts of artwork and illustrations and for designing the front cover.

A special thanks to Mr. Jeffrey McConnell who worked tirelessly as our photographer, photo editor, and videographer.

The use of the vast library resources of the World Life Research Institute are gratefully acknowledged.

Thank you to artist Robert H. Knabenbauer, of Loma Linda, California who has many outstanding illustrations in this book and also to our friend and artist, Yue Ming Chen, in Beijing, China whose work we so proudly share with the readers throughout the color atlas.

Thank you to the fellow researchers who traveled with us on our fact-finding mission. Dr. Ada Garcia, Dr. Francisco Espinosa of La Playa, Baja California, Dr. Ray Baldwin, PA, Grand Terrace, California, and a thank you to our video documenter, Mr. Anthony J. Hilder of Santa Monica, California.

Special thanks to Ms. Joan Lu, Ms. Carrina Lee, Mr. Thomas Chou, and Mr. Haiwei Chen for translating, coordinating, and being endlessly caring and patient with our traveling team.

Particular thanks to all who contributed to our very memorable experiences in Tokyo, Japan. Special acknowledgement and sincere appreciation to Dr. Hiroyuki Abe, Mr. Kenichiro Sakai, president of Kanki Publishing Inc., Mr. Yukio Kurosu president of Health Planning Inc., Mr. Makoto Ide head of sales, Mr. Sartori our primary interpreter, Reiko Ohya and Taeko Iwahara, two lovely ladies who assisted us with interpreting and cultural background, and our experienced drivers Kimio Hara and Youichi Tomizawa. We will never forget our time together!

Special thanks to Dr. Andy Sun and his colleagues in Taiwan and Dr. Hiroyuki Abe in Japan for sharing both their time and their research with our team.

Thank you to the wonderful patients that shared their story either directly or indirectly with us.

Special thanks to the Hong Kong Baptist University School of Medicine and their staff and colleagues. A fond thanks to Ms. Lisa Song, the head librarian, for our visit to their library.

Thanks to Jiuan Judy Liu, Ph.D., and the staff at Development Center for Biotechnology in Taipei, Taiwan for the special presentations and tour on the state of the art investigations being done there.

Thanks to all the other medical researchers, physicians, and scholars we met on our trip (too numerous to list!).

Thanks to Mr. Yan Zhao (China Natural Products, California-Beijing) for donating his services as a translator and guide for us in the majestic city of Beijing where every one of our memories is happy and golden!

All the loving kind hosts and hostesses, students, monks, Master Chen, and assistant Master Jian Teng for our day and special VIP tour in the monastery. And we thank you for your prayers that we have felt everyday since our visit.

We, the authors, wish to particularly acknowledge and thank our families, both immediate and extended, for their love, inspiration, and support. Without all of you, our "true riches" would be lost.

To the Higher Power, who has led, guided and protected us every step of our journey.

To all who have been mentioned and many more we owe our thanks.

## Author's Update

One is never ready to let go of loved ones, and so it was for all of us who knew and dearly loved Dr. Halstead. Dr. Halstead passed away with no warning only weeks after finishing this book. He was 82. This book was very important to Dr. Halstead. It integrated more than two decades of his studies into Traditional Chinese Medicine (TCM). Bruce was most pleased with the final product. He felt it had purpose as well as meaning. Now (2005), as the presses are about to run, I wish to thank several people for their help in bringing this book "to life."

Special thanks to Richard Grossinger, President of North Atlantic Books (NAB). Thank you Richard for embracing this project and lending us so much assistance. Special thanks to Paula Morrison, Layout & Design Artist for NAB, Julie Grant, Project Manager at NAB, Mark Oimet, Sales & Marketing at NAB, and everyone else who is part of the NAB team. Your enthusiasm and helpfulness really made a difference. Thanks to Caitlin McGillicuddy and Duncan McCallum from Spectrum Books. Thanks to Winnie Yueng and her team at Golden Cup Printing Co., Ltd. And an extra thanks to Leonette Medrano and Jeffrey McConnell who worked long hours into the night to proof and finish this book. I am forever grateful to you all.

Terri Lee Holcomb-Halstead
September 2005

# Foreward
## by Daniel Clark, M.D. and Frank Cousineau

Bruce W. Halstead, M.D., distinguished physician, philosopher, scholar, author, and lecturer devoted his life to research and scientific exploration of the environment in relation to life itself. He was the founder and scientific director of the World Life Research Institute, an international documentation center specializing in biological poisons, medicinal plants, pollution, traditional medicine, and nutrition.

Bruce W. Halstead was a world-renowned scientist, concentrating on the areas of global preventive medicine, tropical diseases, marine biotoxicology, toxic plants and animals, global pollution, chelation therapy, traditional medicinal plants, adaptogenic immune enhancement, and nutrition. While well trained in orthodox methods of patient care, Dr. Halstead was deeply involved in the study of oriental herbal therapy on immune deficiency disorders. Like a true pioneer in medicine, he was outspoken in his views of allopathic cancer therapy for which he was criticized and persecuted.

> "I predict that cures can be expected out of the natural products field. Someday we'll discover that some native population had the cancer cure product and was using it...I believe that if we could really do a thorough study of all the naturally occurring materials used by primitive tribes on a world scale, we [the United States] could become a highly productive area of cancer research."
>
> Bruce W. Halstead, M.D.
> February 20, 1970
> *Los Angeles Herald Examiner*

> "In cancer therapy, cytotoxicity, radiation and surgery are the therapeutic hallmarks of oncologists. A cancer victim suffers from the inroads of the carcinogenesis and immunoincompetence and is sold a therapy that is carcinogenic and lowers the immune system. This line of molecular illogic has been successfully sold to both the medical professional and layman alike - - - all at a cost of millions of lives."
>
> Bruce W. Halstead, M.D.
> http://www.forebiddenmedicine.com/main/quotes2.htm

> "What we should be doing instead with cancer is giving the person herbs and nutrients and putting them on a program that will rebuild their immune system."
>
> Bruce W. Halstead, M.D.
> http://www.bowtechforhealth.com/news/Herbs%20vs%20Drugs%20II.htm

A day with Dr. Halstead at World Life Research Institute was unique. Zen gardens, goldfish ponds, the walk down the path to the door, being amongst flora and fauna from around the world, was an experience in itself. Upon entering the

Institute, there are thousands of books in multiple languages. The specimen room housed bottles, jars, slides, and samples of innumerable species of animals and plants. Then, there was Dr. Halstead. All his education and training, Dr. Halstead was just plain "good people". He loved nature, plants, and animals and could communicate on any level with anyone. In the middle of a conversation he'd take time to pet one of the dogs he adored or pull books off one of the many floor to ceiling shelves to give an example of what he was saying.

Dr. Halstead was a consultant to over 40 governmental and international agencies, has authored over 15 books, including his 5 volume work on *Poisonous and Venomous Marine Animals of the World*, published in 1988 which was first published in three volumes by the U.S. Government Printing Office during the 1960s. He has also authored over 300 scientific publiciations some of which have been translated into 8 languages. Dr. Halstead has traveled in over 150 countries in the last 40 years gathering research for his books and publications.

Dr. Halstead's book, *The Scientific Basis of EDTA Chelation Therapy*, was instrumental in the education of thousands of physicians including myself on the value of chelation therapy for the removal of heavy metals from the body. Removal of heavy metals enhances the efficiency of the mitochondria and increases ATP production. This results in the improvement of many chronic diseases by decreasing free radicals.

Dr. Halstead's book, *The Scientific Basis of Chinese Integrative Cancer Therapy*, began in the spring of 2002, after his trip to meet Professor Wang, the developer of the Tien Hsien herbal products. His purpose in writing this book was "to provide the scientific rationale of the Chinese approach to the prevention and treatment of cancer in the context of modern Oriental integrative health care."

Bruce has always had an appreciation of Chinese herbal medicines and their use in chronic disease. This book brings deeper knowledge and understanding of the use of Chinese herbs in the treatment of cancer on a scientific basis.

My good friend and colleague, Bruce W. Halstead, passed away December 5, 2002 at the age of 82 after completion of this publication.

He will be sorely missed by all who knew him.

Daniel G. Clark, M.D.

There are many things one can say about Bruce Halstead, M.D. The obvious ones are: *brilliant physician, outstanding scientist, prolific author* and *preeminent toxicologist,* among numerous others. He was all of those. As one of the world's most knowledgeable toxicologists and marine biologists, he worked with Jacques Cousteau and was a prominent consultant to the *World Health Organization* of the United Nations. Professionally, he was foremost, a clinician with a thriving medical practice. He was also a husband, father, and teacher of youth at his church.

The first time I learned of Dr. Halstead was in the mid-seventies through the printed page of one of the *freedom-of-choice* magazines. Dr. Halstead was ever ready to do battle with the *establishment* over the issue of freedom of health care and the sanctity of the patient-doctor relationship. Whether it was chelation therapy for cardio-vascular disease, or Laetrile and other non-toxic therapies for cancer, he was always at the forefront testifying in front of legislators, giving expert testimony in court cases, speaking in public and with the printed word. On one occasion I was asked to arrange a speaking engagement for him and requested his *Curriculum Vitae.* It emptied my fax machine as it filled over seventy-five pages.

He was all of the things mentioned above, but he was so much more. To me he was not only a friend. He was a mentor. His penchant for scientific integrity was uncompromising. His encouragement for scientific investigation was stimulating, as well as exciting.

He had other yet-to-be-published works on his desk when approached to do this project, which he enthusiastically left behind to take up the task of establishing a scientific basis for what he already knew, based on his life's work. Namely that herbal medicine, in general, and Oriental medicine in particular, offered genuine hope for success in the promethean struggle against the most dreaded disease of the modern age. When he accepted this project, his body was beginning to show the affects of a lifetime of battles with adversaries tremendously inferior to him scientifically and whose intellectual integrity was extremely compromised. The vigor with which he attacked what was to be his ultimate earthly labor was an inspiration to all who accompanied him during an arduous journey through Asia, meeting with the formulator of the unique product discussed in this tome, and the medical professionals who were successfully utilizing it in hospital, clinic, and laboratory.

His raison d'etre was to alleviate suffering and advance scientific knowledge. His hope was that this volume would do both.

All of us who knew and worked with him on his ultimate opus, pray this book will accomplish that purpose.

Frank Cousineau<br>
Vice President, Cancer Control Society<br>
President, International Association of Cancer Victors and Friends

# Introduction

Many books have been written on cancer. It is a popular subject about an unpopular disease. Cancer is a scourge. It is indeed a widespread affliction and the most feared disease of our time. Cancer is on the increase worldwide (Davis, et al, 1990; Marshall, 1990), but more recent cancer mortality statistics suggest that it is on the decline in the United States, but there is no room for complacency. This conclusion can be readily verified by visiting the best cancer hospitals in any part of the world. The cancer problem is far from being solved. However, recent clinical reports from Hong Kong, China, Taiwan, and Japan together with supporting laboratory investigations suggest that a major non-toxic breakthrough in cancer therapy is already available, but is not being utilized to the extent that it should.

One purpose of this book is to examine in some degree of depth the ancient traditional Chinese concepts of cancer therapeutics upon which this new treatment is based. Unfortunately, most Western physicians have had very little exposure to this field and poorly understand these concepts. Let's begin by examining a few basic facts and statistics on the subject of cancer.

## The Bad News—Current Cancer Statistics

According to the World Health Organization during the year 2000 one person died of cancer every 60 seconds in the United States, which amounted to about 1,500, lives a day, or 5.4 million a year in the U.S. alone. Despite this gloomy news, current statistics suggest that these mortality statistics are gradually improving in the U.S. However, the global cancer statistics are anything but encouraging. Much of the cancer mortality statistics can be credited to lifestyle influences such as smoking as well as environmental pollution.

Cancer is considered to be among the most feared diseases of our time. Cancer has in recent decades attracted the attention of most Americans because one out of three persons can expect to develop cancer during their lifetime. It is second only to heart disease in the United States. Cancer is among the fastest growing life threatening diseases of all of the plagues facing Western civilization.

Cancer is more than a disease—it is an economic reality. Cancer is a very big and very profitable business. More people make money from cancer than get sick and die from it. The cancer industry is estimated to generate in excess of $200 billion per year. No one knows the exact amount because the actual cancer statistics are buried in a mass of mortality statistics, which are difficult for even a biostatistician to decipher.

Billions of dollars have been spent in trying to find a cure for this deadly malady, but with only moderately successful results. To determine the success rate in the treatment of cancer one has only to visit any of our finest cancer hospitals in the United States or elsewhere and the failure rate becomes hauntingly obvious. It is obvious that a new approach to cancer therapy is needed.

## The Good News About Cancer

One purpose for writing this book is to present the scientific facts documenting that a completely new approach to cancer therapy is available. This therapy does not have toxic side effects. This therapy is gentle and convenient to use. This therapy also has an unbelievably high rate of reversing cancer of all kinds. This knowledge is a revolutionary opportunity for humankind. It is with great humility and reverence that the authors have written and prepared this manuscript.

Bruce W. Halstead, M.D.
Terri Lee Holcomb-Halstead
July 2002

# Preface

*"For yesterday is already a dream, and tomorrow is only a vision, but today well lived makes yesterday a dream of happiness, and every tomorrow a vision of hope."*

—from Susruta, a 4th century physician of ancient India

This book was born in a climate of complete skepticism. After visiting Hong Kong, Japan, Taiwan, and China and meeting numerous physicians, scientists, and terminal cancer patients we became total believers in the efficacy of the Tien Hsien Herbal Products. Our observations were further strengthened by the meeting of Professor Zhenguo Wang, the primary formulator of the Tien Hsien products, which are produced by the China-Japan Feida Union Corporation (CJFU) in Hong Kong. The Tien Hsien products have now been introduced into 70 countries and to over two million cancer patients. The results, which we personally investigated, included cat scans, X-rays, and other clinical data which supported the fact that terminal cancer patients were getting better. We also independently investigated the phytochemical and pharmacological properties of the various medicinal plant ingredients once we had determined their taxonomic identity—all of which supported the clinical results that we found in the cancer patients. This is a story that needs to be told to the nations and their various regulatory agencies. The personnel of CJFU we met exemplified Susruta's adage.

## About This Book

This book has three sections. **Section One**: ***The Remarkable Tien Hsien Herbal Products*** will highlight the various findings we made as we researched this book first hand in Japan, China, and Taiwan. Also included is a chapter devoted to case histories of twenty cancer patients who treated their cancer with Tien Hsien Herbal Products.

**Section Two**: ***The Scientific and Historical Basis of Chinese Traditional Medicine and How it is Used in Cancer Treatment*** deals with several subjects including: scientific information on the subject of cancer, the immune system, the history of traditional Chinese medicine, the Chinese rationale of integrative cancer prevention and treatment, and lastly the preparation of medicinal herbal products. These subjects all tie together in providing a more complete understanding of the use of Chinese herbal products for cancer.

**Section Three:** ***A Color Atlas of Chinese Anticancer Plants***. The reader will delight in this beautiful color atlas of Chinese anticancer plants. Each botanical plate is accompanied by scientific information on the phytochemistry and pharmacology of the plant.

# Table of Contents

# Section I:

# The Remarkable Tien Hsien Herbal Products

## Chapter 1

# An Overview and Brief Background of the Tien Hsien Medicinal Herbal Products

## Message to Planet Earth

The plant world has been evolving for billions of years. Every living species that has evolved in our present environment has survived by developing its own biochemical defense system. It is really no wonder that from plants we are now witnessing healing therapies that help humans defend against dreaded diseases such as cancers of all types and manifestations. This book covers a broad spectrum of topics, first hand experiences, and scientific data that is woven together by the true life story of a modern day marvel . . . the Tien Hsien Herbal Products.

## A Great Honor is Bestowed on the Authors

We could not be more honored than to be the messengers of the remarkable Tien Hsien Story. In the first portion of our book, we share our first hand experiences researching the Tien Hsien Herbal Products. These medicinal herbal products have their roots in ancient Chinese medicine. The reader will be introduced to various people who are all a part of this Tien Hsien story, in particular, our friend and colleague, Professor Zhenguo Wang, who has formulated these products, and brought a gift of immeasurable value to the world!

The readers will also meet a most unique group of associates who are all part of the China-Japan Feida Union Corporation, more commonly referred to as the CJFU Family. These kind, intelligent, and compassionate people not only made this trip possible, but went way beyond the extra mile to provide us with any and all information possible. We examined everything—leaving no stone unturned. Over and over it was conclusively proven that CJFU was light years ahead of what we anticipated when it came to the scientific validity of their products.

## Highlights of our Research Trip

Our trip to Asia enabled us to document the fact that it is possible for non-toxic medicinal herbal products to be therapeutically effective against cancer. Our

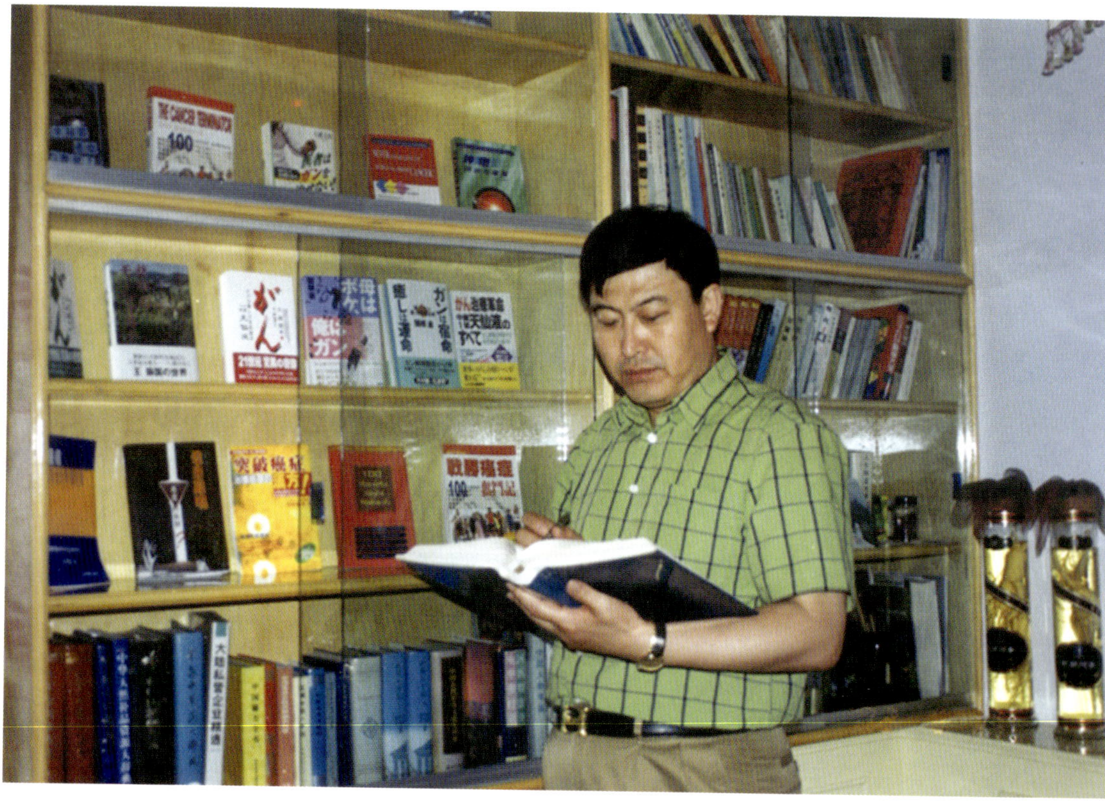

Fig. 1.1. Professor Zhenguo Wang (June 2002, Courtesy of Professor Wang).

findings can be directly credited to the life work of Professor Zhenguo Wang (Fig. 1.1), a truly dedicated researcher. Professor Wang has a fascinating background. Professor Wang devoted much of his life to creating a special line of herbal products best known as "The Tien Hsien Herbal Products". Since early 1975, the Tien Hsien products have been used with remarkable results for cancer therapy in mainland China. The immensity of the contributions to humanity that this dedicated, gentle, and—without question—brilliant man has made will only increase with time and can never actually be measured. Further details on Professor Wang can be found in Chapter Three: Our Visit to China.

In 1985, through a fortuitous set of circumstances, Mr. Sidney Lu (Fig. 1.2) acquired the rights to market and sell the Tien Hsien products outside of China. Mr. Lu, with solid support from his lovely wife and family, shortly thereafter founded the China-Japan Feida Union Corporation (CJFU) and since then has served as the CEO and "guiding light" of the company.

Mr. Sydney Lu has described his years working with the Tien Hsien herbal products as the most important journey in his lifetime. Mr. Lu was born in 1946 in the city of Chung Ching in mainland China where his family had lived for countless generations. In 1947, due to the political situation in mainland China, Mr. Lu's family moved to Taiwan. Sidney was one year of age. In 1970, at age twenty-three, Sidney Lu graduated from the Taiwan Naval Academy. He went on to serve as a captain in the Taiwanese Navy for a total of ten years. Mr. Lu's next career was as an insurance agent in the company AIA Taiwan. Sidney took his work very seriously and consequently earned a worthy financial return. After ten years in the insurance business, Sydney could have retired and lived with his wife and five children very comfortably. However, there was great work still ahead for him.

In 1991 Sydney Lu made a dramatic change in his life path by acquiring marketing rights to the Tien Hsien Herbal Products in all territories worldwide with the exception of mainland China. By this time the word about these health products had begun to spread outside of China, and Mr. Lu set about to create a global marketing company as expediently as he could.

Establishing the foundation and corporate structure was the first step and so it came to pass that the China-Japan Feida Union (CJFU) was born. The initial corporate office was in Hong Kong with sister offices in Taipei, Taiwan and Tokyo, Japan.

Shortly after establishing the mother corporation (CJFU), Mr. Lu asked Mr. Charles Lee (Fig. 1.3) to join him as one of the founding officers of the corporation. This was an offer Mr. Charles Lee accepted with honor. Mr. Lu knew Mr. Lee from their days in the Navy together. They forged a strong and deep friendship that continues to this day.

In February 1992 CJFU established the Greenherb Corporation in Taiwan. In April 1992 CJFU contracted with Tombo Enterprise Company to market Tien Hsien products in Malaysia, Singapore, and Indonesia. A new enhanced formulation of Tien Hsien was introduced into the market (also formulated by Professor Wang) in 1993. In June 1994 the Feida Company was established in Thailand. In March 1995 CJFU acquired the global sole distributorship for a new health product known as Shu Nao Liquid. Then, in November 1997, CJFU contracted with Green and Gold to distribute their products in the Philippines. In March 1998 Tien Hsien was approved as a medicine in Thailand. In January 2000 Tien Hsien was declared by the FDA as a dietary supplement in the United States. In March 2000 CJFU contracted with Dr. Wei-Yi Yang, a research Pharmacologist at the Hong Kong Baptist University Medical Center, to develop Vital Essentials, a new herbal product.

In April 2000 CJFU established the Feida Union Pharmaceutical Manufacturing, a Good Manufacturing Practices (GMP) facility in the United States and the China-Japan Feida Union Ltd. in Australia. In May 2000 the United Medical Development Group in the United States was established. In January 2001 Tien Hsien was classified as a medicine in Australia. In June 2001 CJFU obtained a license to import Tien Hsien liquid from the United States to Taiwan. CJFU then contracted with Innovative Marketing Firm to promote Tien Hsien in the United States in

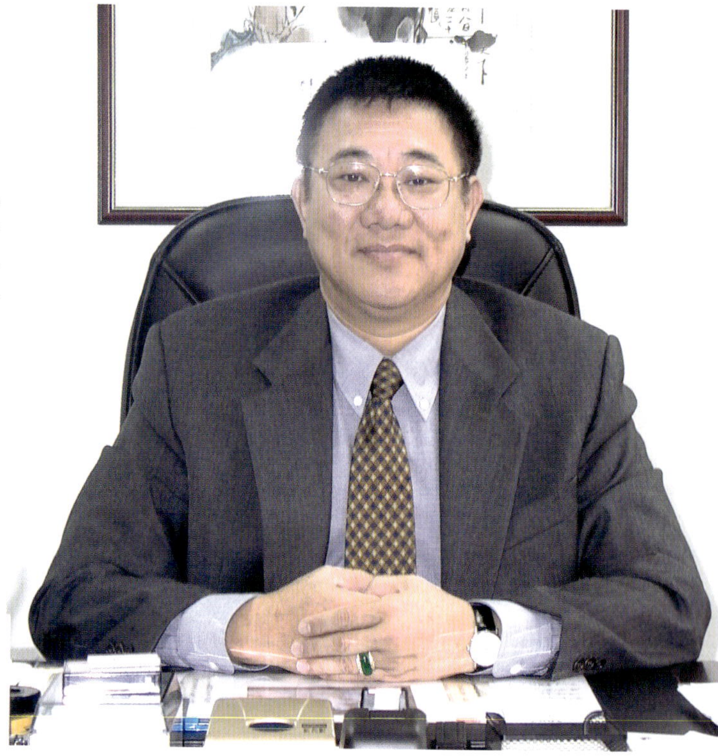

➢ Fig. 1.2. Mr. Sidney Lu, Founder and C.E.O. of China-Japan Feida Union Co., Ltd. (CJFU) (Courtesy of CJFU).

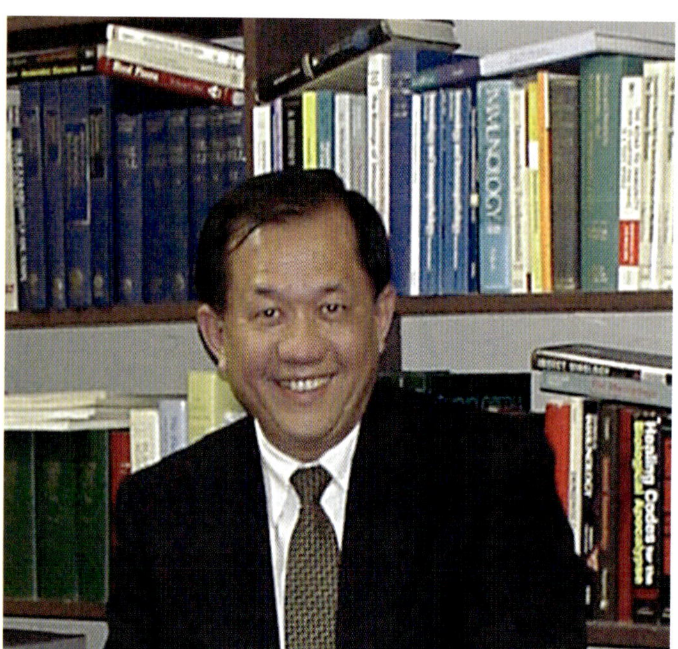

⮜ Fig. 1.3. Mr. Charles Lee, Vice Chairman and Co-Founder of China-Japan Feida Union Co., Ltd. (CJFU). (Taken at the World Life Research Institute in March 2002 by Jeffrey McConnell.)

November 2001. In May 2002 they celebrated their approval of receiving the GMP certification by the Chinese government for their manufacturing plant in Tonghua, China.

In May 2002 we were invited to visit and learn about the Tien Hsien Herbal Products first hand by participating in a seventeen-day fact-finding trip to Japan, China, Hong Kong, and Taiwan. We were accompanied by a western medical team as well as a number of the CJFU family. Mr. Heiwai Chen, Mr. Thomas Chou, Joan Lu, and Corrina Lee were forever providing us translation as well as information. The hospitality was beyond measure. What we learned and saw with our own eyes made this trip the most worthwhile and productive research trip either of us had ever experienced.

In the course of our travels with the CJFU family we found out that Mr. Sidney Lu and his partner, Mr. Lee, have provided herbal medicine to the poor in different countries and have provided substantial financial donations to hospitals and non-profit organizations throughout the world. Mr. Lu and Mr. Lee could both be described as present day humanitarians who unquestionably embrace a global vision of ending needless suffering the world over.

## Investigative Studies of the Tien Hsien Herbal Products

Investigative studies have been conducted in numerous countries at quality research centers including the Hong Kong Baptist University, the Institute of Biophysics in Taipei Taiwan, the Academy Sinica in Beijing, China, and the Guangzhou Tumor Institute in Tonghua, China just to name a few. These institutes have extensive documentation on Tien Hsien products. Their studies have proven the following: Tien Hsien anticancer products have been shown to inhibit free radical activity, enhance the immune system, and have a direct cytotoxic action on cancer cells, while remaining non-toxic to healthy cells. During our trip we had the opportunity of visiting a number of newly equipped state of the art analytical laboratories that verified the potency of the various active ingredients used in Tien Hsien as well as labs where live cancer cell lines were being studied in vitro. In the coming chapters we will discuss these findings as well as those where the subjects were human and the cancer types were from nearly every category and or stage known in oncology.

## Objectives of CJFU

One of our ports of call on our journey into Asia was the fascinating and legendary city of Hong Kong. Hong Kong is home to the corporate offices of CJFU, which is located in the upper floors of a lovely office building in the Kowloon District.

During our four-day stay in Hong Kong, the research team was invited to visit the corporate offices of CJFU. Our meeting began with a presentation by Ms. Joan Lu in their lovely conference room. Joan presented a very informative history and overview of the CJFU Corporation. The following is an excerpt from this presentation that eloquently expresses the mission of the China-Japan Feida Union Corporation.

*"The objective of CJFU is to maintain the infinite value of our health by making the most precious natural supplements available for the people of the world who are health conscious, and who are sensitive to positive and negative changes in their lives. Only by providing the finest quality herbals available can we assist people in maintaining good health in this polluted environment. Only when we maintain good health can we pursue our goals in life. Good health provides everyone with the resources to achieve their dreams. CJFU is committed to providing the health products that will permit your dreams to come true."*

—Joan Lu, daughter and Executive Assistant to President Sidney Lu (May 2002)

So similar were these thoughts to those previously stated in the Preface by Susruta (Circa 4th Century):

*"For yesterday is already a dream, and tomorrow is only a vision, but today well lived makes yesterday a dream of happiness, and every tomorrow a vision of hope."*

# Chapter 2

# Our Visit to Japan

The primary purpose of going to Japan was to meet Hiroyuki Abe, M.D. (Fig. 2.1), founder of the Kudan Clinic in Tokyo, Japan. In 1965 Dr. Abe graduated from the Sapporo Medical University in Sapporo, Japan. Dr. Abe had extensive medical training in the United States, at the University of Pennsylvania, and was a visiting Professor at Stanford University and at the University of California at San Francisco during the 1970's. He was also a visiting professor at the Kyourin University, and a lecturer at the Juntendo University, an Assistant Professor at the Nihon University, and is currently a visiting Professor at the Kyourin University. He is the Chairman of the International Society of Integrated Future Medicine in Japan and serves as an advisor to the International Rehabilitation Cancer Association in Japan.

Our visit to his clinic was an awesome experience (Fig. 2.2). The clinic was divided into several departments: Internal Medicine, Cardiovascular Disease, Gastroenterology, Radiology, Gynecology, Dermatology, Physical Science, and Medical Examination. His clinic was one of the best-equipped clinics that we have ever visited. There were an array of cat scans, radiological equipment, and a wide variety of other diagnostic and automated blood biochemistry analyzers. However, we did not come to see his equipment. We came to meet the man who worked extensively with cancer therapy using both the western methods of treatment and the Tien Hsien products. Dr. Abe is truly an amazing physician. He radiates an intense interest and love for his patients, and has a smiling countenance that reflects sincerity. There was one compelling question that we were most anxious to ask him. "Dr. Abe, we note that you have worked with both Western cancer therapy and have had extensive experience with Tien Hsien for many years in which you have used this product in terminal cancer patients. What do you think of Tien Hsien products in treating terminal cancer patients?" He made it emphatically clear that there was no comparison between using the Western therapy of chemotherapy and radiation and using Tien Hsien. He had used Tien Hsien in patients with lung cancer, cancer of the liver with extensive metastases, cancer of the pancreas, and a wide variety of other types of cancer. In the due course of time, upwards of 80% of his worst terminal patients had recovered. Moreover, none of them had suffered from the toxic side effects of cancer chemotherapy and radiation. All of them had a better quality of life. Some of his patients came to him after they already had chemotherapy or radiation and they improved noticeably after getting on Tien Hsien. The meeting with Dr. Abe was one of the highlights of the entire trip.

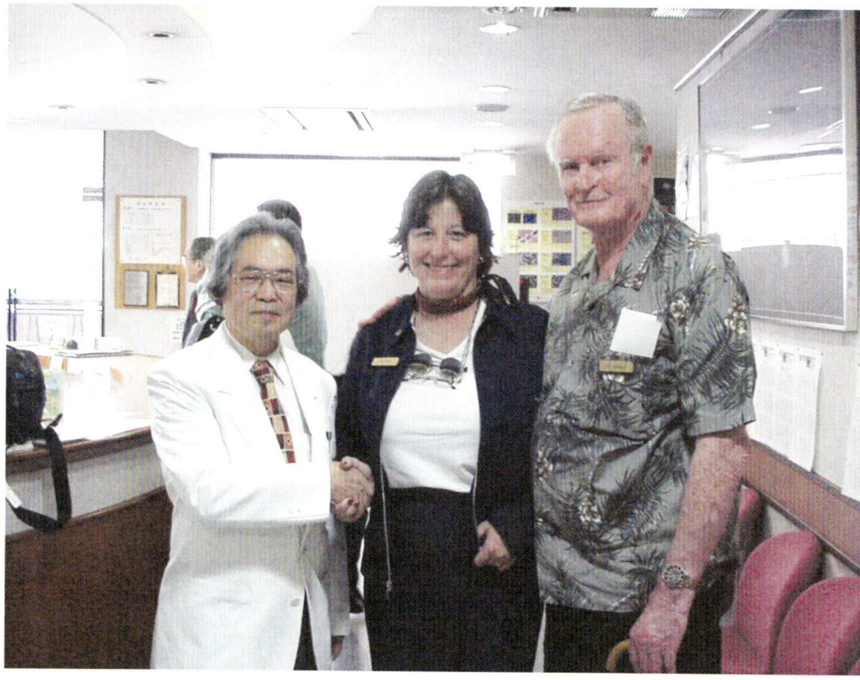

Fig. 2.1. Dr. Hiroyuki Abe, medical director of the Kudan Clinic, meeting Dr. Bruce W. Halstead and Terri Holcomb-Halstead at his clinic in Tokyo, Japan. (May 2002, by Jeffrey McConnell)

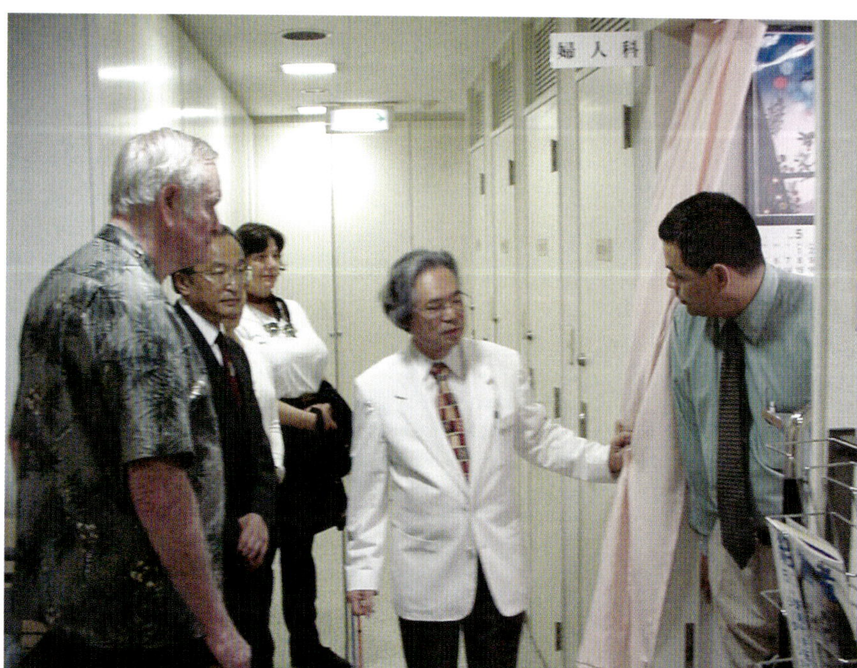


Fig. 2.2. Dr. Hiroyuki Abe giving a tour of the Kudan Clinic in Tokyo, Japan. (From left to right: Dr. Bruce W. Halstead, Mr. Sakurai, Terri Holcomb-Halstead, Dr. Hiroyuki Abe, Dr. Francisco Espinosa) (May 2002, by Jeffrey McConnell)

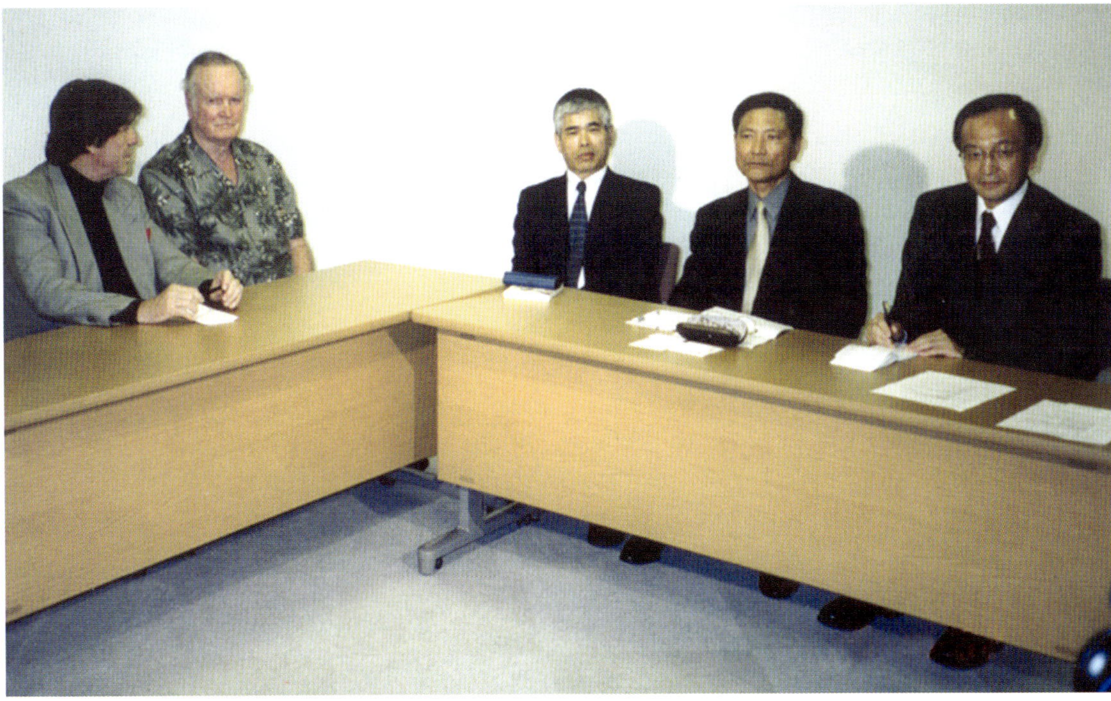

Fig. 2.3. We get to personally interview two of the recovered cancer patients. From left to right: investigative reporter, Anthony J. Hilder; Dr. Bruce Halstead; stomach cancer patient, Mr. Kure; liver cancer patient, Mr. Maeda; interpretor, Mr. Sakurai. (May 2002, by Jeffrey McConnell)

While in Tokyo, the Japanese staff had arranged for a reception in their office. This is where we were introduced to Makoto Ide who had been promoted to Director of Sales due to his level of competence and success. Mr. Ide presented an overview of the sales and distribition of Tien Hsien products in the Japanese market. The products were sold as health supplements, which allows direct sales to the consumer. The Japanese team employed clever strategy to spread the Tien Hsien message. The Japanese have a reputation of being avid readers; the Japanese branch of CJFU used this to their advantage. They published three books in the first five years of marketing efforts. They negotiated a joint venture with Mr. Kenichiro Sakai president and owner of Kanki Publishing Inc. in Tokyo. We had the great pleasure of meeting Mr. Sakai as his guests at a traditional Japanese feast in honor of our research team. Mr. Sakai is as passionate about the Tien Hsien story as anyone could be. It was his guidance into the world of print that optimized CJFU's marketing efforts in Japan. Mr. Sakai is sweet, gentle, and soft spoken; however, the brightness of his mind and the creative gift of publishing shines from him. They placed informative ads and magazine articles in popular publications. They shared true-life stories with the public. They were able to get on several television shows talking about Tien Hsien.

The biggest publicity boost of all came from a popular contemporary actor who recovered from cancer using Tien Hsien products. On his own volition, this celebrity shared his story with enthusiasm. He appeared on talk shows. He also decided to write and published his story in a best selling book. He donated any book proceeds to other cancer patients in need of therapy. Needless to say, sales begin to escalate. Mr. Ide told us that their sales had tripled in the last four years. The final figure for total gross sales from Japan in 2001 was twenty million dollars. The success is a direct result of the positive results experienced by the people who use it.

The next afternoon we were scheduled to meet with two of Dr. Abe's patients who had obtained dramatic results with Tien Hsien (Fig. 2.3). One had liver cancer and the other had stomach cancer. Both patients had been given surgery, chemotherapy and radiation, but they were considered terminal. Their prognosis was bad. In both cases, after taking Tien Hsien for 24 months, their conditions began to improve. That evening the patient with stomach cancer came to dinner with our group and announced that he had just gone to the doctor that very day and his physician was unable to find any evidence of cancer. The patient with stomach cancer ate heartily.

During our short stay in Japan, we were escorted to several fascinating bookstores. This was a particular courtesy for us. I (BWH) am always looking for books on medicinal plants to add to my library. We want to thank and acknowledge all the effort and care that our many Japanese hosts and hostesses from the CJFU family gave to make our trip so wonderful. They would never give up if we were looking for something in particular. One day we walked fourteen blocks until we found a bookstore that I (BWH) remembered from twenty years earlier. We found it by golly! And to make matters even better, I (BWH) located a rare, and magnificent book on medicinal plants. Every page of the book featured a beautiful hand painted medicinal plant. On behalf of CJFU Mr. Charles Lee purchased this book for me (BWH) as a gift. We will never forget the love and kindness that was showered on us by the Japanese branch of CJFU!

## Chapter 3

# OUR VISIT TO CHINA

Our trip to China was of great importance because we met Professor Zhenguo Wang (Fig. 3.1), chief formulator of Tien Hsien Herbal Products, and visited his research laboratory where the Tien Hsien products were first produced. We learned the history of the development of Professor Wang's formulations, which began from his early experiences as a child.

Zhenguo Wang grew up in the province of Jilin in Northeast China (Fig 3.2). His family home was in the foothills of the lovely Changbai Mountain region, an area known for wild ginseng and other medicinal plants. Young Zhenguo had an insatiable curiosity and went about gathering wild medicinal plants at an early age. Although he was too young to be familiar with scientific names, intuitively he seemed to know which plants had significant healing properties. The young boy, Zhenguo, had an inborn "sixth sense" when it came to medicinal plants. By the age of ten, Zhenguo was able to "classify" countless varieties of medicinal plants by tasting them. For example, if he discerned that a certain herb strengthened the body's defense system, he would then classify that herb in the Chinese catagory known as the "tonic" class. Herbs in the tonic classification are considered a "superior herb". These curative plants share the following attributes: adaptogenics of the highest order, very little toxicity, gentle in action, repeated efficacy in therapeutic value. These herbs when properly cultivated and processed, are always effective and always considered good for overall health of the entire body.

Zhenguo Wang began his noble quest of finding answers to sickness from herbs and plants when he was very young. Roaming the woods and mountains, Zhengou conducted his own tests by tasting each plant. His simple methodology has continued to a significant extent until the present time. Once this eager young mind reached the age of reading and writing, he dove into studying ancient herbal manuscripts and everything else he could get his hands on about Chinese medicinal plants. As a young adult, Zhenguo Wang pursued his passion both academically by attending several universities and by practicing his skill in herbal medicine in clinics and hospitals. He received his professorship by age twenty-five. He has spent his entire life in and around hospitals, clinics, and medical research centers. It was when working in a clinic as a young adult, that Zhenguo was inspired to find an answer to cancer. His compassionate heart was touched when he saw first hand the suffering it caused.

When we first learned about the Tien Hsien products our initial request was for a list of all the scientific names of the plants used as ingredients in the Tien

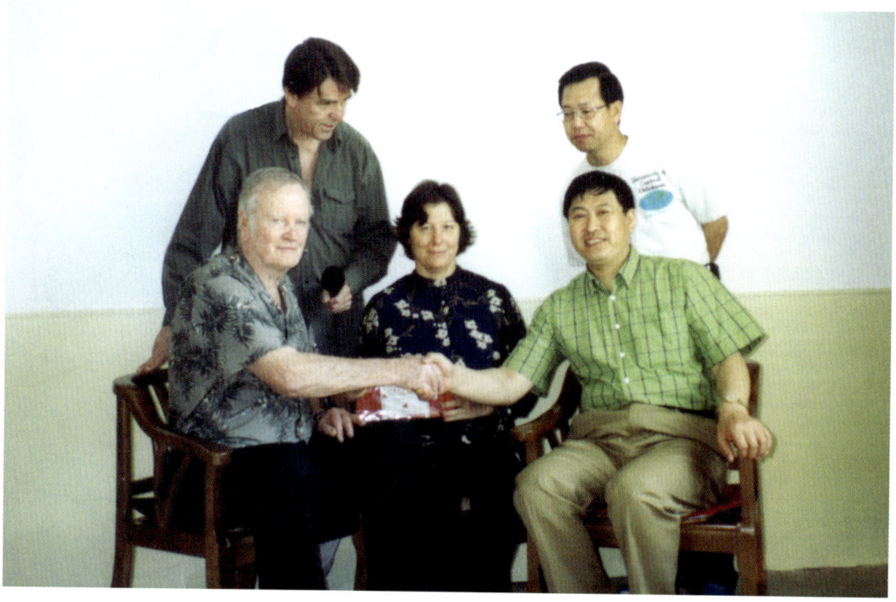

Fig. 3.1. Meeting Professor Wang. Standing are Anthony Hilder (left) and Thomas Chou (right); sitting from left to right are Dr. Bruce W. Halstead, Terri Halstead, and Professor Zhenguo Wang. (May 2002, by Jeffrey McConnell)

Hsien formulation. Professor Wang did not supply these names to us. Instead, we took the scientific names from one of the product containers (Fig. 3.3). Long before meeting Professor Wang we checked out the plants in the phytochemical and Chinese pharmacological literature. To our surprise, he had invariably selected plants that enhanced the immune system and/or possessed anticancer activity. It was obvious that he possessed an insight that was beyond our comprehension.

Professor Wang not only possesses a great deal of curiosity, but he is blessed with an abundance of energy. He is very aware and open-minded. He treats all living things as sacred. He is gentle, warm, clear, focused, and passionate about his mission. Genuine kindness radiates from his being. He is brilliant in his mind.

Professor Wang's entire life has been creative and productive. He has the gift to be continuously creating new research as well as multitudes of projects related to his research. He has worked in hospitals side by side with the best-trained physicians available. Inevitably Professor Wang would end up teaching the physicians and sharing his vast knowledge about medicinal herbal therapies including his own innovations and advancements that he created in this field. These physicians were always amazed at this man's innate ability to heal and cure difficult cases. We feel that Professor Wang is a genius. He also possesses great compassion. We were drawn to the inner soul of this man much like thirsty people are drawn to cool water. It is so evident that every project that Professor Zhenguo Wang invests his talent and energies into prospers and grows. The particulars all fall into place, giving him an excellent track record of success.

# JILIN

Jilin Province, with a population of 26 million, covers an area of a little 187,400 square metres in the centre of northeast China. The Changbai Mountains and the Songhua, Yalu and Tumen rivers are what Jilin's beauty is all about. Vast forests and rich fauna and flora turn the province into an ideal destination for environment-conscious tourists. World-calibre skating and skiing facilities have been established in recent years to accommodate winter sports fans from around the world. The tradition of ethnic culture runs deep in Jilin. The Manchus and Koreans are born singers, and the local folklore sets the stage for a rich variety of tourist activities. Major tourist cities in the province are Changchun, Jilin, Yanji and Tonghua and Baishan.

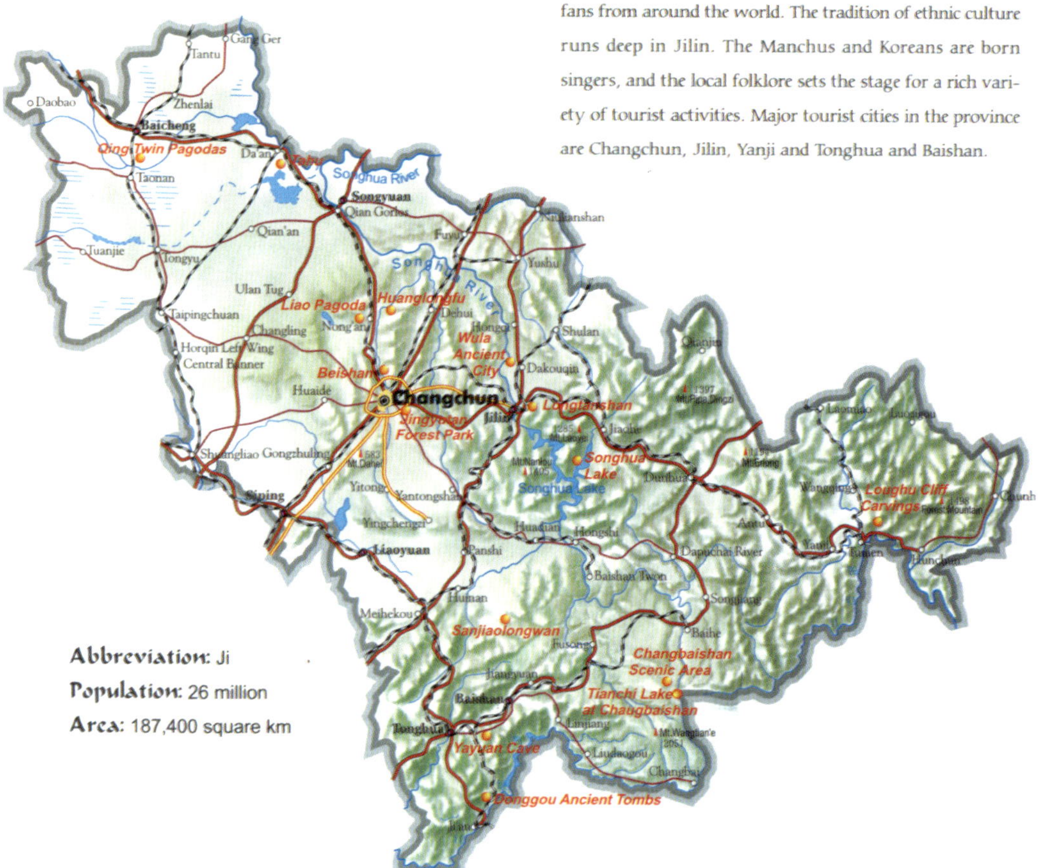


**Abbreviation:** Ji
**Population:** 26 million
**Area:** 187,400 square km

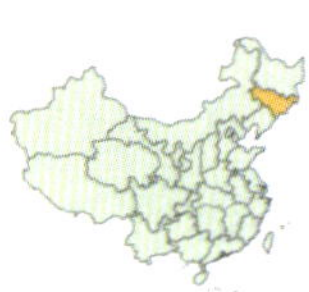

Fig. 3.2. Map of Jilin Province. (Courtesy of China Travel and Tourism Press)

# Fig. 3.3. Ingredients in Tien Hsien.

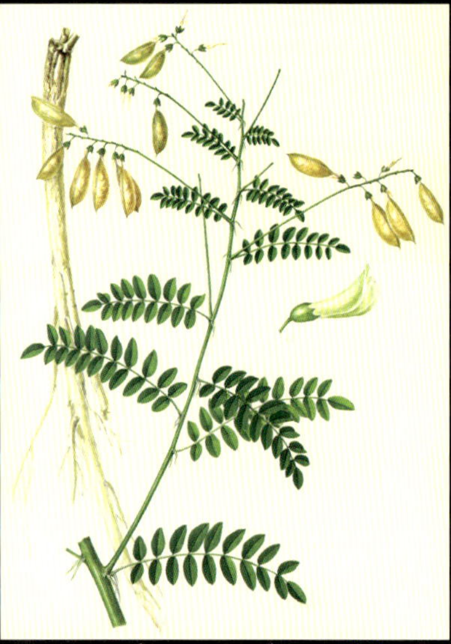

*Astragalus membranaceus*

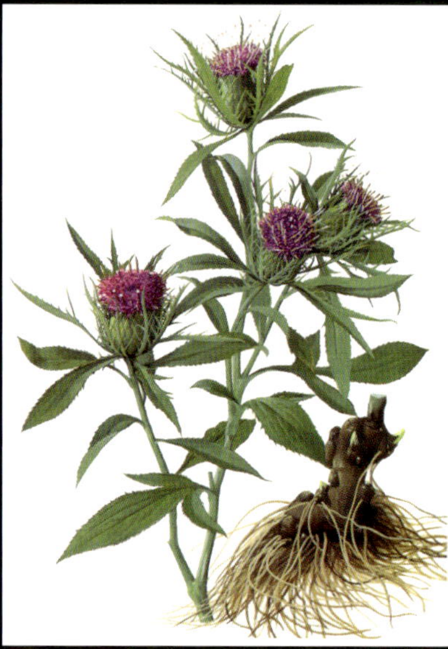

*Atractylodes macrocephala*

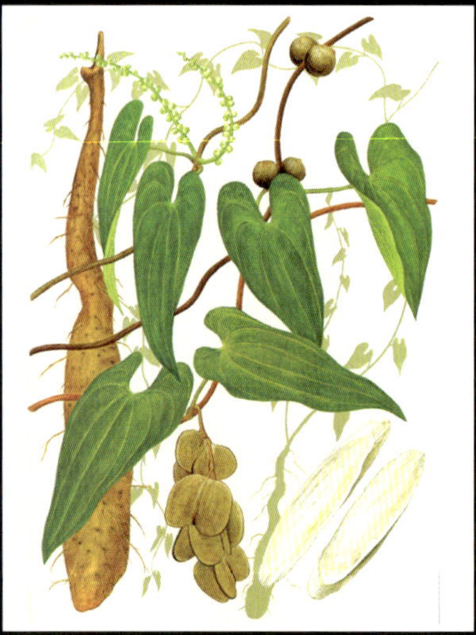

*Dioscorea batatas*

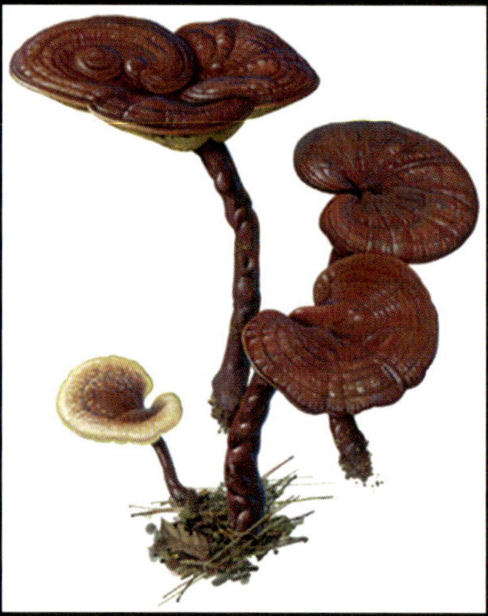

*Ganoderma lucidum*

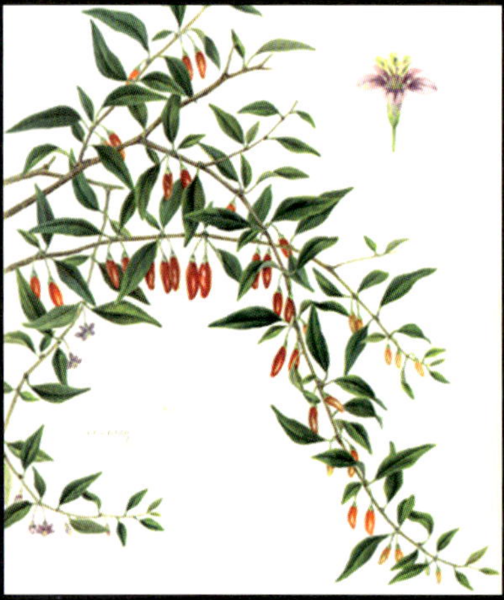

*Lycium barbarum*

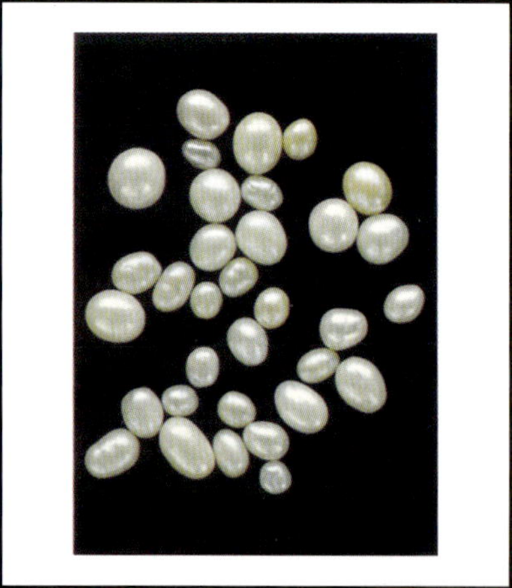

Pearl

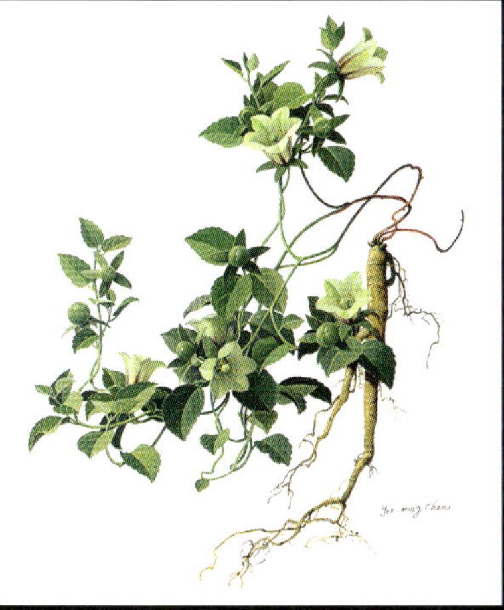

*Codonopsis pilosula*

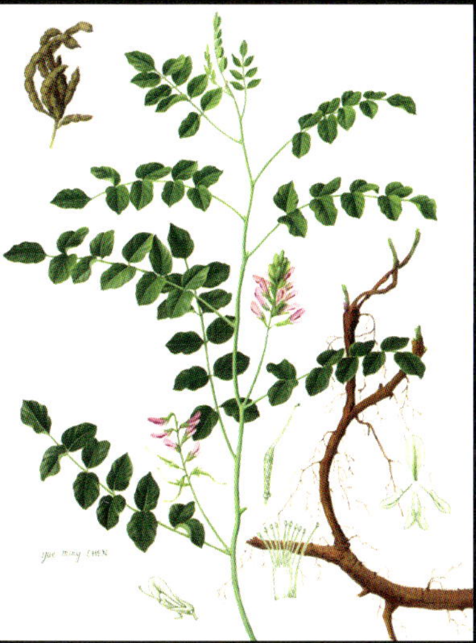

*Glycyrrhiza* sp.

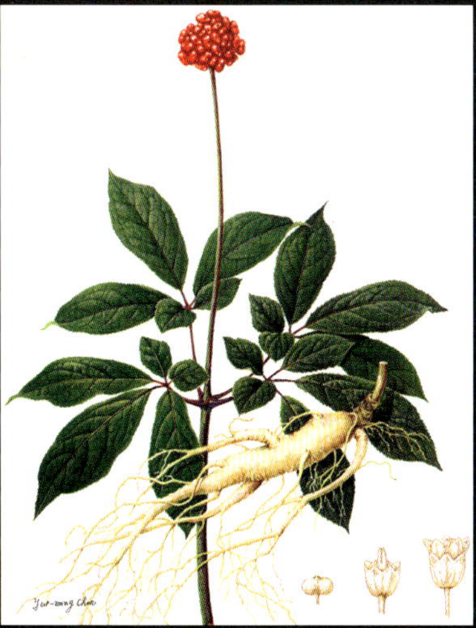

*Panax ginseng*

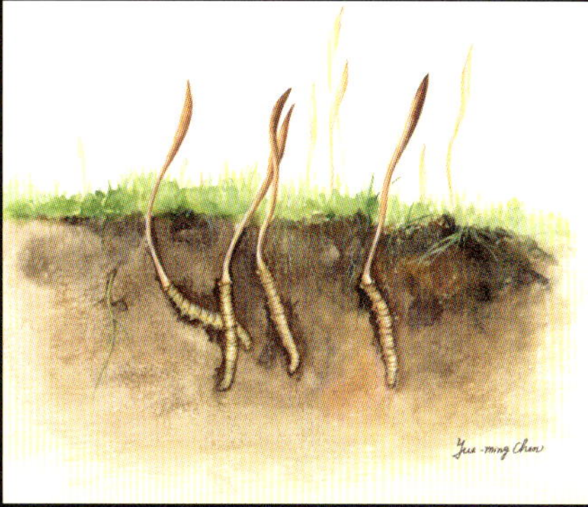

*Cordyceps sinensis*

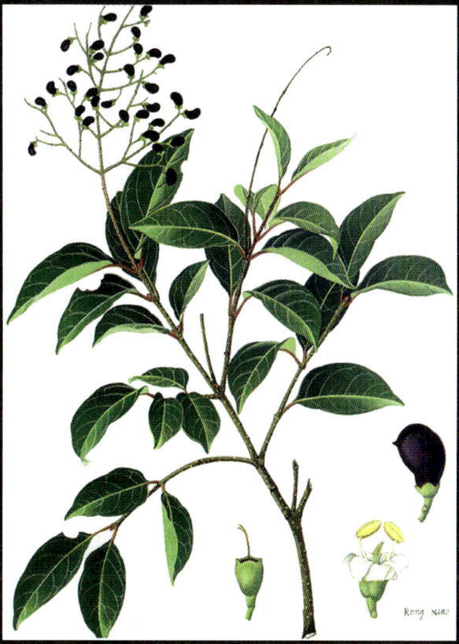

*Ligustrum lucidum*

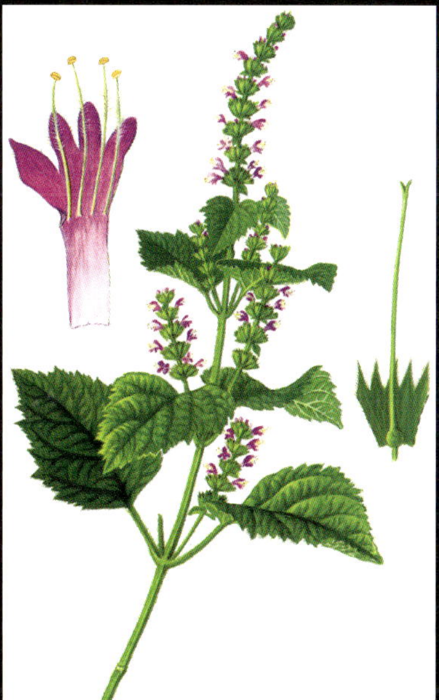

*Pogostemon cablin*

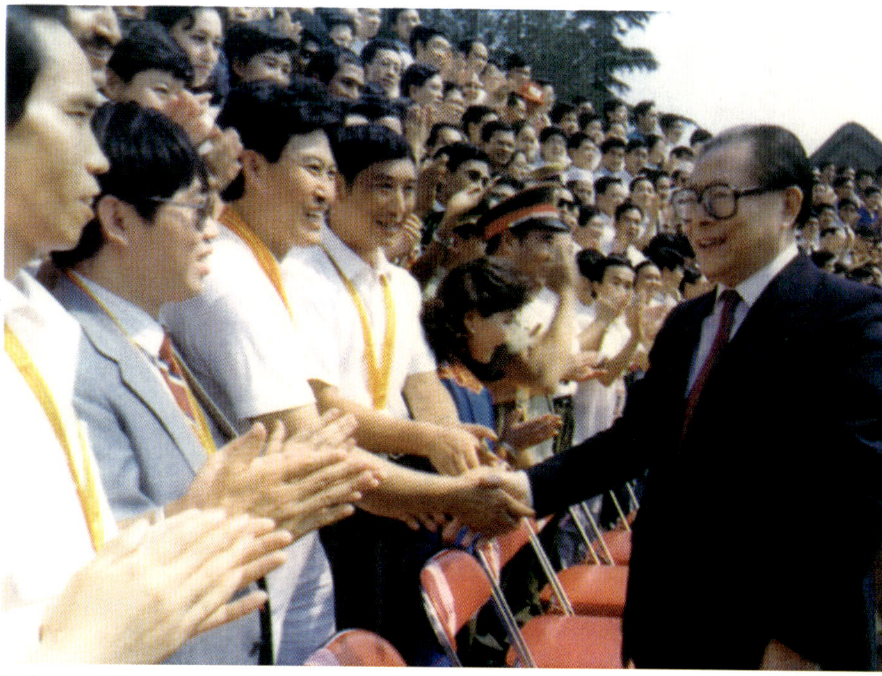

Fig. 3.4. Professor Wang receiving an award from the Premier of China. (Courtesy of Professor Wang)

"Timing is everything," a wise man once said. Professor Wang was yet a young man when the Chinese government changed their policy on private enterprise, making it legal for private citizens to go into business for themselves. This was very fortuitous, as Professor Wang had a natural skill for business. All of his enterprises are in the field of natural medicine.

At age 19, Zhenguo Wang, was elected among the ten most outstanding young people who have made major contributions to China (Fig. 3.4). The Premier of China has presented him with many awards and recognition for his scientific, medical and humanitarian accomplishments. In 1986 the Changbai Mountain Research Institute was established, which we were fortunate enough to visit. The same year Professor Wang founded his first private business, The Zhenguo Industrial Group. The following are but some of the other organizations that Professor Wang has founded: Tonghua Zhenguo Pharmaceutical Co. Ltd., Zhu Hay Zen Medicine Research Institute, Tien Hsien Health Caring Products Co. Ltd., the Shanghai Zhenguo Research Institute for Cancer Prevention and Treatment, the Hong Kong Zhenguo Medicine Industry, Wang Zhenguo Office in Tokyo, Japan, the Long Life Comprehensive Research Institute, in Japan, and the American Zhenguo Research Institute of Science for Life in the United States.

Over the last twenty years, Professor Wang has established more than 300 clinics for the treatment and prevention of cancer in over 70 countries of the world. We were privileged to visit one such hospital, Tonghua Changbai Shan Tumor

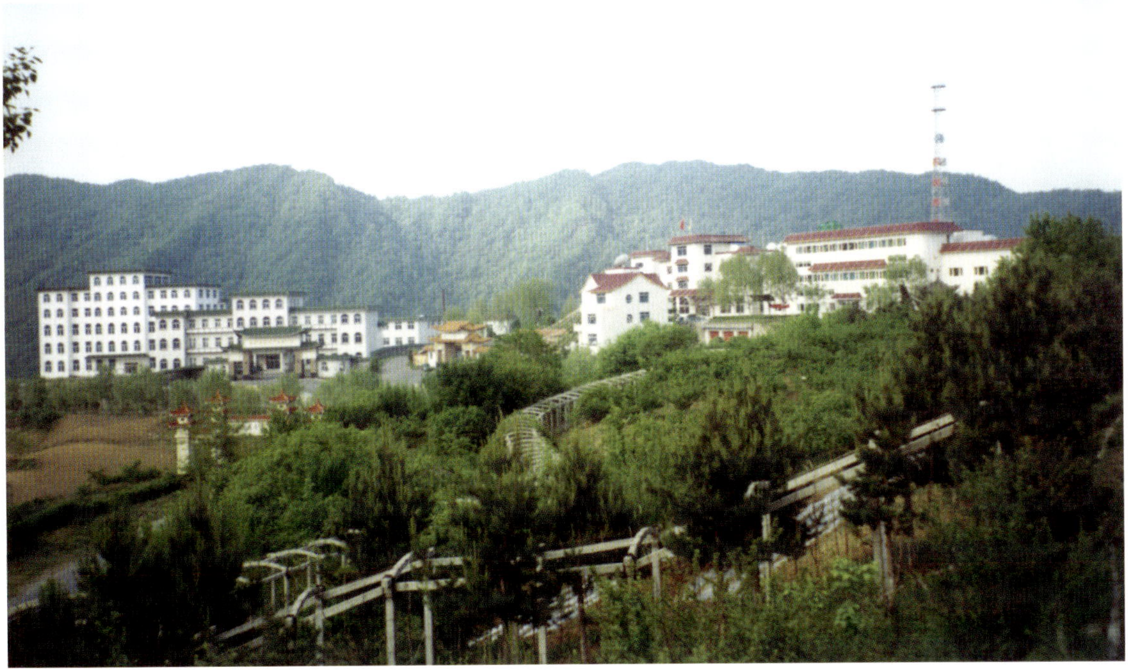

Fig. 3.5. Professor Wang's Changbai Mountain Research Institute. (May 2002, by Jeffrey McConnell)

Hospital in Tonghua, Jilin Province, China. Professor Wang is a recipient of China's award for "practicing good medicine and saving lives". He has also received six international awards for the discovery of Tien Hsien products. His products have been patented in six countries including the United States, China, and Japan.

In order to spend time with Professor Wang at his Institute, we had to make a five hour bus ride through the better part of two provinces. We departed from the city of Shenyang, the largest city in Liaoning Province, and traveled to the outskirts of Tonghua, a mid-sized town in the Jilin Province. Jilin Province is in northeast China bordering North Korea. Wang established his magnificent research facility on a hillside ten miles outside of Tonghua. He named his institute The Changbai Mountain Research Institute. Members of our research team were all looking forward to our trip to the Institue in the mountains. We were not disappointed.

## The Changbai Mountain Research Institute

The Changbai Mountain Research Institute is centered on a hillside that covers over 100 acres of ground overlooking a river with a view of lush green gentle rolling hills and mountains. It had the look of an enchanted kingdom (Figs. 3.5-3.7) and we discovered that indeed it was!

Behind the majestic gates that were wide open to receive our group, was a beautifully designed world to discover. There are three main structures on the prop-

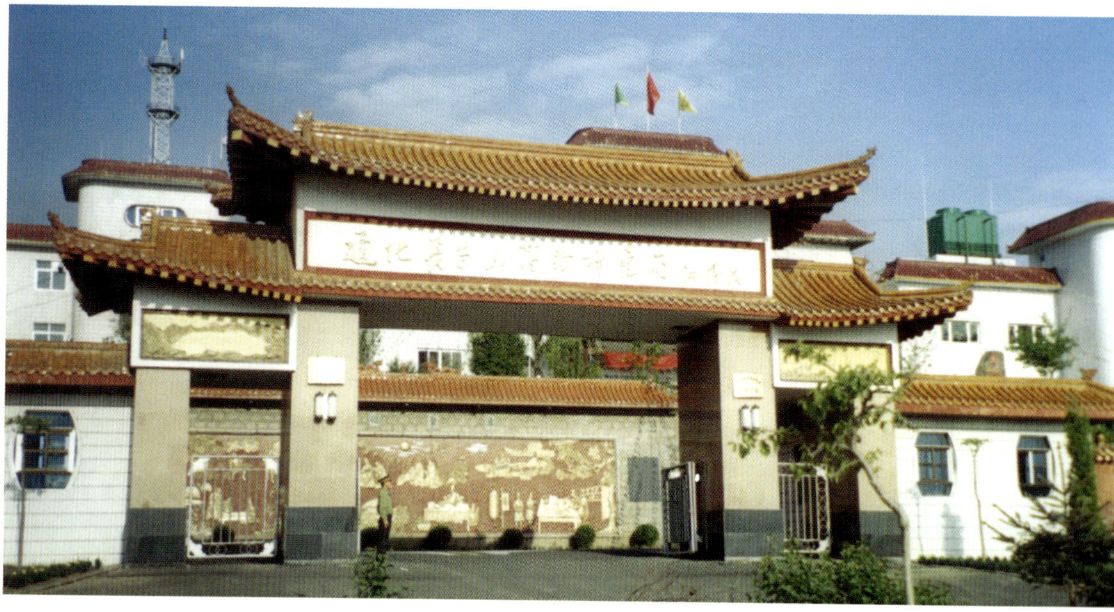

Fig. 3.6. The main gates to the Changbai Mountain Research Institute. (May 2002, by Jeffrey McConnell)

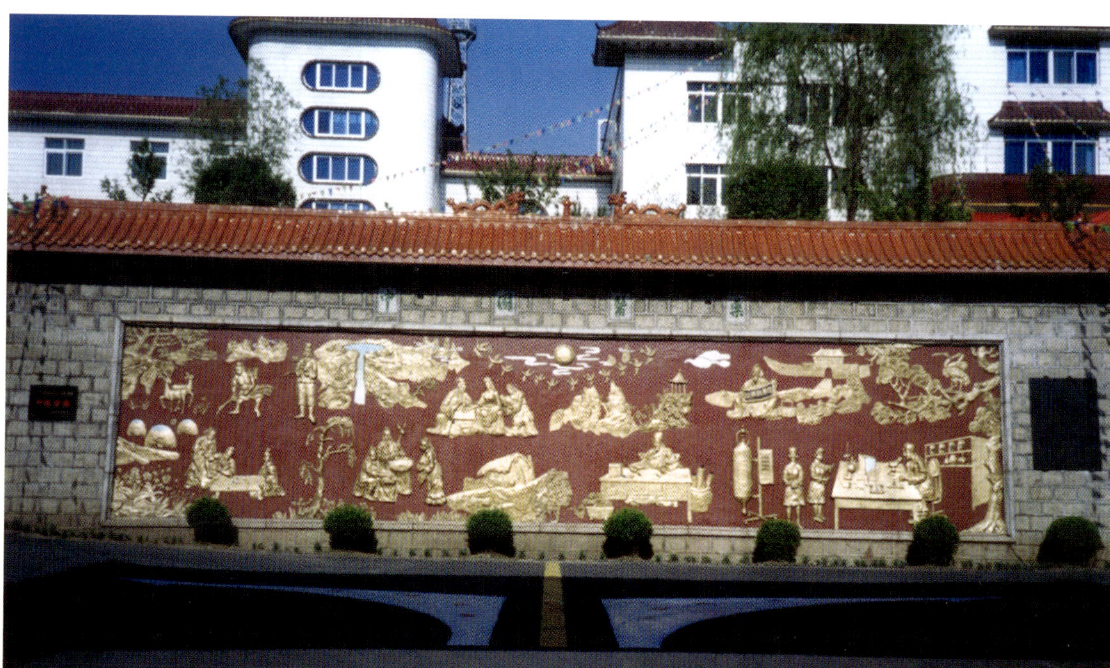

Fig. 3.7. A giant mural just inside the main gate of the Changbai Mountain Research Institute showing the story of Professor Wang's life. (May 2002, by Jeffrey McConnell)

erty and each of them had three spacious stories. The first building we entered upon arriving is a roomy, beautifully designed lodge, primarily for visitors to stay in. However, it also housed one of Professor Wang's private libraries and office. Here we slept for four nights. It was serene, quiet, and every night we enjoyed clear skies and a multitude of stars filling the heavens.

The second structure consisted of two buildings that contained state of the art research laboratories, conference rooms, and an extensive library on medicinal plants. The quality control tests are conducted in these laboratories (Figs. 3.8-3.10). On the second floor of this graciously designed building, was a great auditorium that seated some 200 people. It was here that a ceremony to welcome our research team took place.

The third large building is the manufacturing facility, which contains the grinding, drying, concentrating, bottling, labeling, and other production equipment. This equipment was very new and definitely state of the art. We were given a step by step tour of the herbal manufacturing rooms. The plants were handled very carefully. The process of drying, mixing, and concentrating is a very involved science. Professor Wang has hired experts who are tops in this field. He consults all over China with scientists that are using the latest and most advanced techniques in order to ensure that he provides the end user with the most effective therapeutic products possible. Everything Professor Wang touches has his mark of undisputable quality!

After arriving on a Saturday afternoon, we were treated to an elegant Chinese feast with Professor Wang. The next evening we were part of the celebration for receiving GMP certification. On Monday morning we received a formal reception in the auditorium. Our research team was seated facing the audience of some 200 or so members of Professor Wang's staff. Professor Wang officially welcomed our group. He gave an eloquent aclode to Dr. Halstead (TLH). He said that for so long he has dreamed of a western scientist and physician such as Dr. Halstead who would come to learn first hand about his work at Changbai Mountain Research Institute. It was a wish he had waited for many years to come true. He said it was the greatest honor he could imagine that a prestigious scientist such as Dr. Halstead would make such a long trip at the age of eighty-two! In return Dr. Halstead presented Professor Wang with a beautiful trophy of peace and friendship as a gift from the World Life Research Institute, in Grand Terrace, California. Professor Wang's eyes were full of tears of joy as he accepted the symbolic gift commemorating our union in friendship.

At this formal reception our fellow teammate, Mr. Frank Cousineau, the United States' chapter Vice President of the Cancer Control Society, also presented special awards. Lovely plaques were given in recognition of each recipient's commitment to help further the mission of eradicating the threat of cancer to all people of the world. Mr. Cousineau, together with Mr. Michael Ng, ceremoniously awarded

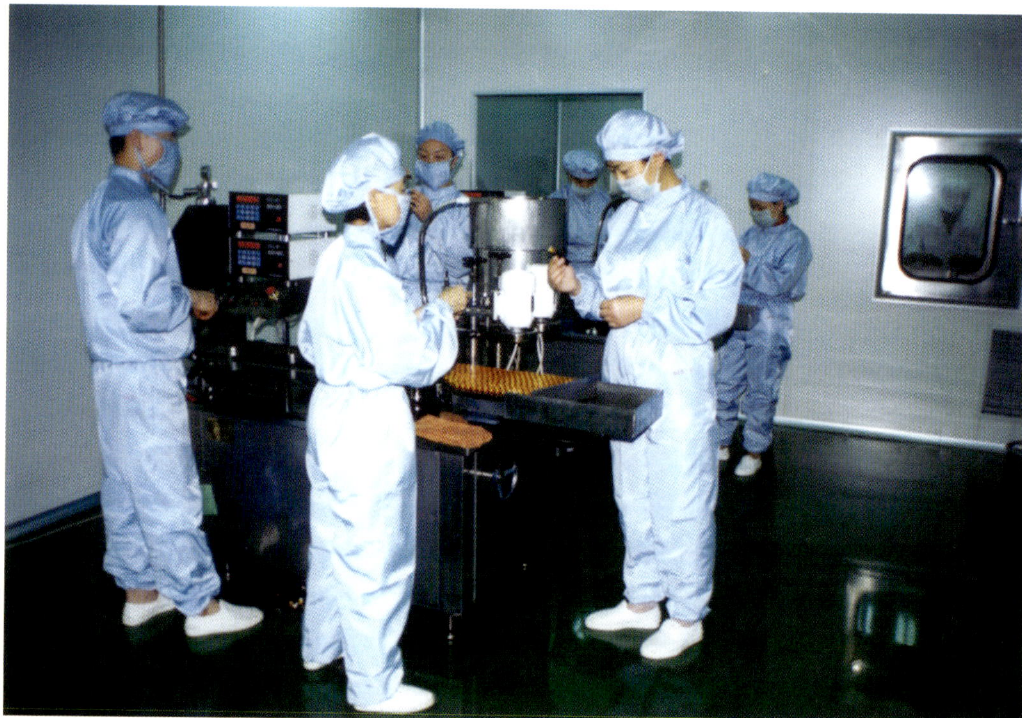

Fig. 3.8. Inspection of the vials of the Tien Hsien Liquid at the Tonghua Zhenguo Pharmaceutical Co. Ltd. in Tonghua, Jilin, China. (June 2002, Courtesy of Professor Wang)

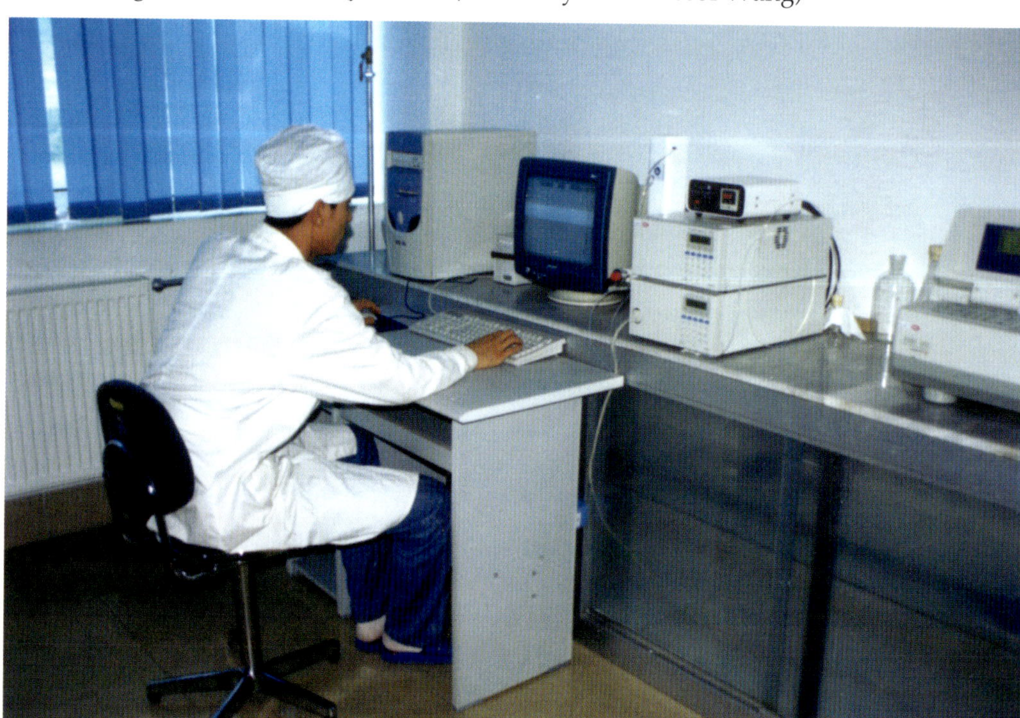

Fig. 3.9. Analyzing chemical constituents and active ingredients in a quality control lab at Tonghua Zhenguo Pharmaceutical Co. Ltd. in Tonghua, Jilin, China. (June 2002, Courtesy of Professor Wang)

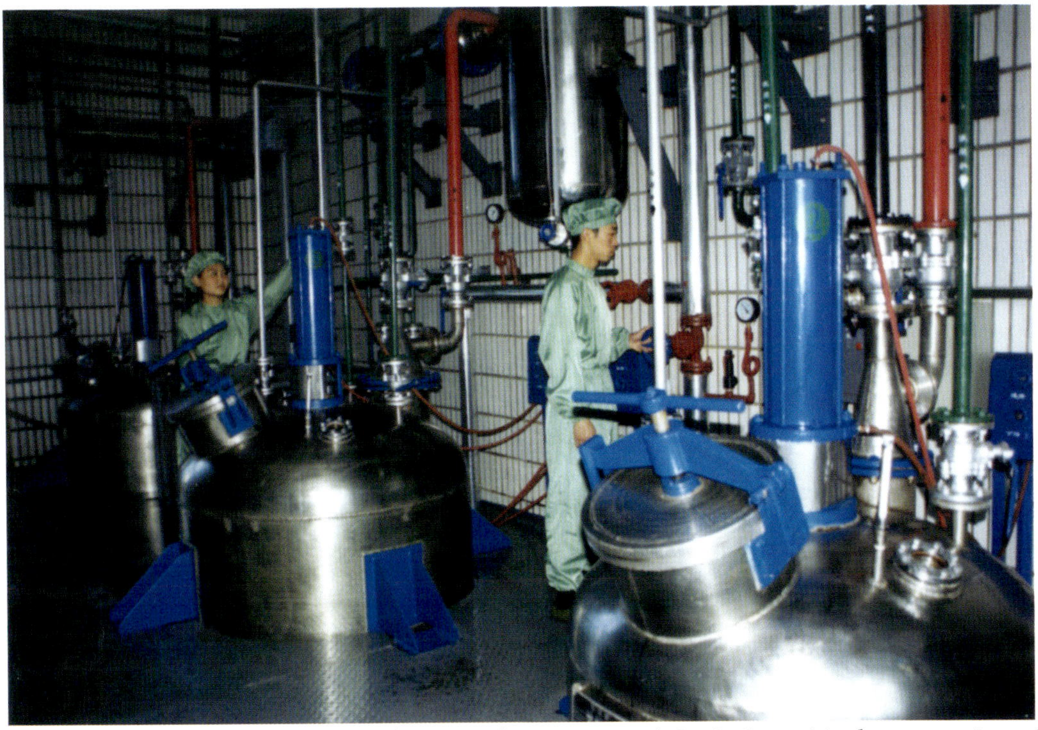

Fig. 3.10. Equipment at the Tonghua Zhenguo Pharmaceutical Co. Ltd. used in the processing of the Tien Hsien herbal products in Tonghua, Jilin, China. (June 2002, Courtesy of Professor Wang)

Professor Wang and each of our team members a plaque. This was one day that felt historically important. We had an inner awareness that this alliance between western and eastern scientists would prove to be of great benefit to all mankind. We believe all nations need to collaborate and work together in order to resolve our common global problems and live in peace.

## The Grounds and Gardens at the Changbai Mountain Research Institute

The outside environment of the Changbai Mountain Research Institute was beautiful and fascinating. We estimated that at least 50 acres were cultivated in a spectacular medicinal botanical garden (Figs. 3.11-3.15). We were informed that there were over two thousand various medicinal plants and trees planted on the grounds. Each specific species was identified by the scientific name on a sign. The landscape flowed with added beautification in the form of pagodas, waterfalls, statues of ancient herbalists, and flower gardens to name a few. When looking in any direction from the institute's grounds, all one sees is beauty and peace. Everywhere there were gentle rolling hills and directly alongside the property ran a lovely

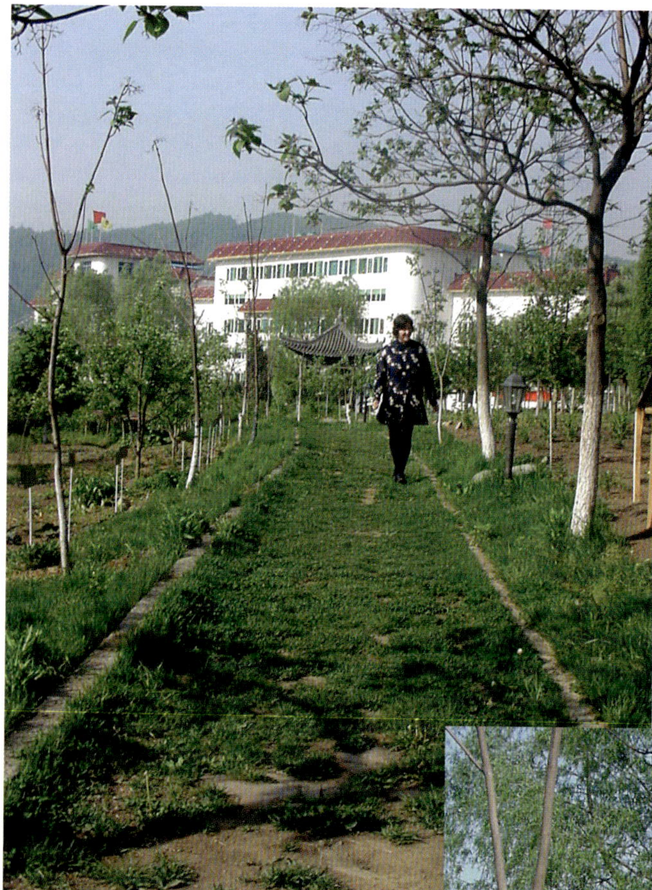

➤ Fig. 3.11. Terri walking through the botanical herbal gardens of the Changbai Mountain Research Institute. (May 2002, by Jeffrey McConnell)

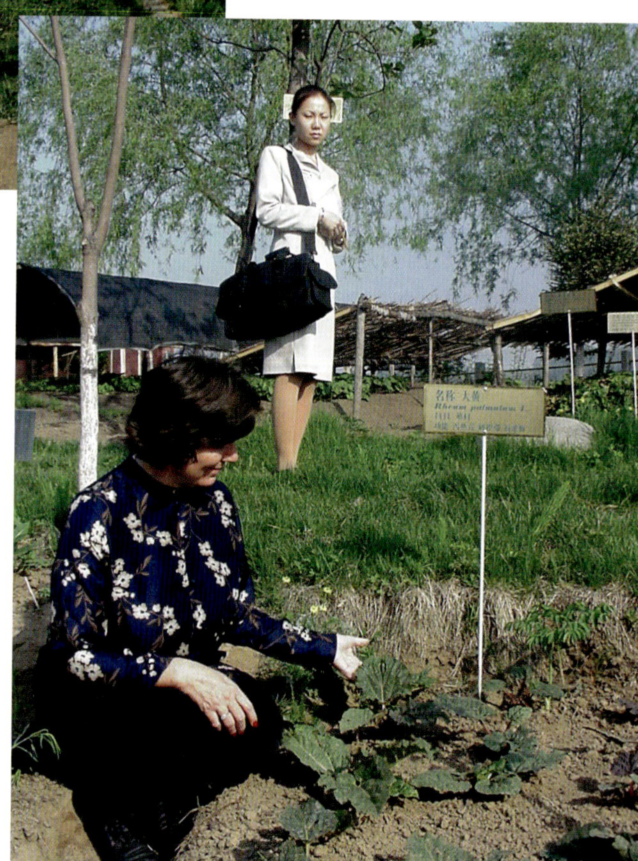

➤ Fig. 3.12. Terri inspecting the herb *Rheum palmatum* L. with Qui Yue one of our three house hostesses. Thanks also to Yuan Ning Ningand Tan Qi (not shown). (May 2002, by Jeffrey McConnell)

➢ Fig. 3.13. Bruce standing next to a statue of Li Ci Zheng. He is considered the father of recording Chinese herbs and their medicinal properties. (May 2002, by Jeffrey McConnell)

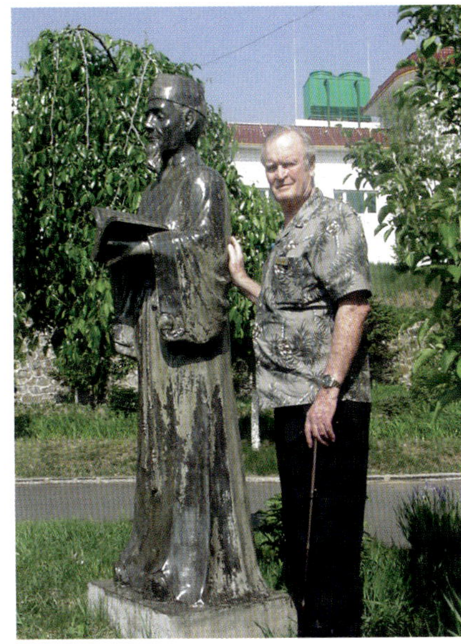

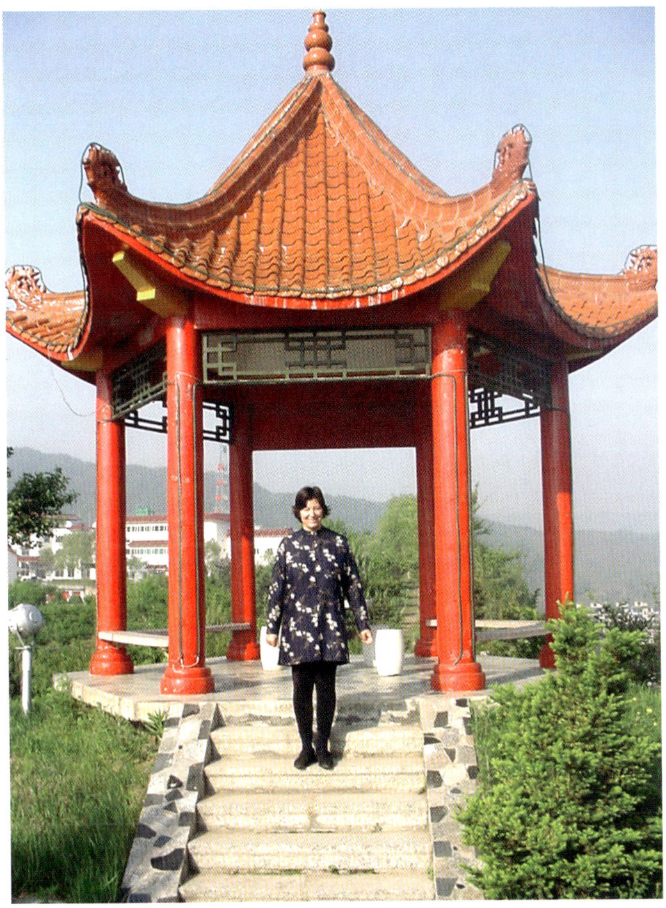

⮝ Fig. 3.15. Terri in a pagoda at the highest point for miles around. Note the commanding view of the Institute in the background. (May 2002, by Jeffrey McConnell)

⮟ Fig. 3.14. Terri sitting at the foot of a statue of Zhang Lang. He is known for having first discovered ginseng growing in this part of China hundreds of years ago. (May 2002, by Jeffrey McConnell)

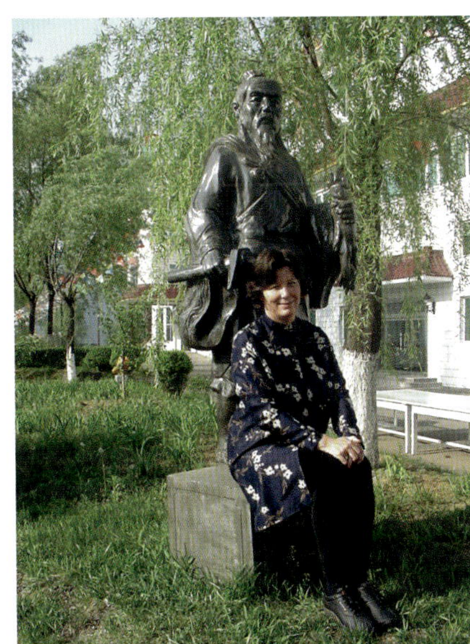

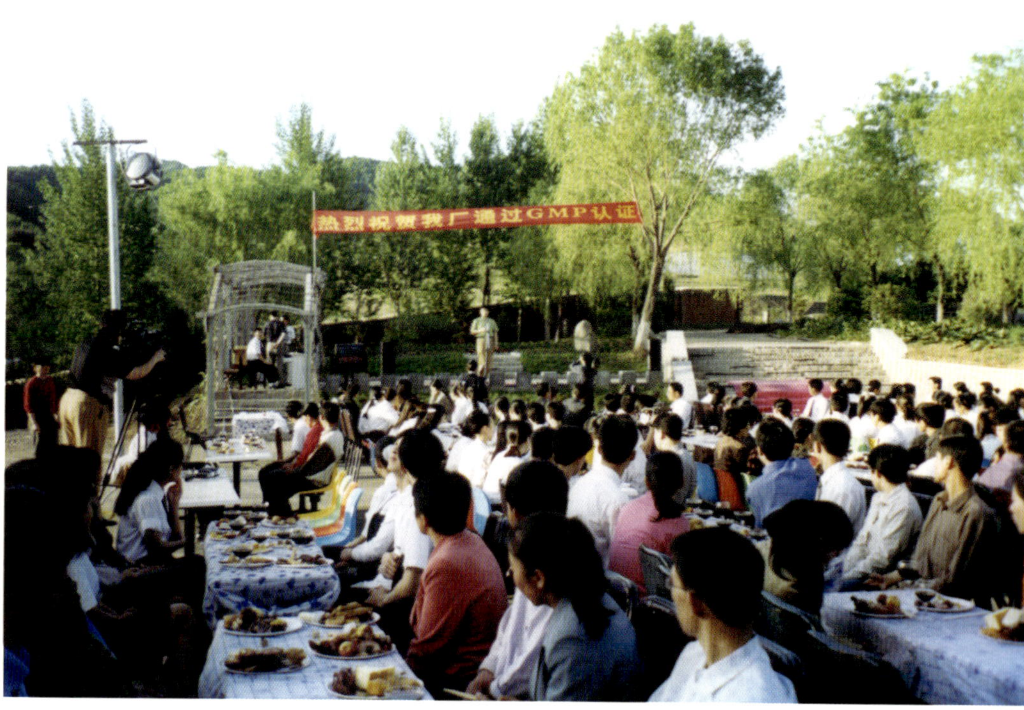


Fig. 3.16. Professor Wang throws a celebration party, thanking all of his employees for their hard work to pass the strict GMP regulatory requirements. (May 2002, by Jeffrey McConnell)

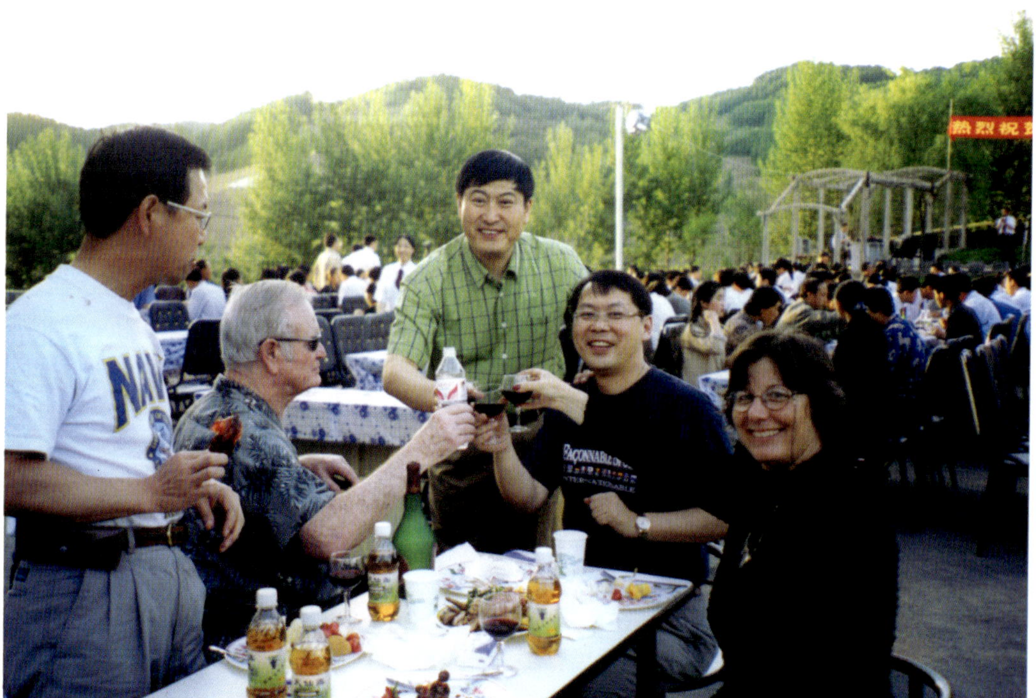

Fig. 3.17. Toasting to the health of the world. From left to right: Thomas Chou, Dr. Bruce Halstead, Professor Wang, Haiwei Chen and Terri Halstead. (May 2002, by Jeffrey McConnell)

river. We all agreed that this was indeed "Shangri La", a place of much beauty, serenity, and charm.

Shortly before our visit, Professor Wang's company had received the Good Manufacturing Practices (GMP) certification from the Chinese government. On Sunday night there was a great celebration taking place among their several hundred employees—for all had sacrificed greatly in making this happen (Figs. 3.16, 3.17). We noticed that as Professor Wang addressed his workers, many of the employees had tears in their eyes. This told us a lot about the caliber of their organization and its leader.

## The Changbai Mountain Herbal Plantation and a Dedication to Dr. Bruce Halstead

While staying at his research institute, we accompanied Professor Wang to his large herbal plantation in the nearby mountain area. We were so impressed with all that we saw and experienced on our journey into the hills with this kind, gentle, extraordinary healer and herbalist. It was so obvious how deeply Professor Wang loved to be in nature among his beloved medicinal plants. He radiated pure joy! We saw a variety of medicinal plants in cultivation. Everything was shades of green as far as the eye could see. These plants were being fed by underground springs fed by waters coming from a large lake some one hundred miles north on the border of Korea and China. This volcanic lake is famous for its beauty and its incredible water. It is named Lake Tianchi (or Heavenly Lake) (Fig. 3.18). The water coming from the lake is believed to contain organic germanium, deuterium and other rare minerals. The soil itself in this region (Changbai Mountains) is highly rich in mineral content.

The soil came from ancient volcanic ash. The water, the soil, and the climate all contribute to producing an incredibly high quality medicinal plant. These are the source of herbs that are used in the Tien Hsien products. Professor Wang has often mentioned that he has never found any other geographical region equal to the Changbai Mountain for growing and cultivating top quality medicinal herbs.

It is important to mention, that the whole process of growing and harvesting these plants must be in the hands of very knowledgably experts. There are countless do's and don'ts in proper cultivation. The Chinese are the world's expert in this subject and without a doubt the crops cultivated by Professor Wang are getting the finest of attention.

Towards the end of our day in the mountainside, we had a delightful surprise. Professor Wang honored me (BWH) by naming a portion of the mountain gardens the "Dr. Bruce Halstead Changbai Mountain Herbal Gardens" (Figs. 3.19, 3.20). I (BWH) considered this kind gesture to be one of the greatest honors in my entire career. We hope to return and enjoy these majestic gardens many more times.

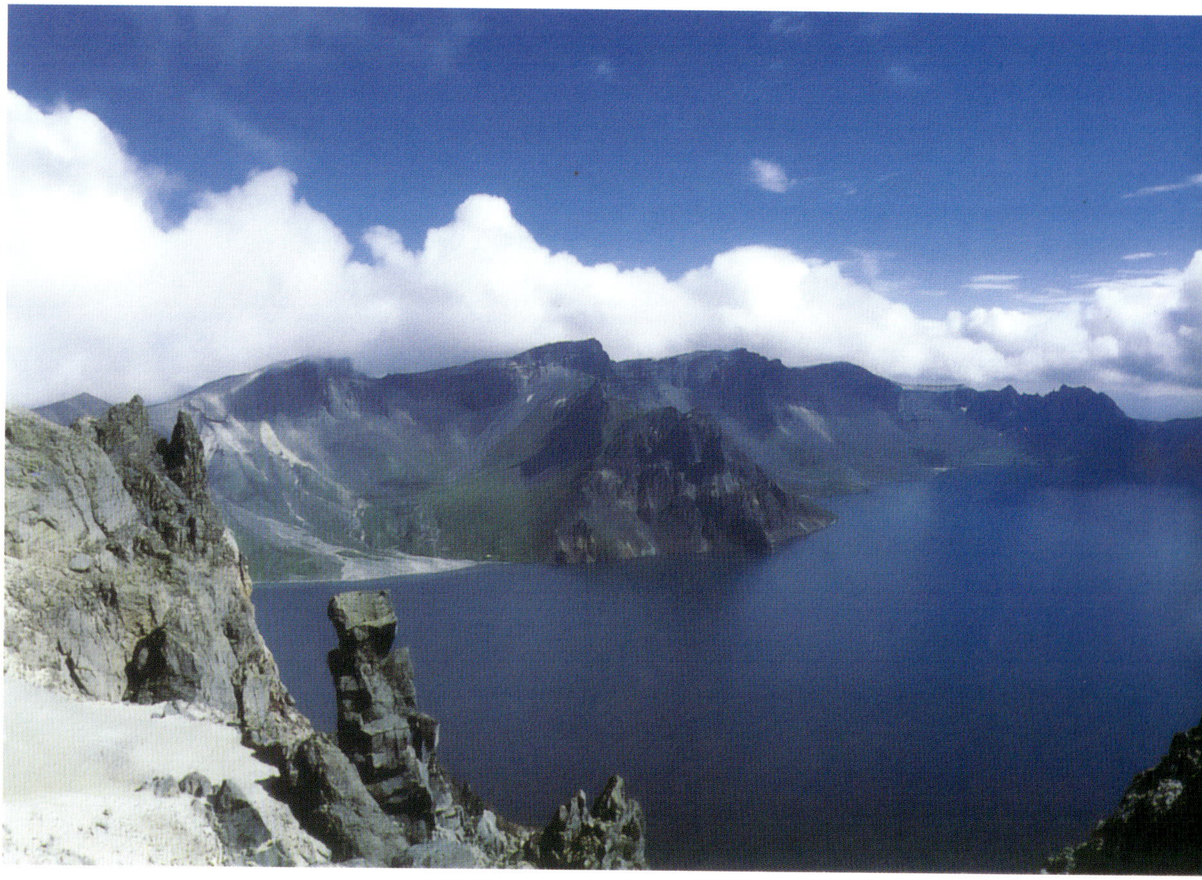

Fig. 3.18. Volcanic Tianchi (Heavenly) Lake in the Changbai Mountains on the boundary line of China and North Korea. (Courtesy of China Travel and Tourism Press)

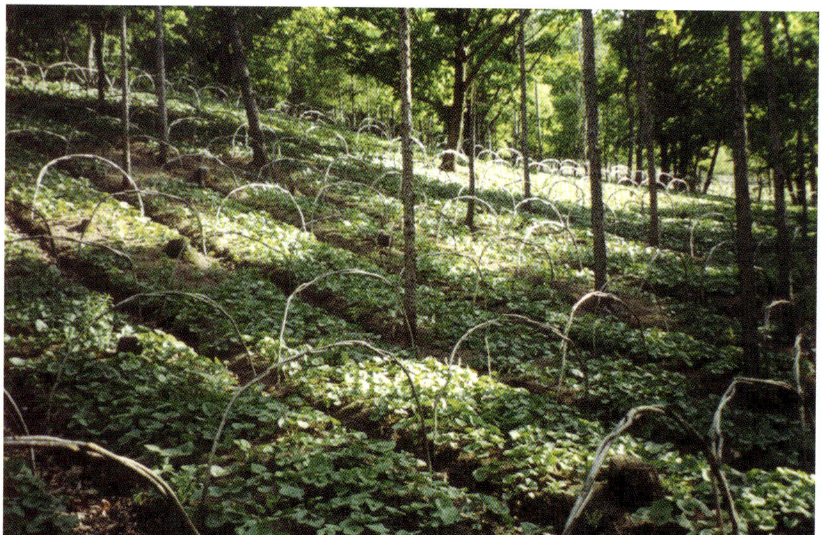

Fig.3.19. The *Dr.Halstead Changbai Mountain Herbal Gardens*. (May 2002, by Jeffrey McConnell)

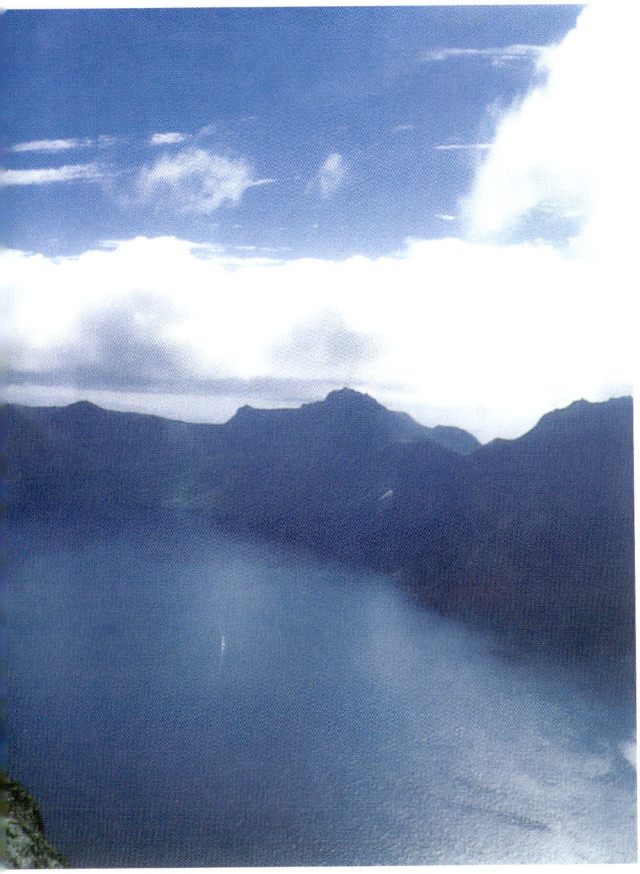

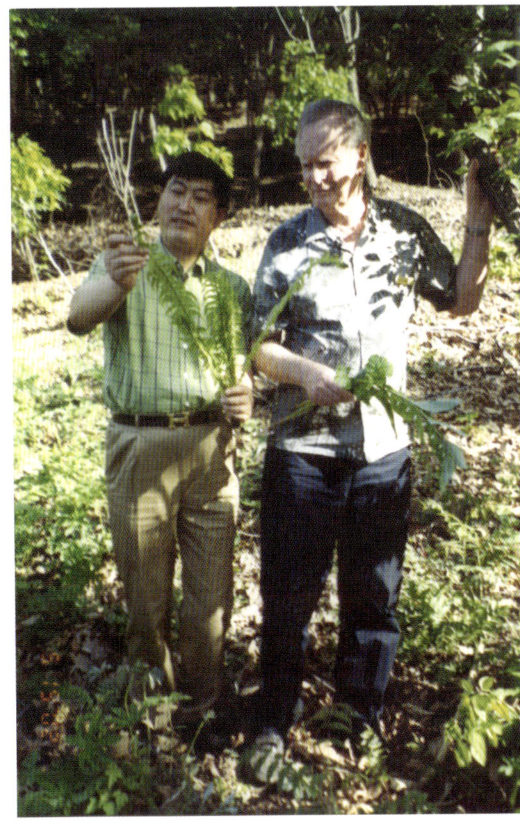

Fig. 3.20. Professor Wang showing Dr. Bruce Halstead some of the many herbs growing on his herbal farms high in the Changbai Mountains. (May 2002, by Jeffrey McConnell)

## Tonghua Changbai Shan Tumor Hospital

On our last day with Professor Wang we visited the Tonghua Changbai Shan Tumor Hospital, which was a short distance from his institute. It is located in the city of Tonghua towards the more central part of town. This was one of the some three hundred hospitals and or clinics Professor Wang helped to open throughout China. This hospital was one of the first that he had started. The patients that walked in the door were all terminal. However, since the beginning, nearly every patient that has come in has walked out healthy and victorious over their cancer.

We were told that the government of China allowed such centers and were supportive of Professor Wang's work. He had permission to operate freely with no limits or government restrictions. Patients who had exhausted their options for conventional treatment such as chemotherapy and radiation were allowed freely to go to this hospital. Therefore, this facility was a compassionate last hope sanctuary. The results have stunned everyone!

It is fortunate that to this day Professor Wang takes time to be actively involved with the many patients who find their way to one of the clinics or hospital facilities that he started. He meets and consults with each patient and their family. We watched him in action as we visited the hospital. He throws his whole being into this work. He always examines each patient, studies the laboratory results, x-rays, microscopic photos of tumors, and all other available information. Some patients are able to pay the costs of treatment; some are not. No one is turned away for lack of financial resources. Professor Wang donates out of his own coffers to make up the financial differences. Professor Wang's knowledge and experience of working first hand with patients is vast. He was able to show us x-ray after x-ray of patient tumors of every type and shape. Time and time again the tumors shrank and ultimately disappeared from the x-rays. When we asked what was the average treatment time he replied, "Six to twenty months depending on the individual case." We asked for an approximate cure rate. The answer: 80-90%. This is virtually unheard of where we come from!

We arrived at the tidy, spacious two-story Tonghua Changbai Shan Tumor Hospital on a sunny spring day with a breeze coming in all the many open windows. When our bus arrived we were greeted by friendly and cheerful doctors and nurses (Fig 3.21). The hospital consisted of 20 beds, an outpatient clinic, X-ray unit, and routine laboratory equipment. The patients were all once considered terminal cancer cases. Most of the patients were all walking around looking surprisingly healthy. One patient we met was a 36-year old female (Fig 3.22). Three years earlier she had been diagnosed with abdominal cancer. Her cancer progressed in spite of conventional treatment. It had spread throughout her body including her brain. For the first two and a half years she had been treated with chemotherapy and radiation, but these had failed to arrest the cancer. When she first arrived at the Tonghua Changbai Shan Tumor Hospital, approximately five months prior to our visit, she was gaunt, had no appetite, and was a shadow of her former self. She was weak and bedridden. Her doctors gave her only a few weeks to live. After evaluation by Professor Wang, and a subsequent protocol of taking Tien Hsien products for five months, the tumors in her abdomen had vanished. One by one the metastases were disappearing including the ones in her brain. Her appetite returned. She had regained a normal healthy weight. To all of us in our team of researchers, she looked healthy, strong, and was radiating good spirits.

This lovely patient was having a treatment when we interviewed her. She was taking the Tien Hsien product intravenously. The solution was sterile and had been prepared to meet pharmaceutical IV standards. Professor Wang elaborated on this. He had found that there are times when a patient who is very ill must take

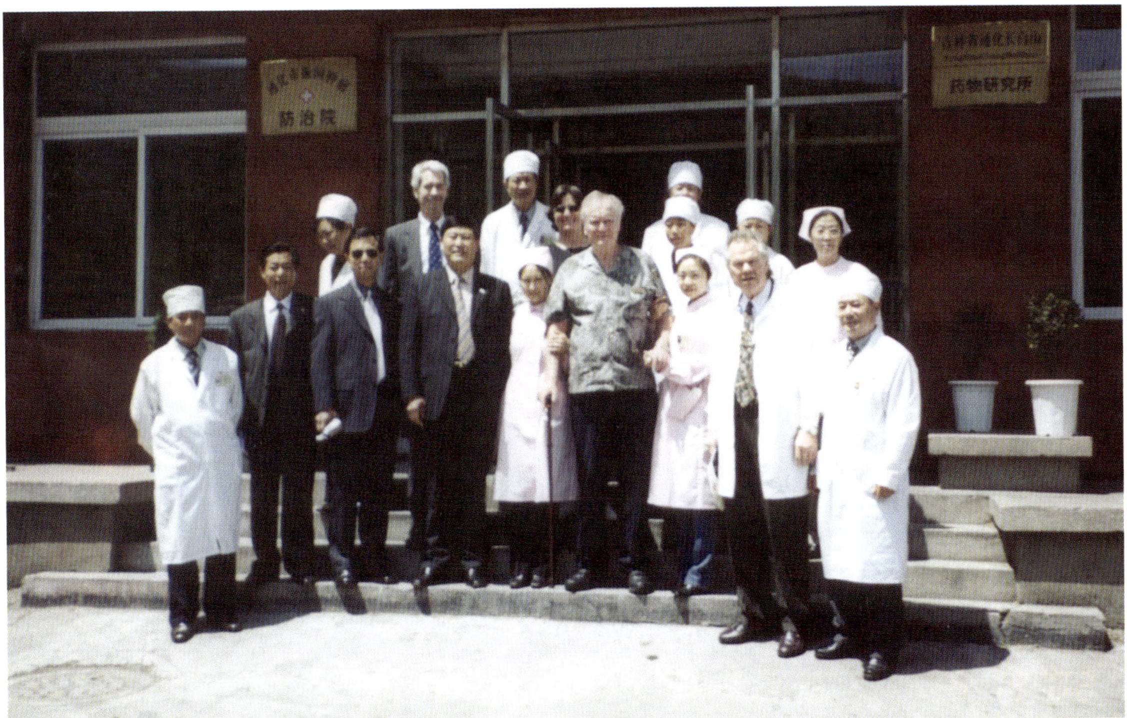


Fig. 3.21. Our group with Professor Wang and the staff of the Tonghua Changbai Shan Tumor Hospital. (May 2002, by Jeffrey McConnell)

Fig. 3.22. The 36-yr old female cancer patient and Anthony J. Hilder. (May 2002, by Jeffrey McConnell)

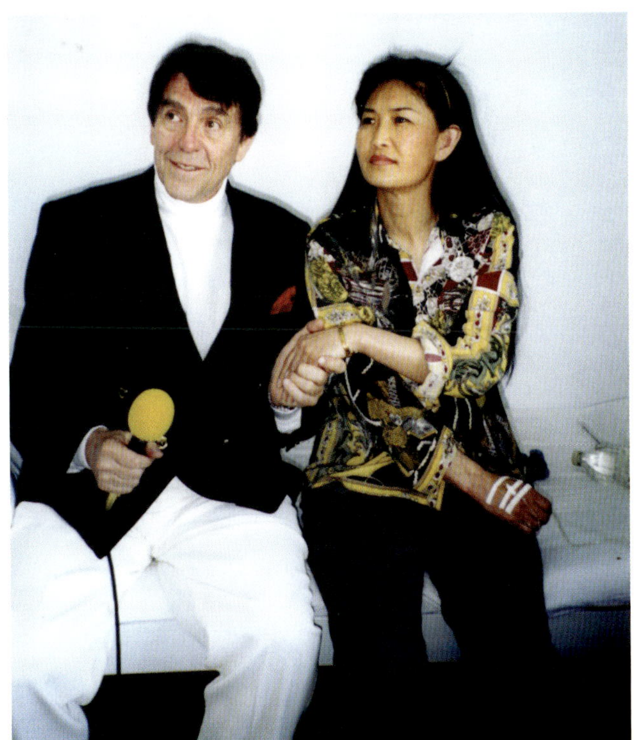

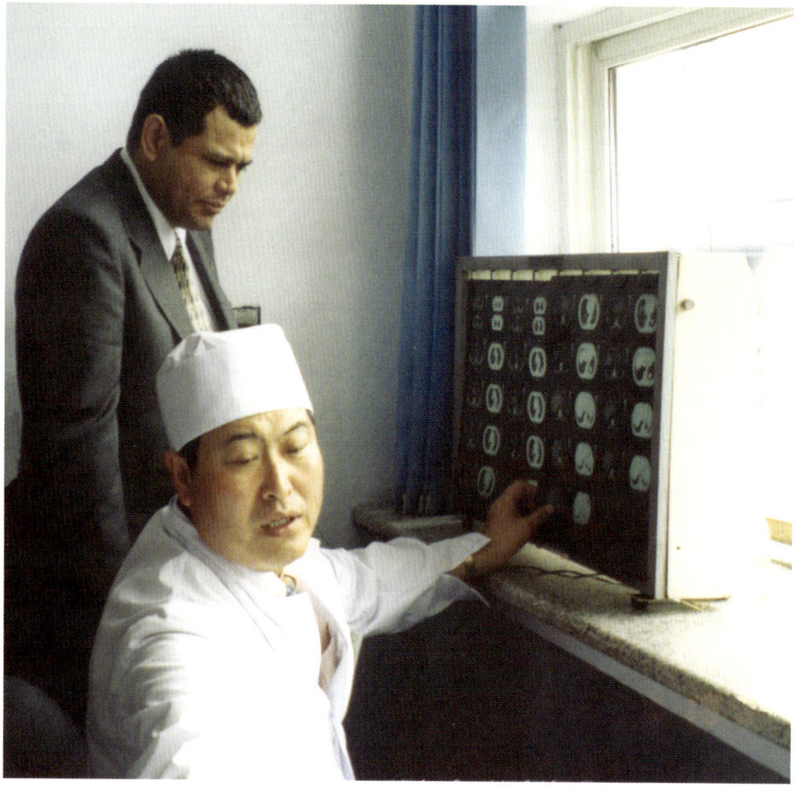

Fig. 3.23. Professor Wang explaining the sequence of x-rays to Dr. Francisco Espinosa showing the regression of a brain tumor utilizing his herbal formulas. (May 2002, by Jeffrey McConnell)

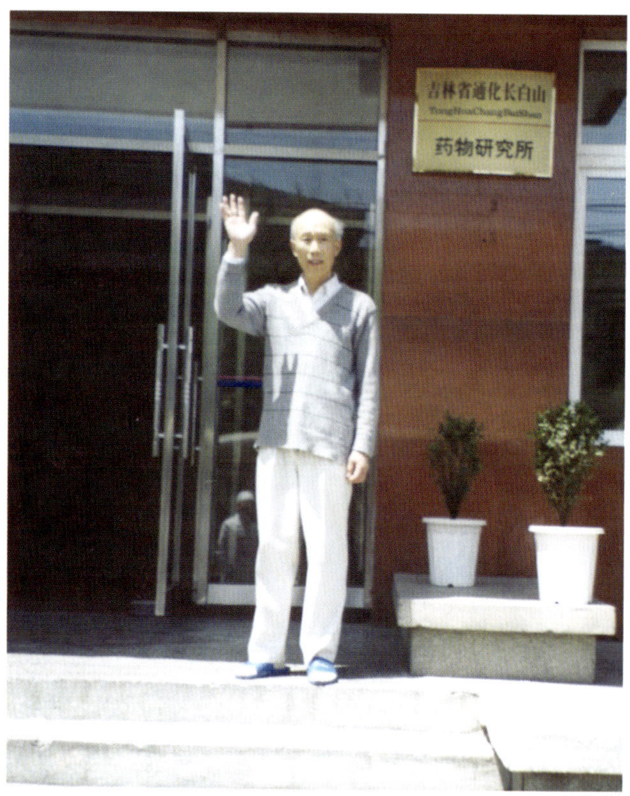


Fig. 3.24. Recovering cancer patient Mr. Chin waving goodbye to our group as we leave the Tonghua Changbai Shan Tumor Hospital. (May 2002, by Jeffrey McConnell)

the herbs in an IV or in some cases the herbs are injected directly into the organ and or tumor. Fascinating! This information was so remarkable to hear. Dr. Francisco Espinosa (Fig. 3.23), our research team oncologist, was unduly impressed! Judging from the results we all concurred that this was a major break through for medicine!

After our four unforgettable days with the remarkable professor Wang we tearfully exited Shangri La (Fig. 3.24)! Again we took a long day trip southeast into Liaoning Province to the city of Shenyang where we caught a flight to Beijing to visit and to do additional research and fact-finding.

## Our Visit To Beijing

There are more fascinating research and educational centers in Beijing than anyone could visit in a lifetime. This was our third research trip that included Beijing on the itinerary. On this particular trip we visited the following people and places:

### PROFESSOR ZONG KUI WEN

Professor Zong Kui Wen (Fig. 3.25) is a long time friend and colleague of ours. Professor Wen is a retired professor from the Institute of Medicinal Plant Development (IMPLAD). IMPLAD is the largest center for medicinal plant development anywhere in the world. It is located towards the outskirts of Beijing. Professor Wen has served as one of the vice-presidents in research at IMPLAD. In recent years, he has established his own medicinal herbal manufacturing plant. He gave us a tour of his facility, which was in full production of herbal products.

### ACADEMY OF CHINESE TRADITIONAL MEDICINE

This very prestigious school and research center hosted an afternoon open house for us, whereby we were able to meet with many of our longtime Chinese friends and scientific colleagues (Fig. 3.26, 3.27). It was an uplifting and productive meeting.

### BOOKSTORES

You have not lived until you go book shopping with Dr. Halstead and Mr. Yan Zhao (Fig. 3.25) in the fascinating city of Beijing (TLH). Mr. Zhao, with his own educational background in botanical pharmagology, knows all to well what kind of books Dr. Halstead is on the lookout for. After all, this was Mr. Zhao's third trip accompanying us inside China. Mr. Yan Zhao completed a special internship in 1992 at the World Life Research Institute and since that time has worked with us on several scientific projects. As in the past, we had to buy another suitcase when the

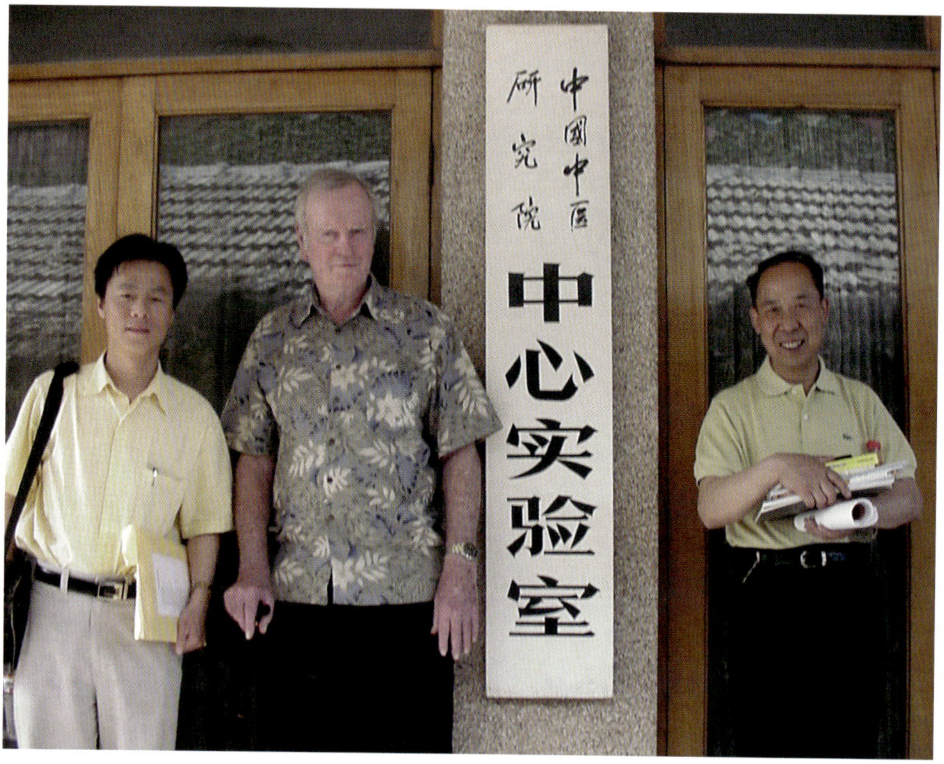


Fig. 3.25. Our long time friends Yan Zhao and Zong Kui Wen with Dr. Halstead Photo taken in front of the Academy of Traditional Chinese Medicine in Bejing China. (May 2002, by Jeffrey McConnell)

shopping spree was over! The books we purchased were beautiful colorful works on medicinal plants. To our surprise, they had some that only recently had become available in English. This was an extra treat for the authors. We want to acknowledge and thank Mr. Yan Zhao for his friendship and his many contributions to our work over the last ten years.

## UNIVERSITY OF PEKING

This was our first visit to the University of Peking, which is one of the most famous learning universities in the world. The entire research team was received like royalty. The arrangements had been made by Michael Ng's niece, April Wong, a student in the University. Once again, we had that feeling of being in a magical kingdom. On our bus driven tour we saw beautiful park like gardens, trees everywhere, large beautiful lakes, a six-story library, sacred pagodas, stunning sculptures, water fountains, and lovely buildings. There was a peaceful serenity and a beauty all around. We felt that this kind of environment and atmosphere was very conducive to learning and creative thinking. We hope to make a return trip to this enchanting university.

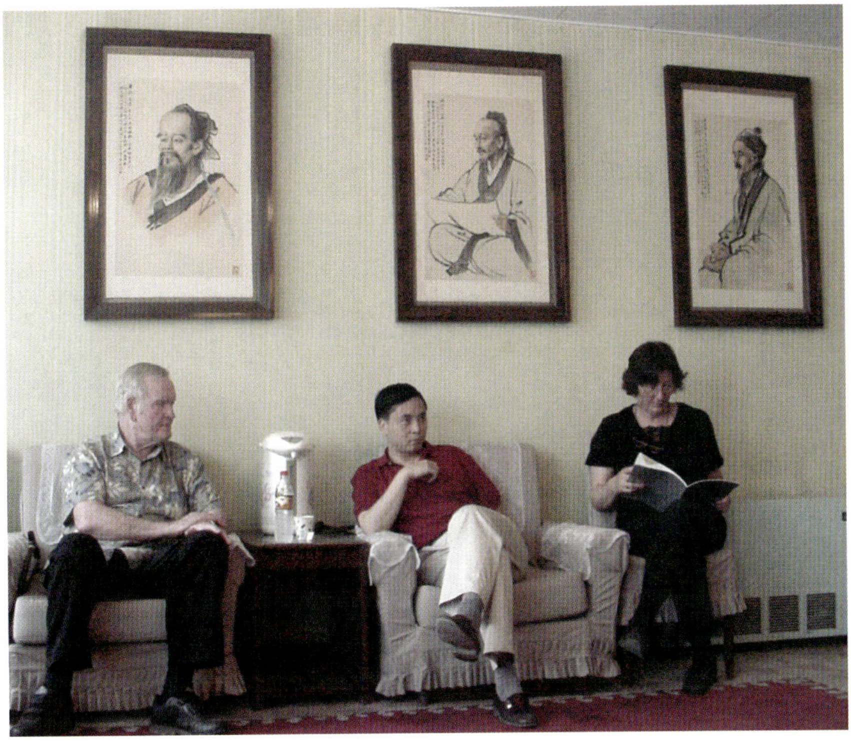

Fig. 3.26. Dr. Bruce Halstead and his wife Terri discussing the history of Chinese herbalogy with Yang Jin Shen under portraits of some of China's most revered historical medicine men. Photo taken at the Academy of Traditional Chinese Medicine in Beijing, China. (May 2002, by Jeffrey McConnell)

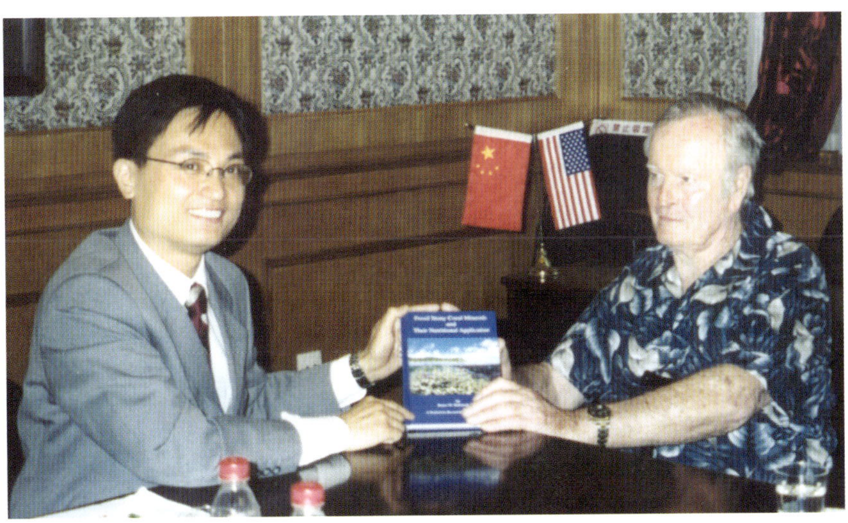

Fig. 3.27. Dr. Halstead presenting his book, *Fossil Stony Coral Minerals and their Nutritional Application* to Program Director of International Relations, Manli Zhou of the University of Peking. (May 2002, by Jeffrey McConnell)

## We Meet More of the CJFU Family

In the Beijing office for Tien Hsien products we met yet another group of dynamic, outgoing staff members. These lovely people were kind enough to arrange interviews with doctors in hospitals and clinics who have been treating cancer patients with Tien Hsien Herbal Products. Dr. Ray Baldwin, Dr. Francisco Espinosa, and Dr. Ada Garcia spent one entire day meeting these physicians and reviewing patients' medical charts, blood work, and x-rays. Again, the results were incredibly positive. Dr. Espinosa, being an oncologist himself, was initially the most skeptical professional member of our team. However, what he saw for himself in Beijing totally convinced him that these products get cancer patients well again. There was no disputing the medical records and the endless x-rays documenting the spectacular results. Dr. Francisco was now significantly in awe of these herbal products. His life had been changed forever. He witnessed first hand what could be considered a major breakthrough for mankind in the field of cancer therapy. Instead of sleeping, that night Dr. Espinosa contemplated the potential impact this therapy could have on the world. Dr. Garcia was moved to tears and Dr. Baldwin was equally moved and impressed.

## Hong Kong Here We Come

After four action packed days in Beijing, our team caught a plane for Hong Kong where the headquarters of CJFU is located (Fig. 3.28). Here we met with their executive staff, which included Sidney Lu, Charles Lee, Thomas Chou, Phillip Chen, Joan Lu, Corrina Lee, and Allan Gao, to name a few. This is when Joan Lu made her outstanding presentation on the overhead projector giving us a historical overview of the company, their mission statement (which we included in Chapter One), and both their short and long term goals and objectives. The presentation included a figure of approximately how many cancer victims have treated their cancer with Tien Hsien outside of those who use it in mainland China. (CJFU has all rights outside mainland China) The figure is estimated to be 2,000,000 people since they began in 1986. The success rate was upwards of 80% recovery. Their marketing strategy included publications, television talk shows, books, and magazine articles. They are experiencing continued growth in every country they have entered for distribution. Their next challange was to open up the markets in Australia, the United States, Canada, and Mexico.

In 2001 the flagship formula also known as Tien Hsien Number One Liquid had received approval as a nutritional supplement by the U.S. Food and Drug Administration. This was accomplished by many months of hard work by Mr. Michael Ng. Mr. Ng, the CJFU consultant in the U.S., and Mr. Frank Cousineau are

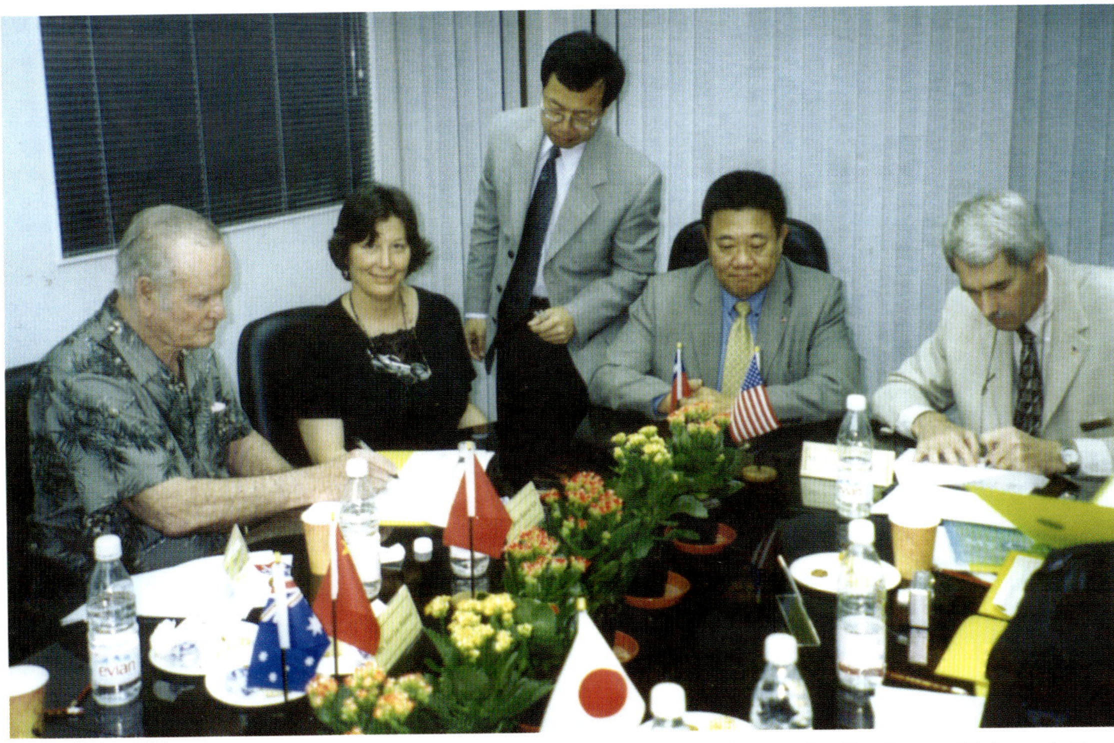

Fig. 3.28. The signing of the contract to write this book. From left to right: Dr. Bruce Halstead, Terri Halstead, Thomas Chou, Sidney Lu, and Frank Cousineau. (May 2002, by Jeffrey McConnell)

CJFU's liscened distributors for Tien Hsien in the U.S., Canada, and Mexico. They formed a company explicitly for this purpose, which they have named Innovative Marketing Firm. Their offices are located in Beverly Hills, California. This was a great step forward. The products can be acquired by contacting their office.

The staff of CJFU arranged for our team to have a special visit and tour of the Hong Kong Baptist University School of Chinese Medicine. At first we wondered why we were going there, but all doubts were removed once we entered the building (Fig. 3.29). The Hong Kong Baptist University received a large grant of money from the Chinese government in 1998 and 1999, and another large grant from the local Jockey Club to build a world-class school, clinic, and research center focusing on traditional Chinese medicine. With this money a new building several stories high was constructed and equipped with the finest analytical equipment available. The objective of this new medical center was to completely modernize Chinese medicine on an international integrated basis. Their library (Figs. 3.30-3.32) contains over 10,000 volumes of Chinese medical books and a complete collection of texts on Chinese materia medicas. This set of materia medicas included over 400 volumes and more than 800 other related works, and over 10,000 individual scientific articles on Chinese medicinal plants. Their electronic Chinese

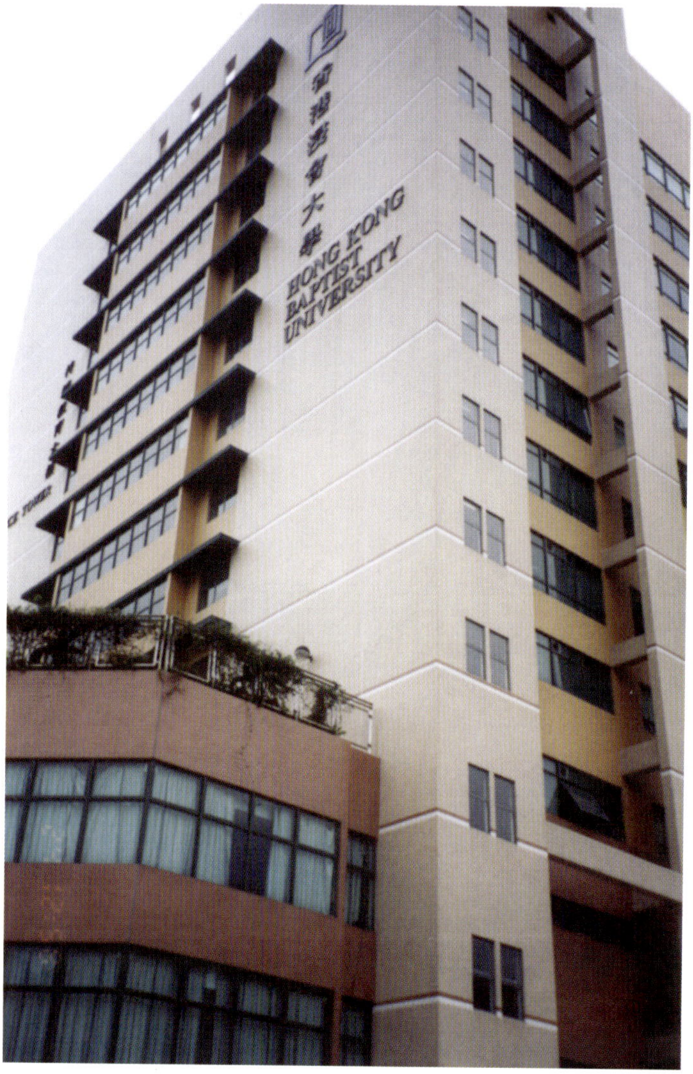


Fig. 3.29. Hong Kong Baptist University. (May 2002, by Jeffrey McConnell)

homepage links them to over 230 internet resources within China and abroad. This is a specialty library, which within its scope compares well with the U.S. National Library of Medicine and the Lenin Library in Moscow. We are grateful to Ms. Lisa Song the head librarian who spent much time sharing information with us.

We want to acknowledge and thank the following staff members who hosted our day at this most amazing school and research center: Professor Wei-Yi Yang, Dr. Zhao-Xiang Bian, Dr. Kelvin S. Y. Leung and Dr. Zhong-Zhen Zhao. It was a tremendous thrill to be introduced and exposed to the advanced research that they were conducting.

One entire floor at the Hong Kong Baptist University School of Chinese Medicine was dedicated to clinical medicine. We toured a spacious, elegant, fully staffed medical clinic, which housed its own medicinal herbal pharmacy (Figs. 3.33,

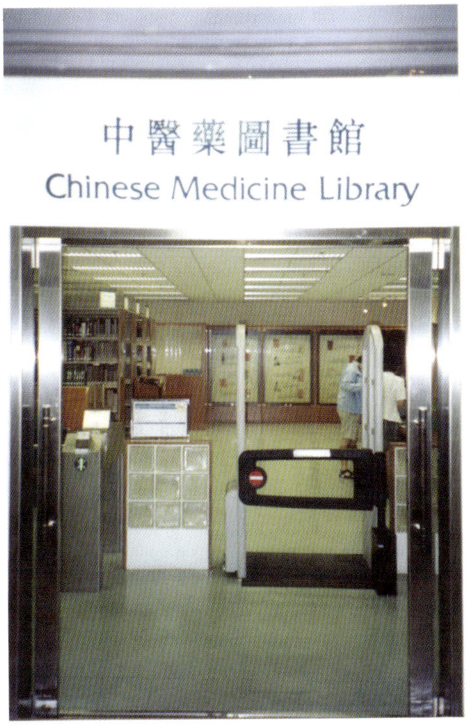


Fig. 3.30. Entrance to the Chinese Medicine Library at the Hong Kong Baptist University. (May 2002, by Jeffrey McConnell)

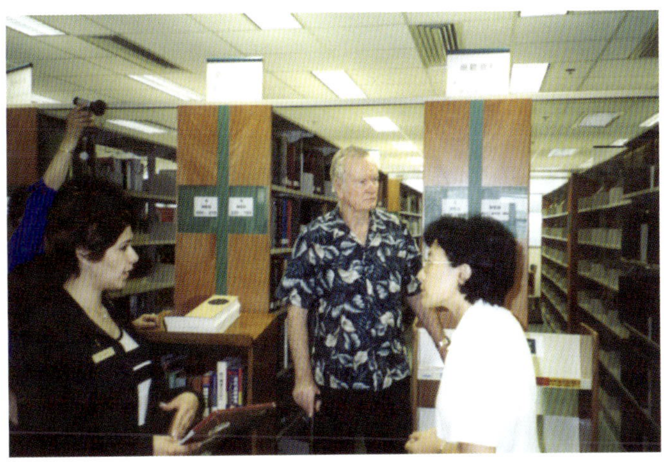

Fig. 3.31. Touring the Chinese Medicine Library. From left to right: Dr. Ada Garcia, Dr. Bruce Halstead, and Lisa L. Song, the Library Coordinator. (May 2002, by Jeffrey McConnell)

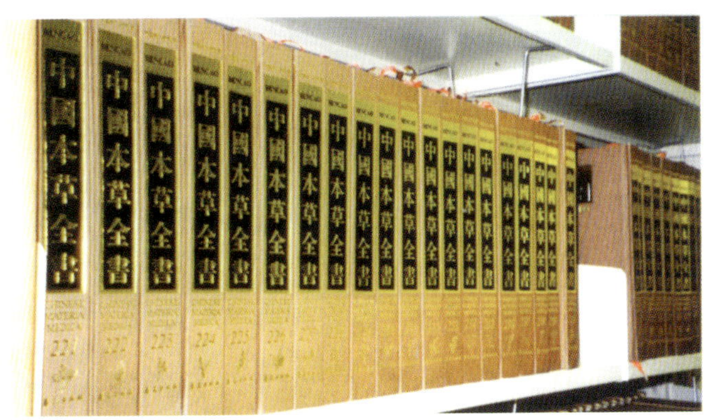


Fig. 3.32. The Chinese materia medicas. (May 2002, by Jeffrey McConnell)

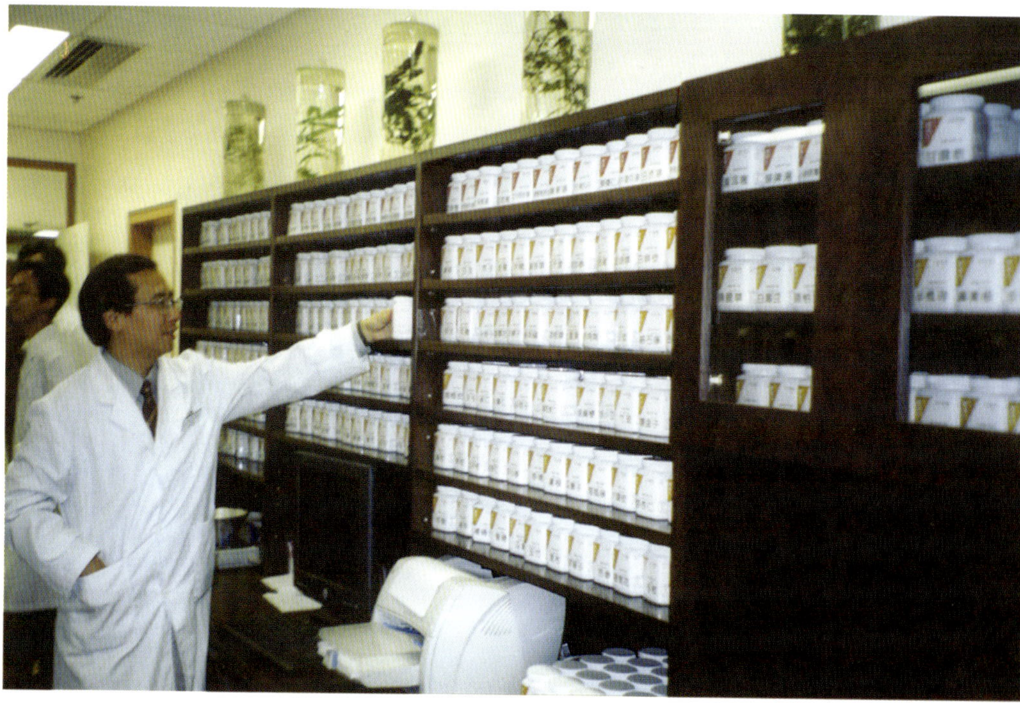

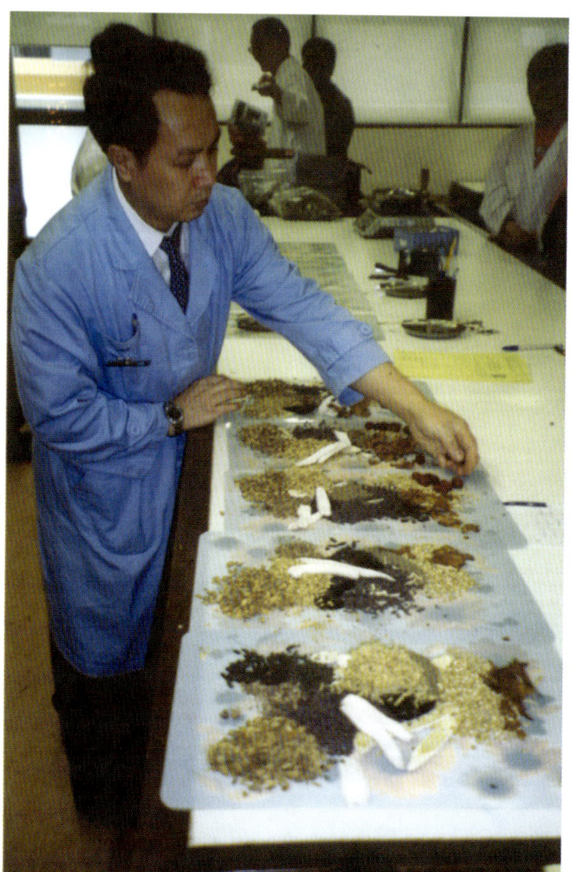

⮝ Fig. 3.33. A doctor from the onsite medical clinic in the pharmacy within the Hong Kong Baptist University. (May 2002, by Jeffrey McConnell)

⮜ Fig. 3.34. A pharmacist filling out a herbal prescription (May 2002, by Jeffrey McConnell)

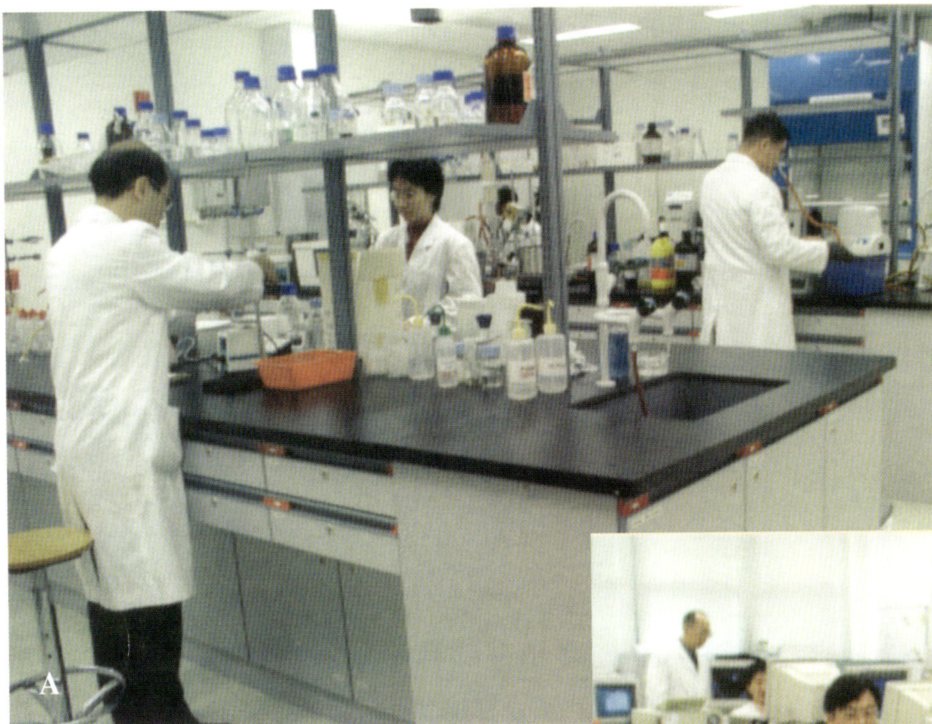


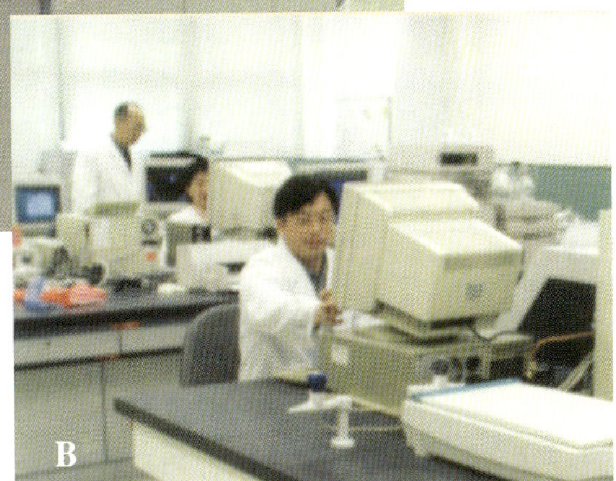


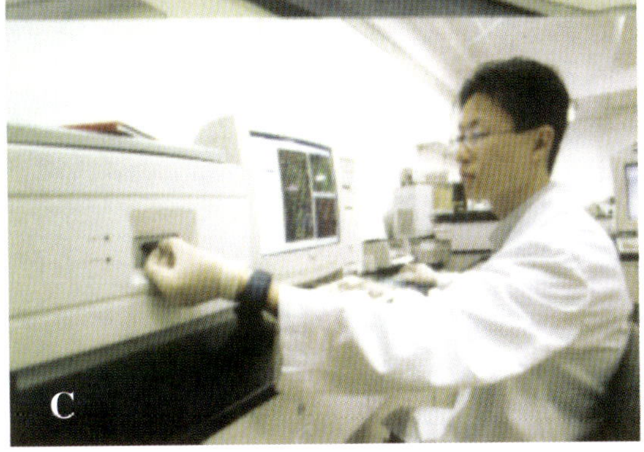


⮝⮞ Fig. 3.35 (A-C). Laboratories at the School of Chinese Medicine. (Courtesy of the Hong Kong Baptist University School of Chinese Medicine)

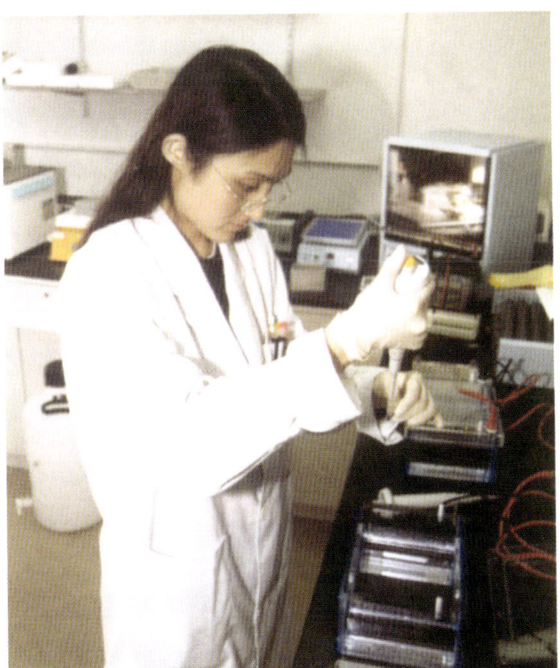

⮜ Fig. 3.36. A lab researcher at the Hong Kong Baptist University studying the DNA fingerprint of botanical herbs. (May 2002, by Jeffrey McConnell)

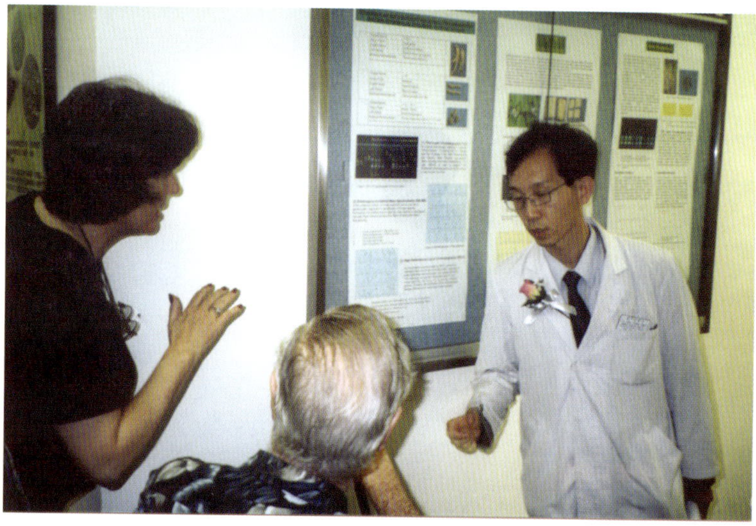

Fig. 3.37. Dr. Zhong-Zhen Zhao explaining to Dr. and Mrs Halstead the format of herbal studies at the Hong Kong Baptist University School of Chinese Medicine. (May 2002, by Jeffrey McConnell)

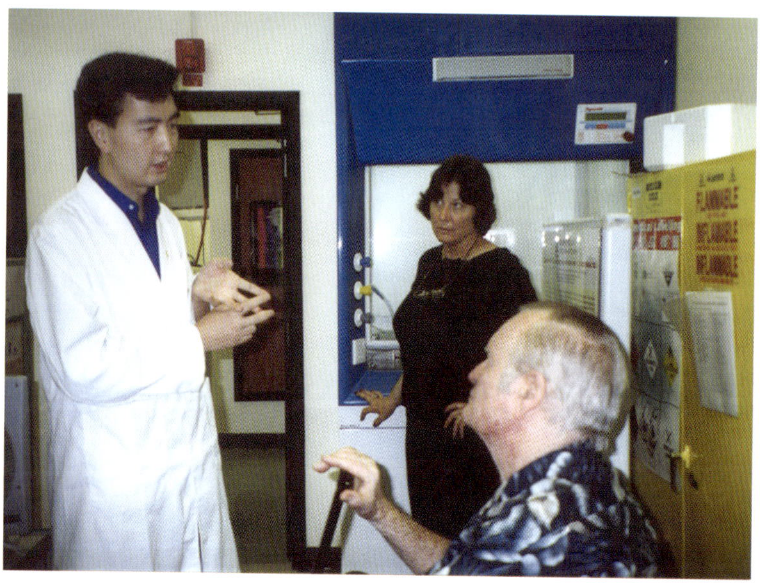

Fig. 3.38. Dr. Kelvin S. Y. Leung answering questions from Dr. and Mrs. Halstead during the tour of the School of Chinese Medicine at the Hong Kong Baptist University. (May 2002, by Jeffrey McConnell)

3.34). Primarily, traditional Chinese medicine is practiced here. This included acupuncture, herbal medicine, acupressure, diet, exercise, meditation, and lifestyle techniques. Western or modern medicine is available as needed. These kinds of physicians and health practitioners integrate western and eastern diagnostics and therapies. They attempt to minimize the patient's exposure to toxic side effects. They strive to work with nature and the body's own immune system. The physicians in this clinic often prescribe Tien Hsien products and have had terrific results with them.

The research laboratories are superb and second to none in any part of the Western world (Figs. 3.35-3.38). They took up two of the floors. At the time of our visit, their scientific staff was working on the authentication of a variety of Chinese

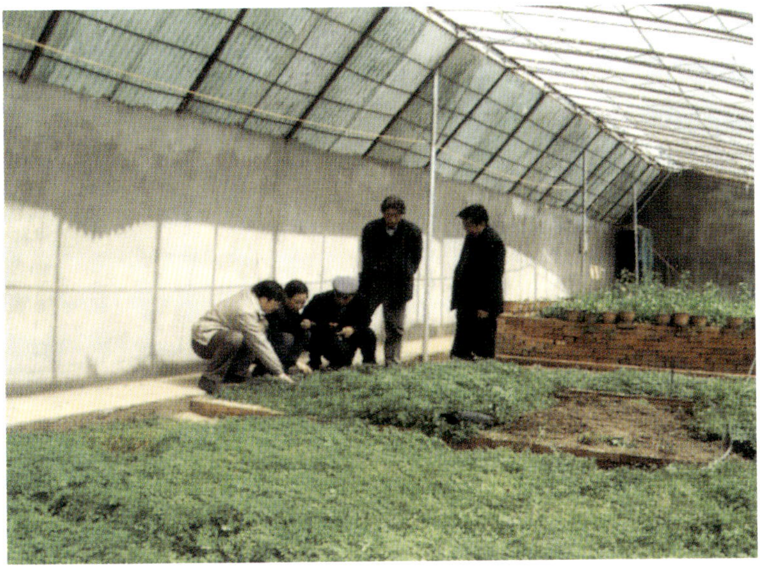

Fig. 3.39. One of the farming beds of the agricultural program at the Hong Kong Baptist University which is used to teach farmers how to grow medicinal plants without the use of pesticides. (Courtesy of the School of Chinese Medicine)

medicinal plants at the genetic level and were doing DNA analysis. They also had an excellent toxicological section that was checking for toxic agents such as pesticides. They also sponsored an agricultural program designed to help farmers raise medicinal plants without contaminating the soil (Fig. 3.39). Some of their scientists are trained in the best American and European universities. We were informed that CJFU is in the process of utilizing some of their excellent resources. Our scientific cup was running over with good things, but more was yet to come. Shortly thereafter we left for Taiwan.

## Chapter 4

# Our Visit to Taiwan

Our trip to Taiwan was the last part of our trip, and proved to be among the best. We had the good fortune of visiting the Development Center for Biotechnology (DCB), which is located in Taipei (Fig. 4.1). DCB is a unique organization. It provides a pre-clinical testing service for investigational new drugs (IND) that is acceptable to the U.S. Food and Drug Administration (FDA). The financial support of the organization largely comes from the Taiwanese government. They are very similar to the U.S. FDA in that they deal with the safety and efficacy of Chinese medicinal plants that are in the process of seeking new drug status. They also deal with the safety of chemical agents of all types, cosmetics, and medical devices. An independent Quality Assurance Unit in compliance with Good Manufacturing Practices audits all of their tests. Their toxicological tests are accepted by most foreign regulatory agencies including the U.S. FDA. The executives of the CJFU informed us that they were in the process of working with the DCB prior to approaching the U.S. FDA. However, these matters will be discussed in a second book.

DCB also has a function similar to the U.S. Environmental Protective Agency in that they deal with pesticides and environmental wastes. They are housed in several buildings with over 350 employees and have a staff of scientists who have been trained in the United States and Europe. Our guide, Dr. Jiuan Judy Liu (Fig. 4.2), received her Ph.D. in immunology from the University of Illinois.

While visiting Taipei, we had a very educational visit to the National Taiwan University College of Medicine Hospital established in 1897. Located in the center of Taipei, this enormous complex is one the largest and oldest hospitals in Taiwan. The older part of the hospital, which has now been renovated, was originally built in 1903 during the later part of the Chiang Dynasty. The newer additions have increased the total size considerably, creating a very impressive medical center, many stories high. The facility not only treats patients but is also a teaching and research facility. At the hospital we were introduced to a team of dedicated researchers (Figs. 4.3-4.5), who have conducted many scientific studies using Tien Hsien liquid. The head of the team was Dr. Andy Sun. Dr. Sun has a very extensive curriculum vita. He received his D.D.S. in Dentistry in 1978 and in 1992 a Ph.D. in immunology; both degrees were earned at the National Taiwan University. He has taught and lectured at numerous universities and research centers both in Taiwan and mainland China. He has published an extensive number of scientific papers as well as a several books. Dr. Sun's scientific work is well known in both Mainland China and Taiwan. He is also well known for being a political advocate for tradi-

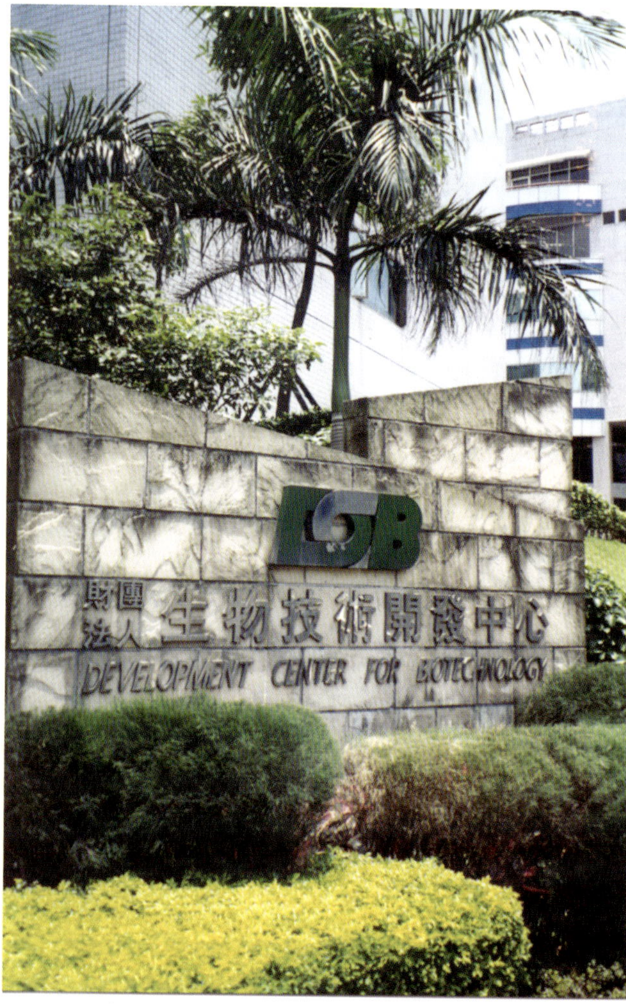


Fig. 4.1. The Development Center for Biotechnology (DCB) entrance in Taipei, Taiwan. (May 2002, by Jeff McConnell)

tional Chinese medicine. It is his firm belief that modern Western medicine should be integrated with traditional medicine so that everyone has the opportunity to benefit from both. As a result of advocates like Dr. Sun, the government of Taiwan is now integrating traditional medicine into all their medical schools and hospitals. This has been a positive change for everyone.

The other members of the research team included Dr. Chun-Pin Chiang, Dr. Jean-San Chia, and Dr. Won Bo Wang. Dr. Sun presented a slide show that demonstrated the results of their studies using Tien Hsien liquid. The researchers have completed a series of both patient studies and cell line studies. They had compared the efficacy of Tien Hsien to a variety of other herbal cancer therapies. In every case, the results showed that Tien Hsien far exceeded any of the other preparations.

Our final visitation was to the Chung Tai Monastery, the largest Buddhist temple in the world (Fig. 4.6). Joan Lu, the daughter of Sydney Lu, is a Buddhist and she thought we might enjoy visiting the temple and indeed it proved to be a spiritual blessing to all of us. The story behind the temple was awesome. The structure eclipses the Vatican in Rome both in size and architecture.

In the early 1970's Master Wei Chueh (Fig. 4.7) began his austere practice of Buddhism under very primitive conditions. He was very poor, but he practiced his religion with joy. He was eventually discovered by some passerby and gradually developed many followers. Eventually, he became known as the master who had revived Buddhism in Taiwan. It soon became evident that they needed a much larger place to worship and so he set about raising the necessary funds to build a new edifice. This proved to be a long and arduous task and thus began the work of

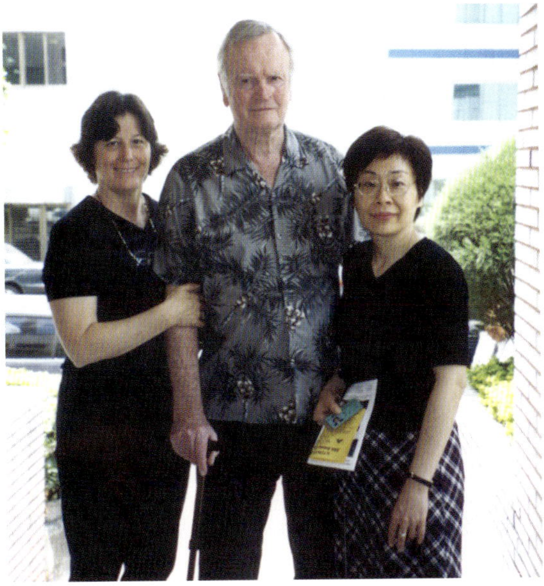

⮜ Fig. 4.2. Senior researcher, Jiuan Judy Liu, Ph.D., with Bruce and Terri Halstead after the tour of the Development Center for Biotechnology. (May 2002, by Jeff McConnell)

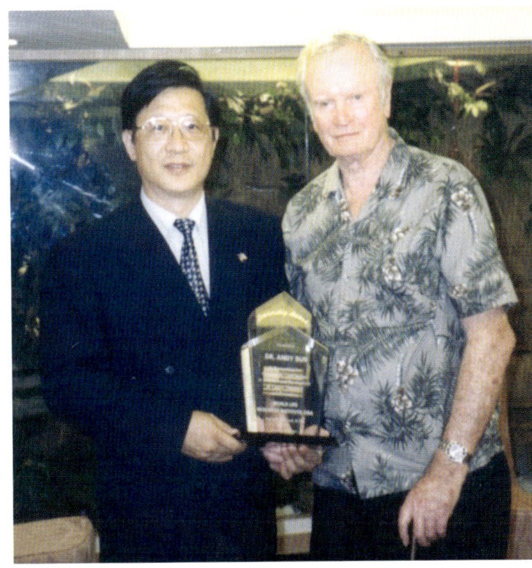

➢ Fig. 4.3. Dr. Halstead presenting an honorarium from the World Life Research Institute in Grand Terrace, California, to Dr. Andy Sun for his research in Chinese herbs for the benefit of mankind. (May 2002, by Jeff McConnell)

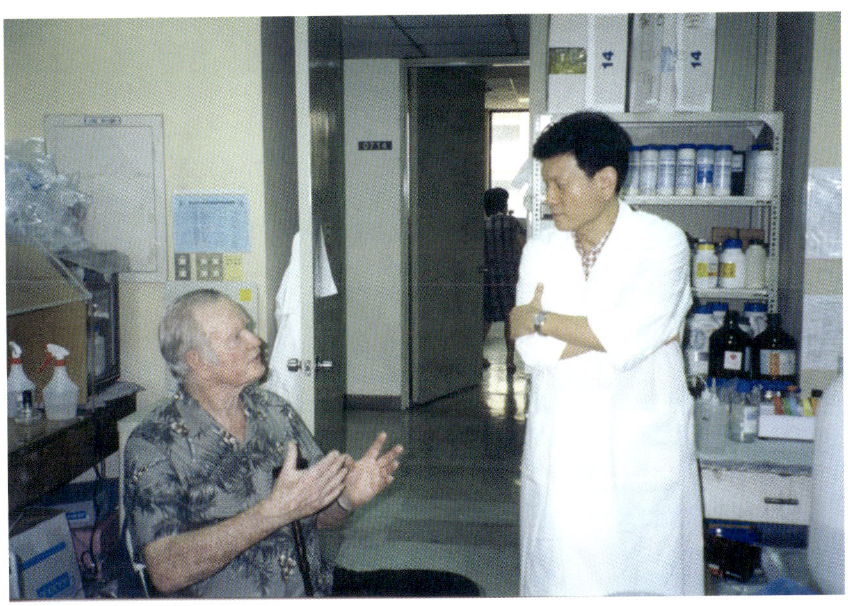

Fig. 4.4. Dr. Bruce Halstead with Dr. Won Bo Wang discussing the various medical applications of their work at the National Taiwan University College of Medicine and Hospital. (May 2002, by Jeff McConnell)

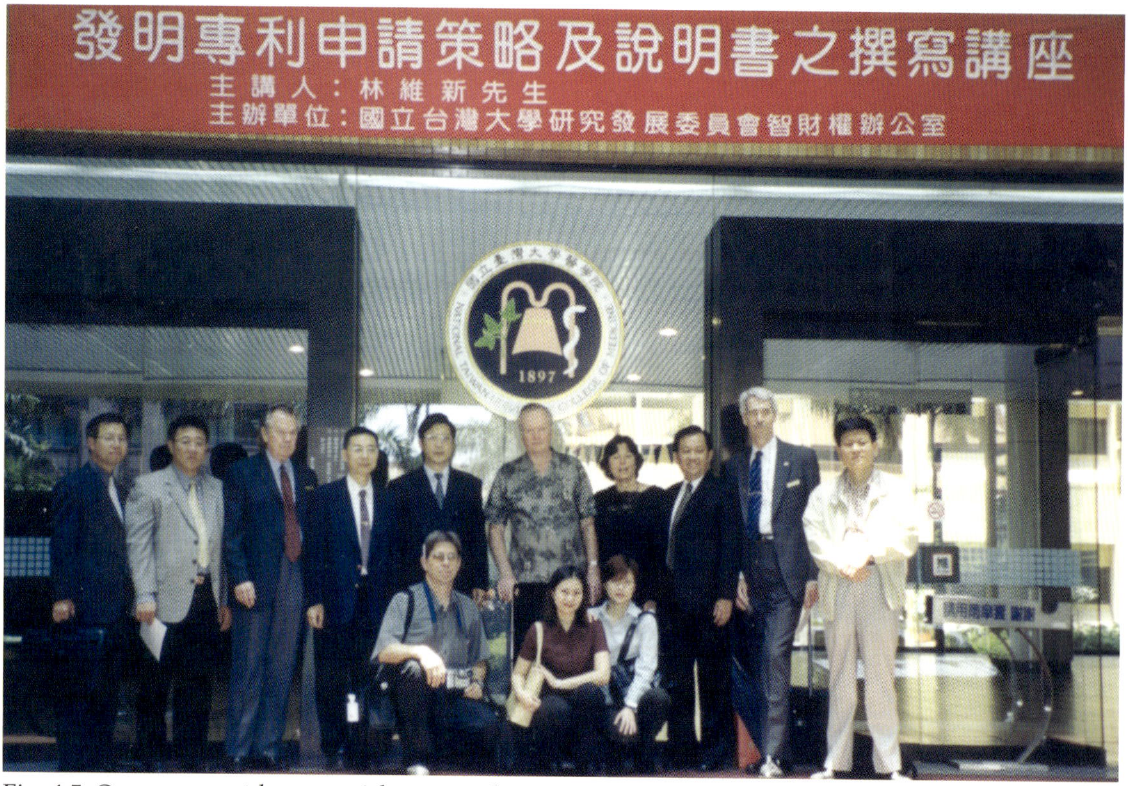
發明專利申請策略及說明書之撰寫講座
主講人：林維新先生
主辦單位：國立台灣大學研究發展委員會智財權辦公室
1897

Fig. 4.5. Our group with some of the research doctors from the National Taiwan University College of Medicine Hospital in Taipei, Taiwan. (Courtesy of CJFU)

building the Chung Tai Chan Monastery. The monastery was designed by a world-renowned Buddhist architect, C. Y. Lee. The cost of the construction is estimated at over $100 million U.S. dollars and it is still growing. The building is 37 stories high. Viewed from afar the temple appears as a person sitting in peaceful meditation in a mountain setting of beautiful trees and flowers. The Great Chant Hall holds over a thousand people for worship. They have a very sophisticated communication and computer system, a sound studio, a photographic studio where they produce films, videos, CDs, internet programs, etc. They operate a very large kitchen that produces Chinese, Japanese, and western style vegetarian foods of all types. The temple is located in the mountains of central Taiwan in a garden of flowers and trees, many of which have been imported from all over the world. They also operate a clinic that provides medical and dental services of all types free of change to their clients. Within the monastery there is the Chung Tai Buddhist Institute, which operates a graduate school, a high school, and an elementary school.

We were very fortunate to see their excellent library, which contains an enormous collection of all of the Buddhist sayings; each Tripitaka may amount to over 100 huge volumes, some of which have been written over 1,000 years ago. Leaving the Monastery (Fig. 4.8) we headed back to the airport and for home.

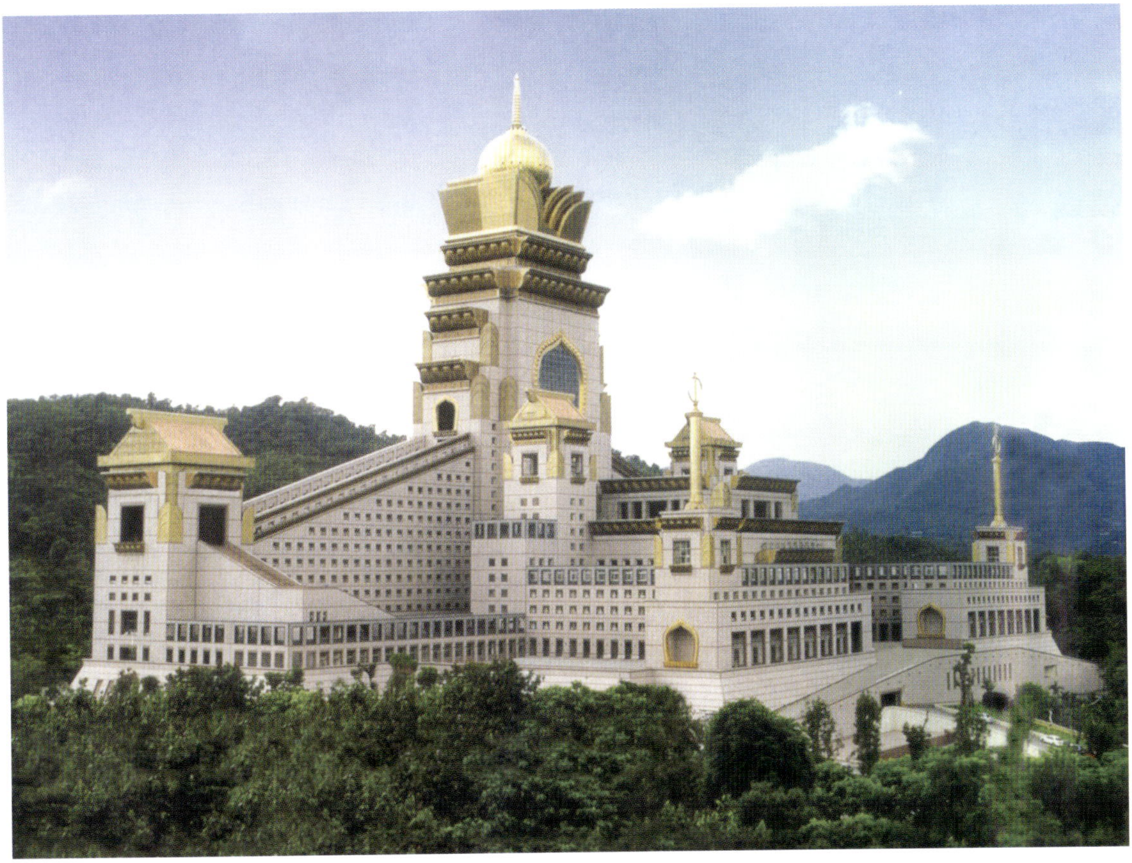

Fig. 4.6. The Chung Tai Monastery. (Courtesy of the Chung Tai Monastery)

Fig. 4.7. Master Wei Chueh, the Head Abbot and founder of the Chung Tai Monastery. (Courtesy of the Chung Tai Monastery)

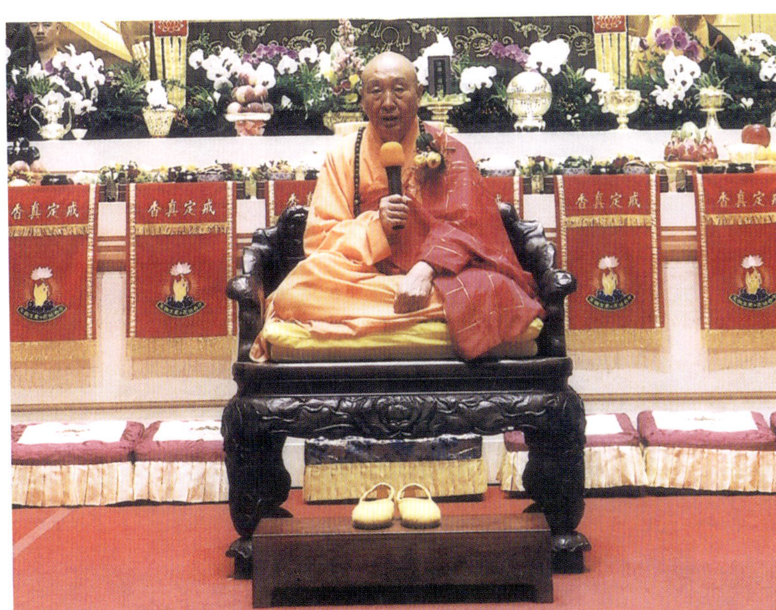

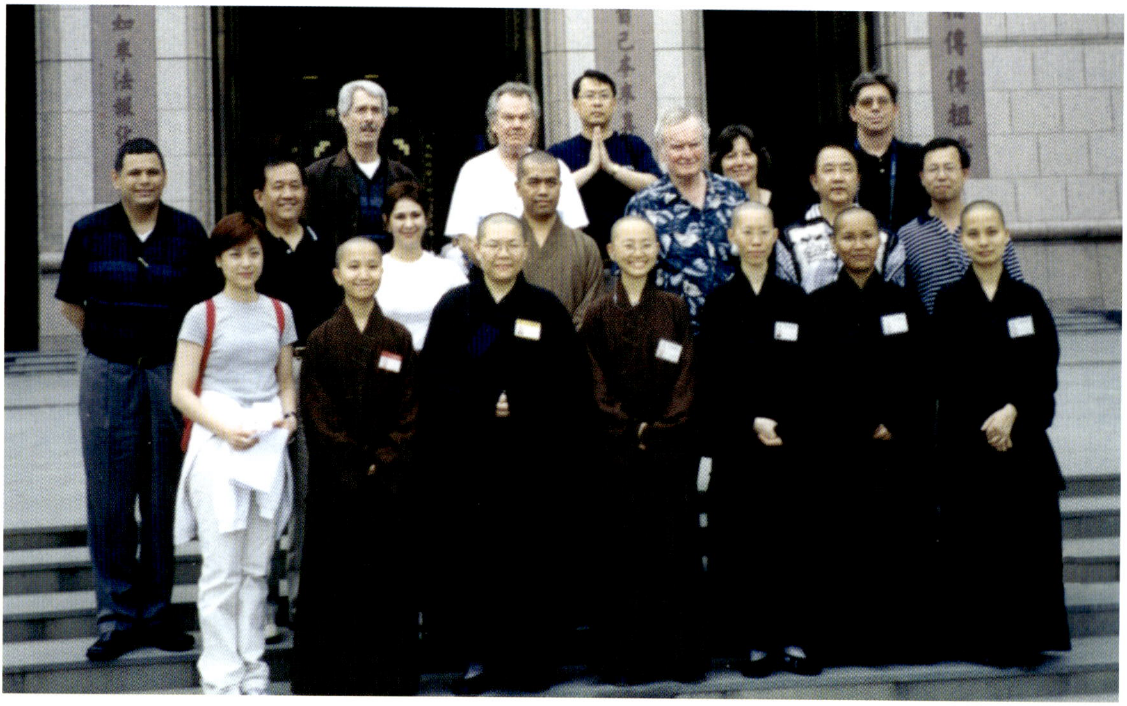

Fig. 4.8. Our group in front of the Chung Tai Monastery with several monks including Master Jian Teng standing in the second row wearing a brown robe. (May 2002)

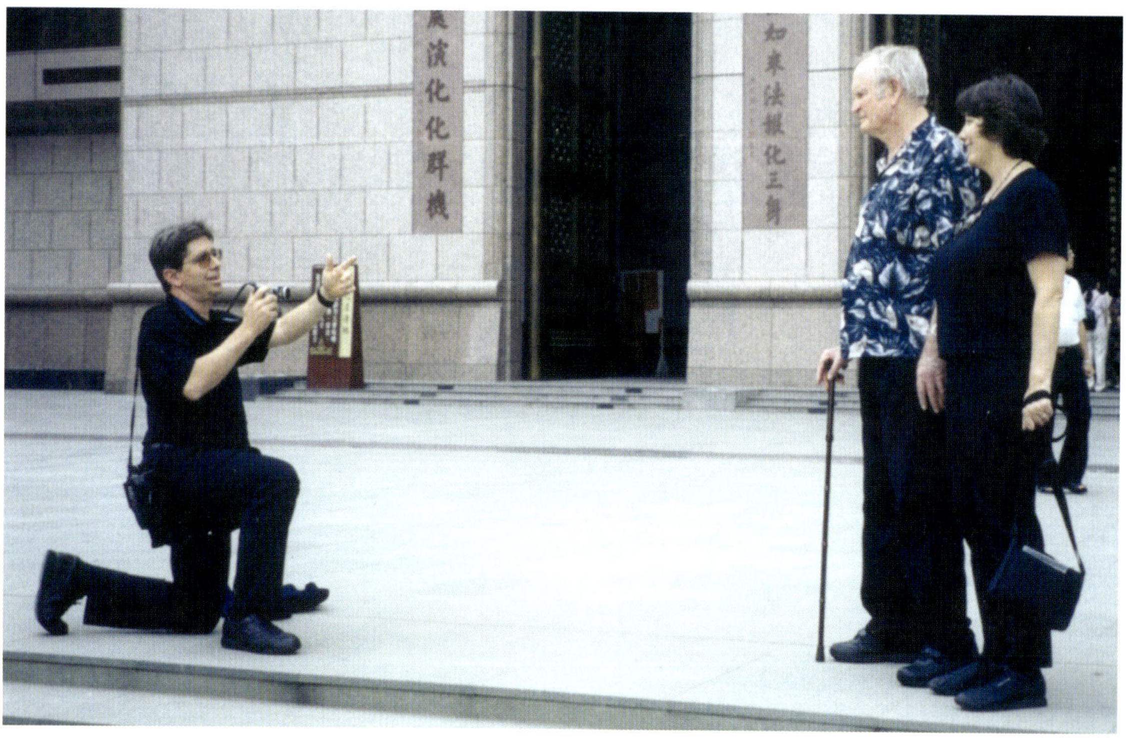

Fig. 4.9. Jeffrey McConnell taking a picture of us in front of the Monastery. (May 2002, by Haiwei Chen)

## A Summary of Our Trip

The trip to Japan, China, Hong Kong and Taiwan was 17 days in duration, from the 12th of May to May 29, 2002. Over the years I (BWH) have traveled in over 150 countries of the world, on my own, with the military, on Cousteau expeditions, with the World Health Organization, and the Food and Agriculture Organization, under the best of conditions and under the worst, but never have I been exposed to a finer group of people, and a greater learning experience than the one I have just encountered. The trip was intense and highly focused. We were there for one purpose—to gather information on the book that needed to be written on the *Scientific Basis of Chinese Integrative Cancer Therapy*. Reaching our goals was not a problem. Fortunately, we took Jeff McConnell along to handle our photographic needs (Fig. 4.9). We now have an abundance of excellent photos for the book. We were more than pleased with the technical information we obtained about Tien Hsien.

## Author's Update

Dr. Andy Sun, together with several associates, recently had English translations of their research papers (Sun, Chia, Wang & Chiang, 2004, 2005; Sun, Chia, Chiang, et al, 2005) published in Western peer-reviewed medical journals. These studies provide reliable, scientific data regarding the effectiveness of Tien Hsien Liquid. It is encouraging and significant that such high quality scientific research involving Chinese Traditional Medicine (CTM) is beginning to reach Western medical journals.

Terri Holcomb-Halstead
September 2005

## Chapter 5

# DOCUMENTED CANCER CASES IN WHICH TRADITIONAL ADAPTOGENIC PLANTS HAVE BEEN SUCCESSFULLY USED

Numerous claims have been made about cancer cures but few turn out to be successful. After 40 years of working in the cancer field I (BWH) have found nothing that remotely compares with the clinical results that I personally observed in terminal cancer patients that have been on Tien Hsien. Tables 5.1 and 5.2 provide some of the therapeutic results of cancer patients treated with Tien Hsien based on data taken from Wang's (2001) *The Cancer Terminator*.

**Table 5.1**
(After Wang, 2001)

| Name of Cancers | Number of Cases | Number of Effective Cases | Number of Ineffective Cases |
|---|---|---|---|
| Esophagus Cancer | 225 | 201 | 24 |
| Stomach Cancer | 376 | 334 | 42 |
| Intestines Cancer | 95 | 85 | 10 |
| Lung Cancer | 94 | 73 | 21 |
| Liver Cancer | 34 | 25 | 9 |
| Breast Cancer | 78 | 56 | 22 |
| Brain Cancer | 46 | 28 | 18 |
| **Summary** | **948** | **802** | **146** |

**Table 5.2**
(After Wang, 2001)

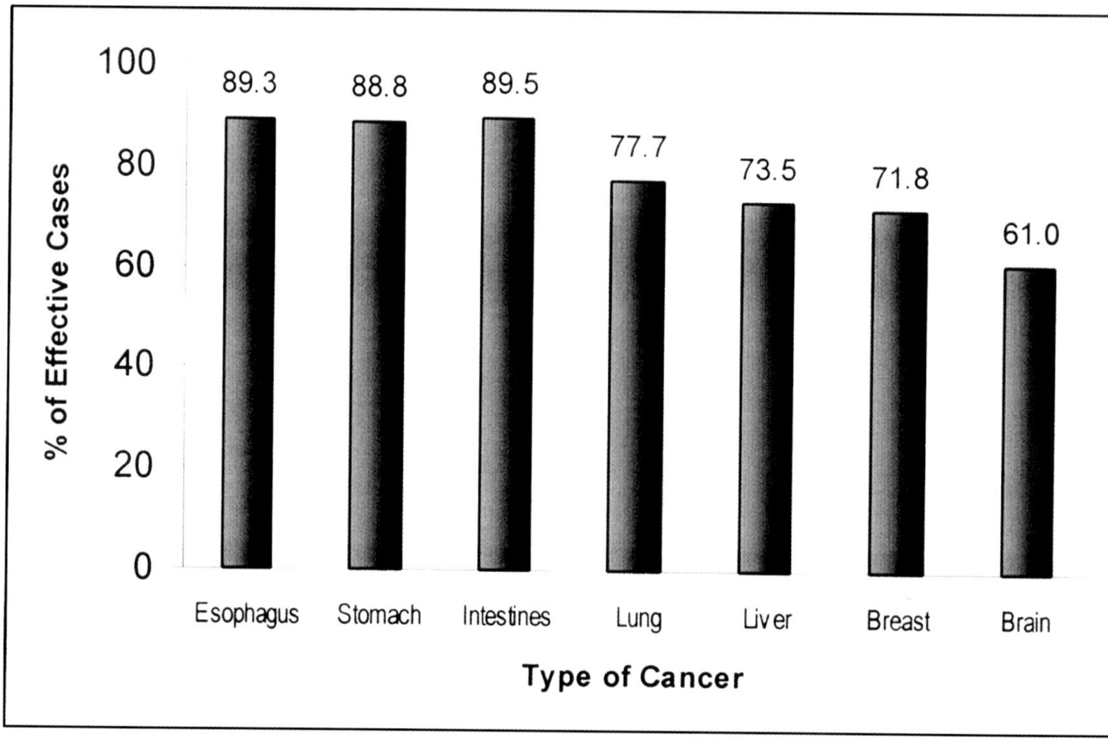


Although the clinical results were very impressive, the big question to be answered was: What were the ingredients contained in the Tien Hsien products that produced these clinical results? A study of the phytochemistry and pharmacology of these plants provides the scientific basis as to why Tien Hsien works. This information appears in Chapter Eleven. A few representative case histories have been taken from Wang's book as follows:

## Case Histories

Case 1. E.S. immigrated from Taiwan to San Francisco, California; housewife; age 49. In October 1977 she was diagnosed with cancer of the uterus and the breast and was informed she had only five years to live. The doctor recommended having a cervical operation, but she refused. Later she started bleeding and so she decided to go ahead with the cervical surgery, but retained her uterus and ovaries. About a month later after her surgery she returned to Taiwan. She got a second opinion and the Taiwanese doctors told her it was unnecessary to have her uterus and ovaries removed. After returning to the United States she discovered a hard lump in her right breast, which turned out to be cancer. She had a partial mastectomy and was then given radiation. After the operation she started taking Tien Hsien. She has responded well and as of this writing is still alive.

Case 2. M.S. from Japan; unemployed; age 44. In 1998 she was diagnosed as having an ovarian cancer with metastasis to the lungs. She was given chemotherapy, which was to be followed by surgery. The chemotherapy proved to be ineffective. Her physical condition only worsened. Further studies revealed that both lungs had cancer and she had a large mass on her right ovary. About that time she started taking Tien Hsien. After taking Tien Hsien for six months her appetite returned and her physical condition improved. She is presently enjoying a life of good quality.

Case 3. L.S.Y. from Hong Kong; housewife; age 65. She was diagnosed in 1996 with a uterine cancer. Part of her uterus and ovaries were removed in order to prevent metastasis. After the surgery she was given radiation to prevent metastasis. Then in the spring of 1997 they found that the cancer in the uterus had returned to the uterus and had spread to her lungs and brain. She was then informed that she should take chemotherapy and radiation, but she refused. She then started taking Tien Hsien. She remained on the product for six months and then went back to her doctor for examination. To their surprise they were unable to find evidence of cancer. Further studies revealed that the metastatic cancer had almost disappeared and the uterine cancer was completely gone.

Case 4. L.B.C. from Taiwan; housewife; age 62. The patient started loosing weight from 50 kg to 45 kg. She went to the hospital and was diagnosed as having a third stage uterine cancer. She remained in the hospital for six months during which time she received chemotherapy. Finally, she was released from the hospital at which time she started taking Tien Hsien which she continued taking for one year and two months. She later returned to the hospital and the doctor reported he was unable to find any evidence of cancer.

Case 5. L.A. from the Philippines; housewife; age 53. In June 1997 the patient went into the hospital for a breast examination. It was found that she had cancer of the breast (which breast not stated). She was advised to have an operation and chemotherapy. She refused. She started taking Tien Hsien in October. After taking Tien Hsien for one week the lump in her breast started softening and there was some drainage from the nipple. In January she went into the hospital and the doctor examined the breast and found that the lump had disappeared.

Case 6. L.S. from Thailand; teacher; age 45. About 1973 the patient was diagnosed with cancer of the right breast. She was given a mastectomy. Two years later the cancer metastasized to the left breast. She was then given chemotherapy and radiation, which resulted in serious side effects. She became bedridden and was unable to walk. In December 1999 she started taking Tien Hsien. After several months she regained her strength and appetite and was able to walk again without any help.

Case 7. M.K. from Japan; company employee; age 69. The patient was diagnosed with cancer of the right lung in March 1999. He was given only six months to live. The tumor had spread and his doctors were only able to remove part of the tumor. He was given chemotherapy and radiation. He started taking Tien Hsien in May 1999 after the surgery, chemotherapy, and radiation. Shortly thereafter the side effects from the treatment began to disappear. When he was released from the hospital in June the tumor had reduced to about half its size. His appetite and energy has returned. The last examination he received in March 2000 failed to reveal any evidence of the cancer.

Case 8. M.K. from Japan; company employee; age 45. The patient was diagnosed with cancer of the lungs with metastases to the bones in the spring of 1999. He was given chemotherapy and radiation and suffered many side effects, including a decrease in his white blood cells. In October he discontinued taking the chemotherapy and started taking Tien Hsien. His physical examinations in January and February 2000 showed no evidence of the cancer. His appetite and energy had returned and he went back to work.

Case 9. L.N. from Japan; housewife; age 62. Patient was diagnosed in early 1999 with cancer of the right breast. She received a mastectomy. She was also given chemotherapy. In April 1999 she learned that the cancer had metastasized to her lungs. She started taking Tien Hsien in September. In January 2000 her examination failed to show any evidence of cancer.

Case 10. W.Z. from Malaysia; shop owner; age 63. Diagnosed with cancer of the left lung in March 1997. The patient was given chemotherapy. Shortly thereafter he started taking Tien Hsien. One month after taking Tien Hsien the tumor reduced to half the size. By October 1997 the tumor had completely disappeared. His coughing was gone.

Case 11. M.H. from Japan; company employee; age 70. Patient was diagnosed with hepatitis C. In June 1999 he was diagnosed with cancer of the liver. At that time he was given three months to live. He was not able to have surgery because of the involvement with the portal vein. He was given chemotherapy, but it did not help. After being released from the hospital he started taking Tien Hsien. In January 2000 he returned to the hospital; the doctor found evidence of improvement in his cancer. In February he was again examined and there was no evidence of cancer.

Case 12. M.I. from Japan; company employee; age 51. Patient was diagnosed with advanced cancer of the liver. He was informed that he had only about two months to live. He started taking Tien Hsien. Five years later he has no evidence of liver cancer.

Case 13. L.N. from Japan; housewife; age 78. In November 1995 the patient was diagnosed with cancer of the liver. She was given an "embolism treatment" but they were unable to operate. She was not given chemotherapy or radiation. She started taking Tien Hsien in April of the following year. By June her appetite and complexion had improved. An examination in January 1996 failed to reveal any evidence of cancer in her liver. There was no indication of cancer in the following three years.

Case 14. L.E. from Japan; housewife; age 51. Patient had cancer of the breast with metastasis to the uterus. Patient was given a mastectomy. Three years later the cancer had metastasized to her lungs and then to her liver. She was given chemotherapy, but it was useless. After taking Tien Hsien for several weeks her appetite had returned to normal, and the liver tumor had reduced from 3 cm to 1 cm, and she has continued to improve.

Case 15. M.F. from Japan; unemployed; age 74. Patient was diagnosed with stomach cancer in March 1998. The doctor removed $^{2}/_{3}$ of his stomach. In January 1999 he was reexamined and the doctor informed him that he did not have long to live. About that time he started taking Tien Hsien. In January 2000 he was reexamined and they were unable to find any evidence of cancer. He has been on Tien Hsien since that time and there has been no return of the cancer.

Case 16. L.T. from Japan; housewife; age 58. Patient was diagnosed with stomach cancer. Received an operation in which $^{3}/_{4}$ of her stomach was removed. The cancer metastasized to her pelvis, surrounding lymph glands, and ovaries. She was then given cancer chemotherapy. She then had her ovaries removed. She was only given one year to live. After the surgery she started taking Tien Hsen and is now doing very well.

Case 17. M.K. from South Africa; college professor; age 57. In April 1995 the patient was diagnosed with a malignant myeloma. In August he started taking Tien Hsien. In May 1997 an examination failed to reveal any evidence of cancer.

Case 18. W.R. from Malaysia; student; age 13. The patient was diagnosed with bone cancer of the left leg in October 1998. The patient was given chemotherapy, which was ineffective. In December 1998 his left leg was amputated. In March 1999 they discovered the cancer had metastasized to both his lungs. In late April they operated on his lungs and removed seven small tumors from the left lung and nine from the right lung, but there still remained evidence of cancer. He was then placed on chemotherapy. Shortly after he was released to go home, but he only got progressively worse. He was placed on Tien Hsien in December 1999. In June 2000 he underwent a comprehensive physical examination and they were unable to find any evidence of cancer in his body, and his physical condition had dramatically improved.

Case 19. M.W. from Japan; fire fighter; age 56. Patient was diagnosed with stomach cancer in May 1999. He shortly thereafter underwent an operation and had the cancer removed. The doctor informed him that within two years the cancer would probably return. Shortly after the operation he started taking Tien Hsien. One year later his stomach returned to normal condition and so did his appetite. Three years later his examination failed to show any evidence of cancer.

Case 20. C.W. from Taiwan; age 60. The patient was diagnosed with stomach cancer in June 1998 and had the stomach removed. Shortly thereafter he started taking Tien Hsien. Three years later he is feeling great.

# Section II:

# The Scientific and Historical Basis of Chinese Traditional Medicine and How It Is Used In Cancer Treatment

## Chapter 6

# WHAT IS CANCER?



---

Cancer is the result of an abnormal growth from otherwise healthy cells. This biotransformation is at first undetectable and insidious in its growth, seemingly growing without restraint, and finally leading to death. Cancer is a potentially fatal disease complex the therapy of which continues to be elusive despite the billions of dollars that have been spent attempting to find a cure.

A brief overview will be presented of cancer therapy as practiced by Western medicine, but the main thrust of this book is to provide the reader with the scientific rationale of the Chinese approach to the prevention and treatment of cancer in the context of modern Oriental integrative health care.

## Cancer Terminology

First, we need to review some of the terminology that is used by the cancer establishment because it can become quite confusing to the layman. The medical specialty that deals with cancer is referred to as **oncology**. It appears that there is no single definition of cancer that is completely satisfactory to everyone, which in itself is a commentary on the complexity of the disease. **Cancer** is sometimes defined as a disease entity characterized by uncontrolled cell proliferation. Cancer has also been defined as a cellular tumor, the natural course of which is fatal. Cancer is a malignant tumor, or neoplasm. The term **neoplasm** refers to a progressive, uncontrolled new growth of tissue. In the case of solid tumors the term cancer and neoplasm are used interchangeably. Cancer is not a single disease but a complex or a family of over 100 different diseases. There are about 270 different cell types of human cancers that have been recognized and histologically described. Cancer has also been defined as a group of diseases of unknown and multiple causes that occur in most human and animal populations, and arise in tissues that are composed of cells capable of dividing. Sharks are largely an exception to this statement, because they have an immune system that is about 600,000 times more active than a human. Cancer is a rarity in sharks.

The term **tumor** is frequently used to designate an abnormal growth of cells, which may be either benign or malignant. **Malignancy** is a state in which there is progression in the virulence of the cancer, which ultimately leads to death. Malignancy is in contradistinction to **benign**, which refers to a **nonmalignant** tumor. It is not recurrent and can generally be treated and is favorable for recovery. An **adenoma** is a benign tumor arising from glandular epithelium.

The term **metastasis** refers to the spread of cancer cells to distant body sites. If the cancer has metastasized it indicates that the cancer is worsening. Metastasis is one of the characteristics of malignancy. Tumor cells may originate in one part of the body, which is known as the **primary tumor**, and suddenly appear in some other organ or distant part of the body, known as a **secondary tumor**.

The pattern and incidence of cancers may vary with sex, race, environmental conditions, and geographic locality. Cancer is a disease of tissue organization. For many years it was believed that cancers were by definition irreversible, but it is now known that some cancers under certain conditions can be reversed (Fauvet, Roujeau & Piet, 1964; Boyd, 1966; Everson & Cole, 1966; O'Regan & Hirschberg, 1993).

## Types of Cancer

Cancers can be divided into two general categories: carcinomas and sarcomas. **Carcinomas** are malignant growths of epithelial cells, which are found in the breasts, digestive tract, uterus, skin, prostate, bladder, oral cavity, and pancreas. An **adenocarcinoma**, for example, is a carcinoma arising from glandular epithelium. A **basal cell carcinoma** is a common type of skin cancer, which can be readily treated if caught early. A **squamous cell carcinoma** is a cancer of flat epithelial cells found in the skin and other parts of the body. A **melanoma** is a cancer of the pigment-producing cells of the skin, which is a very malignant form of cancer.

Another group of malignancies are the **sarcomas**, which are cancers derived from and involve such connective tissue as bone, muscle, nerves and lymph glands. Hodgkin's disease and melanomas are types of sarcomas. Most brain tumors are

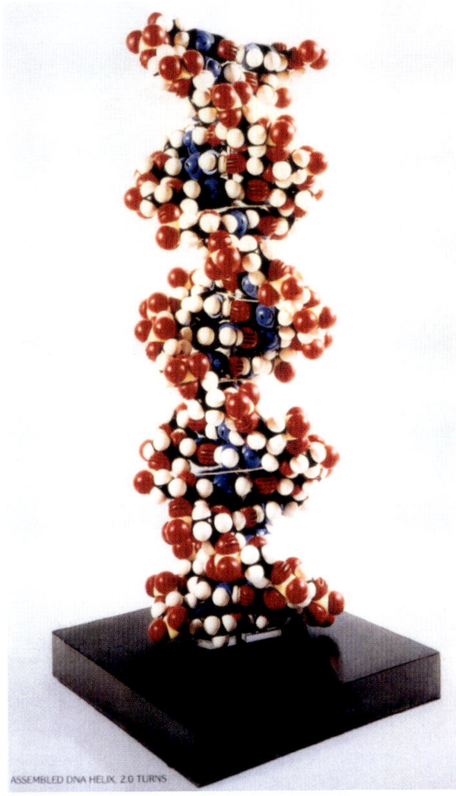


Fig. 6.1. The Harvard DNA double helix model. DNA is an elegantly simple structure that resembles a gently twisted ladder. The rails of the ladder are made of alternating units of phosphate and the sugar deoxyribose. The steps of the ladder are each composed of a pair of nitrogen-containing nucleotides adenine, cytosine, guanine, and thymine. DNA has been referred to as the master molecule of the body because it contains all of the genetic material necessary for the functioning of the living organism. (Courtesy Cambridge Apparatus Company)

neoplasms of the interstitial tissue and are referred to as **gliomas**, of which there are several different types. Generally, tumors are classified according to their cell type. Some tumors contain both epithelial and connective tissue elements. Tumor cells may not mature properly in which case the pathologist may refer to them as "anaplastic" or "undifferentiated", which means that the cells do not have the appearance of the tissues from which they originated.

**Leukemias** are another type of connective tissue malignancies that involve a progressive proliferation of the blood forming organs of the bone marrow or white blood cells of the body. Leukemias are sometimes referred to as cancers of the blood. There are many types of leukemia each of which is designated according to the white blood cell involved.

## Carcinogenesis

**Carcinogenesis** may be simply defined as the production of cancer. The factors involved in the production of cancer are multitudinous, insidious, and generally defy adequate quantitation. The primary target in the process of carcinogenesis is the DNA molecule, which is concerned with the genetic mechanism of the cell (Fig. 6.1).

Carcinogenesis is an extremely complex subject which has attracted the scientific attention of thousands of scientists involving an ever increasing number of scientific disciplines, especially in the fields of oncology, epidemiology, immunology, biology, genetics, virology, molecular biology, bacteriology, parasitology, organic chemistry, bioinorganic chemistry, ecology, medical geography, toxicology, biophysics, atomic physics, enzymology, botany, zoology, mathematics, psychoneuroimmunology, biostatistics, economics, herbology, ethnopharmacology, environmental sciences, preventive medicine, and other disciplines.

No one has found the complete answer. The search for all of the elements in carcinogenesis continues to challenge some of the finest minds that the world has produced. Nobel Laureates and those of a lesser ilk have failed to decipher the complete carcinogenic enigma. The following are some of the basic elements of carcinogenesis according to current thinking. For a review of some of the theories of carcinogenesis see: Searle, 1984; Ruddon, 1987; Waring & Ponder, 1987; Iversen, 1988, 1993; Sarma & Sarma, 1988; Colburn, 1989; Waxman & Sikora, 1989; Sikora, et al, 1991; Higginson, Muir & Muñoz, 1992.

## Causes of Cancer

The causation of cancer is an age-old question that does not have a single answer. It has been estimated that about 90% of the cancers are caused by environmental factors. The factors involved are multitudinous. Substances that cause cancer are termed **carcinogens** and defy quantitation. Carcinogens may be chemical, physical, or biological in nature.

**Chemical carcinogens** are chemical agents that have the capability of causing cancer. It is estimated that there are over 7 million chemical agents in the environment, many of which are carcinogenic. The exact number of chemical carcinogens is unknown. Examples of chemical carcinogens include aflatoxin, benzidene, benzopyrene, bischloromethylether, nitrosamine, napthylamine, nickel carbonyl, nitrogen mustard, and some of the cancer chemotherapeutic and immunosuppresive drugs, to mention just a few. Cancer drugs are notorious producers of free radical pathology, producing lipid peroxidation, destruction of cellular homeostastasis, and damage to the DNA molecule, which is concerned with normal protein synthesis. (See the following section on Free Radicals in this chapter for more information.) These are the destructive processes that ultimately lead to further carcinogenesis and immune impairment. Also included within this group are the chemical carcinogens that may be found in certain dietary products, fats, alcohol, and tobacco.

**Physical carcinogens** include solar radiation, ionizing radiation from such sources as X-rays and radiation produced by the decay of radioactive particles, such as uranium, radium, and radon gas.

**Biological carcinogens** include cancers produced by living organisms such as viruses and helminth parasites. Some viruses have been found to be extremely potent carcinogens. These tumor-producing viruses are referred to as oncogenic viruses. Experimentally it has been found that when these viruses are introduced into cultures of normal cells they then acquire the altered growth properties of cancer cells by means of a process known as cellular transformation.

Parasitic helminths, such as the blood fluke, *Schistosoma hematobium*, can cause inflammation of the bladder, which can later cause a malignant squamous cell epithelioma. The Chinese liver fluke, *Clonorchis sinensis*, produces inflammatory changes within the bile ducts of the liver and has been associated with cholangiocarcinoma and hepatocarcinoma of the liver, but the nature of carcinogensis has not been clearly defined (Katz, Desommier & Gwadz, 1982). Cancers produced by parasitic trematodes occur in tropical and subtropical regions of the world in which these trematodes are endemic. Parasitic trematodes are generally not a problem of temperate zones.

**Heredity** may also play a role in the development of cancer; however, cancer is not generally considered to be an inherited disease. The vast majority of cancers has not been inherited and is not passed on to the offspring. Probably less than 2% of the cancers are inheritable. The predisposition to cancer is similar to any other genetic disorder. In cases where there is a genetic predisposition toward cancer, it is transmitted from parent to child, and the development of the cancer is inherited like any other genetic trait such as facial features, hair or eye color. Examples of some of these inherited cancers include retinoblastoma, Wilms' tumor, colon carcinoma, Li-Fraumeni cancer family syndrome (sarcomas, breast carcinoma, brain tumors, leukemia, adenocortical tumors), pheochromocytoma, neuroblastoma, neurofibrosarcoma, and others (Carney & Sikora, 1990; Cooper, 1992; Higginson, Muir & Muñoz, 1992). Although heritable cancers are largely independent of environmental factors, it is believed there is nevertheless an interplay of one's genetic background, lifestyle, environmental carcinogens, and nutritional factors which may modify the process of carcinogenesis.

Another group of factors that play a role in carcinogenesis are those that depress immune function. This includes a wide variety of chemical agents, radiation, lifestyle, and one's mental attitude. This is an area where the use of immunomodulating adaptogenic herbs and dietary nutrients can exert a positive effect in inhibiting carcinogenesis.

## FREE RADICALS

Free radicals play an important role in the body, both in health and disease. Toxic agents of many types may adversely affect the molecules in the body by producing free radicals. Free radicals have been implicated in over 100 diseases,

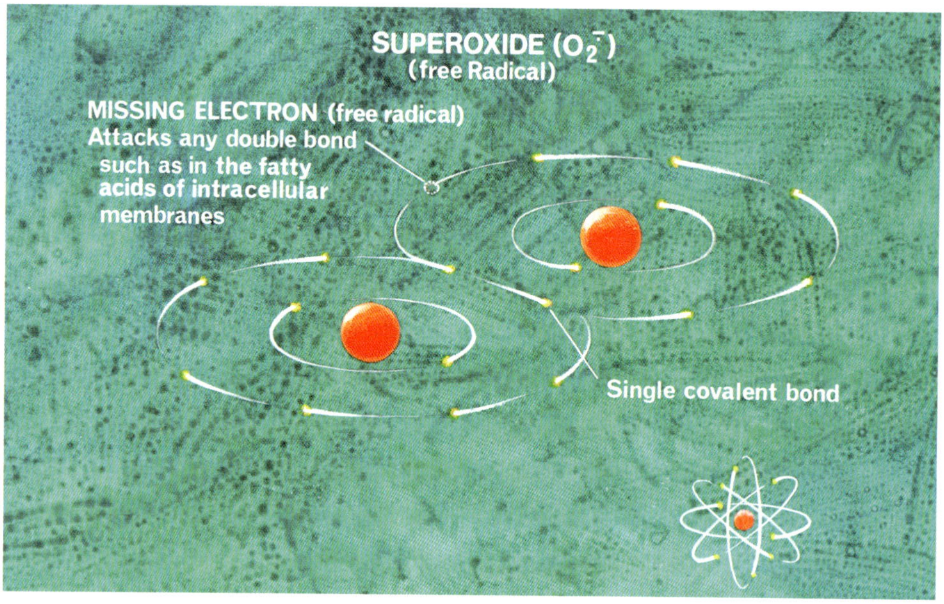


Fig. 6.2. Superoxide is used to illustrate the structural nature of a free readical. Under the conditions shown within a single covalent bond and a missing electron, a free radical is highly reactive. In the lower right corner the electrons are symbolized revolving around the oxygen nucleus. (R.H. Knabenbauer)

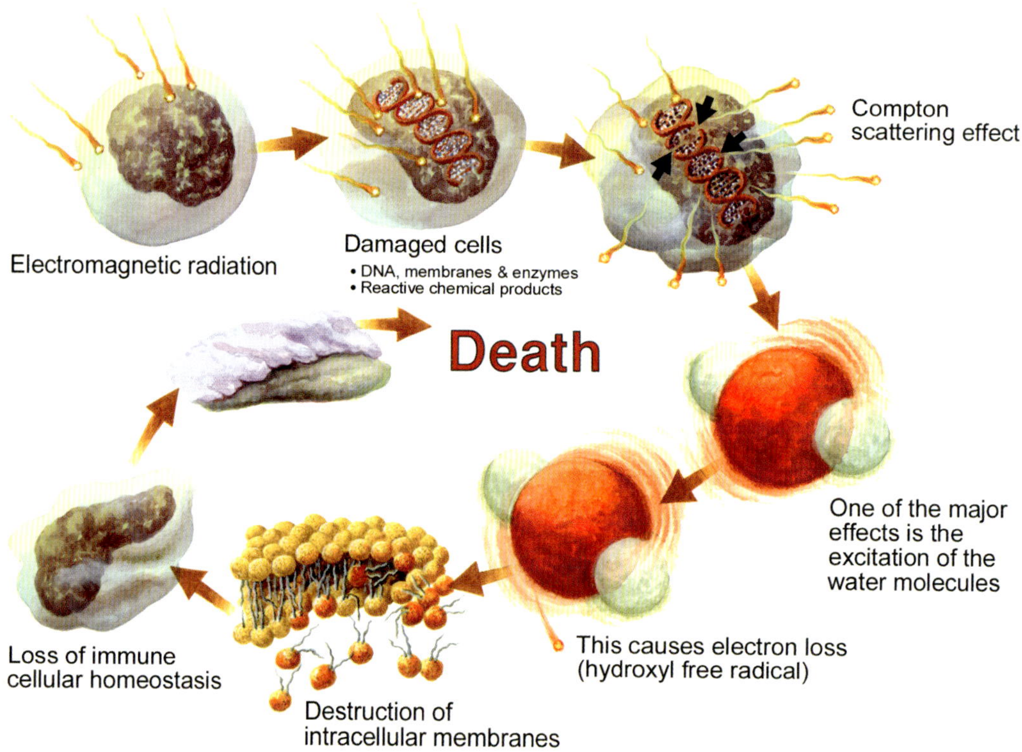


Figure 6.3. Ionizing radiation, illustrating the development of hydroxyl free-radicals and their effects on DNA and intracellular membranes. (R.H. Knabenbauer)

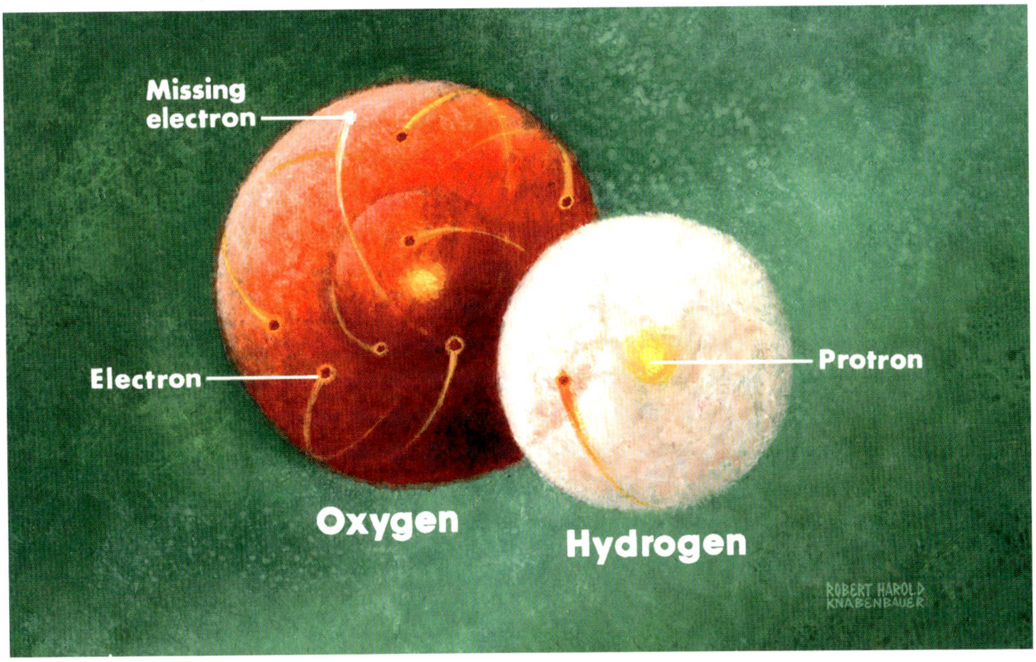


Figure 6.4. Hydroxyl radical. This is one of the most reactive and dangerous species of free radicals. The hydroxyl radical is carcinogenic and the most potent oxidant known. (R.H. Knabenbauer)

including cancer, radiation sickness, and AIDS. A free radical, also known as a reactive oxidant species (ROS), is a chemical species capable of existing independently having one or more unpaired electrons. Thus a free radical is defined as a chemical species having an odd number of electrons and a single unpaired electron in the outer orbital ring (Fig. 6.2). Free radicals may be either of endogenous or exogenous in origin. Endogenous free radicals are generated intracellularly, acting within the cell. Exogenous sources of free radicals include irradiation, chemicals, chemotherapy, and many medications. Exposure to ionizing radiation is a major cause of free radical production (Fig. 6.3). When water is irradiated, an electron from the molecule is removed. The damaging free radicals are H· and OH· The hydroxyl free radical (Fig. 6.4) is highly reactive and extremely carcinogenic. Other important free radicals include superoxide, hydrogen peroxide, peroxyl radicals, and singlet oxygen. Free radicals also play an important role in the body's microbial defense system. Free radicals are terminated or neutralized by nutrient antioxidants

For further discussion on free radicals and carcinogenesis see McBrien and Slater (1982), Waring and Ponder (1987), Sarma and Sarma (1988), Halliwell and Gutteridge (1989), Levine and Kidd (1994), and Halstead and Rozema (1997).

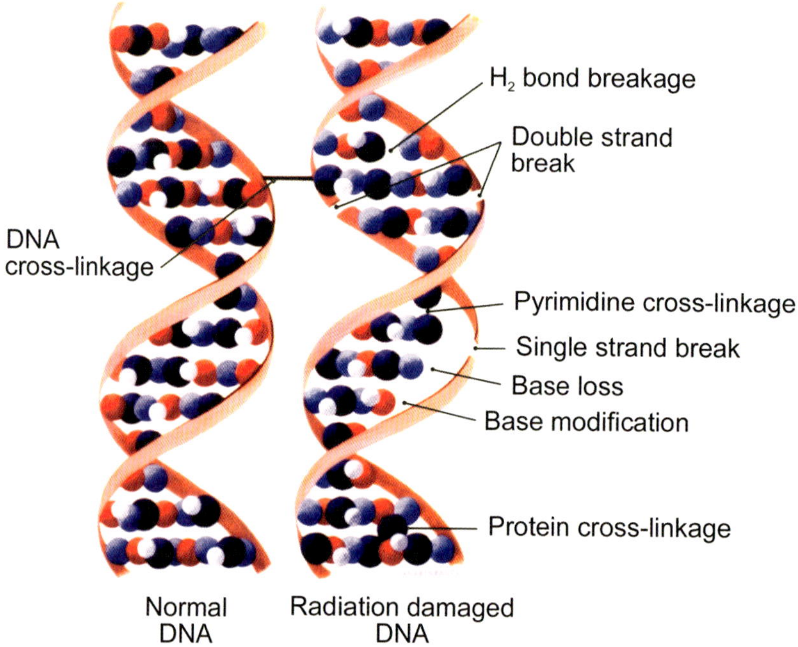


Fig. 6.5. A diagrammatic hemi-section through the DNA molecule showing the normal DNA (left) and a damaged DNA molecule (right), with a single strand and double strand break. (R.H. Knabenbauer)

## The Process of Carcinogenesis

The multistage process of carcinogenesis involves genetic mutation and the selection of rapid cell growth having invasive and metastaic potential.

**Tumor Initiation** is the first step in carcinogenesis. Cancer develops as a consequence of damage to the cell's genetic material, namely the DNA molecule (Fig. 6.1). Many carcinogens react with DNA to induce genetic mutations (Fig. 6.5). These carcinogens are referred to as initiating agents since the induction of critical mutations are generally thought to be the initial events leading to cancer development.

**Tumor Proliferation** is the second step in carcinogenesis. Some carcinogens are believed to contribute to the development of cancer by promoting cell proliferation rather than inducing mutations. Carcinogens of this type are referred to as promoting agents. These agents are required for the initial development of a population of proliferating cancer cells.

Many carcinogens have been found to possess both initiating and proliferating properties, but some of the more dangerous carcinogens are those that primarily promote cell division. Examples of important proliferative agents are hormones such as estrogen and certain dietary fats (Searle, 1984; Castegnaro & Sansone, 1986; Iversen, 1993; Spitz & Newell, 1992).

## Regulatory Mechanisms Governing Cell Growth

The unregulated proliferation of cancer cells is the result of defects in the molecular mechanisms that control the basic elements of cell growth and differentiation. The nature of this regulatory mechanism that controls cell division in the body is genetic. It has now been determined that cell growth is controlled by genes. There are three broad classes of genes that are involved in the progression from a normal cell to a cancer cell.

**Oncogenes** are genes which are related to normal cellular genes, but when altered can induce cancer characteristics into normal cells. Oncogenes arise from proto-oncogenes due to genetic alterations that can either increase gene expression or lead to uncontrolled function of the oncogene-encoded proteins. The products of most proto-oncogenes serve to stimulate normal cell proliferation, but the unregulated action of the corresponding oncogene proteins may lead to the proliferation of cancer cells.

**Tumor Suppressor Genes** are genes that normally act to control cell proliferation, such as the p53 gene. In cancer cells the tumor suppressor cells are inactivated. The action of tumor suppressor genes is opposite to that of oncogenes. It has been found experimentally that the introduction of tumor suppressor genes into cancer cells results in a loss of their tumorigenicity (Cooper, 1992; Culotta & Koshland, 1993).

**DNA Repair Genes** are a group of genes that under normal circumstances can repair DNA damage, but when these genes are altered they can predispose a person to cancer (Farmer & Walker, 1985; Colburn, 1989; Franks & Teich, 1991; Cooper, 1992).

It has also been found that other genes encoding proteins, such as proteinases, and other enzymes capable of disrupting tissues and vascularity may be involved in carcinogenesis.

Experimental evidence suggests that in the majority of cases cancers arise from a single cell that has acquired some heritable form for growth proliferation. The initiation of this process is due to either a chemical or physical carcinogen. The cells at this stage appear to be genetically normal even though the DNA molecule has been altered. Because of damage to the regulatory genes governing cellular growth there emerges clones of cells having the propensity for further cancerous growth. Finally, additional changes in the regulatory mechanism allows for cells having metastatic potential. With each succession of cancerous cells there is an increasing potential for instability of the cells and increased potential for malignancy and metastasis (MacDonald & Ford, 1991; Cooper, 1992).

**Adaptogenic Regulatory Substances.** There are nontoxic adaptogenic plant substances that appear to have a regulatory mechanism in the body that need to be evaluated for use as cancer therapeutic agents. There is reason to believe that immunomodulary adaptogens may be useful in normalizing the regulatory machinery governing cell growth.

## Nutrition and Cancer

During recent years there has been a growing recognition of an association between nutrition and cancer. High consumption of fat and animal protein has shown a definite correlation with cancer of the breast and colon death rates. Studies dealing with a variety of dietary factors as contributory agents in the causation of cancer have been well documented. Until recent years the importance of nutrition in the prevention and treatment of cancer has been either minimal or largely ignored. Fortunately, the importance of nutrition as a chemopreventative measure is beginning to be recognized on an international scale as never before.

The interrelationships between nutrition, immunology, and cancer have come under serious scrutiny only during the past decades. When dealing with cancer it is therefore necessary to discuss the nutrition of the immune system. Any nutrient deficiency or excess that adversely affects DNA synthesis, cell division and replication, differentiation of immune cells, synthesis of complement, lymphokines, and endogenous mediator proteins, or the process of normal cellular metabolism may affect immune function and cancer metabolism.

Cancer-induced anorexia and cachexia are major factors in the development of malnutrition which generally leads to a loss of immune competence. Cachexia and anorexia are further aggravated by surgery, chemotherapy, and radiotherapy. A patient suffering from anorexia also suffers from mental depression, which further depresses immune competence by negative psychoimmunologic processes. (See Chapter Seven on the subject of Psychoneuroimmunology.) A depreciated immune system leads to secondary infections and increased morbidity and mortality rates. Thus, a vicious fatal cycle is activated.

The body's defense system is an extremely complex chemical communication network whose competence depends upon its ability to recognize foreign antigenic or aberrant molecules, which includes malignant cells, and to react in an appropriate manner with specific responses.

It has been found that nutritional deprivation or depletion caused by inadequate nutritional intake, increased protein catabolism due to injury, medication, surgery, or disease, may adversely affect protein synthesis—all of which may result in increased carcinogenesis. Determination of the health status of the immune system can be accomplished with the use of sophisticated immune panels that are able to determine both the numbers of immune cells and their functionality.

# Phytochemical Inhibitors of Carcinogenesis

There is a substantial body of scientific information that demonstrates that there are a number of plant constituents that have the ability to inhibit carcinogenesis (Duke & Wain, 1981; Luoh, 1981: Yang, 1981). This information includes both epidemiological studies in humans and laboratory studies in animals. The following is a brief review of the chemical nature of some of these plant compounds. Unfortunately, the precise mechanisms of action of these chemical agents as to how they inhibit cancer are not completely understood.

The cruciferous, family Cruciferaceae, which includes the vegetables cabbage, brussel sprouts, cauliflower, broccoli, and related vegetables, are especially rich in carcinogenic inhibitory substances.

**Indoles.** One of the groups of anticancer agents in cruciferous vegetables are the indoles, such as indole-3-acetonitrile, 3,3"-diindoly-methane, and indole-3-carbinol. These indoles have been found to inhibit the production of malignant tumors in mice. All three of these indoles have been found to alter microsomal monooxygenase oxidase activity in laboratory animal studies as part of a protective activity against carcinogenesis. These three indoles also demonstrated increased glutathione-S-transferase activity, which is a major detoxification system in the body. (Wattenburg & Loub, 1978; NRC, 1982).

**Isothiocyanates.** The isothiocyanates are among the more important carcinogenic inhibitors. These are a group of substances that are chemically characterized as an organic alkyl or aryl compound containing the anion -HCS. These thiocyanates are widely distributed in nature and are found in numerous plants, including cruciferous plants of the genus *Brassica*. Thiocyanates may exert thyroid-inhibiting effects by interfering with iodine uptake.

**Cyanogenic glucosides.** The widely distributed cyanogenic glycosides may be transformed to thiocyanates in mammalian metabolism. Probably the best-known member of the cyanogenic glycosides is amygdalin. A glycoside is any natural product derived from a plant or animal that contains a sugar. A cyanogenic glycoside is a sugar-containing compound capable of producing a cyanogen or hydrocyanic acid. The chemical structure of amygdalin is D(l)-mandelonitrile-$\alpha$-D-glucosido-6-$\alpha$-D-glucoside. Amygdalin is an herbal constituent derived from the kernel of various fruits of the genus *Prunus* which includes the plum, prune, almond, apricot, cherry and peach.

Amygdalin is found in over 1,200 plant species involving at least 13% of all plant families. Amygdalin is one of the most ancient of all plant products used in the treatment of cancer (Halstead, 1977). The toxicity of amygdalin when given parenterally, ranges from only slightly toxic to almost non-toxic ($LD_{50}$ in rats IP is 9.5 g/kg). Amygdalin is more toxic when administered by mouth because of hydrolysis by the gastric juices. Amygdalin does not contain sodium cyanide or hydrocyanic acid. When properly administered amygdalin is completely safe. Unfortunately, there is a great deal of misinformation that has been released to the general public and believed by the medical profession at large concerning the toxicity of amygdalin.

The metabolic degradation of amygdalin in mammals ultimately results in the production of thiocyanate. The precise mechanism of action is unknown, but it is believed to inhibit carcinogensis as a blocking agent and stimulates glutathione-S-transferase production. Amygdalin also produces benzaldehyde, which has an analgesic effect and thereby reduces the pain in some cancer victims. This feeling of well-being promotes psychoneuroimmunological mechanisms which contribute to immune enhancement, a subject which is discussed in the section of Psychoneuroimmunology in Chapter Seven.

**Sulforaphane** [1-isothiocyanato-4-(methyl-sulfinyl) butane] is another isothiocyanate compound which has been isolated from the florets of broccoli. It has been shown to possess potent anticancer activity. Sulforaphane is one of more than 100 different hydrolysis products known as glucosinolates that have been isolated from various plant tissues. It has been determined that the ability of a cell to render certain carcinogenic agents harmless depends upon the level of activity of certain protective enzyme systems within the cell. It is currently believed that by altering these carcinogens before they interact with DNA or other cellular structures they can prevent carcinogenisis and other cellular damage. The protective detoxification enzymes that appear to be induced through the action of sulforaphane include glutathione transferases, NADPH, quinone reductase, UDP-glucuronsyltransferases, and epoxide hydrolase. These enzymes play an important role in protecting the cells of the body against toxic substances and carcinogenesis. Thus, broccoli is an important cancer preventive vegetable and should be in the diet of cancer patients (Prochaska, et al, 1992; Zhang, et al, 1992, 1994).

**Dithiolthiones** are also an important group of protective substances found in cruciferous vegetables such as cabbage. Dithiolthiones are characterized by a pentacyclic ring consisting of two adjacent sulfurs with a third sulfur attached to a carbon and an aromatic ring attached to another carbon.

Dithiolthiones have been found to be potent free radical scavengers and have a protective action against certain chronic degenerative diseases. During World War II a group of American prisoners of war in Germany were fed largely cabbage juice. A medical evaluation of these prisoners at the end of the war revealed that they had a very low incidence of arthritis, atherosclerosis, bursitis, and other chronic degenerative diseases.

Though work on the chemistry of dithiolthiones dates back to the work of Jirousek (1958; Jirousek & Starka, 1958), who found large quantities of dithiolthiones in cabbage, little is known regarding these important biochemical substances.

Preliminary work by Ernest Bueding at the School of Hygiene and Public Health, Johns Hopkins University, demonstrated that the dithiolthiones of cabbage had a number of unique properties as anticancer and radioprotective agents, and in liver protection against toxic substances such as carbon tetrachloride. He found that the cabbage dithiolthiones were able to protect normal tissues in rats with cancers that were exposed to lethal gamma radiation. Cancerous tissues were not protected from radiation, but the normal tissues were protected. Strange to say Bueding was unable to obtain financial support from the National Cancer Institute for his investigations on the cabbage dithiolthiones. Bueding was hoping to continue work on the chemical structure of these dithiolthiones and their mechanism of action, but he died before completing his great work.

The mechanism of action of the dithiolthiones is not completely known, but some of the preliminary work with mice and rats clearly indicates that the oral administration of dithiolthiones results in a significant increase in elevations of tissue levels of glutathione and in the activities of such protective enzymes as glutathione-S-transferases and NADH quinone reductases, catalyzing the inactivation of carcinogens and other toxic agents. These effects are associated with chemoprotective and radioprotective actions as well as with the inhibition of carcinogenesis (Ansher, 1983; Ansher, Dolan & Bueding, 1983; Bueding, 1983-personal communication; Bueding, Ansher & Dolan, 1985).

**Bioflavenoids, Flavones, Flavonoids, and related compounds** are a major source of the natural blue, red, and some yellow pigments, which were formerly referred to as vitamin P. They are widely distributed in vegetables, fruits, flowers, and grains. Bioflavenoids are abundant in the rinds of citrus fruits, rose hips, and black currents. Bioflavenoids are synergistic in their action with natural vitamin C.

The bioflavenoid chemical nomenclature is confusing. Several different systems of chemical classification of these compounds are in use. Included within the family of compounds known as bioflavenoids, depending upon the chemical authority one follows, are the flavones, flavanones, flavonols, isoflavones, anthocyanidins, chalcones, catechins, epicatechins, isoflavanones, isoflanols, benzopyrones, coumarins, flavans, flavanolols, leucoanthocyanidins, dihydrochalcones, aurones, proanthocyanidins, procyanidins, prodelphidins, profixtinidins, prorobinotidins, and proquibourtinidins.

There are about 20,000 bioflavenoids that have been reported. Much of the nutritional research dealing with bioflavenoids has been concerned with their function relating to capillary fragility and permeability, their antiinflammatory properties, and antioxidant properties, but they have a wide range of other pharmacological properties. Bioflavenoids are said to serve as active antioxidants in preventing lipid peroxidation. Probably the best known of these antioxidant bioflavenoids in nutritional circles is "pycnogenol" which is discussed in the following section. They also play an important role as chelating agents in metalloenzyme systems and in maintaining cellular membranes. Bioflavenoids possess significant bacteriostatic properties. Bioflavenoids have also been shown to have anticarcinogenic properties (Kühnau, 1976; Hayatsu, et al, 1988).

The two bioflavenoids quercetin and rutin are widely distributed in plants and induce aryl hydrocarbon hydroxylase, which has been found to suppress carcinogenesis. It is believed that some of the bioflavenoids stimulate protective conjugating enzymes, including glutathione S-transferase. Certain bioflavenoids have been found to have antiviral properties. Some of the bioflavenoids are immunomodulators (Farkas, et al, 1974; Cody, et al, 1985; Lesser, 1977; NRC, 1982; Ensminger, et al, 1983; Merck, 1989; Harborne, 1994).

**Protease inhibitors.** One of the characteristics of malignant cells is their ability to secrete enzymes known as proteases which have the ability to digest other proteins. The process of metastasis involves the spread of cancer cells through the walls of tissues and blood vessels, which are composed of insoluble proteins. For example, the extracellular matrix of connective tissue, is composed of collagen which is a protein secreted by fibroblasts. Cancer cells are able to penetrate through the surrounding normal tissues by secreting protease enzymes which are able to dissolve the extracellular substances, and thereby assist in the spread of the cancer. The metastatic potential of a particular cancer is dependent upon the amount of proteases that they are able to secrete.

Thus protease inhibitors play an important role in controlling the spread of cancer. Protease inhibitors are widely distributed throughout the plant world and are particularly abundant in seeds. A variety of protease inhibitors are found in soybeans and lima beans. Studies have reported that protease inhibitors not only inhibit protease enzymes, but also inhibit carcinogenesis, and reduce the incidence of breast cancer in irradiated rats. Part of the mechanism of action of cancer protection by protease inhibitors is believed to be due to their free radical scavenging and antioxidant properties (Troll, 1980; NRC, 1982; Cooper, 1992).

**Beta-Sitosterol.** This is a common sterol that is present in many different plants and vegetable oils, and has been found to have an inhibitory effect on carcinogenesis. Sitosterol is found in wheat germ, corn oil, soybean, cottonseed, and numerous other plant oils (Cohen & Raicht, 1981; NRC, 1982).

**Phenols.** Another group of carcinogenic inhibitors includes the phenols, which are various derivatives of cinnamic acid. They are present in a large variety of plants, such as members of the plant families Styracaceae, Hamameliaceae, Meliaceae, and others. Many of these plants are consumed by humans (Wattenberg, et al, 1979; Hsu, Chen & Hong, 1980; NRC, 1982; Hayatsu, et al, 1988). The inhibitory effects of phenols are believed to be due to the production of a coordinated enzyme response that results in increased detoxification. One such example is the enhancement of glutathione-S-transferase activity and increased glutathione tissue levels. Glutathione is an important sulfur-containing tripeptide found throughout plant and animal tissues that is vital to the oxidative and protective processes of organisms. There are undoubtedly other anticarcinogenic activities of glutathione, but not all of them have been fully delineated.

One of the best sources of polyphenols having anticancer activity is found in the Chinese green tea, *Camellia sinensis*, the Lung Ching variety, which is grown in the Yunnan Province of China. Green tea extracts have been found to act as a free radical scavenger, inhibiting the production of malondialdehyde, possesing antimutagenic and anticancer activity ( Mukhtar, et al, 1992, 1994; Wu, 1993; Gao, et al, 1994; UCB, 1994).

**Kombucha Tea.** This is an ancient fungus tea, which dates back to about the Tsin Dynasty (221 - 207 BC). The tea apparently originated in ancient China, and eventually spread throughout the Orient, into Russia and eastern Europe, and is currently popular in the United States and western Europe. The tea is comprised of various species of yeast fungi of the genus *Saccharomyces*, *Torula*, and bacterial cultures. Kombucha is flavored with tea derived from *Camellia sinensis*, which provides a variety of polyphenols having anticancer activty (Fasching, 1994; Frank, 1994).

**Fibers.** The role of dietary fibers as protective agents against colon cancer has been under extensive investigation since the 1970's. It is generally accepted that the fibers found in grains, fruits and vegetables have a protective effect against colon cancer, but it is not known for certain whether all of the anticancer activity is due specifically to the fiber content or to other phytochemical constituents that may be present. At any rate the eating of high fiber content foods is encouraged in nutritional cancer therapy.

## Evaluation of Traditional Anticancer Agents

### THE USE OF MULTIPLE PLANTS IN A PRESCRIPTION

The two most widely used types of traditional medicine practiced throughout the world utilize primarily plant products. Chinese and Ayurvedic traditional medicine employ multiple plant products that are used in a variety of combinations. Many of these plants have adaptogenic and immunomodulating properties. Chinese medicinal herbs, for example, are generally used as a polypharmaceutical in which there are a number of plants and their active phytochemical constituents are concurrently at work. Chinese herbalists believe that their best therapeutic results are obtained from a synergism of active phytochemical constituents rather than from a single plant product. See Chapter Eight for further details on this subject.

A single Chinese prescription may have a combination of plants containing numerous phytochemical constituents having anticancer, antiradiation, antiviral, immunomodulating, tonic, and adaptogenic properties. At the present time there is no western anticancer screening procedure that deals with all of these combined therapeutic elements. Cancer is a multifactorial disease process and it requires a multifactorial therapeutic solution. Failure to adequately address this complex therapeutic issue is one of the primary reasons for the failure to win the war against cancer.

Unfortunately, modern western pharmaceutical science is not equipped to handle this type of therapeutic analysis. Consequently, the critics of traditional medicine tend to sweep this type of ethnobotanical research under the pharmacognostic rug and categorize this research as anecdotal and "poor science", which is merely an excuse for their our own scientific inadequacies. Unfortunately, modern science is still unable to cope with synergisms either in the field of therapeutics or in toxicology.

## THE USE OF A SINGLE PLANT IN A PRESCRIPTION

A second type of traditional medicine practiced throughout much of the ethnic world utilizes a single plant product in the treatment of a disease. Although a single plant species may be employed there are multiple phytochemical constituents, but there may be only a single primary biodynamic constituent that is exerting the desired therapeutic action. Although a single plant may be used it is essentially a polypharmaceutical product.

Farnsworth, et al (1985) conducted a valuable study on the use of medicinal plants as therapeutic agents in which they documented a high correlation between the traditional use of certain plants and the pharmacological action of 119 substances isolated from these plants. They concluded that a study of traditional plant uses was a good approach for discovering new therapeutic drugs. They further concluded that a random screening of plant samples for biological activity was a less effective method in the search for new drugs.

The Farnsworth group suggested that the use of safe galenical plant products, i.e. crude plant extractives, that have proven to be effective in humans in many developing countries may be a practical economic necessity even though the active principles have not been chemically purified or identified.

Most Chinese herbalists are of the opinion that the chemical purification of plant products may also result in a loss of therapeutic activity and an increase in the toxicity of the substance. The use of crude plant prescriptions is unacceptable to the modern pharmaceutical industry, but is nevertheless culturally acceptable to about 80% of the world's population.

## Western Medicine Cancer Therapy

The type of cancer therapy as practiced in the Western world consists largely of surgery, chemotherapy, and radiation. Each of these modalities has their advantages and their disadvantages. All of them have their limitations. It should be noted that the role of nutrition in cancer prevention or therapy was not generally recognized in the United States until about the 1980's.

If the cancer can be surgically removed then surgery should be employed. However, if the cancer has metastasized, surgery may not be effective.

Chemotherapy has been found to be effective in only about 8% of the advanced systemic cancer cases. The difficulty with chemotherapy is that the chemical agents used in the treatment are extremely toxic and fail to differentiate between healthy cells and cancer cells. Moreover, cancer chemotherapeutic agents produce cancer and lower the immune system. Cancer chemotherapy follows a line of molecular illogic. In many cases, chemotherapy only lessens the cancer patient's chance for survival.

Radiation both kills cancer cells and causes cancer. Unfortunately, radiation can also produce a lethal scattering effect, which may result in a worsening of the existing cancer. The use of the proton accelerator is the single exception to this statement.

Both chemotherapy and radiation have several things in common. They are notorious producers of free radical pathology, causing lipid peroxidation, destruction of cellular homeostasis, and damage to the DNA molecule—the master molecule of the body that engineers protein synthesis.

The primary purpose of this book is to present a nontoxic Chinese form of cancer therapy that is not well known to most Western physicians. Western cancer therapy has not been a total failure. Unfortunately, there has been so much marketing hype it takes a biostatistician to sort out the therapeutic facts from the therapeutic fancy.

The Chinese side of the cancer therapy coin presented in this book is relatively inexpensive, non-toxic and the clinical studies that have been documented thus far have shown this form of therapy to be highly effective because it neither lowers the immune system nor is carcinogenic. We will begin by discussing the philosophical and scientific rationale in Chapters Eight & Nine, but first an overview of the immune system will be presented.

## Chapter 7

# IMMUNOLOGY & CANCER



---

## Introduction

Most cancer patients suffer from immune impairment to some degree. Consequently the health of the immune system is of major concern in the prevention and treatment of cancer and other immune disorders and affects the general health and quality of life of every person, and most vertebrate animals on this planet. A critical study of the immune system has shown that immunocompetence depends upon the availability of certain nutrients. It has also been shown that certain natural products have the ability to enhance the activity of various components of the immune system. The immune system is extremely complex. The science of immunology is still in its infancy; sorting out the pieces, attempting to comprehend its morphological and chemical nature, and the vast importance of its operations in our body is a matter of vast importance.

Before reviewing some of the basic elements as to the nature of the immune system there are a few sobering considerations on the health of our immune systems here in the United States. The U.S. is generally considered to be a nation having one of the better health care systems in the world. The following information presented by the National Coalition on Immune System Disorders (NCISD) leaves no room for complacency on the health of the nation's immune system. We are a sick nation! They estimate that one out of four Americans are suffering from a secondary immune disorder due to various causes. This amounts to about 80 million immune dysfunctional Americans (Bellanti, 1978).

Immune deficiencies set the stage for a wide range of microbial diseases, including AIDS, cancer, and a large number of metabolic disorders. Immune dysfunction, primary and secondary, are at the cutting edge of some of the greatest medical disasters facing mankind today on a worldwide basis. A review of some of the causes of secondary immune disorders is most illuminating. Consider the following partial list in Table 7.1 of threatening factors that are contributing to a significant degree in the causation of immunoincompetence in the general population.

## Dangerous FDA Approved Drugs

The matter of iatrogenic disorders resulting from FDA approved drugs, which are certified by the Government as "safe and effective", is not an incidental matter in the causation of secondary immune disorders and other serious disorders. There are about 2 billion drug prescriptions written annually in the United States. The bad news reported in June 1990 according to the U.S. Congressional watchdog agency, the General Accounting Office (GAO), was that more than half of the new drugs approved for marketing by the FDA in the United States had severe or fatal side-effects which had not been discovered during the clinical trials of the drug approval process. Unfortunately, their disastrous side effects did not become evident until years after their release into the market place (Culbert, 1994).

The matter of nosocomial infection during hospital stays is another matter of frightening proportions. In December 1992, the Centers for Communicable Diseases and Prevention (CDCP) in Atlanta, Georgia, released statistics to the effect that more than 2 million patients entering hospitals and clinics in the U.S. had developed bacterial and viral infections at a cost of $4.5 billion in 1992 (Culbert, 1994).

**Table 7.1**
Causative Factors in Immune Dysfuntion

| | |
|---|---|
| **Diseases** | Malignancies<br>Diabetes<br>Autoimmune disorders (e.g., lupus erythematosis, rheumatoid arthritis)<br>Cirrhosis of the liver<br>Microbial infections (viral, bacterial, fungal)<br>Protein-losing disorders (nephritic syndrome) |
| **Lifestyle** | Alcoholism<br>Recreational drug use<br>Nicotine addiction<br>Lack of exercise<br>Malnutrition |
| **Environmental Factors** | Chemical pollution<br>Radiation<br>Burns |
| **Iatrogenic and Nosocomial Factors** | Excessive drug medication<br>Chemotherapy<br>Radiation therapy<br>Hospital infections from antibiotic resistant microbes |

The patients were leaving the hospital with an immune system that was much worse than when they entered.

This infectious disease situation is part of an extremely serious health problem that is emerging worldwide and points up the importance of disease organisms and the immune system. For an excellent general summary on the emerging microbial plague, see Garrett's (1994) *The Coming Plague*.

Excessive drug medication, the use of recreational drugs, and drug resistant infections are significant factors contributing to America's immune incompetence. In addition, excessive exposures to toxic chemical agents such as pesticides, industrial pollutants, and ionizing radiation are taking their toll on our immune systems. Examination of these causal factors in producing immune dysfunction makes it obvious that the health of a person's immune system is a matter of immense importance when dealing with such disorders as cancer.

The following basic information is presented in order to provide some insight as to the nature of the immune system and how it relates to the prevention and therapy of cancer. This chapter is not intended to be an in-depth review in immunology, but it will provide some of the basic vocabulary that is helpful in dealing with the subject matter of this book.

## Definition of Immunity

The term **immunity** derives from the Latin *immunis*, originally referring to exemption from public service, or state burdens, such as taxes. During the last century the term immunity has denoted a health condition in which there is resistance to an infectious agent attacking the body.

Immunity has been further defined as the combined physiological mechanisms that provide the body with the capacity to recognize materials as foreign to itself and to neutralize, eliminate, or metabolize them with or without injury to its own tissues. Succinctly stated, the science of immunology deals with the understanding of how the body distinguishes between what is "self" from what is "non-self".

Bellanti (1978) has defined immunity thus: "The immunologic response may be viewed as an adaptive system in which the body attempts to maintain homeostasis between the internal body environment and the external environment."

Excellent reviews on basic and clinical immunology are presented in the text by Stites, et al (1987), Benjamini and Leskowitz (1991), Roitt, et al (1993), Roitt (1994), and the less technical publication by Schindler (1988) of the National Cancer Institute.

Although the science of immunology is thought to be relatively new by most western immunologists, observations of an immunological nature are very ancient and date back to old China.

## History of Immunology

The history of immunology and the role of ancient China in the discovery and use of immunomodulating adaptogenic herbs is important to this discussion because it is a matter that is generally overlooked or has received minimal attention in the history of Western medicine.

The earliest evidence of terminology having immunological implications in ancient China appears in the Yellow Emperor's Classic *Huang Ti Nei Ching Su Wen*, traditionally credited to the early Han Dynasty (206 B.C. - 23 A.D.). In the second chapter of the classic entitled *Szu Chi Tao Shen Talun*, or *Simple Questions on the Great Treatise on the Harmony of the Atmosphere of the Four Seasons with the Spirit*, the statement is made that "it is better to prevent disease than to treat it."

The book *Shang Han Lun* (Treatise on Febrile Diseases), written during the Han Dynasty, contains important observations on the symptoms of various diseases and the various herbs used in their prevention. Although the semantics having immunological significance described in the *Shang Han Lun* are different, a careful evaluation of the diseases and the symptoms discussed clearly indicates that they were dealing with what are now the modern immunological terms of "inflammation", "immunology", and "allergy".

Both the *Shang Han Lun* and the *Huang Ti Nei Ching Su Wen* discuss microbial disease organisms which they termed "evil agents" that are now recognized as viruses, bacteria, fungi, and allergens. Despite the difference in semantics it is quite evident that immunological phenomena were recognized in ancient China.

It is a well-established fact that most Chinese herbal medicines, whether they consist of single herbs or combined formulations, are adaptogenic and tonic immunostimulants. These herbs stimulate blood flow, increase microcirculation, enhance phagocytosis, and generally affect metabolism and the endocrine system—all of which affect the immune system.

During the Chou Dynasty (1030 - 221 B.C.) physicians practicing nutrition were placed at the highest level in the ranking of physicians. Surgeons were placed at the lowest level. Foods were considered as medicines when properly used. Prevention was considered the highest priority, and treatment was looked upon as a necessity, but secondary to prevention. During the Han Dynasty (206 B.C. - 23 A.D.) there was a saying (Wong & Wu, 1977) that "a skilled physician cures illness when there is no sign of disease, and thus the disease never comes."

Needham (1980) reviewed the subject of immunology in ancient China dealing largely with mankind's battle against smallpox during the early Sung Dynasty (960 - 1128 A.D.). Although 1000 A.D. is usually the date given as the beginning of the use of smallpox inoculations in China it is believed by Chinese historians that vaccinations were secretly in practice several hundred years prior to that time. Actual documentation on the use of smallpox vaccinations did not appear until about the Ming Dynasty (1368 - 1644 A.D.). As knowledge about smallpox vaccinations began to emerge from the cloak of secrecy there began to appear detailed accounts about the selection of scabs to be used in the vaccinations, their color, shape, and methods of application to the skin. Some of these accounts appeared in the *Tou Chen Shih I Hsin Fa,* written in 1549 A.D., in a work about smallpox and measles. Later Chinese physicians learned to attenuate the virulence of the smallpox scabs by steaming them in plant mixtures using the crow onion, *Scorzonera albicaulis,* and licorice, *Glycyrrhiza glabrus.*

During the 1500's there was a steady increase in the Chinese literature beginning with words '*Chang Tau...*', or 'transplanting the smallpox...' Gradually information on the methodology of performing smallpox vaccinations made its way into India, Turkey, south to Africa, and on to Europe, following the old silk trade routes by Taoist traders.

The Turkish practice of smallpox variolation, which was clearly of Chinese origin, was introduced into England, about 1700, and then made its way into Europe. The technique of variolation, which is the intradermal application of powdered scabs obtained from active cases of smallpox, was used throughout the Middle East during the 18th century.

It is generally recognized that this primitive form of smallpox immunization was first brought to the attention of Western Europe by two Greek-Italian physicians, Emanuele Timoni and Jacob Pylarini, in 1714 in a series of letters addressed to the Royal Society of London. The letters called attention to the technique of variolation as it was then practiced and popularized in Constantinople. The timing of these letters was a little late, but nevertheless of major importance because smallpox had been pandemic throughout Europe in 1614 and epidemic in England during the period of 1666 - 1675, claiming the lives of over 20 million people.

One of the foremost discoveries in the early development of immunology was made by the English physician Edward Jenner (1749 - 1823). While still a medical student, he observed that cow maids that developed cow pox never developed smallpox. He came to the conclusion that cow pox provided the same degree of protection from smallpox with much less jeopardy to the patient. He published his findings in 1798. It should be noted, however, that safe inoculation procedures for smallpox had been in practiced in England and other parts of Europe for almost a century prior to Jenner's work, and the medical profession was already aware of the fact that a smallpox inoculation conferred life-long immunity. Nevertheless, Jenner's studies are generally recognized as an important benchmark in the history of immunology.

The Russian zoologist Eli Metchnikoff (1845 - 1916) studied the role of motile cells of transparent starfish larvae and their protective role against foreign intruders at Messina, Italy, in 1882. He demonstrated that leukocytes were capable of ingesting bacteria by a process known as phagocytosis. Metchnikoff joined the Pasteur Institute in Paris in 1887, where he promoted the concept that the inflammatory process was the result of enzymatic activity due to ingestion of a noxious agent by motile phagocytes. His work is considered to be the starting point of cellular immunology.

Metchnikoff's theory of cellular immunology came under sharp criticism by a group of German investigators who observed immunological activity in the absence of cells. In 1890 Robert Koch (1843 - 1910), Emil von Behring (1854 - 1917), and Shibasburo Kitasato (1852 - 1931) while working at Koch's Institute in Berlin discovered that immunity to diphtheria and tetanus was due to antibodies against the exotoxins of these bacteria. Their work was instrumental in developing the humoral theory of immunology.

These events led to a major controversy between the French school of cellularists and the German school of humoralists. History has shown that both sides were dealing with truth, but unfortunately at that point in time more adrenaline than immune substance was clouding the intellectual atmosphere. The remainder of the history of immunology in Western medicine has been well documented in numerous texts and will not be discussed further in this present work. An excellent and very detailed history of the various theories and development of immunology has been written by Silverstein (1989).

## A Brief Overview of the Immune System

The basic operation of one's immune system is designed to protect the body against environmental agents that are foreign to the body. These agents may comprise a vast array of microorganisms such as bacteria, fungi, viruses, or their toxic products, foods, chemicals, drugs, pollen, hair, dander, ad infinitum. The immune reactions employed by the body may be either innate or acquired and are detailed as follows:

**Innate Immunity:** Innate immunity consists of those immunological elements with which the individual is born. These elements consist of body surfaces such as skin and mucous membranes, the cough reflex, hydrogen ion concentration of skin and membranes, and secreted fatty acids. There is also a complex of inner elements consisting of leukocytes comprised of phagocytic cells such as granulocytes, macrophages, and microglial cells of the central nervous system that are concerned with the elimination of foreign materials that have penetrated the physical and chemical barriers of the nervous system. There are numerous other immune responses which include fever, interferons, a variety of nonspecific substances released by white blood cells, lysozymes, polyamines, kinins, $\alpha$-lysin, and others which comprise innate immunity.

**Acquired Immunity:** Acquired immunity supplements the protection provided by innate immunity, and is more specific and complex. Acquired immunity is not exhibited unless that individual has had prior contact with that agent. The initial contact with a foreign agent such as in the immunization process triggers a chain of events that activates lymphocytes, which leads to the production of antibodies (immunoglobulins) (Fig. 7.1). Once this process takes place the individual acquires the immunity to withstand any subsequent attack by the same offending agent (antigen). Acquired immunity may be defined as a specific immunity attributable to the presence of antibodies and to an increased reactivity of antibody-forming lymphoid cells and of phagocytes following prior exposure to an infectious agent or its antigens.

The discovery of the phenomenon of acquired immunity had been known for many centuries, but was rediscovered by Edward Jenner in 1798 when he experimentally induced immunity to smallpox in a small boy by vaccinating him with pus from a dairymaid who had cow pox.

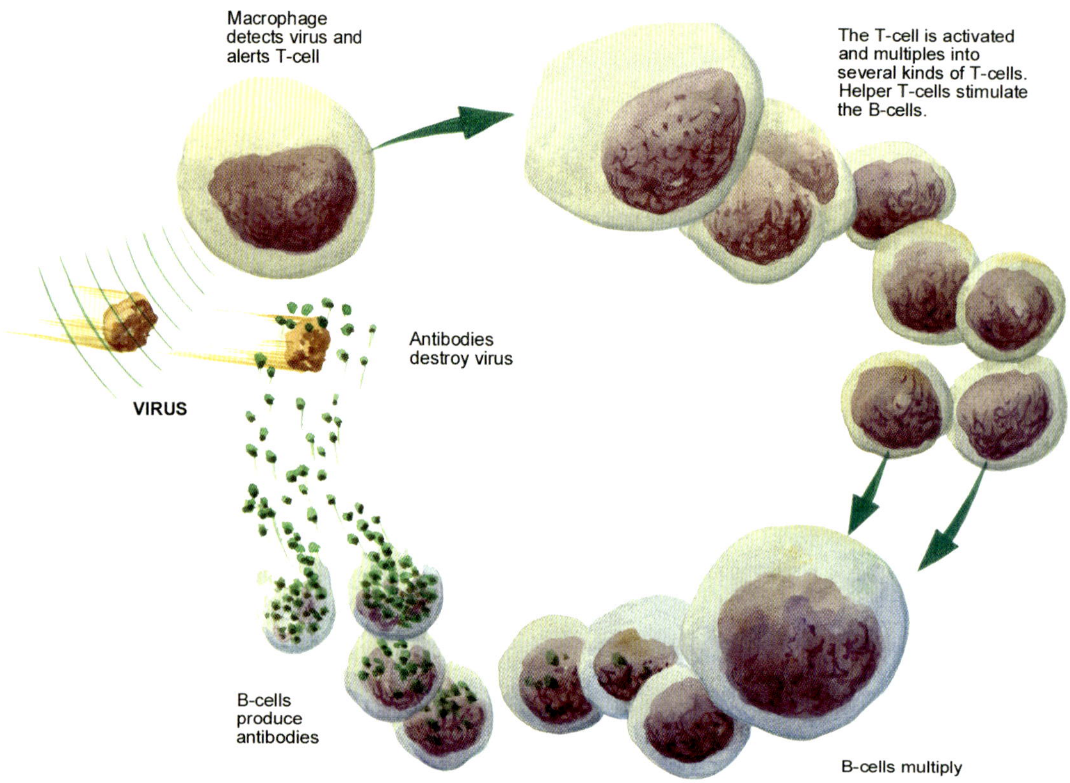


Fig. 7.1. The sequence of events in a typical antigen-antibody reaction resulting in the production of antibodies, which are comprised of immunoglobulins. (R.H. Knabenbauer)

## Types of Acquired Immunity

Acquired immunity may be induced by several different means.

1) **Active Immunization** - refers to immunization of an individual by means of an antigen such as is used in smallpox vaccinations.
2) **Passive Immunization** - refers to immunization by means of a transfer of a specific antibody or immunoglobulin from an immunized individual to a nonimmunized individual.
3) **Adoptive Immunization** - refers to the transfer of immunity by the transfer of immune cells.

## Unique Characteristics of the Immune Response

The acquired immune response has several generalized features that distinguish it from all other physiological responses in the body. They are as follows:

**Specificity:** One of the unique characteristics of the immune system is to be able to discriminate between different molecular entities presented to it, and respond only to those specific entities, rather than making a random undifferentiated response.

**Adaptiveness:** The immune system has the unique ability to respond to the unknown molecules which may have never before been encountered.

**Ability To Discriminate Between Self and Non-self:** A major feature of the specificity of the immune system is its ability to recognize and respond to molecules that are foreign (non-self) and avoid making a response to those molecules that are self.

**Memory:** The immune system has the ability to recall previous contact with a foreign molecule and respond to it in a more rapid fashion. The nervous system has similar recall ability.

The following sections will deal with the subject of immune system function and responses in greater detail.

## General Work of the Immune System

The immune system is a vastly complex chemical communication system that helps to maintain the total metabolic processes and harmony of the body in an orderly manner (Fig. 7.2). The success of this system in maintaining the health of the body is an incredibly elaborate and dynamic regulatory cellular and chemical communications network. Countless millions of cells and complex chemical substances pass information back and forth like ants in an anthill.

Immune system functions are concerned with defense against foreign invaders such as microorganisms, maintenance of homeostasis, and surveillance, (i.e., perception of malignant or mutant cells and foreign invaders). The immune system is also involved in allergic and hypersensitivity reactions.

**Defense** against invasion by microorganisms (bacteria, fungi, viruses and parasites) has long been recognized as a major function by immunologists. The various antigen-antibody mechanisms involved are extremely complex and will only be briefly touched upon in this writing.

**Homeostasis** involves chemical balance within the cell and is an important immunologic function when dealing with radiation sickness. The chemical balance within the cell is determined to a large extent by maintaining the integrity of the intracellular and outer cell membranes (Fig. 7.3-7.6). Cell membrane integrity is further dependent upon the availability of the proper nutrients. It appears that not only vitamins and minerals play a vital role in membrane integrity, but homeostasis may also be assisted by a variety of plant and animal chemical constituents the

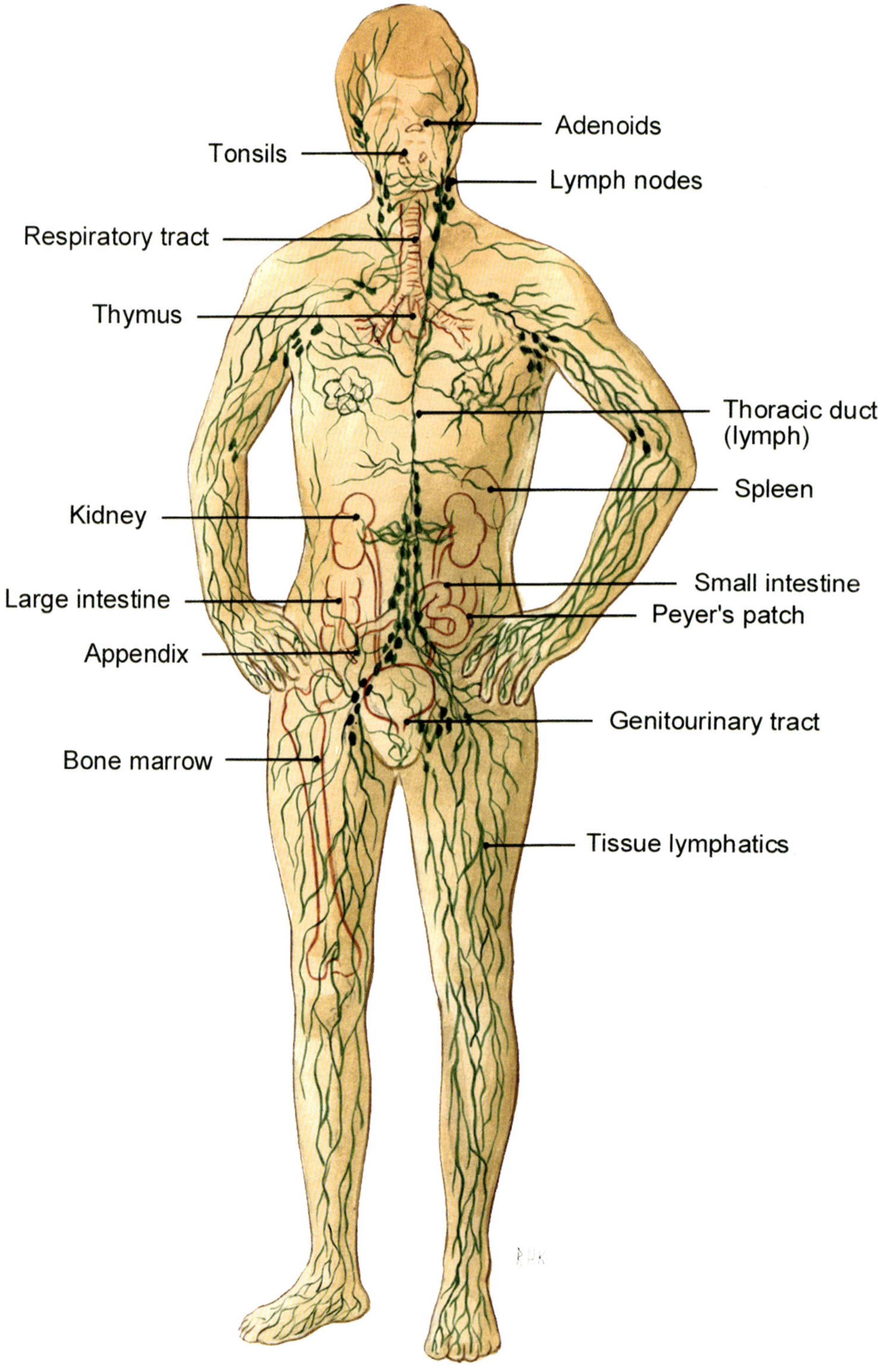


Fig. 7.2. Lymphatic system of the body, showing the distribution of the major lymph channels throughout the body. (R.H. Knabenbauer)

precise chemical nature of which has not been clearly defined. Some of the radioprotective and anticancer activities of the various substances discussed in this book may be due to their role in cell membrane protection or possibly some other homeostatic mechanism that is not fully understood.

**Surveillance** is concerned with the monitoring of abnormal cells by the immune system. Abnormal cells are constantly arising in the body under normal conditions, but the process is greatly accelerated when the body is exposed to radiation and many chemical pollutants. Thus the immune system is charged with the recognition and the disposal of these abnormal cells. Surveillance is the body's tracking system. Malfunction of the surveillance process is a significant factor in the development of malignancies and other forms of degenerative diseases. The immune system is able to recognize many millions of distinctive non-self molecules and can potentially produce molecules and cells to match up with and to counteract each one of them. Thus a competent immune system maintains a ready arsenal of weapon systems that is accurate, prompt, effective, and self-limiting.

**Allergic and hypersensitivity reactions.** Allergies are immune reactions to nonpathogenic antigens which lead to inflammation and deleterious effects to the host. Hypersensitivity is a state of reactivity to an antigen that is greater than normal for the antigenic challenge. The term hypersensitivity is regarded as the same as allergy, but denotes a deleterious outcome rather than a protective one.

## Immune Responses

There are two types of immune responses: nonspecific and specific. **Nonspecific responses** involve the skin and mucous membranes by cells that are capable of ingesting foreign substances, by inflammatory reactions, by elevation of body temperature (fever), and through the action of a large number of antimicrobial substances such as fatty acids, bile salts, heme (porphyrins), polysine (basic polypeptides), protamine, lysozyme, phagocytin, betalysin, properdin, opsonin, and complement. When microorganisms enter the body after trauma or injury to the epithelial surfaces, they are immediately confronted by a secondary defense mechanism consisting of these antimicrobial substances (Hokama & Nakamura, 1982). The nutritional status of the individual has a direct effect on the efficacy of these nonspecific responses and the immune system at large.

**Specific responses** differ from nonspecific resistance in that it is designed to attack specific microorganisms or foreign proteins. The specific resistance of the body is comprised of two distinct but completely integrated systems, the cell-mediated system and the humoral system. This brings up the subject of the structure of the immune system.

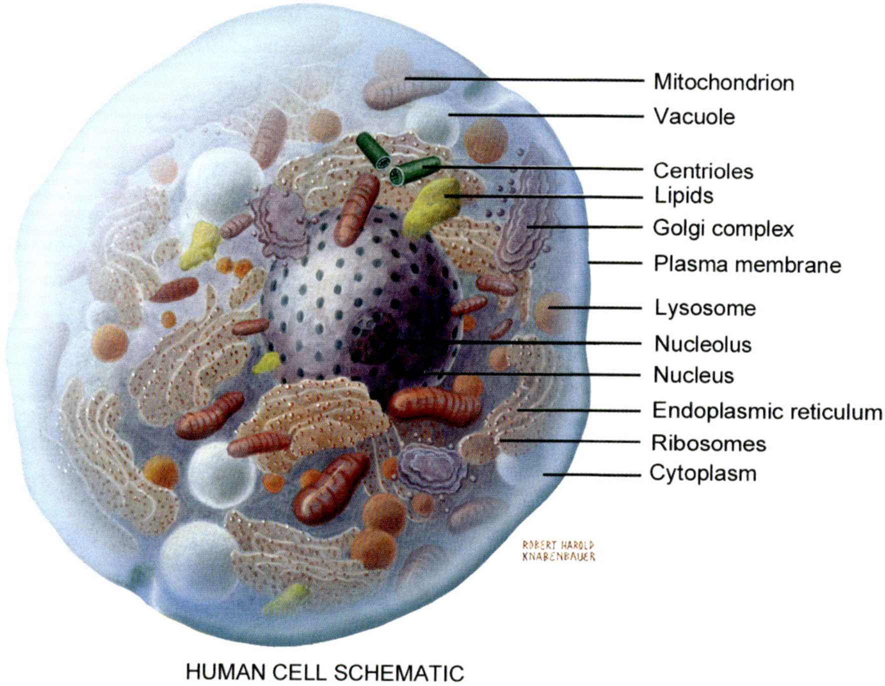


Fig. 7.3. A hypothetical cell showing the various subcellular components or organelles which are involved with the various metabolic functions of the cell. (R.H. Knabenbauer)

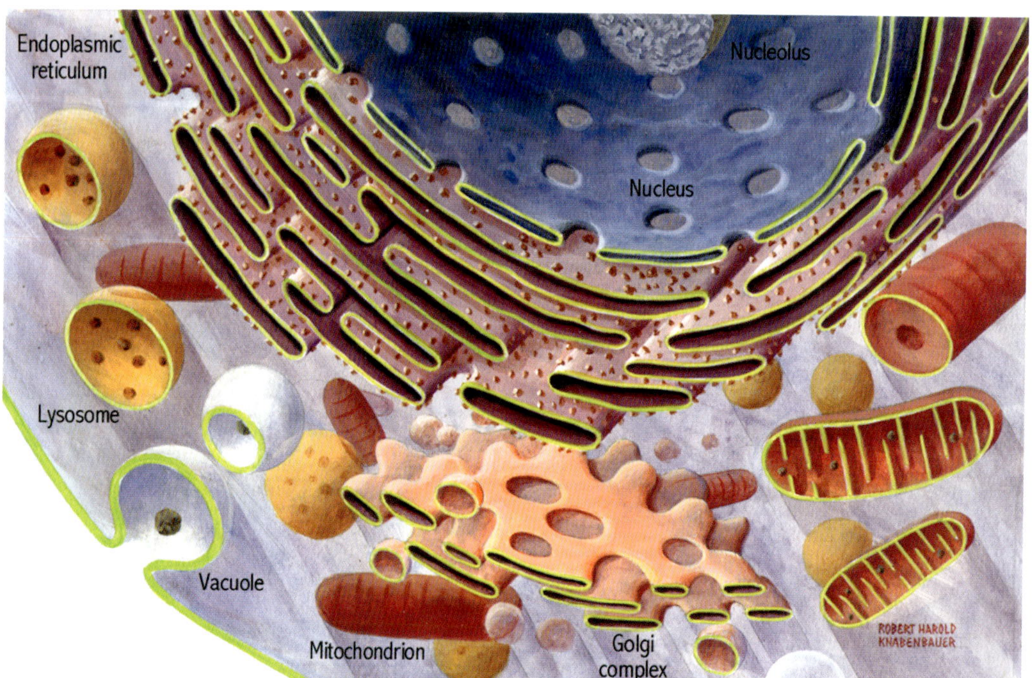


Fig. 7.4. Enlargement of the organelles showing the relationship of their intercellular membranes to the cell at large. (R.H. Knabenbauer)

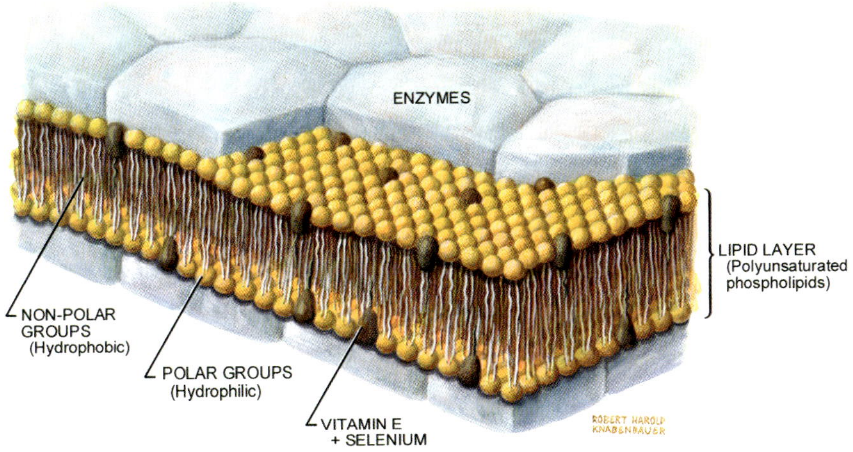


**NORMAL MEMBRANE**

Fig. 7.5. A more detailed view of the theoretical structure of a biological membrane. Membranes are bimolecular and capable of dealing with both lipids and aqueous substances. Membrane proteins may interact with membrane lipids to produce biochemical reactions, sending a series of chemical messengers to other membrane-bound structures within a cell, resulting in a physiological reponse. The general topography of membranes includes well-defined structural and functional sites, including ion pumps, antigens, neurohumeral receptors, intracellular junctions, immunoglobulins, etc. This is why damage to intracellular membranes can ultimately result in a biochemical disaster, causing a health catastrophe. (R.H. Knabenbauer)

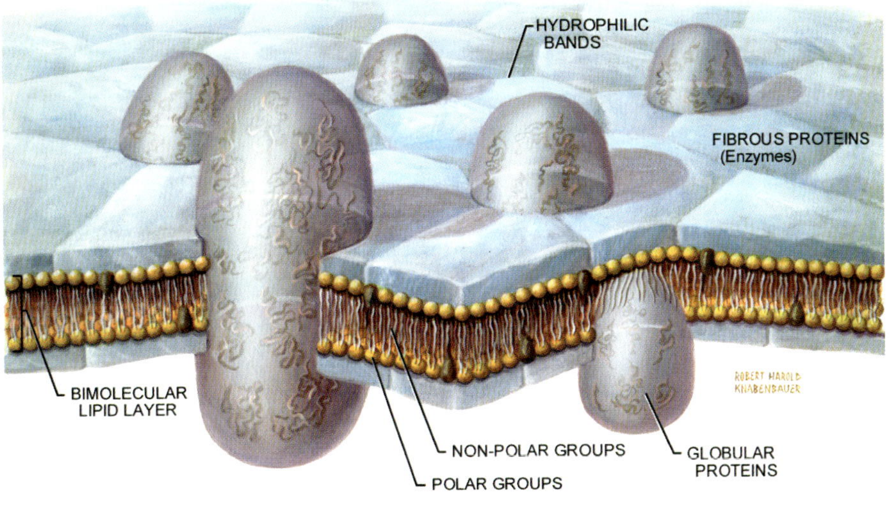


Fig. 7.6. Modified Singer-Nicholson model of a generalized biological membrane which is theoretically representative of intracellular membranes in general. Spectroscopic and ultrastructural evidence suggests that extrinsic and intrinsic proteins of these membranes float on a sea of lipids. Many of the important biological communications between cells and their environment are transduced by proteins intimately associated with membranes. Alteration of these membranes can seriously affect the enzyme functions of the organelles with which they are associated. (R.H. Knabenbauer)

## Structure of the Immune System

The organs of the immune system, generally referred to as lymphoid organs, are widely scattered throughout the body, and are concerned with the growth and development of lymphocytes. The **lymphoid organs** include the bone marrow, thymus, spleen, tonsils, lymph nodes, adenoids, appendix and Peyer's patches in the small intestine. The **lymphocytes** are an important group of mononuclear white blood cells that participate in both cell-mediated and humoral immunity. The blood and lymphatic vessels serve as the conduit through which the lymphocytes are transported to the various parts of the body (Fig. 7.2).

The lymphocytes and other blood cells are all produced in the **bone marrow**, the soft tissue within the hollow shafts of the long bones of the arms and legs. The primary cells within the bone marrow are the **stem cells**. Some of the descendants of the stem cells become erythrocytes (red blood cells), or various types of leukocytes (white blood cells), which include lymphocytes, neutrophils, basophils, monocytes, macrophages, eosinophils, mast cells, and platelets. The major classes of lymphocytes are T-cells and B-cells, the functions of which will be elaborated upon shortly.

The T-cells migrate to the **thymus** (Figs. 7.7, 7.8.), a multi-lobed organ that lies behind the breastbone and in front of the heart, where they are programmed for specific immune functions. The thymus also produces several hormones, one of which is thymosin, a hormone that stimulates the production of peripheral lymphoid tissue. The thymus is especially active during early life and then gradually declines with age. The decline of the thymus gland is one of the reasons for the diminished immunocompetence that accompanies aging. T-cells are referred to as thymus-dependent or mediated cells.

Once the lymphocytes leave the bone marrow and thymus, some of the cells congregate in other immune organs such as lymph nodes, whereas others circulate throughout the body via the blood and the lymphatic vessels. The **lymph nodes** (Fig. 7.9) are small bean-shaped structures that are widely scattered over the body. Each lymph node is a compartmentalized structure that houses large numbers of T, B and other white blood cells capable of enmeshing antigens (foreign invaders) and presenting them to T-cells for destruction. The lymph nodes thus serve as central clearing houses that are capable of bringing together the components needed for an immune response and the destruction of foreign invaders.

Another organ involved in the mobilization of immune defenses is the **spleen**. The spleen varies in size depending upon the age and a variety of conditions, generally about 12 cm in length by 7 cm in breadth and 4 cm in width and is located in the left upper aspect of the abdomen under the rib cage. The spleen diminishes in size in the elderly. The spleen serves as a staging area for immune cells. The red

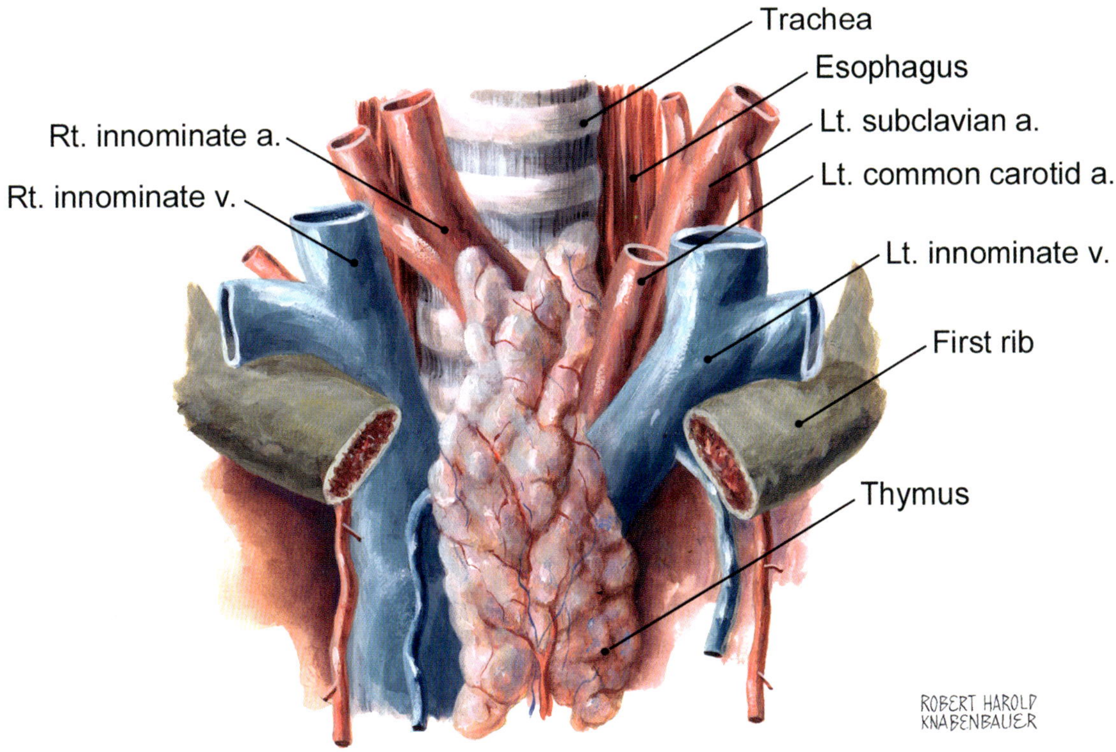


Fig. 7.7. Thymus gland. The thymus is concerned with important immune functions, including the programming of T-cells as shown in Figure 7.8. The thymus produces the hormone thymosin, which stimulates the production of peripheral lymphoid tissue. (R.H. Knabenbauer)

pulp portion of the spleen is where the worn-out blood cells are disposed of, and the white pulp contains the lymphoid tissue.

Clusters of lymphoid tissue are also found in other parts of the body such as the tonsils and adenoids lining the respiratory tract and the appendix and Peyer's patches in the digestive tract.

The **lymphatic vessels** (Fig. 7.2) serve as the main conduit through which the clear lymph fluid carries the lymphocytes, macrophages, and foreign proteins (antigens). These substances are then transported to lymph nodes where the antigens are filtered out and presented to immune cells for disposition. Additional lymphocytes reach the lymph nodes via the blood stream. The lymphatic vessels join larger and larger vessels and eventually merge into the main thoracic duct, which finally empties into the subclavian vein near the base of the neck thereby discharging its contents into the blood stream.

The immune system functions primarily through specialized cells and a complex of chemical substances. Thus, the immune system is said to have a dual nature comprised of a cell-mediated portion and a humoral portion comprised of the various immunoglobulins.

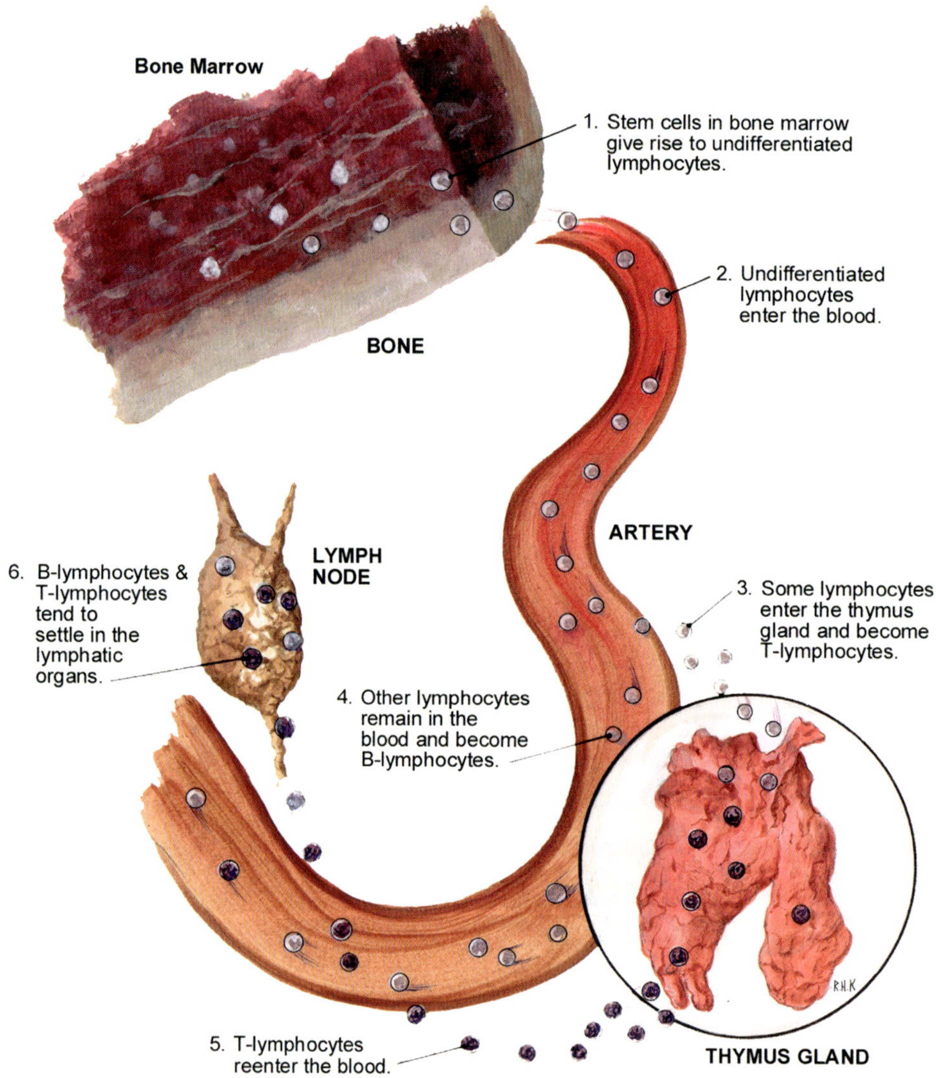


Fig. 7.8. Showing the process of T-cells through the thymus gland. (R.H. Knabenbauer)

# Cell-Mediated Immune System

The cell-mediated immune system is responsible for defense against bacteria, viruses, fungi, protozoans, helminths, transplanted tissue, and cancer cells. The cell-mediated portion of the immune system involves the use of specially designed leukocytes or white blood cells, all of which are derived from stem cells in the bone marrow.

One of these major groups of white blood cells is the **lymphocytes.** There are two basic types of lymphocytes, the T-cells and B-cells. The T-cells are processed in the thymus gland. The processing of B-cells takes place in the bone mar-

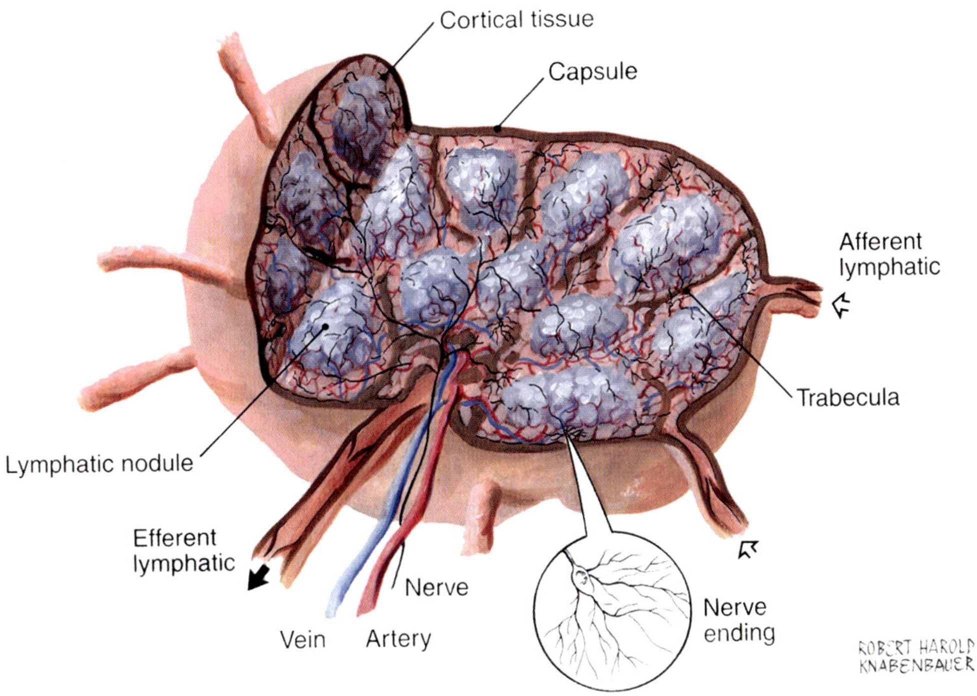


Fig. 7.9. The lymph nodes are scattered throughout the body and are an important part of the lymphatic system. See Figure 7.2. The thymus produces the hormone thymosin, which stimulates the production of peripheral lymphoid tissue. (R.H. Knabenbauer)

row, liver, and associated lymphoid tissues of the gut tract, tonsils, appendix, and lymphoid tissues of the intestines. After processing, both T- and B-cells migrate to lymphoid tissues, which are found in the lymph nodes, spleen, gastrointestinal tract, and the bloodstream. The T-cells are said to be thymus-dependent cells. The B-cells are referred to as thymus-independent cells.

Further appreciation of the work of the cell-mediated immune system can be obtained by examining the functions of the T- and B-cell lymphocytes.

## T-Cells

**Stem cells,** or T-lymphocyte precursors (prethymic cells), from the bone marrow seed the thymus where they become thymocytes and participate in the development of the thymus. The thymocytes proliferate from the outer layer or cortex at a rapid rate and move inward to the innermedulary portion of the thymus where they undergo maturation.

The immature T-cells develop the important ability to recognize the difference between self and non-self, or the detection of foreign proteins. When the mature thymocytes move into the circulating pool of lymphocytes they are termed **T-**

**lymphocytes** or **T-cells**. They comprise about 80% of the circulating lymphocytes of the blood.

When a circulating T-cell encounters the antigen that its cell surface receptors have been programmed to recognize, it becomes activated. T-cell function is associated with cell-mediated immunity, which includes delayed hypersensitivity reactions, surveillance against malignant cell transformations, and protection against microbial infections. T-cells are also involved in tissue transplant reactions. T-cells neither transform into plasma cells nor do they elaborate immunoglobulins such as in the case of B-cells.

Activated T-cells proliferate rapidly producing various subset populations as follows:

**T-helper cells (CD4 cells).** T-cells are also known as inducer, or effector T-cells, which will take part in repelling foreign invaders and they are able to concentrate specific antigens for presentation to the B-cells, which are stimulated to produce their antibodies. Helper cells may also enhance certain aspects of other T-cell activities. The exact role a T-helper cell will play in the body's defense system depends on the programming it receives in the thymus. Some T-helper cells participate directly in the destruction of targeted cells, whereas, others participate indirectly by producing message molecules that help organize the activities of other immune system cells such as B-cells or macrophages of the nonspecific immune system.

**T-suppressor cells (CD8 cells).** These T-cells have the specific function of suppressing the production of antibodies by the B-cells. The lack of appropriate suppressor cell activity can lead to the overproduction of antibodies, as is seen in autoimmune disorders in which the immune system attacks the body's own normal cells. The balance of powers between helper and suppressor cell activity is vital to the maintenance of health and the normal functioning of the immune response. In the Acquired Immune Deficiency Syndrome (AIDS), the helper-suppressor balance in the T-cell population becomes severely disturbed and the normal ratio is reversed.

**T-memory cells.** These are T-cells that retain the capacity to rapidly respond to future invasions by a particular foreign protein or organism by remembering a previous antigenic encounter in the body.

**T-killer cells.** These are T-cells that can recognize either virus-infected or tumor cells which they are able to destroy by releasing a toxic substance or by punching holes in the target cell membrane, which results in its destruction.

**Lymphokines.** When sensitized T-cells come in direct contact with target antigens, they are activated. This activation then initiates the release of a variety of substances that affect macrophages, polymorphonuclear neutrophils, lymphocytes, and other cells. These substances are called **lymphokines.** The amounts of lymphokines are small, but they have a profound effect on target cells. Lymphokines play a significant role in a wide range of immunological processes (Hokama & Nakamura, 1982).

**Interferons.** The interferons are one of the lymphokine groups, which are heterogeneous low molecular weight glycoproteins elaborated by virus-infected cells. They have been grouped into three major groups, alpha, beta, and gamma types. Immunologists have identified 14 different types of **alpha interferons** that are produced by leukocytes. **Beta interferons** are produced by fibroblasts and probably all types of cells. **Gamma interferons** are produced by lymphocytes.

The interferons work collectively to cordon off healthy cells from the spred of an invading virus. Interferons have multiple properties, which include potent antiviral activity, enhancement of phagocytosis, inhibition of cell division, affecting cell membranes, and influencing the response to ionizing radiation (Baron & Dianzani, 1977). Interferons play an important role as regulators of the immune system since they are produced in response to antigenic stimuli (Merigan & Friedman, 1982; Taylor-Papdimitriou, 1985). Interferons also assist in the healing process. Viruses may stimulate the production of interferon in the body (Roitt, 1994).

Interferon production is controlled by the genetic machinery of the cell and when this is damaged by irradiation, interferon production can be diminished.

## B-Cells

**B-cells** are lymphocytes which also originate from stem cells in the bone marrow. B-cells may be distributed directly to the spleen, lymph nodes, and other lymphoid tissues. However, some of the B-cells may traverse or be regulated in the bone marrow, liver, appendix, intestines, or tonsils to become functional B-lymphocytes. The B-cells are found in the germinal centers of lymphoid follicles within the lymph nodes and spleen.

When B-cells are activated by the presence of an antigen, some of the B-cells enlarge, divide, and change into clones of plasma cells. The plasma cells are involved in antibody synthesis which is elaborated into the blood and serous fluids. The plasma cells found in the endothelial areas of the respiratory tract, nasal cavities, secretory glands, and gastrointestinal tract are associated with the synthesis of the immunoglobulins IgA and IgE.

## Phagocytes

A second major group of white blood cells of the cell-mediated portion of the immune system are sometimes referred to as **phagocytes**. These are large leukocytes which can engulf and digest microorganisms, and other antigenic materials. The phagocytes include large white blood cells such as the **monocyte-macrophages** and the **granulocytes** comprising the polymorphonuclear neutrophils, eosinophils, and basophils. There is an interworking between lymphocytes and phagocytes in that some of these large white cells are able to present antigenic materials to lymphocytes.

## Natural Killer Cells (NK Cells)

There is another group of specialized cells known as the **natural killer cells** (NK cells), which are lymphoid cells that are antigenically distinct from T- or B-cells. They exhibit cytolytic activity against a wide range of tumor target cells.

## Humoral Immune System

The **humoral immune system** is chemical in nature consisting of **immunoglobulins (antibodies)** which are elaborated by plasma cells following the transformation of antigen-stimulated B-cell lymphocytes. The humoral immune system is responsible for defense against microbial organisms which act as antigens in body fluids.

An **antigen** is a substance, usually a foreign protein, which when introduced into the body provokes an immune response with the formation of antibodies or sensitized lymphocytes. Antigens are generally foreign to the molecular structure of the host, which the immune system recognizes as non-self. When the body fails to recognize self, antibodies may be produced which attack the body itself, such as in autoimmune disorders. Once an antibody or sensitized lymphocyte has formed, subsequent or continuing exposure to the same antigen results in modification, neutralization, or elimination of the antigen.

There are myriads of antigens in the environment, which include bacteria, viruses, pollens, foreign proteins in foods, and many xenobiotics, i.e., synthetic chemical substances. An **antibody** is a protein created by the body in response to the presence of an antigen and is part of the body's effort to destroy the challenging antigen.

## Immunoglobulins

Antibodies are also known as immunoglobulins. **Immunoglobulins** belong to a group of proteins called globulins, named after their globular shape (Figs. 7.10, 7.11). There are five classes of immunoglobulins: IgG, IgM, IgA, IgD, and IgE.

**IgG** - represents about 80 to 85% of the antibodies in serum. It is found in blood and lymph. IgG provides naturally acquired immunity to the newborn, neutralizes toxins, and enhances phagocytosis.

**IgM** - comprises about 5 to 15% of the antibodies found in blood serum. IgM is the first antibody to arrive following injection of antigenic substances. IgM is very effective against microorganisms, among other things.

**IgA** - comprises about 14% of the immunoglobulins. IgA is found in tears, mucus, intestinal contents, milk, blood, and lymph. The function of IgA is to protect mucosal surfaces from pathogens.

**IgD** - Only about 0.2% of serum antibody is IgD. It is found in blood and lymph and on B-cells. IgD may be concerned with the differentiation of B-cells, but very little is known about the function of this immunoglobulin.

**IgE** - Constitutes 0.002% of the serum antibody count. IgE is found throughout the body in the blood and is bound to mast cells (cells which contain histamine and other substances that stimulate vasodilation). IgE is involved in allergic reactions and may also play a part in protecting the body from protozoan parasites.

Although the various components of the immune system have been discussed as separate entities, they all interact in harmony with each other in attempting to maintain the body in a state of optimum health. Exposure to irradiation and certain toxic chemical agents can have disastrous effects to the immune system due to destruction of the stem cells in the bone marrow. Therefore, one of the objectives in both the prevention and treatment of diseases such as cancer and radiation sickness is in the use of nutrients and adaptogenic agents that can exert a positive modulatory effect on the immune system.

## Immunomodulation

The term **immunomodulation** refers to the process of producing a change or an effect in immune responsiveness by whatever means. The use of immunomodulating herbs dates back to ancient times in Chinese traditional medicine. The fabled founder of Chinese medicine Emperor Shen-nung (ca. 2700 B.C.), who is credited with starting the *Pen Tsao* system (*Great Materia Medicas of China*), is believed to have been the first to employ immunomodulating herbs in the treatment of disease. Herbs affecting the immune system have been discussed by numerous other herbalists of antiquity. See Chapter Eight for further details.

The use and clinical efficacy of these immunomodulating plants were well known to ancient Chinese practitioners and continue to be employed by modern herbalists as well. The useful properties of these plants are unfortunately viewed by modern western practitioners with unfounded skepticism.

In some of the more recent reviews dealing with immunomodulators, for example, Gottlieb, et al (1985), Gomatos, et al (1992), Benjamini and Leskowitz (1991), no mention is made of the largest collection of immunomodulators known to the science of biological modification, namely, Chinese adaptogenic nutritional plant

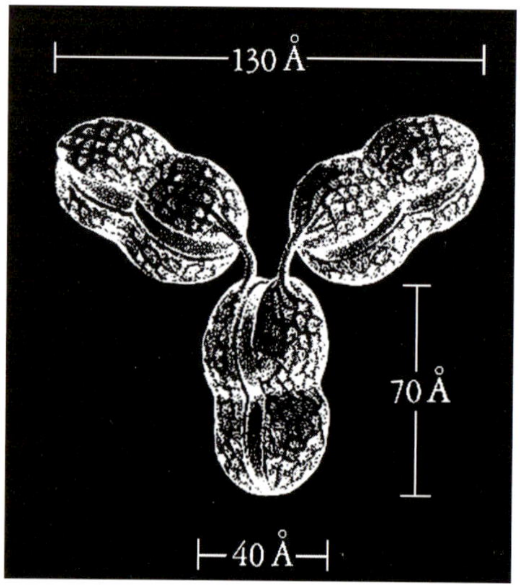


Fig. 7.10. Showing the structure of a three dimensional model of the IgG immunoglobulin. This model is based on studies involving X-ray crystallography and elecron microscopy.

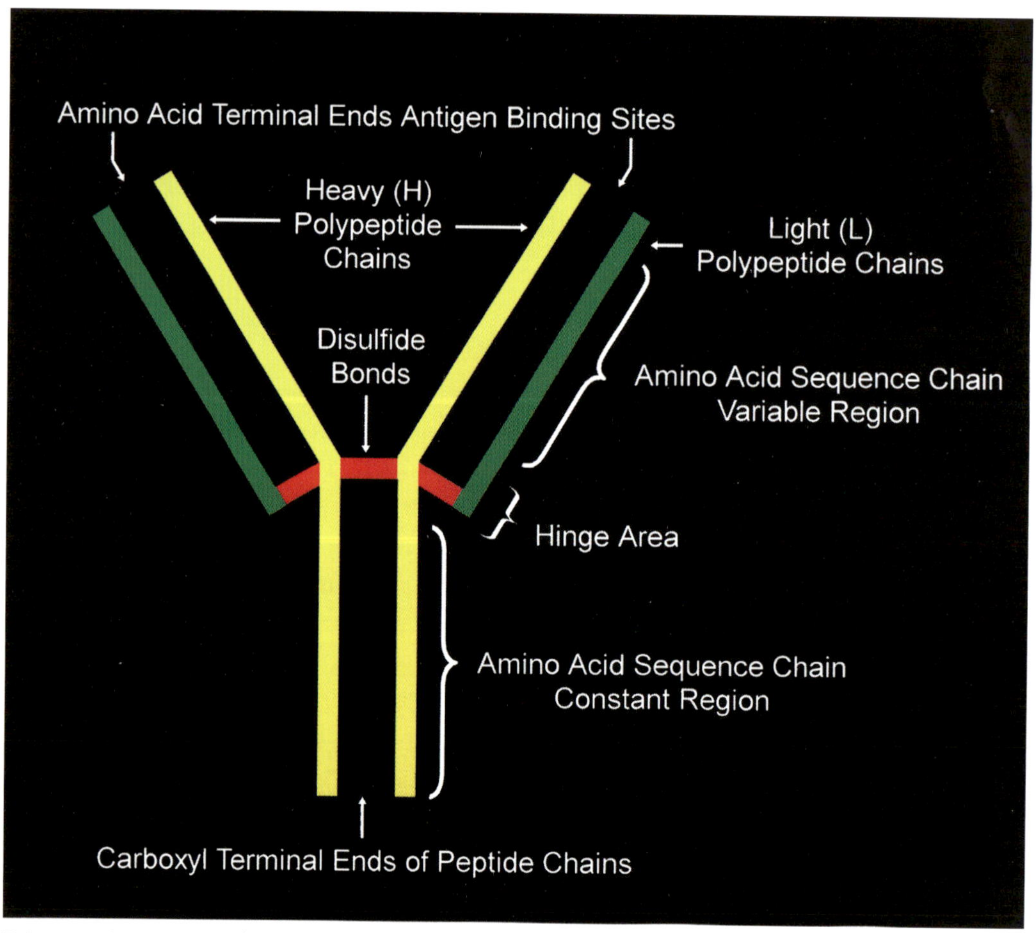


Fig. 7.11. Antibodies are characteristically Y-shaped. This stylized drawing shows some of the component parts of the structure of an antibody. Antibodies are proteins that are produced as a result of stimulation by antigens that react specifically with that antigen. All antibodies are immunoglobulins, of which there are five main classes: IgG, IgA, IgM, IgE, and IgD. (L. C. Medrano)

substances. This is a classical example of Western medicine's failure to explore the treasures of Chinese traditional medicine—all at a cost of millions of lives.

There is compelling scientific evidence that many of the immunomodulators that western immunologists are eagerly seeking are waiting to be rediscovered today in ancient Chinese materia medicas. There is a growing amount of scientific evidence derived largely from Oriental traditional medicine and confirmed by modern analytical methodology that it is clinically feasible to orchestrate the immune system as a practical non-toxic therapeutic modality in chronic disease management and in tissue transplantation. Most of which is unused by the Western world.

## Immunostimulants

Some biodynamic substances are capable of serving as **immunostimulants** or immunopotentiators which may lead to a non-specific stimulation of the immune defense system. These substances may possess either antigenic or non-antigenic properties. This section will touch only briefly on this topic.

Another group of compounds are known as **mitogens**, which are polyclonal activators of T- and/or B-lymphocytes. Concanavalin A and phytohemaglutanin are sometimes used as T-cell stimulators. Lipopolysaccharides and pokeweed are mitogens used for B-cell stimulation. Mitogens have been found to have varying potency and to some extent specificity. Immunostimulants may also stimulate T-suppresser cells and thereby reduce immune responsiveness.

**Immunoadjuvants** are substances that enhance the production of antibodies without acting as antigens themselves. The effects of adjuvants are frequently thymus-dependent and their primary targets appear to be macrophages (Wakeman, 1980; Wagner & Proksch, 1985). Several different adjuvants may be administered concurrently.

Immunostimulants have been found to be effective perorally, intravenously, or intraperitoneally, depending upon the situation. Non-specific immunostimulants do not seem to affect the immune memory cells and since their therapeutic efficacy fades comparatively quickly, they have to be administered either in intervals or continuously. This is one of the reasons for using adaptogenic nutrients on a continuous basis as food products.

Research on natural-occurring immunomodulating substances clearly indicates that it will someday be possible to fine-tune the human immune system on a customized basis to fit the individual needs of the patient's disease condition. Moreover, this therapy is simple, nontoxic, and can be done on an oral basis without the assistance of a physician once the individual learns the basic principles of the use of adaptogenic tonics.

## Mechanism of Immunomodulation

The mechanism of immunomodulation has been discussed at length by Wagner and Proksch (1985) to wit: Immune defense and the resulting cellular homeostasis in the body is the result of a complicated interplay between non-specific and specific cellular and humoral responses, stimulation and suppression of immunocompetent cells, and the influence of hormonal and other mechanisms with the immune system.

It is believed, however, that regardless of the primary targets of immunostimulants the increase in phagocytosis by macrophages and granulocytes plays a central role in immune enhancement. The activation of macrophage activity is thought to be due to a binding process resulting from contact between the cell and the immunostimulating substance. The activated macrophage is said to display not only increased phagocytosis, but is also converted into a secretory cell and acts as a cytotoxic effector cell.

According to Hadden and Stewart (1981) the major role in the amplification of the non-specific immunological defense system is played by lysosomal enzymes secreted by activated macrophages, the components of complement, interferon, lymphokines, macrophage migration inhibition factor (MIF), colony-stimulating factor (CSF), prostaglandins, leukotrienes, and other substances. The second most important role is said to be the stimulation of T-lymphocytes, which are achieved directly or indirectly via macrophages.

Terrestrial and marine polysaccharides constitute some of the principle substances in traditional Chinese herbs, which serve as immunostimulants. The function of these polysaccharides includes stimulation of the reticuloendothelial system, intense phagocytosis by means of macrophages, activation of T-lymphocytes, and activation of the complement system (Tsung, 1987, 1989).

Immunostimulation by exogenous mitogens or antigens may also be achieved indirectly by stimulating the body's own steroid hormones or biogenic amines (serotonin and histamine). Unfortunately, many of the details of the molecular processes of immune cell activation are still unknown.

It is obvious that the immune system plays a paramount role in health maintenance. Restoration of the immunocompetence of the body is a vital element in cancer, radiation sickness therapy, and the maintenance of general health.

## Injuries to the Immune System

At the beginning of this chapter a partial listing was provided of some of the causative factors which induce immune dysfunction. This subject will now be explored further.

The immune system can be injured by a number of mechanisms, which includes exposure to toxic chemical agents, diseases, microbial organisms, lifestyle, ionizing radiation, and environmental, iatrogenic, and nosocomial factors, all of which were previously listed in Table 7.1.

One of the most serious of these immune destructive processes is ionizing radiation. Lymphoid tissue, which involves the immune system, is in the same range of radiosensitivity as the hematopoietic organs (bone marrow). Whole body irradiation at relatively high levels results in rapid death of large numbers of lymphocytes and inhibits cell division of many other cells.

Repeated irradiation at low dose rates is generally believed to have a lesser effect on the immune system than a single acute dose. However, the safety of low-dose radiation is a subject of great concern, and the concept of a safe dosage of any radiation is now a subject of great controversy. Whole body irradiation of the order of 500 Rads causes rapid degeneration of lymphoid cells.

Active proliferation of lymphoid cells begins about four weeks after irradiation and the lymph nodes begin to appear normal shortly thereafter. If an antigen is introduced after irradiation, the formation of antibodies is delayed until the capacity for cell reproduction has recovered.

If antigenic stimulation has caused cellular proliferation just prior to irradiation, the lymphoid cells may continue their differentiation and eventually produce antibodies. However, the time interval between the introduction of antigen and the appearance of antibodies in the blood will be prolonged and the amount of antibody production will be reduced.

Cells that are actively synthesizing antibodies may continue to be active for a period of time even though massive doses of irradiation have been received (Pizzarello & Witcofski, 1975). One of the major problems in radiation sickness is the susceptibility of the victim to diseases by both pathogenic and nonpathogenic organisms. If the immune system is not restored, disease susceptibility may be fatal. Consequently, the restoration of the immune system is a matter of vital importance.

## Restoration of the Immune System

Various modalities have been used to restore the immune system in victims who have been exposed to irradiation, such as bone marrow transplants and injection of spleen and lymph node cells. The injection of nucleic acid degradation products concurrently with a suitable antigen has also been found useful in restoring antibody production after irradiation.

There is an ever increasing amount of scientific evidence that the proper use of radioprotective nutrients, free radical scavengers, anticancer and anti-viral adaptogenic herbs can provide radioprotection, cancer protection, virus protection, and assist in the restoration of immunoincompetence. Adaptogenic immunomodulators act as biological response modifiers. The mechanisms of action of biological response modifiers have become a matter of immense interest in the field of immunology (Torrence, 1985). The chemical spectrum of these modifiers range from ancient Chinese adaptogenic herbal nutrients to some of the newer synthetics, and involves most of the known minerals and vitamins that are recognized in human health. In the section on immunomodulation authors Gottlieb, et al (1985), Gomatos, et al (1992), Benjamini and Leskowitz (1991), and others, have reviewed or made reference to the subject of immunomodulators, but none of them have made reference to a large body of scientific literature on adaptogenic plants, which have appeared in both the Russian and Chinese literature. A cursory review of some of this literature on immune enhancement has been published by Halstead and Hood (1984a,b).

Kojima, et al (1984), obtained a U.S. Patent No. 4,469,685 on September 4, 1984, for a process of producing water-soluble interferon inducers from plants of the genera *Aralia, Asparagus, Astragalus, Atractyloides, Bupleurum, Cimicifuga, Cocculus, Cnidium, Datura, Euchresta, Evoida, Gastroida, Heracleum, Notopterygium, Panax, Pinellia, Polygala, Sinomenium, Sophora, Stephania, Rheum*, and other varieties. The authors reported that the phytochemical constituents of the plants to be of potential value in the prevention and treatment of humans and animals suffering from various virus infections by stimulating interferon production in their bodies. See also Halstead and Hood (1984a,b). Also, Aso, et al (1985), have suggested the use of organic germanium as an interferon inducer.

Axelrod (1971), Beisel (1975, 1979, 1980, 1981a,b, 1982), Beisel, et al (1981), Chandra (1980, 1981, 1992), Cheung and Harrison (1983), Flavin and Kolbe (1982), Geng, et al (1989), Good (1981), Graber, et al (1981), Halstead and Hood (1984a,b), Tsung and Hsu (1986), Tsung (1989), Tuoto (1982), Zhan, Liu, and Zhou (1989), and numerous others have published on the use of vitamin, mineral, and herbal nutrients and their importance in the enhancement of immune function.

## Nutrition and Immunity

It has been clearly established that nutrition does influence immune function. The matter of nutrition and its influence on immune responses is rapidly becoming a matter of great interest in Western health care and immunological research. It is noteworthy that the importance of nutrients in health maintenance was an immunological phenomenon that was clearly observed and documented in ancient China many centuries ago.

The role of nutrition in populations suffering from malnutrition and its negative impact on immuncompetence has long been recognized in the Western world.

However, during the last ten years an increasing amount of attention is being directed to the importance of nutrition and immunocompetence in populations having only mild nutritional deficiencies. There has been a dramatic shift toward the investigation and recognition of the role of single and other complex nutrient deficiencies in human sub-populations worldwide. The recognition of immune nutrients is of particular importance with an ever increasing destruction of the environment due to toxic chemical pollutants, exposure to ionizing radiation, emerging microbial agents, and the growing evidence of secondary immune deficiency disorders in the general population.

The cancer plague is a health consequence of secondary immune disorders resulting from exposure to an emerging plague pandemic of highly virulent microbial organisms, carcinogenic chemical agents, and ionizing radiation.

## Psychoneuroimmunology

### GENERAL BACKGROUND

The general concept that ones thinking, behavior, and the body's defense system operate as an integrated whole is not a new one. The ancient Chinese concept of Qi, or adaptive energy, clearly reflected the fact that this energy can be positively affected by one's lifestyle, which includes the use of exercise, good nutrition, positive thinking, and the use of adaptogenic medicinal herbs. Exposure to toxic agents, poor lifestyle, sedentary habits, negative thinking, and a host of other adverse environmental factors can reduce Qi, the quality of life, produce illness, and decrease one's longevity. The Chinese writings dealing with this general concept are about 5,000 years old.

Soloman, in Proverbs 17:22 in the Bible, states, "A merry heart doeth good like a medicine, but a broken spirit drieth the bones."

At the turn of the century White (1905) expressed the view in the book *Ministry of Healing* that: "The relation that exists between the mind and the body is very intimate. When one is affected, the other sympathizes. The condition of the mind affects the health to a far greater degree than many realize. Many of the diseases from which men suffer are the result of mental depression. Grief, anxiety, discontent, remorse, guilt, distrust, all tend to break down the life forces, and to invite decay and death. Courage, hope, faith, sympathy, love, promote health and long life. A contented mind, a cheerful spirit, is health to the body and strength to the soul."

It is obvious that the concept of an intimate relationship of the psyche, behavior, and the body's defense system had its origin in antiquity, but it is only recently that medical scientists have been able to determine the anatomical and chemical mechanisms involved.

In recent years recognition of psychosomatic illness began to emerge and clinicians began to realize the impact of the mental attitude of the patient and behavior on the course of such diseases as peptic ulcer, ulcerative colitis, hyperthyroidism, regional enteritis, essential hypertension, rheumatoid arthritis, bronchial asthma, cancer, and even infectious disease processes. In the due course of time it was recognized that even in infectious diseases in which a specific etiological microorganism was involved the response varied from one individual to the next. It was obvious that there were multiple factors that were influencing the clinical course of the disease, in addition to the causative disease agent. Some of these factors included nutrition, mental attitude, behavior, the environment, and the immune response of the patient.

Serious studies on the relationship of the mind, body and disease began with the early investigations of such workers as Dunbar's (1943) book entitled *Psychosomatic Diagnosis,* Alexander's (1950) *Psychosomatic Medicine,* Dubos' (1961) *Mirage of Health,* and the work of Engel (1954, 1977) on the multifactorial etiology and biopsychosocial factors in disease.

One such doctor who noted the relationship between attitude and disease was Dr. Carl O. Simonton. Dr. Simonton, an internationally renowned American oncologist who is known to be one of the earliest pioneers of psychoneuroimmunology, first began his work in this field in 1971. At that time his wife, Stephanie Simonton, a psychologist, worked with Carl to integrate his ideas into the field of psychology. They were able to show in clinical trials that through emotional intervening cancer could be slowed down and often conquered. The therapy included such things as using funny movies to invoke laughter, positive visualization and above all, using music with visualization. Dr. Simonton thoroughly understood that the brain controls the immune system and developed a large portfolio of programs and tools for patients to incorporate into their recovery. In recent years, Dr. Simonton founded a center in California that he named the Simonton Cancer Center. The center works directly with patients and serves as a training center for other doctors and health practitioners who want to learn his techniques. His unique programs for patients and doctors have gained worldwide recognition and have been incorporated at cutting edge medical treatment centers the world over. It is foreseeable that all cancer treatments will someday be using these techniques.

The extensive classical animal studies of Selye (1946, 1973) dealing with stress and the general adaptation syndrome provided an important experimental background for much of the clinical work in psychosomatic and behavioral medicine during this period, both in this country and in Russia. According to Selye the general adaptation syndrome linked environmental stress to a nonspecific adrenocortical response. Selye believed that this hormonal response accounted to a significant extent for the survival of the animal.

An excellent overview of the scientific literature of psychoneuroimmunology is presented in the publications of Plaut and Friedman (1981), Locke, et al (1985), Ader (1981), and Ader, et al (1991).

Norman Cousins, formerly the editor of the *Saturday Review,* was one of the best known advocates of psychoneuroimmunology. His interest in this field came about as a result of his own illness in which he suffered from a serious case of ankylosing spondylitis in 1964, possibly precipitated by adrenal exhaustion due to severe stress. When all other therapeutic measures seemed to have failed he began to take charge of his recovery. He decided to take larger doses of vitamin C, and began watching old comedy films that stimulated mirthful laughter. Gradually he began to recover. During his recovery process he became convinced of the important role that his emotional state played in his recovery.

Later, in 1980, Cousins suffered a serious heart attack, and once again he took charge of his case with the use of exercise, good nutrition, and a positive mental attitude, which once again paid excellent therapeutic dividends.

The experience gained in his skirmishes with illness provided Cousins with a first hand experiential basis, which resulted in his literary contributions in this field (1979a,b, 1981, 1983a,b). Cousins undertook a serious investigation of the healing process as a layman examining the importance of taking control of one's health by a positive mental attitude, good nutrition, and exercise. Cousins did much in his later life to stimulate both medical scientists and the general public in the importance of the mental attitude of patients in disease therapy, and the fledgling field of psychoneuroimmunology.

The following is one of Cousin's most noteworthy statements: "I have learned never to underestimate the capacity of the human mind and body to regenerate—even when the prospects seem most wretched. The life-force may be the least understood force on earth."

There is an interesting relationship between the findings of Selye's animal work and the observations of Cousins involving humans. Both men developed great respect for the role of negative stress in both mice and men in the causation of disease on one hand, and the value of positive stress, sometimes referred to as eustress, in health maintenance on the other.

It is appropriate at this point to interject the fact that Selye's work in Canada had a pronounced influence on the conceptual development of adaptogenic medicine as it entered the English-speaking world. Although the Chinese were the first to utilize adaptogenic medicinal plants, it was the Russians that propagated the adaptogenic concept via the use of *Eleutherococcus senticosus*. The English term *adaptogen* is one that the Russians adopted from Selye (Brekhman, 1982 - personal communication).

As time progressed psychiatrists, neuroscientists, and immunologists have discovered that these psychosomatic disorders and recoveries were not merely a series of mystical events, but were based on solid physiological, anatomical and chemical processes, much of which can be quantified. Thus, was born the science of what is now known as psychoneuroimmunology.

## CURSORY REVIEW OF PSYCHONEUROIMMUNOLOGY

**Psychoneuroimmunology** is that branch of medical science that deals with the interactions of the mind, neurotransmitters, hormones, and the body's immune system. This is an immensely complex integrated science involving the nervous system, endocrinology, neurochemistry, and immunochemistry. The parameters of our knowledge in this field are rapidly expanding with the advent of modern analytical technology.

Human behavior, stress, and a multitude of environmental factors, all play important roles, which are able to bring about health or disease. One soon learns from the study of psychoneuroimmunology that the immune system is not an autonomous entity as was previously believed. The mind and the immune system actively communicate with each other by means of their common chemical language of neurotransmitters and hormones.

## MIRTHFUL LAUGHTER—EFFECTS ON THE IMMUNE SYSTEM

Clinical laboratory tests have shown that when people are being exposed to hilarious comedy movies resulting in mirthful laughter, there were quantitative cellular and chemical changes in the peripheral blood of the test subjects (Berk, Tan, Fry, et al, 1989; Berk, Tan, Napier & Enby, 1989). The following is a summation of some of these blood changes.

**T-cell Changes:** Mirthful laughter stimulates the activation of T-lymphocytes. Under ordinary circumstances there appears to be a large number of T-cells in the blood that are inactive, but when the individual is involved in mirthful laughter there is suddenly an increase in T-cell activity. It has also been found that moderate exercise produces a similar activation effect. It has been suggested that perhaps this is one of the reasons why people who consistently follow a moderate exercise program have a lower incidence of certain types of cancers and cardiovascular disease.

Mirthful laughter was also found to produce an increase in T-cells having helper or suppressor receptors. Each cell in our body has numerous receptors that neurotransmitters or other modulators such as cytokines are able to plug into which results in an alteration of cellular metabolic activity. The stimulation of T-helper cells is an important aspect of treatment in AIDS.

**Natural Killer (NK) Cell Changes:** Mirthful laughter was also found to increase the numbers of natural killer (NK) cells. These cells play an important role in the immune surveillance system of the body, which is vital to the eradication of malignant cells. NK cells also attack virus-infected cells. When the immune system is functioning properly, NK cells are able to detect aberrant or abnormal cells and are able to bring about their destruction. Thus, mirthful laughter modifies the physiology and the chemicals that affect natural killer cells and increases their number and activity.

**Immunoglobulin Changes:** A positive mental attitude laced with humor has also been found to increase the activity of the humoral immune system by increasing the **IgA** immunoglobulin fraction. This increase has been found to appear both in the peripheral blood and the saliva. The IgA fraction plays an important role in the mucosa of the upper respiratory tract in combating pulmonary infections. One observation that has been made in marathon runners is that because of the negative stress resulting from their strenuous exercise they suffer a greater number of respiratory infections.

Humor has also been found to increase the **IgG** fraction. This is the major immunoglobulin fraction of the humoral immune system, which provides naturally acquired immunity to the newborn, neutralizes toxins, and enhances phagocytosis.

The **IgM** fraction was also increased with humor. This is one of the first immunoglobulin fractions to arrive with the initiation of a microbiological infection. After the initial work of the IgM fraction, the IgG fraction takes over and provides long-term immunity.

**Cytokine Changes:** Berk (1993) and his associates also examined the response of the cytokines of the immune system to humor, namely, gamma interferon. They found that humor also increased the release of gamma interferon. This is an important finding because gamma interferon tends to activate other parts of the immune response in the body.

They also found that humor produced a positive response by increasing **Complement 3**, which assists antibodies by piercing infected, damaged and dysfunctional cells, thereby aiding in their removal.

The **complement system** serves as the primary humoral mediator of antigen-antibody reactions. It consists of at least 20 chemically and immunologically distinct serum proteins that are capable of interacting with each other, with antibodies, and with other cell membranes. The activation of the complement system results from the lysis of various cells, bacteria, viruses, and the mediation of inflammatory processes. There are 9 major complement components which have been designated as C1-C9, each of them having specific functions (Fudenberg, et al, 1980).

**Neuroendocrine Changes:** Berk's group also measured the effects of humor on neuroendocrine responses with positive results. There are three catecholamines produced by the adrenal glands: **epinephrine, norepinephrine,** and **dopamine**. Since dopamine is metabolized very rapidly they decided to test for dopac, which is the major serum catabolite, the breakdown product of dopamine in the peripheral blood. Dopamine is involved in the flight or fight response, and produces vasoconstriction and immunsuppression. Dopamine is not a desirable substance to have available in large quantities in the blood stream over an extended period of time. Dopamine is sometimes administered when a patient's blood pressure is dropping. Berk's group found that when the test subjects were exposed to mirthful laughter that epinephrine and dopamine blood levels dropped.

**Lymphoid Organs and the Nervous system:** The lymphoid organs of the body, i.e., bone marrow, thymus, lymph glands, are composed of a reticular stroma that forms a meshwork which provides support and compartments for the varying populations of cells of the immune system, many of which are mobile. These compartments provide a basic support system for the various functions of the immune cells. There are also chemically specific nerve endings that are associated with these compartments that are believed to regulate the numerous specific functions at these sites. They found that the cell traffic into these organs is via the capillary system, which is supplied with a large variety of nerves and several neurotransmitters, including norepinephrine and the neuropeptides designated merely as NPY, SP, CGRP, and VIP (Ader, Felten & Cohen (1991)).

These compounds are vasoactive and control blood flow, perfusion pressure, blood volume of the organs, and lymphocyte movement. These compounds are thought to determine the direction or specific target lymphoid organ to which the various lymph cells are to go. There are areas where T-lymphocytes, B-lymphocytes, macrophages, and other cells are mixed. These areas are associated with large blood or lymph sinuses where antigen presentation takes place, such as the marginal zone of the spleen and the medullar cords of the lymph nodes. It was also found that these areas are inervated largely by noradrenergic/NPY-containing nerve fibers.

Authors Ader, Felten and Cohen (1991) concluded that chemical signals released from the nerves initiate or modulate some functions of target cells such as lymphocytes, macrophages, and granulocytes. These cells possess adrenoceptors as well as other receptors. The investigators believed that when a neurotransmitter is released into the microenvironment of a lymphoid cell containing a suitable receptor, the cell will respond through appropriate identified second messengers and will initiate metabolic or molecular processes. It should be noted, however, that lymphoid cells also secrete signal molecules known as lymphokines or interleukins that may also be potential candidates for communication back to the nervous system, which may be localized, or more distant, by fleeing back to the central nervous system.

The essence of these findings is that there is direct neural innervation between the nervous and immune systems. Moreover, there is a direct functional signaling in both directions suggesting that these two great memory and communications systems are poised to respond to internal and external challenges for the protection and preservation of the individual, and are inter-dependent. Thus, the immune system is not autonomous. Behavior and neural responsiveness is affected by the immune status of the organism. One of the striking observations to be derived from these findings is the commonality of signaling mechanisms that are used throughout the body, which are specific and yet pliable, and convergent enough to meet new challenges.

These findings are of profound importance in dealing with the therapeutics of patients suffering from cancer, and a host of other disabling diseases. This cursory review provides only a small glimpse of the growing and exciting science of psychnoneuroimmunology. The reader is urged to examine the basic works of Ader (1981), Locke, et al (1985), and Ader, Felten and Cohen (1991) for further information on this important subject.

## Chapter 8

# History of Traditional Chinese Medicine
# The Origin of Herbal Medicine In Ancient China



---

When attempting to understand the rationale of Chinese medicine it is helpful to understand its history. The use of herbal medicine originated in ancient China with some of the greatest herbalists of ancient times. Although there were many great herbalists only three of the most renowned will be discussed.

## Shen Nung—The Father of Traditional Chinese Medicine

Shen Nung (Fig. 8.1) has also been designated as the "Divine Ruler" and acquired the titles of "the God of Agriculture and the Father of Chinese herbal Medicine". The exact dates of the birth and death of Shen Nung have never been verified, but it is believed that he was born about 3494 B.C. Shen Nung was first referred to by the great Chinese philosopher Meng-tzu, also known under his latinized name of Mencius (372 - 289 B.C.) who lived during the Chou Dynasty. Regardless of the dispute about his birth date, medical historians are in agreement that he was the founder of Chinese traditional medicine. It has been said that prior to the advent of Shen Nung the ancient Chinese people were without a system of medicine and were unable to treat their diseases.

Shen Nung is alleged to have tested large numbers of herbs and determined their medicinal properties. He is said to have tested over 70 herbs in a single day. In this regard it can be accurately stated that Shen Nung was also the father of the infant sciences of pharmacognosy and pharmacology during ancient times.

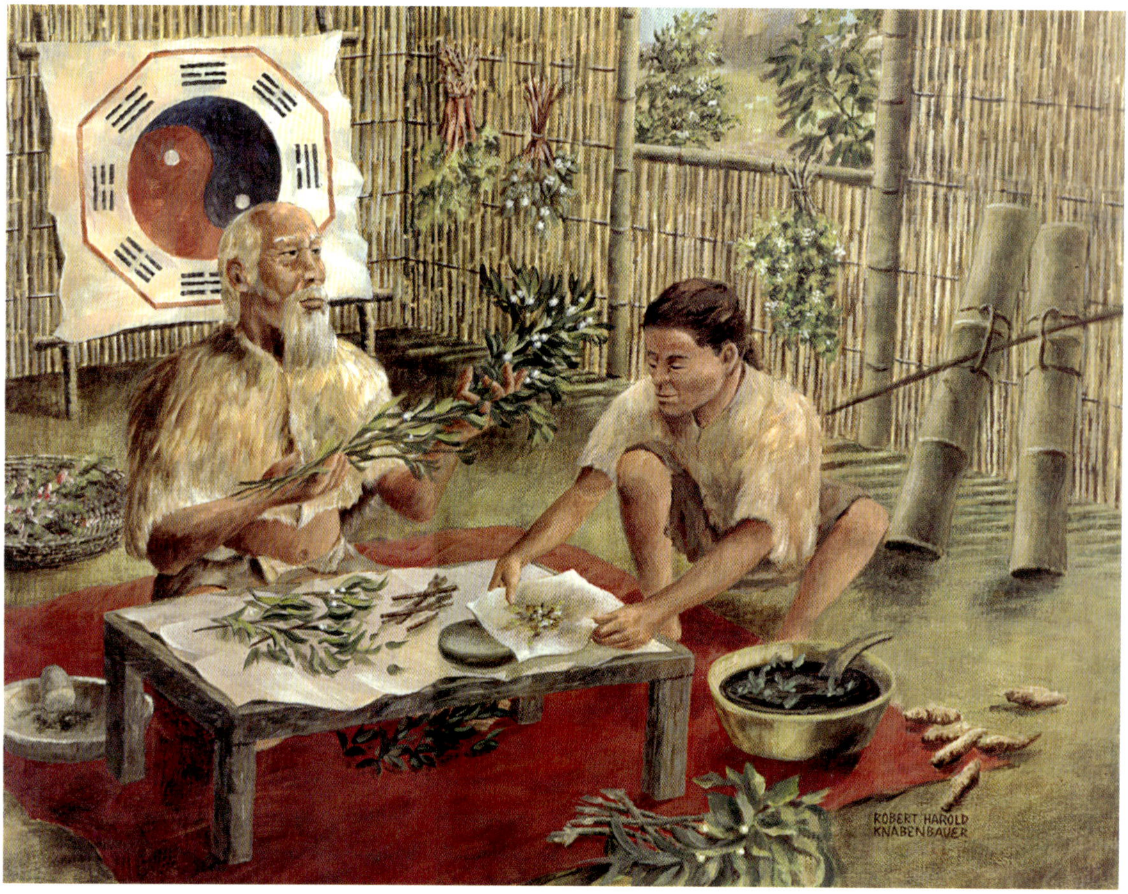


Fig. 8.1. Shen Nung (ca 3494 B.C.). He is known as the "Divine Ruler" and has acquired the titles of the "God of Agriculture" and the "Father of Chinese Herbal Medicine". Shen Nung is said to have tested large numbers of herbs and is credited as being the first to establish a system of medicine for the Chinese people. (R. H. Knabenbauer)

Shen Nung's system of medicine taught that there were five elements in the human body: *metal, wood, fire, water,* and *earth,* and if any of these elements were out of balance it would result in illness. His approach to treatment was to use a natural substance having the opposite characteristic as the disease. The various herbs, animal and mineral products used in his system of medicine were ascribed one of these elemental characteristics and were prescribed according to the characteristics of the illness. This is essentially the same system that is used in Chinese herbal therapy at the present time. If for example, there was an inflammation or an infection (i.e., "fire"), then he would prescribe a herb having a "water" characteristic. Water puts out fire.

Shen Nung is said to have been a highly productive worker and critically documented his observations. His work provided the foundation for the Great Materia Medicas of China, usually referred to as the *Pen Tsaos* of which there have been probably hundreds of editions and modifications over millenniums of time.

The term *Pen Tsao* is used in the context of one who possessed knowledge of how to use herbs and other substances in the treatment of illness. *Pen* refers to "knowledge" in the use of *Tsao*, or "herbs". In the due course of time the term was later adopted to designate materia medicas or medical writings dealing with pharmaceutics, plant, animal, and mineral substances

Unfortunately, most of Shen Nung's work was done prior to China's written history and none of his original work is extant today since all of it was handed down verbally. It is believed that incomplete reports of Shen Nung's work may have been put into writing some time during the Eastern Han Dynasty (25 B.C. - 220 A.D.), or possibly earlier. At present the oldest written commentary on the *Shen Nung Pen Tsao* extant is the *Shen Nung Pen Tsao Ching* (sometimes shortened to *Pen Ching*), or the *Divine Husbandman's Classic of the Materia Medica*, which apparently was a revision of Shen Nung's earlier work written by Tao Hung-ching (452 - 536 A.D.), and revised by other authors during the Liang Dynasty (500 - 557 A.D.), written ca. 500 A.D.

## Huang Ti—The Yellow Emperor

The Yellow Emperor, Huang Ti (Fig. 8.2), is believed to have lived during the period from 2698 - 2598 B.C. Genealogies of Chinese dynasties list him as the third of China's first five rulers. However, some historians believe him to be a mythological character. Nevertheless, he has claimed a position in Chinese medical history as one of their greatest legendary rulers.

Huang Ti's personal name is said to have been Yu-hsiung, named after his hereditary principality. The Yellow Emperor is said to have taught his people how to build wheeled vehicles, ships, develop armor, produce pottery, wood and metal utensils, and a variety of other useful products.

Su-ma Chien, the great Chinese historian of the second century, names the Yellow Emperor as the founder of the Chinese civilization and the first human ruler of the empire. Regardless of his historicity, Huang Ti is credited with the authorship of the *Nei Ching Su Wen*, the classic treatise on internal medicine, which is considered to be the oldest medical book extant. The date of writing of this treatise is in dispute as is the authorship according to some scholars, whereas others insist that it was the work of the Yellow Emperor. For a more detailed discussion on the authorship of this medical classic the reader is referred to the excellent work by Veith (1966) entitled *Huang Ti Nei Ching Su Wen* or *The Yellow Emperor's Classic of Internal Medicine*. Regardless of the controversy over the authorship it is generally agreed by medical authorities familiar with the topic that this classic provides an influential basis for most of the traditional medical writings of China.

# *Huang Ti Nei Ching Su Wen*— The Yellow Emperor's Classic of Internal Medicine

The *Huang Ti Nei Ching Su Wen*, sometimes referred to as the *Canon*, of the Yellow Emperor consists of about 44,000 Chinese ideographs that amounts to about 120,000 English words. The extant edition of this *Canon* consists of 24 books, divided into 81 chapters, and owes its present form largely to the work of its most famous commentator Wang Ping, who lived during the Tang Dynasty (618 - 906). The Yellow Emperor's treatise was subsequently edited again during the Sung Dynasty (960 - 1126) by Kao Pao-heng and Lin I during the decade of 1068 - 1078 in the reign of Shen Tsung. As a result of these revisions it is doubtful that the present document contains much of the text in its original form.

## THE FORMAT OF THE *NEI CHING SU WEN*

Huang Ti presents his *Canon of Internal Medicine* in the form of a dialogue between himself and his minister, Chi Po, in which the emperor generally poses the question and the minister replies in the form of long discourses. This form of writing went beyond that of ordinary medical texts. Consequently, the *Canon* takes on the form of a treatise on general ethics and a regimen of life, which included the prevailing religious beliefs of that period. It should be noted that early Chinese medical concepts were a part of philosophy and religion, all of which propounded a wholeness, or oneness with nature. This concept might be viewed as an ancient forerunner of the modern idea of holistic health care. This is where integrative health care had its beginning.

## PHILOSOPHICAL FOUNDATIONS

It is not the purpose of this present work to delve into the intricate philosophical details of the Yellow Emperor's *Canon*, but a brief comment on this subject is pertinent. To understand the foundations of modern integrative Chinese medicine and the use of their healing herbs it is essential to note the role of cosmogony or philosophy of the world in the context of Taoism. Tao is the key to understanding the intermingling of heaven and earth. Tao is the means of shaping earthly conduct to conform to the demands of heaven or the other world.

The ancient Chinese derived their livelihood from agriculture and thus developed a relationship with nature, and the use of healing herbs as part of their lifestyle. Tao, which originally meant "the way", was a crystallization of this concept. The earth was dependent upon heaven. Tao as its dual role of the supreme regulator of the universe and as the highest code of conduct played an important

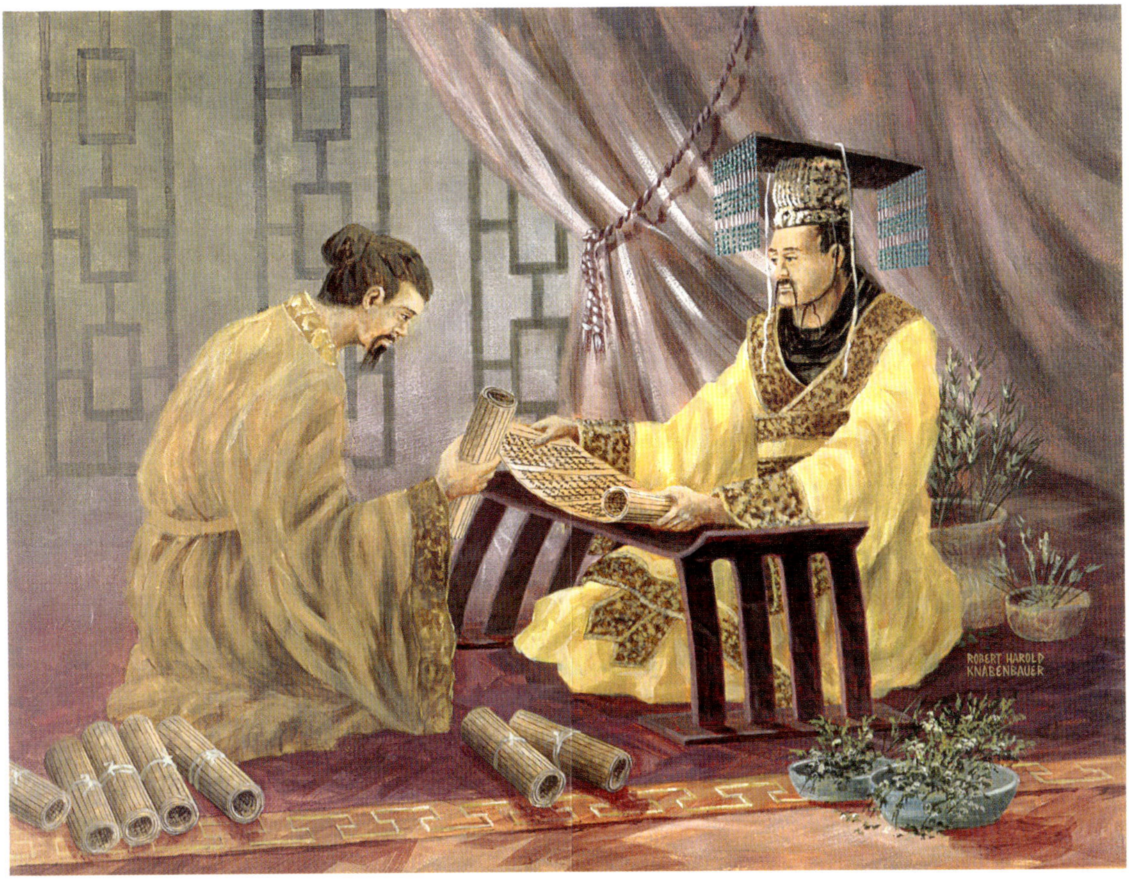


Fig. 8.2. Huang Ti (2598 - 2596 B.C.). The Yellow Emperor is depicted in dialogue with his minister, Chi Po. This dialogue has been historically recorded in the *Nei Ching Su Wen*, or the *Yellow Emperor's Classic of Internal Medicine*, which is considered to be the oldest medical book in existence. Huang Ti is credited as providing the philosophical basis for the concept of the Yin and the Yang. (R. H. Knabenbauer)

part in early Chinese medical thinking. The principles and basis of Chinese medicine and the use of healing herbs are drawn directly from the traditional Taoist philosophy. The Chinese believe that the human body is a microcosm of the grand cosmic order. The same principles that apply to the grand cosmic order apply directly to the human body.

The *Canon* is a repository of Chinese classical medical theory and practice. It deals with an ancient and great people and how they dealt with their medical problems over centuries of time. The *Canon* presents an integrated perspective of moral and physical conduct and foreshadowed by many centuries the modern concept of holistic health care. Moreover, it affected the destinies of the peoples of the Orient, constituting over one fourth of the world's population, and their medical care for thousands of years. The reader is referred to the *Canon* for further details.

The Chinese generally arrive at their medical conclusions based on their empirical observations and experiences. They have little faith in rigid systems based on abstract theories. The *Nei Ching Su Wen* discusses some of this basic Taoist thinking, generally in reference to the two component parts of the universe, the Yin and Yang, the Five Elements, various diseases, diagnostic concepts, acupuncture and moxibustion. Some of these concepts and their applications will be explored in greater details in Chapter Nine.

## Li Shih-chen—<br>Author of *The Great Chinese Materia Medica*

Another outstanding writer of the *Pen Tsaos* was Li Shih-chen (Fig. 8.3), who lived during the Ming Dynasty (1368 - 1644). He was born in 1518 in Slate Dam village outside the east gate of Chichow, Hupeh. His grandfather and father were both physicians and he became familiar with the names, properties, and uses of many medicinal herbs at an early age. Li Shih-chen became an ardent student of natural history, and developed a knowledge of a wide variety of plants and animals largely because of the influence of his father who took him on numerous treks through the fields and woods.

During the Han Dynasty (202 B.C. - 220 A.D.) all medicinal plant and animal discoveries had been compiled into one comprehensive work known as the *Shen Nung Pen Tsao Ching* (also known as the *Pen Ching*) or the *Emperor Shen Nung's Materia Medica*. Later, numerous supplements and commentaries were written about this great herbal. This was the primary edition of the *Pen Tsao* in use during Li Shih-chen's time. While practicing medicine and conducting his investigations on medicinal plants he became convinced that there were numerous errors in the *Shen Nung Pen Tsao Ching* and set about to rectify the matter.

Li Shih-chen is said to have spent many years of his life traveling throughout China observing the various methods and substances that were being used by herbalists in the treatment of various illnesses. Li Shih-chen became a very renowned physician and people traveled from all parts of China in order to have him treat their most difficult diseases. It is said that he read over a thousand manuscripts dealing with a variety of topics having a bearing on herbal medicine and natural history in preparation for the writing of his great herbal magnum opus.

In 1552 when Li Shih-chen was 35 years old he began to write his great Materia Medica, the *Pen Tsao Kang Mu*. This enormous work was more than merely a compilation of the writings of previous authors. Li Shih-chen based his writing on numerous expeditions into the fields throughout China and collected biological specimens, all of which provided a fresh perspective for his writings.

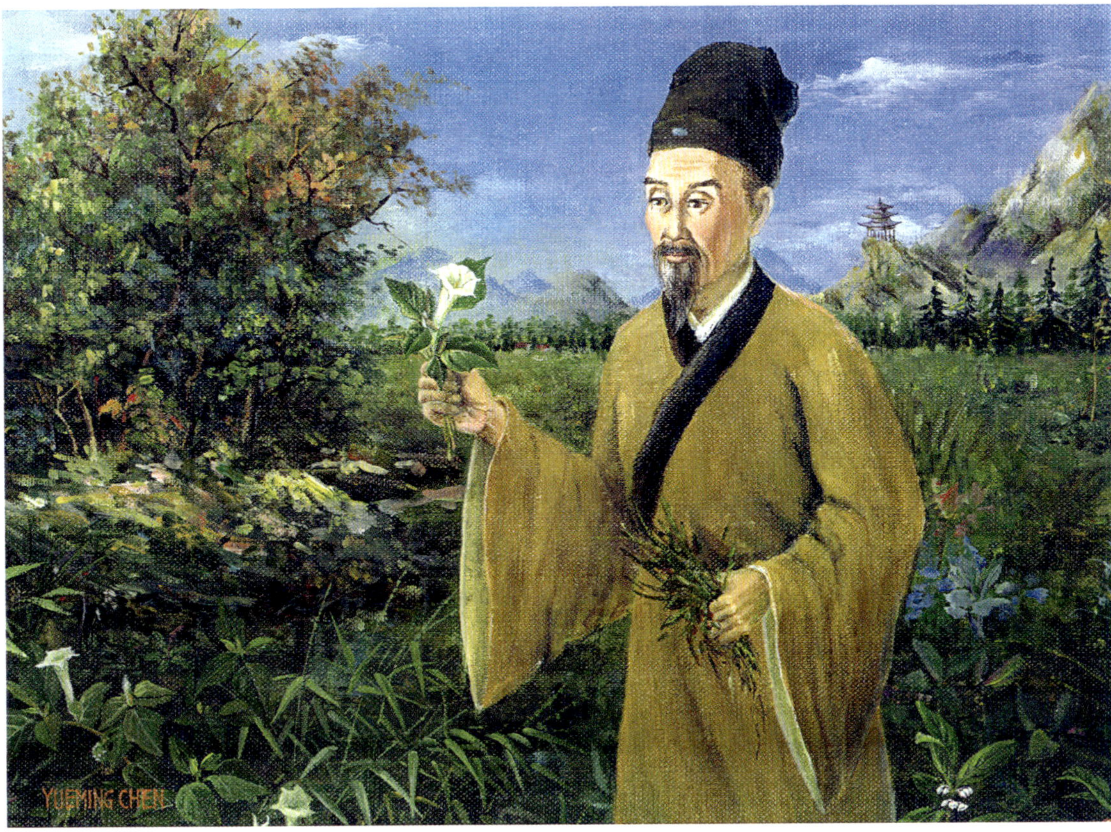


Fig. 8.3. Li-Shih-chen (1518 - 1593) is the author of the *Pen Tsao Kang Mu, 8,* which is also known as *The Great Chinese Materia Medica*. This work was not just another compilation of previous works, but entailed numerous field expeditions and a review of over a thousand manuscripts. He added 374 herbs not included in previous herbals, and corrected numerous mistakes in some of the earlier *Pen Tsaos*. The writing of his magnum opus took 26 years to accomplish. He developed a binomial system of nomenclature not unlike the Linnean system that is currently used today. (Yue-ming Chen)

Li Shih-chen finally completed his initial writing of the *Pen Tsao Kang Mu* in 1578 after 26 years of intensive effort. In the years that followed he continued to revise and update the work, which finally covered 52 volumes of material. Many medicinal substances were regrouped, or reclassified, and some of the doubtful items were eliminated.

One of the unique contributions of Li Shih-chen's work was his arrangement of the various organisms that he dealt with into an orderly system involving what might be termed families and genera and a binomial system of taxonomic nomenclature not unlike the Linnean system that is followed by systematists today in the naming of plants and animals. Moreover, he added 374 herbs not included in previous herbals by other authors, thus making a total of 1,892 herbal, animal, and mineral species that were listed, and included 8,160 prescriptions.

The first edition of the *Pen Tsao Kang Mu* was published in Nanking in 1590, but the actual printing was not completed until shortly after his death in 1593. Only four copies of this first edition are said to be in existence. See Halstead and Hood (1980) for a more detailed account on the *Pen Tsao Kang Mu*, the Great Herbal of China.

Chapter 9

# The Chinese Rationale of Integrative Cancer Prevention and Therapy



## Introduction

Western medicine tends to look upon the history of medicine as merely a subject of academic interest, but of no great value to a practicing clinician. Chinese physicians take historical medical classics very seriously because they feel that they are important to their medical practice. The great classics of Chinese traditional medicine represent an accumulation of clinical observations made by innumerable critical observers over more than five millenniums of health care (Ching-wei, 1999).

The Chinese deal with the prevention and treatment of cancer in the same manner as any other chronic disease complex, namely, in a holistic fashion. Evidence of the difference between the Oriental approach to disease therapy and that used by Western physicians is seen in their drug prescriptions. Western physicians use a monopharmaceutical approach, usually a single drug for a single disease, whereas Chinese physicians use a polypharmaceutical approach, multiple drugs for a single disease. Chinese traditional herbology has a documented history of more than five-thousand years using thousands of medicinal plants. A good scientific Chinese herbalist is reputed to be knowledgeable about the medicinal value of about 10,000 plant species, a good clinical herbalist about 5,000 plant species, whereas the average practitioner uses about 500 plant species.

The following sections will present the philosophy behind Chinese medicine, the rationale behind the use of herbs, and the classification and properties of Chinese herbs.

## Yin and Yang

The terms **Yin** and **Yang** express the Chinese concept of a dual power. They are elementary terms that convey the idea of the polar quality of all effects. These terms and the concepts they represent are basic to the Taoist philosophy of life and to Chinese health care. The Chinese believe that the balance between these two primordial cosmic forces is the key factor in all natural phenomena and life processes. The Yin-Yang theory pervades every aspect of Chinese life, the cosmos, medicine, and the application of healing herbs.

The Yin and the Yang were looked upon as cosmic regulators. The ancients noted that day changed into night, light unto darkness, spring and summer into fall and winter. Nature was constantly changing and influencing human, animal, and plant life under these regulators. They came to the conclusion that neither of the components ever existed in an absolute state. Within the Yin there was some Yang and within the Yang there was some Yin. When the Yin reached its zenith the Yang was in its dependency, and vice versa.

The polar nature of the Yin-Yang is expressed in Fig. 9.1. The definition of the two Chinese characters depicting the Yin and Yang has been given a great variety of interpretations. A literal translation of Yin refers to "the shady side of a hill", whereas Yang refers to "the sunny side of a hill". There are a variety of variations of this same theme, but are logically derived from this same idea. Yin is always placed before Yang in the word order. They are mutually dependent forces. When Yin increases Yang diminishes accordingly, and the reverse is true, but the net total remains constant. It will also be noted in the drawing that both Yin and Yang contain the germ of their own opposite within themselves as symbolized by the white and black dots.

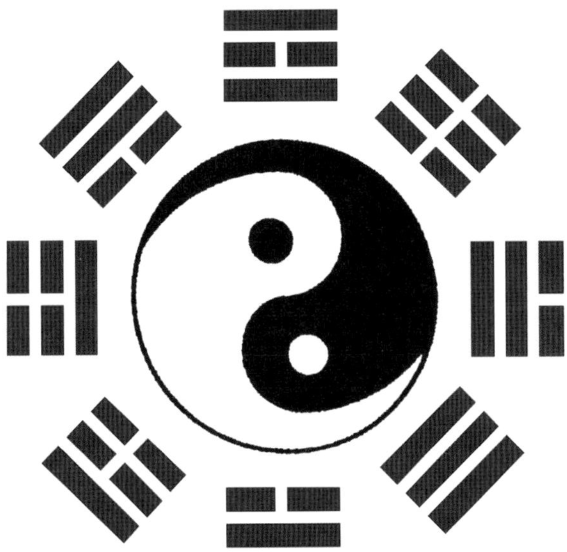

Fig. 9.1. This figure shows the eight Kua, or trigrams, derived from the Yellow Emperor's ancient classic *I. Ching*, known as *The Book of Changes*, written by four holy men, Fu Hsi, King Wên, Duke of Chou, and Confuscius. The eight trigrams surround the elemental forces Yin and Yang. The eight trigrams are symbols standing for changing transitional states. The eight trigrams do not represent things as much as they represent tendencies in movement. Together they represent the evolution and eternal changes in nature. In the center of the diagram is seen the dark colored Yin flowing into the light colored Yang even as Yang approaches its zenith, while Yang flows into Yin as Yin approaches its zenith. Yin and Yang are mutually dependent forces, one cannot exist without the other. The Yin and the Yang are in a constant state of balance. Each of them contain a germ of the other as indicated by the black and white dots. The ideal state of health requires a harmonious balance between the Yin and the Yang. (After the *I. Ching*)

Yin is female in nature, and represents a passive, negative force, dark, cold, low-lying, contractive, descending, a downward, inward flow, represented by the moon, earth, night, moisture, and symbolized by water.

Yang is male in nature, an active positive force, lightness, expansive, high-flying, ascending, upward, outward flow, represented by the sun, heaven, heat, dryness, and symbolized by fire.

The Taoists believe that Yin is the stronger of the two forces pointing out that although fire will flare up, providing a momentary show of strength and power, it can be quickly extinguished by water. Water is indestructible. Water can be heated, and brought to the boiling point—if the fire continues. Yin can retain Yang energy for a prolonged period of time.

Yin signifies something sustaining and preserving. Yin implies that the support involves an act of maintenance, a static condition. Yang signifies something that nourishes, promotes, and enhances. Yang implies an element of growth. Yin represents standstill and death. Yang represents motion and life.

The duality concept exists within the natural world. The modern disciplines of mathematics, physics, chemistry and biology provide a plethora of examples in which duality is always present, viz.: plus and minus, addition and subtraction, positive and negative charges, north and south poles. Computers function on the basis of these dual physical principles. There are positively charged protons and negatively charged electrons, positive ions and negative ions, materials that gain electrons become negatively charged while materials losing electrons become positively charged. Other examples are to be found in biological systems such as male and female, immune T-helper cells and T-suppressor cells, to cite just a few examples of the duality of the natural world.

The Yin-Yang concept was applied to the application of Chinese healing herbs and health. To understand the basis of the Yin-Yang theory as it relates to health care it must be understood that the Chinese do not believe in absolutes or ideals. They believe that everything is relative, and in a continual state of flux. There is a constant waning and waxing of the two forces. Change is the only thing that is constant in the body. This brings up the concept of relative balance.

## RELATIVE BALANCE—CELLULAR HOMEOSTASIS

A more technical modern scientific term describing relative balance as it relates to cellular metabolism would be **cellular homeostasis**, or chemical balance within the cells of the body. The chemical balance within the cells is constantly changing. The chemical balance within cells is never constant, and is at best only in a relative state of balance. The only constant in the chemistry of cells is change. Health is a metabolic biochemical reflection of the Yin-Yang concept of health, which is a further reflection of the electromagnetic energy state of the body, which deals with bioenergetics, or as the late Nobel Laureate Albert Szent-Györgyi might have termed it electronic biology.

## SEASONAL ENERGY BALANCE OF THE YIN AND YANG

The Yin-Yang concept can be further illustrated by the energy balance in the body during the various seasons of the year. During the summer the body may be in a satisfactory state of balance, but would not be suitable for the winter. Since the cold Yin-forces dominate the environment during the winter, the body would require extra Yang-warming forces. In the case of the summer months the body would require the Yin-cooling forces. Thus, the appropriate food or herb would be administered accordingly. Under normal circumstances the body can adjust itself within a reasonable range of conditions. However, when the body's energy resources exceed its normal buffering mechanism utilizing ordinary nutrition, additional herbal supplementation may be required.

## APPLICATION OF YIN AND YANG TO HERBOLOGY

The Yin-Yang theory plays an important role in Chinese therapeutics. An excellent example of this is in the use of Yin and Yang tonics.

The Yin tonics are used to treat those disorders suffering from Yin emptiness in such organs as the stomach, kidneys, liver, and lungs. The symptoms in these cases include: stomach-Yin deficiency, red lips, dark red tongue, peeling tongue coating, thirst, and loss of appetite; kidney-Yin deficiency, afternoon fever spells, nocturnal sweats, spermatorrhoea; liver-Yin deficiency, dry eyes, blurry vision, dizziness, headaches; lung-Yin deficiency, dry coughs, blood in sputum, "empty fever", thirst, and irritability. Most Yin tonics are sweet, cold, moist, and sticky. Examples of these tonic plants include *Adenophora tetraphylla* (four-leaf bellflower), *Eclipta prostrata* (prostrate Eclipta), *Liriope spicata* (spiked Liriope), and *Lycium barbarum* (Chinese wolfberry). The Yin tonics should be used sparingly.

Yang tonics are used to treat disorders having a Yang-deficiency. The primary target organs of Yang-energy are the kidneys, which are believed to house primordial Yang-energy. Most Yang-deficient disorders involve the kidneys. Most Yang-tonics tonify and warm the kidneys. The symptoms of kidney Yang-deficiency include: cold hands and feet, fear of cold, impotence, spermatorrhoea, nocturnal emissions, premature ejaculation, etc. Since sexual potency involves the kidney and adjacent adrenal glands, Chinese aphrodisiacs belong to the Yang-tonic category. Chinese herbalists state that aphrodisiac tonics should only be used by people with Yang-deficiency. If these tonics are used by people with Yang-excess and/or Yin-deficiency, they may further aggravate the Yin-Yang imbalance.

Yang-deficiency may also affect other organs such as the spleen and the heart. Spleen Yang-deficient symptoms are fatigue, poor appetite, lumpy diarrhea, abdominal discomfort, hernias, prolapse of the rectum, etc. Heart Yang-deficiency symptoms are profuse cold sweats, pallor, weak irregular pulse, etc. These conditions should be treated with herbs that warm the blood and with energy tonics. The liver and lungs are said to rarely display Yang-deficient symptoms, Yang-excess is the usual imbalance in these organs. Yang-tonics are considered to be warm and drying and should be used sparingly in persons with chronic deficiency or fire excess. The ultimate goal is to obtain a Yin-Yang balance within the body.

Healing herbs are used in Chinese medicine to manipulate these natural relationships in order to adjust energy imbalances caused by either an excess or a deficiency of these forces in the body. This is the central core of Chinese traditional herbology.

## HERB TONICS

Herbs that are capable of restoring the normal tone or strength of a muscle, enhancing the immune system, or restoring the feeling of well-being are referred to as tonics. Many of these plants are adaptogens, and capable of restoring normalcy. The Chinese use the term "empty" when the body is in need of a tonic. Many of these plants are classified as superior herbs and can be used over an extended period of time as foods without untoward effects. There are disorders in which there are deficiencies or "emptiness" causing a weakened condition in the body's defenses due to an excess of "evil-qi". Chinese herbalists will correct the condition by using herbs that will dispel the evil-qi, combined with herbs that act as a tonic to stimulate "pure-qi". The use of these herbs helps to restore the primordial energies of the person.

Tonics are used in four types of deficiency states: 1) energy deficient, 2) blood deficient, 3) Yang-deficient, and 4) Yin-deficient. The corrective tonics are named after the condition, as energy tonic, blood nourisher, Yang-tonic, and Yin-nourisher. Although the terms "tonic" and "nourisher" are somewhat interchangeable, a "tonic" is generally used to describe energy and Yang herbs, whereas "nourish" refers to blood and Yin herbs.

## YIN AND YANG DOMAINS WITHIN THE BODY

The Yin and Yang forces have their own domains within the human body. However, the spheres of influence intersect. The Yin controls the lower, internal, and front portions of the body. The Yang controls the upper, external, and back portions of the body. The vital organs of the body are equally divided between the Yin and the Yang. Yin controls the blood, and Yang governs energy-qi. Yin descends, and Yang ascends the body. Innate instinct are Yin in nature, whereas learned skills are Yang.

## FIVE ELEMENTS AND THE SYSTEM OF NUMBERS

The Yin and the Yang is further developed in the *Nei Ching* into other more tangible components. These include the theory of the five elements, a subject which is also discussed in other ancient Chinese medical writings. These elements were subdivided into water, fire, metal, wood and earth. They believed that everything on earth is dominated by one of these elements. The constant interplay of these elements, combined with the Yin and the Yang, explain all change and activity in the natural world. This is a symbolism that they have also applied to the functions of the human body.

The Five Elements represent the primeval forces of the body interacting in set patterns according to their natural relationships. Each force has a creative (generative) and a subjugate influence on another force which in turn is generated or subjugated by a different force. This is said to be a cyclic phenomenon where one force drives another one.

The *Nei Ching* explains the victories of the various elements in the following manner: *Wood* brought in contact with metal is felled; *fire* brought in contact with water is extinguished; *earth* brought in contact with wood is penetrated; *metal* brought in contact with fire is dissolved; *water* brought in contact with earth is halted. This basic concept was expanded and applied in many directions.

The sequence of creative force is: Metal creates water, water creates wood, wood creates fire, fire creates earth, earth creates metal. The sequence of subjugation is: Metal subjugates wood, water subjugates fire, wood subjugates earth, fire subjugates metal, earth subjugates water. The negative subjective cycle is complementary to the positive generative one.

The essence of the Five Elements, and other Chinese descriptions of the world, is that they are symbolic representations of fundamental natural forces. The interactions or interplay of these forces is the most important aspect of the subject.

In order to understand the connection between the Five Elements and the use of healing herbs it is necessary to explain the relationship of the concept of these Elements to the human body. Each vital organ in the body belongs to one of the Five Elements. If one understands the fundamental relations of the Five Elements then the interactions of the vital organs and their influence upon each other become clear. The generative-subjective cycle explains how external environmental factors affect individual organs and the body as a whole.

Healing herbs are used in Chinese medicine to manipulate these natural relationships in order to adjust energy imbalances caused by either an excess or a deficiency of these forces in the body. This is the central core of Chinese traditional herbology.

The *Nei Ching* attempted to schematize the functions of the universe and the human body by using a series of numbers through a complex system of parallelism, and thereby explain how the total scheme of things function.

The numbers and their multiples constitute the law for the growth and decline of a human. The number five was selected because the basis of this system was the five elements. The *Nei Ching* developed a concordance that included each of the elements, seasons, flavors, odors, climates, musical notes, grains, animals, and other factors, which affected the physical body. Since the interrelationships of these various factors go beyond the scope of this present work the reader is referred to the *Nei Ching* (Veith, 1966) for further information on this topic.

## Chinese Approach to the Use of Healing Herbs

These early Chinese herbal practitioners were not so much concerned with the specific ability of a plant substance to "cure" a particular disease, but rather the ability of the substance to strengthen the body's defense system and to protect the person from illnesses of all kinds by acting in a nonspecific or *adaptogenic* manner. Herbs having this biodynamic property are referred to as *adaptogens*. One might conclude that even during ancient times the Chinese had already developed an appreciation of the use of adaptogenic nutrients in the maintenance of a healthy immune system. This is a profound concept which is still not understood by Western medicine.

## CONCEPT OF ADAPTOGENIC MEDICINE

Most of the Chinese medicinal plants have adaptogenic properties. The term *adaptogen* appears to have originated in the Russian herbal literature during the late 1950's. The Russian pharmacologist Nikolay V. Lazarev is credited with introducing the term adaptogen into the field of herbology. However, the introduction of the term to the western medical world is largely the work of his pupil Professor Israel I. Brekhman of the Far Eastern Science Center in Vladivostok. The first major publication to deal with this topic in depth in the United States appeared in a book by Halstead and Hood (1984a) entitled *Eleutherococcus senticosis: An Introduction to the Concept of Adaptogenic Medicine*, published by the Oriental Healing Arts Institute, Long Beach, CA. An "adaptogen" is a substance of natural origin which when ingested or injected has a normalizing effect on the body. An adaptogen tends to normalize pathological conditions. However, it should be recognized that the normalization process has limitations. Normalization has to do with altering a chemical metabolic processes. Adaptogens are biodynamic chemical substances derived from plants or animals which assist the body in bringing it into a state of metabolic harmony with its environment by inducing chemical and cellular homeostasis. The Russians constantly refer to this process in their scientific literature as "increasing the nonspecific resistance of the body" in an immunological sense. The Russians have used Siberian ginseng to increase the stamina and physical endurance in their athletes, military, and cosmonauts.

If one traces the adaptogenic concept back in scientific ethnobotanical history, it soon becomes obvious that adaptogenic nutritional thinking had its primordial roots in ancient Chinese traditional herbology. A preponderance of Chinese medicinal plants have adaptogenic properties. Unfortunately, the medical science behind adaptogenic nutrition is little known in the United States, despite the fact that hundreds of scientific articles have been written on various aspects of the subject in Chinese, Japanese, and Russian. Critics of the use of adaptogens complain of the lack of research and quality control of the products being sold in the United States and elsewhere.

*Eleutherococcus* serves as a model for plants having similar properties. *Eleutherococcus* is a member of the ginseng family Araliaceae, which includes about 84 genera and a large number of species that are endemic to Asia, Malaysia,

Polynesia, Europe, North Africa, and the Americas. I (BWH) first proposed the English vernacular term Siberian ginseng in a meeting with I. I. Brekhman and VO Medexport officials in Moscow in 1970. *Eleutherococcus* is a member of the ginseng family and was found in Siberia and that was how it was given its vernacular name "Siberian ginseng". While the senior author was in Vladivostok he found that the Russians had produced a popular cola-like health drink that was sold in the local restaurants made from *Eleutherococcus* called "Bodrust", which was anglicized as "vigoro". The drink was so popular they could never produce enough to keep up with the demand.

Brekhman (1968) has summarized an adaptogen as a plant product having the following properties:

a) Low toxicity, causing minimal disturbance of the normal physiological functions of the body.

b) A nonspecific ability to enhance the resistance of the host to disease processes. It must have a broad therapeutic effect.

c) It has an overall normalizing effect on the entire body.

Davydov and Krikorian (2000) have prepared an excellent critical review on the subject of adaptogens in which they have compared the chemical and pharmacological properties of *Eleutherococcus senticosus* and *Panax ginseng*. They found that although both of the genera are from the family Araliaceae their phytochemical constituents are quite different, but have similar pharmacological and therapeutic properties. Their chemistry and pharmacology are summarized in Table 9.1.

## Classification and Properties of Chinese Herbs

In Western medicine drugs are classified into various categories according to their pharmacological and therapeutic properties. A good example of drug classifications can be found in the *Physicians Desk Reference*, where drugs are classified as allergens, amebicides, bronchial dilators, cardiovascular agents, central nervous system stimulants, laxatives, hormones, sedatives, etc.

Traditional Chinese drugs are founded on an accumulation of empirical human experience rather than on animal research. Most of this information is recorded in a series of materia medicas known as the *Pen Tsaos* that were written over a period of thousands of years.

Chinese herbalists have traditionally classified drugs in a system that reflects the toxicity, safety, and rejuvenative properties of the substance. For example: a **superior**, or **upper class drug**, can be taken safely for extended periods of time and has rejuvenative properties. A **medium**, or **middle herb**, is regarded as a **tonic** whose toxicity varies according to the dosage and may be taken for variable peri-

**Table 9.1.**
Comparisons of the chemistry and pharmacology of the adaptogens *Eleutherococcus senticosus* and *Panax ginseng*.

| *Eleutherococcus senticosus* | *Panax ginseng* |
|---|---|
| **CHEMISTRY** | |
| Syringin<br>Sesamin<br>Hedersaponin B<br>β-sitoserol and some of its analogs<br>Isofraxidin<br>Caffeic acid<br>Coniferyl aldehyde | Ginsenosides $Rb_1$, $Rg_{3, e, f, g, h}$<br>Protopanaxadiol<br>Ginsenoside $Rh_{1, 2}$ |
| **PHARMACOLOGY** | |
| Protects against radiation.<br>Protects against DNA damage.<br>Improves white blood cell count.<br>Enhances immune system.<br>Contains antioxidative, antimicrobial, anti-inflammatory, anti-senility, anti-atherosclerotic, & anti-cancer effects. | Contains antioxidative, anti-cancer, anti-melanoma, & anti-ovarian cancer effects. |

ods of time. The term "tonic" generally implies an immune enhancement substance of some type or a substance of some other type of stimulating beneficial effect.

**Inferior**, or **lower herbs**, are regarded as poisonous and are used only for limited periods of time. Most of the FDA approved drugs used in Western medicine would fit into this category.

Chinese medicinal herbal properties are further characterized as to their four essences, five flavors and four directions of actions. These terms will be explained in the following sections.

## The Four Essences (Energies)

The four **Essences**, also referred to as **Energies**, or Si Qi, cold, hot, warm and cool. These are four properties of medicinal herbs that refer to their therapeutic effects and the body's reaction. In actuality, cool and cold are in the same general category, varying in only degree, just like warm and hot. Balanced or neutral herbs which do not lean toward either warm or cool, are termed "bland". Of the 365 herbs found in the *Shen Nung Pen Tsao Ching*, 131 of them are classified as bland herbs. There are only 17 warm herbs.

Chinese traditional physicians follow a differential diagnosis that classifies all diseases by their symptoms into the broad categories of Yin and Yang. Chinese herbologists divide all healing herbs into Yin or Yang plants. The clinical application of healing herbs employs the fundamental principles of balance and opposites in which Yin herbs are used for Yang disorders, and Yang herbs are used to treat Yin illnesses.

As one proceeds with some of the other properties or characteristics of healing herbs it will be observed that a single herb usually does not satisfy all of the therapeutic requirements of a disease. Consequently, other herbal properties may be required necessitating the use of additional herbs. Another group of herbal properties include the Five Flavors which are discussed below.

## Five Flavors

The Five Flavors are pungent, sweet, sour, bitter, and salty. Flavor is that quality of a substance that affects the sense of taste. The Chinese use the designation of Five Flavors in reference to the effects certain healing herbs have on the body. The Five Flavors are mentioned in the *Shen Nung Pen Tsao Ching* and other editions of the *Pen Tsaos*. The *Nei Ching* mentions a sixth flavor designated as tasteless or bland.

The Five Flavors have been shown to have specific effects in the body. For example:

**Pungent** herbs exert dispelling and promoting effects. They assist in driving away or dispersing various effects, beneficial or otherwise. Pungent herbs such as ginger (*Zingiber*), perilla (*Perilla*), and mentha (*Mentha*) may dispel external pathogens.

**Sweet** herbs exert tonifying and regulating effects. They tend to have a soothing effect. Many of the adaptogenic herbs are found in this category. Examples of the sweet herbs are gingseng (*Panax*) and licorice (*Glycyrrhiza*) both of which nourish ch'i and relieve pain. They also enhance the immune system.

**Bitter** herbs have a dampness-drying and a purging action. Examples of bitter herbs are coptis (*Coptis*), bitter melon (*Cucumis*), and rhubarb (*Rheum*).

**Sour** herbs soften, fortify, and moisten. Examples are *Portulaca, Hovenia*, and *Polygonum*.

**Salty** herbs such as kelp are used to treat stagnant phlegm and tuberculosis. Salty herbs soften hard masses, dissolve lumps, and have a purgative effect. Other examples of salty substances are the plants *Sappan, Rostellularia*, and various animal products. In reading a Chinese materia medica it will be noted that there are comparatively few salty substances listed.

**Bland** herbs such as hoelen (*Poria*) and *Akebia* are diuretics.

Chinese herbalists combine two or more flavors in a prescription for the purpose of producing several therapeutic effects simultaneously. This is accomplished by selecting the flavors that are capable of producing the desired functions in the body based on the key herbal actions as noted in the preceding paragraphs.

## Formulating Healing Herbs

Knowledge concerning the formulation of Chinese healing herbs is the result of thousands of years of empirical experience by Chinese physicians using trial and error methods in treating human diseases. The properties of the herbs consisting of the essence and flavor of the herbs in the context of the Yin-Yang philosophy provided the general guidelines in the use of these herbs. They learned over a period of time that the addition or deletion of herbs having certain properties altered the clinical effects. The medieval Chinese physician Li Tung-Yuan, also known as Li Kao (1180 - 1251) compiled herbal formulations according to the compatibility of their properties. He found that essence and flavor were interrelated. Flavors may differ, but different herbs may fall in the same essence category, or an herb may fall in one essence category, but possess several different flavors. In order to properly apply healing herbs skillfully it is necessary to understand the properties of the four essences and the five flavors.

For examples of how some of these combinations are used see Hsu (1979) and Hsu, et al (1986).

## Seven Effects of Herbs

Many Chinese herbal formulations utilize from four to twelve individual herbs, all of which are interacting with each other. Consequently, any attempt to analyze an individual herb on the basis of its pharmacological properties in a Chinese formulation would be a difficult—if not an impossible—task. It should be further noted that because of these multiple herbal formulations any other type of pharmacological evaluation is also difficult to obtain.

There are two basic types of herbal interactions or synergisms:

1) Interactions between the phytochemical constituents within a single herb.
2) Interactions between the phytochemical constituents of each of the other herbs in a formulation.

It is these various synergistic interactions that compound the problem for Western pharmacologists attempting to evaluate the pharmacokinetic properties of Chinese herbal formulations. Chinese herbologists have become quite skilled in putting together the proper herbal formulations in treating a wide range of maladies.

The epicenter of the beneficial actions of traditional Chinese herbs is to be found in the synergisms of their actions in which the overall therapeutic effects are greater than the sum of their individual parts. These synergistic actions in the body may proceed in several ways as follows:

1. When two or more phytochemical constituents are mixed this may result in a **synergistic action** such as a multiplication or enhancement of a pharmacological action. This is considered as an additive or pharmacological **potentiation** by use of multiple herbs in a formulation.
2. There may be an **antagonism** in the synergistic action in which the mixing of the phytochemical constituents may cancel out one or more of the biodynamic effects of other constituents within the formulation.
3. A **transition** effect may occur when the combination of two or more herbs changes the effects of the individual herbs.

Chinese herbalists refer to the pharmacological effects derived from the combination of two or more herbs as the "seven effects of herbs". In actuality this is an expansion of the overall concept of synergism. Chinese physicians have learned after centuries of empirical clinical experience with herbs that the effects of a particular herb on the body change with the molecular environment in which it is used. Some combinations enhance a biodynamic activity whereas others reduce it. For example, in some cases toxicity may be enhanced or reduced. Chinese herbalists have described seven different types of herbal effects (Hsu, et al, 1986) as follows:

1. **Single effect.** This occurs when the formulation contains only a single herb. For example, ginseng contains several different phytochemical constituents that work synergistically within a single plant and exert only one effect.
2. **Additive effect.** This occurs when two or more kinds of drugs having similar properties used in combination can mutually reinforce the therapeutic actions. For example, gypsum and *Anemarrhena* reduce internal heat; *Rheum* and mirabilitum have a purging action.

3. **Synergistic effect.** When their are two or more ingredients in a prescription, one acts as the principle substance while the others play a subsidiary role reinforcing the action of the principle ingredient. For example, the combination of *Astragalus* and *Poria* enhances the diuretic action and strengthens ch'i and the spleen.
4. **Mutual restraint or antagonist effect.** Two or more ingredients in a prescription can weaken or neutralize each other. For example ginger (*Zingiber*) may weaken the action of *Pinellia* and *Arisaema*.
5. **Counteraction or inhibitive effect.** The action of one drug may inhibit the action of another. For example, ginger (*Zingiber*) may counteract *Scutellaria*.
6. **Destructive or neutralizing effect.** One drug or ingredient may neutralize the toxicity of another. For example, *Ledebouriella* neutralizes the toxic effects of arsenic.
7. **Incompatible effect.** When two herbs such as *Aconitum* and *Pinellia* are used together they are toxic. Incompatible drugs cannot be used together.

Chinese physicians have discovered over the centuries the importance of using these synergisms to therapeutic advantage.

## The Four Directions of Herbs

The four directions of herbs refer to the different disease locations in the body which serve as targets for herbal actions. The terms ascending, descending, floating and sinking represent four additional qualities used to categorize herbs. Diseases that are externally manifested as situated in the upper part of the body require herbs that have ascending or floating qualities. Ma huang (*Ephedra*) and cinnamon (*Cinnamomum*) are two such examples of herbs that are used to treat external wind and cold disorders that have these properties. Diseases that are manifested internally in the lower part of the body require descending and sinking herbs such as rhubarb (*Rheum*) and the mineral mirabilitum (magnesium sulfate), which are used to treat constipation due to dry intestines. If a disease develops causing an upward motion in the body then a sinking type of herb is needed, whereas a downward condition will require an ascending or floating herb. These are additional examples of the Yin and Yang principle.

Herbs that are hot, pungent, and sweet have ascending and floating actions, whereas cold, cool, sour, bitter, and salty have sinking and descending actions. The various parts of a herb have varying actions. For example, flowers and leaves usually possess ascending and floating qualities (Reid, 1987).

## The Relationship Between Foods, Drugs, and Poisons

The quest of the ancient Chinese for edible foods led them into the world of biodynamic substances that involved not only foods, but therapeutic agents and poisons as well. In the course of these activities they learned that it was sometimes difficult to draw distinct lines between foods, drugs, and poisons. The great Swiss physician, Philippus Aureolus Paracelsus (1493 - 1541), succinctly stated this fact when he said, "All substances are poisons; there is none which is not a poison. The right dose differentiates a poison and a remedy." Dosage of any given herb, animal or mineral was a matter of concern in ancient China and they attempted to use dosages judiciously.

Chinese herbalists observed that foods and medicinal herbs possess different metabolic actions according to their ingredients and the amounts ingested. They found that if they were to maintain good health, it was necessary to eat and drink in a balanced and temperate manner utilizing a variety of nutrients that help to maintain a biochemical harmony within the body. They came to the conclusion that one must avoid excesses in any direction. These ancient Chinese observations were in accord with the later Paracelsus dictum.

## Chinese Herbal Formulations

Chinese herbal formulations are generally comprised of eight to twelve formulations of different herbs. However, in some cases the formulations may also contain animal or mineral products. The science that deals with the composition, actions, indications, dosage, and clinical uses of these herbal formulas is called *herbal pharmaceutics*. In order to develop an effective formula the herbalist must develop a working knowledge of the composition and properties of these herbs.

More than half of the formulations in use today were developed over 1,800 years ago, and some of them have been in use for over thousands of years. The literature on the origin of Chinese herbal formulations is vast, but much of this literature has been referenced in Unschuld's *Medicine in China. A History of Pharmaceutics* (1986). Hsu and Hsu (1980) have published an excellent bibliography on the Chinese and Japanese literature on Oriental formulations of antiquity. This section will provide only a few brief highlights on some of the complexities of Chinese herbal formulations.

A Chinese herbal formulation is generally comprised of four classes of herbs:

**Imperial Herb.** The imperial herb is the chief component of the formulation.

**Ministerial Herb.** A ministerial herb is an ancillary herb that assists in the biodynamic activity of the imperial herb.

**Assistant Herb.** An assistant herb may either augment the activity of the two preceding herbs, or may assist in diminishing any of their side effects.

**Servant Herb.** The servant herb coordinates the actions of all of the herbs in the formulation.

Skilled herbalists over the centuries have modified certain basic formulations, but most of them continue to be in use up to the present time.

## Dosage Forms of Traditional Chinese Drugs

Chinese herbalists have developed a number of different dosage forms which are used to facilitate processing, administration, and storage of the herbs. These herb forms are as follows:

1. **Slices.** Herbs are cut into slices for use in preparing decoctions.
2. **Powders.** Herbs that are combined with one or more herbs which are pulverized and homogenized into a dry powder which can be used either externally or internally.
3. **Pills.** Herbs are pulverized into a fine powder, mixed with appropriate adjutants and binders and made into pills. There are several types of pills such as honey pills, water pills, gruel pills, waxed pills and honey-water pills. For further details on the formulations of these pills see Hsu, et al (1986).
4. **Plaster.** There are a variety of forms of plasters that may be used internally or externally.
5. **Tan.** This is a form of medication that is made by sublimating or melting minerals. It may be formulated into a pill, powder, or pellet.
6. **Medicated Liquor.** This is an alcoholic preparation made by extracting the active ingredients of an herb with the use of a liquor which acts as a solvent and is used as a drink.
7. **Herb Distillate.** The active ingredients of the herbs are obtained by distilling the herbs in water.
8. **Pellets.** Drug powders are bound together into solid forms in a variety of shapes: spindles, cubes, cylinders, and other forms.
9. **Glue.** This is made by boiling animal skin, bones, or horns into a solid mass that is then dried and cut into cubes or bars.
10. **Tea.** This is produced from an herbal formula that is prescribed by the physician. The herbs are ground into a coarse powder that is combined with a binder to form a mass and then decocted by immersion in boiling water.
11. **Tablets.** Tablets are similar to pellets, but in recent times are now formed by compression using special tableting machinery. They may be coated with a variety of substances such as sugar.

12. **Capsules.** Herbs or their concentrates are now placed in either hard or soft gelatin capsules.
13. **Tinctures.** This is a clear aqueous solution that is made by extracting the active principles of an herb using various concentrations of ethanol.
14. **Extracts.** A fluid extract is prepared by extracting the active principles from a herb by using a variety of different solvents and then evaporating the solvents and adjusting the concentration of the active principles to the desired dosage.
15. **Instant Granules.** Active principles of herbs or their extract are powdered and made into granules. The granules are than placed in hot water to form an instant decoction.
16. **Ointments.** Herbs or their extracts may be added to a suitable base such as lanolin to form a semisolid preparation for external application.
17. **Creams.** Herbal extracts may be emulsified into a cream base for application to the skin.
18. **Miscellaneous Forms.** In recent times a large variety of other delivery systems are being used including suppositories, ampoules, douche powders, syrups, troches, and other methods that are now being used by the pharmaceutical industry.

## Herbs and Their Therapeutic Actions on Channels

### ENERGY—SI QI

The Chinese believe that at the time of birth each individual is endowed with a specific amount of Si Qi or adaptive energy. This energy can be affected positively by one's lifestyle, which includes the use of exercise, good nutrition, positive thinking, and the use of medicinal herbs. Exposure to toxic agents, poor lifestyle, sedentary habits, negative thinking, and a host of other adverse environmental factors can reduce Si Qi, the quality of life, produce illness, and decrease ones longevity. The proper utilization of environmental factors can extend this adaptive energy, and improve quality of life, longevity, and health.

The term Si Qi refers to the essential or adaptive energy that flows through the meridian complex of the body. The Chinese consider these meridians to be a biological energy system centered around one of the vital organs of the body. These meridians are also referred to as channels. Meridians can be electronically determined when vital points in these meridians are stimulated by acupuncture. The precise anatomical or physiological nature of this system has never been fully elucidated and is difficult for most western medical practitioners to understand. They do not completely follow the usual anatomical relationships known to western physicians, but involve primarily the energy flow in the body, which has been studied in great detail over the centuries by Chinese practitioners.

There is said to be 59 meridians, of which 12 are thought to be of a primary nature, which dominate the others. Each of the main meridians represent a biological energy system centered around one of the twelve vital organs. Si Qi energy flows from one meridian to another in a specific order throughout the entire meridian network, delivering vital energy to every part of the body.

Stimulating one of the twelve meridians with acupuncture or herbs has a specific effect on the connected organ as well as a more general effect on the entire system. The task of the physician is to determine the most effective meridianal connections that will provide maximum essential energy and health to the body. The herbs may be applied in the form of poultices, or by moxibustion over a particular meridian.

## ACTIONS ON CHANNELS

Ancient Chinese herbalists classified every herbal formulation according to the channels or meridians (kwei ching) that they affect. This concept dates back to the Shen Chin-ao's book *Yo Yao Feng Chi* of the Ching dynasty (1644 - 1911). In his book he classified herbs according to the five viscera, six bowels, three Yin and three Yang channels, and the four fundamental substances.

The *Chen Chu Nang* from the Chin-Yan dynasty (1115 - 1368) and the *Pen Tsao Kang Mu* (Ming Dynasty 1590) classified herbs into the following twelve meridians or channels:

1. The **heart channel** (Shao-yin). Examples of herbs that enter this channel are *Coptis* and *Asarum*.
2. The **small intestine-hand channel** (Tai-yang). Examples of herbs entering this channel are *Ligustrum* and *Phellodendron*.
3. The **kidney-foot channel** (Shao-ying). Examples of herbs entering this channel are *Anemarrhena, Cinnamomum* and *Asarum*.
4. The **urinary bladder-foot channel** (Tai-yang). Example of an herb entering this channel is *Angelica*.
5. The **lung channel** (Tai-yin). Examples of plants entering this channel are *Platycodon, Cimicifuga, Allium*, and *Angelica*.
6. The **large intestine-hand channel** (Yang ming). Examples of herbs entering this channel are *Angelica, Cimicifuga*, and the mineral gypsum.
7. The **spleen-foot channel** (Tai-yin). Examples of herbs entering this channel are *Cimicifuga, Atractylodes*, and *Pueraria*.
8. The **stomach-foot channel** (Yang-ming). Examples of herbs entering this channel are *Angelica, Cimicifuga, Pueraria*, and the mineral gypsum.
9. The **pericardium channel** (Chueh-yin). Examples of herbs entering this channel are *Bupleurum* and *Paeonia*.

10. The **gall bladder-foot channel** (Shao-yang). Examples of herbs entering this channel are *Bupleurum* and *Citrus*.
11. The **liver foot channel** (Chueh-yin). The herbs entering this channel are *Citrus, Evodia, Cnidium*, and *Bupleurum*.
12. The **triple warm-hand channel** (Shao-yang). The herbs entering this channel are *Forsythia* and *Bupleurum*.

The classification of medicinal herbs according to their therapeutic actions on channels involves the Yin-Yang concept to a large degree, and derives from the theories of the viscera, bowels, and meridians. The herbal actions may extend to the physiology of different internal organs according to ancient Chinese medical thought. Moreover, an herb can affect various channels at one time as can be seen by examining the listing above. This therapeutic method is called "selection of drugs according to the channels". Chinese herbalists have found this method of therapeutics to be important and effective.

The actual practice of Chinese medicine is very complex and ponderous, and it is not the intent of this book to deal with this broad subject in any degree of depth. See the works of Wallnöfer and von Rottauscher (1965), Porkert (1979), Xie and Huang (1984), and Reid (1987) for additional information on the practice of Chinese traditional medicine.

## General Concepts of Chinese Health Care

There is a distinct difference in the rationale of Western medicine and that employed by the Chinese. Western-trained physicians generally employ a medicinal agent consisting of a single synthetic chemical ingredient or a single natural extractive. This is termed **monopharmacy**. Most of these drugs have a high degree of toxicity and an alarming number of them have carcinogenic, mutagenic, or teratogenic properties and may depress the immune system. One has only to read the *Physicians Desk Reference* to confirm this fact.

In contradistinction, Chinese traditional physicians employ a combination of herbs which have had centuries of use in humans and which, for the most part, do not have harmful side effects, and a large number of them enhance the immune system. This is termed **polypharmacy**. In one study of 200 commonly used Chinese herbs, they were found to have an exceptionally safe acute toxicity range of $LD_{50}$ values of 5.0 to 8.0 gm/kg (Hsu, et al, 1986). By comparison with the average western FDA approved drugs, this is a safety factor of several orders of magnitude greater than that of western legal pharmaceutical drugs.

Western medicine emphasizes diagnosis, establishes the name of the disease, and then prescribes specific treatment. Chinese medicine pays special attention to the patient's symptoms and prescribes a general treatment on a subjective basis that considers the lifestyle and physical constitution of the patient and the cause of the problem. Chinese physicians tend to emphasize treatment and employ nontoxic corrective measures. Although Western medicine has made enormous technical advances in the field of acute medicine, advances in the areas of chronic degenerative disease medicine have not achieved their therapeutic expectations.

A global reflection of this fact is the resolution in 1977 by the Thirteenth World Health Assembly (WHA 30.49) urging governments to give adequate importance to the utilization of traditional health systems. This suggestion was made in recognition of the fact that global health goals to be achieved by the year 2000 were not going to be met utilizing only the current Western medical modalities. The World Health Organization publication *Traditional Medicine and Health Care Coverage* (1983) was produced as a general guide for use in exploring traditional health care. The Burton Goldberg Group has published a compilation entitled *Alternative Medicine: The Definitive Guide* (Goldberg, 1993), which provides additional insight as to the scope of alternative health care including the use of herbal medicines.

Although there are no accurate statistics as to the use of herbs on a worldwide basis, it is safe to say that an excess of 85% of the world's population use herbs or their extractives to a greater or lesser extent in health care.

The threatening catastrophic diseases such as cancer and the combined destructive effects of pesticides, environmental poisons, excessive use of prescribed drugs, illegal recreational addictive drugs, industrial pollutants, radiation, and the emerging viruses emphasize the importance of re-examining other approaches to health care. It will be found that there are less expensive, less dangerous, and more effective methods in achieving desirable therapeutic results. One of the most encouraging of these therapeutic areas is that of the use of ancient Chinese healing herbs. They represent a vast assemblage of healing substance that have largely been lost to modern Western medicine. It is important that Western medicine takes time to re-discover them.

There is a vast array of other ancient herbal documents that could be used to embellish the empirical use of medicinal plants in China. However, neither time nor space will permit a further literary excursion into antiquity. The point of this brief review is that these adaptogenic plants were not just dug out of the garden yesterday, but have enormous documentation of safe usage in humans covering a span of thousands of years.

China has a completely awesome medical history and a very complex system of therapeutic herbology that has produced results worthy of investigation by modern analytical chemistry and pharmacology. Modern health care experts will do well to explore the subject in much greater depth.

For more information on the use of Chinese medicinal plants see Ying, et al (1987), Yeo-runn (1994), Pharmacopeia Commission of the Ministry of Public Health P.R.C (1998), Chung (1996-2001), Wiart (2000), and Li (2002).

Chapter 10

# THE PREPARATION OF PLANT EXTRACTS



---

## Preparation of Plant Extracts

There are a variety of methods that are used for extracting bioactive substances from medicinal herbs. The following is a brief overview of the techniques commonly employed and a brief discussion of some of the newer methods that have been found to be safer and more effective. The matter of plant extraction is of extreme importance to the entire subject of clinical pharmacology and the therapeutic results.

Phytopharmaceuticals are prepared from fresh or dried plants, or parts of plants by expression, distillation, and other methods. The primary objective is to obtain the bioactive ingredients for high quality therapeutic results. The results vary greatly with the methods used. Historically water and alcohol have served as the primary extractants.

## Traditional Processing Methods

**Herbal Teas** are the simplest and most ancient method of drug extraction. Herbal teas are aqueous infusions from one or a mixture of ground or intact medicinal plants. They may be used straight or flavorings and other medicinal agents may be added. One of the limitations of teas is the lack of controlled dosage. This problem can be solved by concentrating the tea into a powder and encapsulating or tableting it.

**Tinctures.** This is a clear aqueous solution made by extracting the active principles from the plant by using various concentrations of ethyl alcohol.

**Extracting with Solvents.** A fluid is prepared by extracting the active principals from an herb by using a variety of different solvents. Some of the hydrocarbon solvents, such as hexane and acetone, may be toxic and if the residues are not completely removed they may be harmful. The solvents are then evaporated and the concentration of the active ingredients are reduced to the desired dosage. Unfortunately, residues of these toxic agents may remain. This method is in the process of becoming obsolete because of its potential toxicity.

**Water Distillation Extraction.** The raw herbs are first dried, then they are cut into slices or they are ground into a coarse powder. Often a binder is added to the powder to create a larger mass. The raw herbs are then immersed into water that is heated at low temperatures. After a period of time the thick paste-like residue is slowly decocted. Some manufacturers dry this paste into powder using a variety of methods such as freeze dry or spray dry, etc., and a liquid oral product is produced from the paste.

**Simple Maceration** of a medicinal plant is a slow process so many manufacturers have employed a process known as vertical turbo extraction, which is accomplished with a high speed homogenizer. The shearing and cutting process is a more effective and time saving process than simple maceration. However, turbo extraction must be done with caution because it increases the heat within the container. Anything that increases the temperature may be destructive to the bioactive substances being extracted. This can be controlled by stopping the process periodically or by chilling the container. Turbo extraction has been shown to be superior to simple maceration.

**Percolation Extraction.** Percolation is the most widely used extraction procedure next to maceration. Prior to percolation the medicinal plant is rendered into a suitable form, which is done by comminution or pulverizing, as is done in maceration with use of a shredding mill. However, the material must not be too finely ground.

**Ultrasound Extraction** is accomplished with the use of magnetostrictive or piezoelectric transmitters. Ultrasound is defined as frequencies above 20,000 Hz. The principle effects of ultrasound extraction increases the permeability of the plant cell walls and the release of the bioactive constituents. Ultrasound extraction is more effective when conducted at a temperature of 50°C rather than at boiling temperatures. Ultrasound extraction should be kept at the lower range.

**Extraction by Electrical Energy.** Electrical energy has been used by establishing an electromagnetic field, or using electric discharges. A steel plate is used as a cathode placed at the bottom of the extraction vessel and several carbon electrodes serve as anodes at the top. The extraction proceeds when the electric current is applied.

**Countercurrent Extraction.** In continuous countercurrent extraction a moving solution, emulsion or solid mass is extracted by a liquid phase flowing against it. Continuous countercurrent extraction can be used to advantage when large quantities of material have to be processed. Countercurrent extraction can be used 24 hours a day when the proper equipment is employed.

**Extraction with Supercritical Gases.** The physical properties of a gas are altered when the conditions go beyond the critical point. At the lower density a supercritical gas behaves more like a gas, but when the density is increased it behaves like a liquid. It is the changes in the properties of the gases that permit them to dissolve numerous substances from a medicinal plant. Only those gases, which can be converted into the supercritical state at attainable pressures and temperatures, can be used for extraction purposes. Low temperatures are essential.

For further details on the various methods of extraction see List and Schmidt, 1990.

## Pesticidal Contamination

The contamination of soils by pesticides has become a major problem worldwide, especially in China and India, both of which are major exporters of medicinal plants. Consequentially, medicinal plants are now being routinely screened for pesticidal content. See Tab. 10.1 for a sample quality control test used to screen herbal products for pesticides and insecticides. Most pesticides are carcinogenic and can adversely affect cancer patients that are being treated with contaminated medicinal plants.

The cultivation of medicinal plants has become big business on a global scale. However, this has not solved the problem unless the farmers are properly educated. Ignorant farmers will use pesticides and artificial fertilizers which in turn will contaminate the soils and the plants. Wijesekera (1991) has written an excellent book that discusses this subject in detail. There is such a growing demand for medicinal plants that natural growth can no longer keep up with the demand. Fortunately, there are newer technologies that can be utilized in solving this problem. Furthermore, these technologies need to be exported to developing countries where they can assist them in developing their local economy. The cultivation of Tien Hsien medicinal plants is a matter of special concern as noted in Chapter Two on our visit to China.

## New Technologies Applied in Herbal Concentrating

### NON-TOXIC COMPREHENSIVE EXTRACTION PROCESS

A non-toxic comprehensive extraction process has been developed by Dr. John Pierce. Dr. Pierce received his Ph.D. in analytical chemistry at the University

**Table 10.1**

A sample quality control test of an herbal ingredient.
This test has the capacity to screen for 173 pesticides and insectides.

Page 1 of 2

Method : PAM 242.1 Detection Limit: 0.05 ppm

| COMPOUND | QUANTITY ppm | COMPOUND | QUANTITY ppm |
|---|---|---|---|
| Halogenated Pesticides | | Halogenated Pesticides cont. | |
| Alachlor | ND | Fluchloralin | ND |
| Aldrin | ND | Flucythrinate | ND |
| Anilazine | ND | Folpet | ND |
| Atrazine | ND | Heptachlor | ND |
| Benzoylprop-ethyl | ND | Heptachlor Epoxide | ND |
| BHC (alpha, beta, delta) | ND | Hexachlorobenzene | ND |
| Bifenox | ND | Imazalil | ND |
| Bifenthrin | ND | Iprodione | ND |
| Butachlor | ND | Lambda-Cyhalothrin | ND |
| Captafol | ND | Lindane | ND |
| Captan | ND | Linuron | ND |
| Chlordane | ND | Metalochlor | ND |
| Chlordimeform | ND | Methoxychlor op/pp | ND |
| Clorfenson | ND | Mirex | ND |
| Chlomitrofen | ND | Monolinuron | ND |
| Chloroneb | ND | Myclobutanil | ND |
| Chlorobenzilate | ND | Nitrofen | ND |
| Chlorothalonil | ND | Nuarimol | ND |
| Chloroxuron | ND | Ofurace | ND |
| Chlorpropham | ND | Oxadiazon | ND |
| Cyanazine | ND | Oxyfluorfen | ND |
| Cyfluthrin | ND | PCNB | ND |
| Cypermethrin | ND | Permethrin | ND |
| Cyproconazole | ND | Perthane | ND |
| DCPA | ND | Phosalone | ND |
| DDD | ND | Procydimone | ND |
| DDE | ND | Pronamide | ND |
| DDT | ND | Propanil | ND |
| Deltamethrin | ND | Propiconazole | ND |
| Dichlobenil | ND | Simazine | ND |
| Dichlofluanid | ND | Simetryn | ND |
| Dichlobutrazol | ND | Tebuconazole | ND |
| Dicloran | ND | Terbacil | ND |
| Dicofol | ND | Tetradifon | ND |
| Dieldrin | ND | Thiobencarb | ND |
| Dimethachlor | ND | Tolyfluanid | ND |
| Endosulfan I, II,III | ND | Toxaphene | ND |
| Endrin | ND | Tralomethrin | ND |
| Esfenvalrate | ND | Triadimefon | ND |
| Etaconazole | ND | Triadimenol | ND |
| Ethylan | ND | Vegadex | ND |
| Fenson | ND | Vinclozolin | ND |

Method : PAM 242.1 Detection Limit: 0.05 ppm

| COMPOUND | QUANTITY ppm | COMPOUND | QUANTITY ppm |
|---|---|---|---|
| **Organophosphates** | | **Organophosphates cont.** | |
| Acephate | ND | Methidathion | ND |
| Azinphos-ethyl | ND | Methyl Trithion | ND |
| Azinphos-methyl | ND | Mevinphos | ND |
| Bensulide | ND | Moncrotophos | ND |
| Bromophos | ND | Naled | ND |
| Bromophos-ethyl | ND | Omethoate | ND |
| Cadusafos | ND | Parathion | ND |
| Carbophenothion OA | ND | Parathion Methyl | ND |
| Carbophenothion | ND | Phorate | ND |
| Chlorfenvinphos | ND | Phosmet | ND |
| Chlorpyrifos | ND | Phosphamidon | ND |
| Chlorpyriphos-methyl | ND | Piperophos | ND |
| Chlorthiophos | ND | Pirimiphos-methyl | ND |
| Coumaphos | ND | Profenophos | ND |
| Crotoxyphos | ND | Propetamphos | ND |
| Cyanophos | ND | Prothiofos | ND |
| DEF | ND | Prothoate | ND |
| Demeton-O + S | ND | Quinalphos | ND |
| Demeton-S-Sulfone | ND | Ronnel | ND |
| Dialifos | ND | Sulprophos | ND |
| Diazinon | ND | Terbufos | ND |
| Dichlorvos | ND | Tetrachlorvinphos | ND |
| Dicrotophos | ND | Thiometon | ND |
| Dimethoate | ND | Thionazin | ND |
| Dioxathion | ND | Triazophos | ND |
| Disulfoton | ND | **Methyl Carbamates** | |
| Disulfoton Sulfone | ND | Aldicarb | ND |
| Edifenphos | ND | Aldicarb Sulfone | ND |
| EPN | ND | Aldicarb Sulfoxide | ND |
| Ethion | ND | Aminocarb | ND |
| Ethoprop | ND | Bendiocarb | ND |
| Etrimfos | ND | Bufencarb | ND |
| Fenamiphos | ND | Carbaryl | ND |
| Fenitrothion | ND | Carbofuran | ND |
| Fensulfothion | ND | 3-keto-Carbofuran | ND |
| Fenthion | ND | Ethiofencarb | ND |
| Fonofos | ND | Fenobucarb | ND |
| Formothion | ND | Methiocarb | ND |
| Heptenophos | ND | Methiocarb Sulfone | ND |
| Iprobenfos | ND | Methiocarb Sulfoxide | ND |
| Isazophos | ND | Methomyl | ND |
| Isofenphos | ND | Oxamyl | ND |
| Leptophos | ND | Propoxur (Baygon) | ND |
| Malathion | ND | Thiodicarb | ND |
| Methamidophos | ND | | |

of California at Riverside, California and has spent many years researching non-toxic extraction methods that retain the active ingredients' extractable constituents in their entirety rendering a more bioactive final product. In one step of this process fat-soluble and water-soluble constituents are separated in order to maintain their integrity. These components are reunited in the final step of the process. This research shows great promise for future manufacturing.

## FULL SPECTRUM STANDARDIZED HERBAL EXTRACTS

There is a fundamental principle that needs to be considered when preparing herbal extracts for the market and that is that the medicinal value of a plant is greater than the sum of its phytochemical parts. This statement is making reference to the ancient Chinese concept of synergism. In the medicinal herbal industry "full spectrum" refers to the entire range of phytochemical constituents that are naturally occurring in whatever plant species and particular part of the herb being used. There are some manufacturers who have developed a method of extracting both measurable "standardized" levels of the active ingredients and the full range of constituents from an herb, resulting in a final product that is both high in total active ingredients and that retains the original constituent mix in the original plant.

Research and years of trials have shown that it is best not to isolate a single active ingredient as a medicine. The rationale for this is that through natural selection plants have finely tuned over millennia the chemical balance of their constituents so they could thrive and survive competition. Plants have hormones that control their growth, antibiotics to fight disease, and built-in biological defenses to fend off predators. Each plant has a chemical arsenal that enables them to carry out the complex life processes required for survival. It has been understood by herbalists for many centuries that it is better to trust in the wisdom of this balanced synergy of the plant then to upset it by isolating the individual herbal components.

# Section III:

# A Color Atlas of Chinese Anticancer Plants

# Chapter 11

# A Color Atlas of Chinese Anticancer plants

The phytochemistry and pharmacology of the medicinal plants discussed provide the scientific basis of why these plants work in the treatment of cancer. The plants are listed in alphabetic order according to their scientific generic name.

*Acanthus ilicifolius* Linn. (Fig. 11.1)
*Aconitium carmichaeli* Debx. (Fig. 11.2)
*Acorus gramineus* Soland. (Fig. 11.3)
*Acronychia pedunculata* (Linn.) Mig. (Fig. 11.4)
*Actinidia chinensis* Planch. (Fig. 11.5)
*Adina rubella* (Sieb. & Zuc.) Hance (Fig. 11.6)
*Agaricus arvensis* Schaeff. ex Fr. (Fig. 11.7)
*Agrimonia pilosa* Ledeb. (Fig. 11.8)
*Agrocybe praecox* (Pers ex Fr.) Fayod. (Fig. 11.9)
*Ailanthus altissima* (Mill.) Swingle (Fig. 11.10)
*Akebia trifoliata* (Thunb.) Koidz (Fig. 11.11)
*Allium sativum* Linn. (Fig. 11.12)
*Amanita caesaria* (Scop. Ex Fr.) Pers. ex Schw. (Fig. 11.13)
*Amorphophallus konjac* Belval (Fig. 11.14)
*Ampelopsis brevipedunculata* Trautv. (Fig. 11.15)
*Andrographis paniculata* (Burm f.) Nees (Fig. 11.16)
*Arisaema consanguineum* Schott. (Fig. 11.17)
*Aristolochia debilis* Sieb. et Zucc. (Fig. 11.18)
*Artemesia annua* Linn. (Fig. 11.19)
*Astragalus membranaceus* (Fisch.) Bunge (Fig. 11.20)
*Atractylodes macrocephalus* Koidz. Baizu. (Fig. 11.21)
*Auricularia mesenterica* (Dicks ) Pers. (Fig. 11.22)
*Baphicacanthus cusia* (Nees) Bremek. (Fig. 11.23)
*Berberis poiretii* Schneid. (Fig. 11.24)
*Bjerkandera fumosa* (Pers. ex Fr.) (Fig. 11.25)
*Bolbostemma paniculatum* (Maxim.) Franquet (Fig. 11.26)
*Boletus erythropus* Pers. ex Fr. (Fig. 11.27)
*Brassica oleracea* Linn. (Fig. 11.28)
*Brassica oleracea* var. *italica* Plenck. (Fig. 11.29)
*Brucea javanica* (Linn.) Merr. (Fig. 11.30)

*Camellia sinensis* (Linn.) Kuntze (Fig. 11.31)
*Camptotheca acuminata* Decne. (Fig. 11.32)
*Cantharanthus roseus* (Linn.) G. Don. (Fig. 11.33)
*Cantharellus cibarius* Fr. (Fig. 11.34)
*Carthamus tinctorius* Linn. (Fig. 11.35)
*Cephalotaxus harringtonia* K. Koch (Fig. 11.36)
*Chelidonium majus* Linn. (Fig. 11.37)
*Cimicifuga heracleifolia* Kom. (Fig. 11.38)
*Clematis chinensis* Osbeck (Fig. 11.39)
*Clitocybe nebularis* (Batsch. ex Fr.) Qué (Fig. 11.40)
*Codonopsis pilosula* (Franch.) Nannf. (Fig. 11.41)
*Coix lacryma* Linn. (Fig. 11.42)
*Coprinus atramentarius* (Bull.) Fr. (Fig. 11.43)
*Coptis chinensis* Franch. (Fig. 11.44)
*Cordyceps sinensis* (Berk.) Saccardo (Fig. 11.45)
*Coriolopsis occidentalis* (Kl.) Murr. (Fig. 11.46)
*Coriolus versicolor* (Linn. ex Fr.) (Fig. 11.47)
*Cortinarius violaceus* (Linn.) Fr. (Fig. 11.48)
*Crocus sativas* Linn. (Fig. 11.49)
*Crotalaria sessilflora* Linn. (Fig. 11.50)
*Croton tiglium* Linn. (Fig. 11.51)
*Curcuma aromatica* Salisb. (Fig. 11.52)
*Daedaleopsis tricolor* (Fr.) Band. et Sing. (Fig. 11.53)
*Daphne genkwa* Sieb. et Zucc. (Fig. 11.54)
*Dictyophora indusiata* (Vent. ex Pers.) Fischer (Fig. 11.55)
*Dioscorea bulbifera* Linn. (Fig. 11.56)
*Duchesnea indica* (Andr.) Focke (Fig. 11.57)
*Dysosma pleiantha* (Hance) Woodson (Fig. 11.58)
*Echinops latifolius* Tausch. (Fig. 11.59)
*Eclipta prostrata* Linn. (Fig. 11.60)
*Eleutherococcus senticosus* (Rupr. et Maxim.) Maxim. (Fig. 11.61)
*Engleromyces goetzi* P. Henn. (Fig. 11.62)
*Euphorbia kansui* T. N. Lion ex T. P. Wang (Fig. 11.63)
*Ficus carica* Linn. (Fig. 11.64)
*Flamulina velutipes* (Curt. ex Fr.) Sing. (Fig. 11.65)
*Fomitopsis officinalis* (Vill. ex Fr.) Bond et Sing. (Fig. 11.66)
*Ganoderma lucidum* (Leys. ex Fr.) Karst. (Fig. 11.67)
*Gardenia jasminoides* Ellis (Fig. 11.68)
*Gloeophyllum trabeum* (Pers. ex Fr.) Murr. (Fig. 11.69)
*Glycyrrhiza uralensis* Linn. Gancao (Fig. 11.70)
*Gossypium hirsutum* Linn. (Fig. 11.71)

*Grifola frondosus* (Dicks. ex Fr. ) S. F. Gray (Fig. 11.72)
*Gymnopilus liquiritae* (Pers. ex Fr.) Karst. (Fig. 11.73)
*Gyrophana lacrymans* (Wulf.) Pat. (Fig. 11.74)
*Gyroporus castaneus* (Bull. ex Fr.) Quél. (Fig. 11.75)
*Hericeum erinaceus* (Bull. ex Fr.) Pers. (Fig. 11.76)
*Hibiscus mutabilis* Linn. (Fig. 11.77)
*Hordeum vulgare* Linn. (Fig. 11.78)
*Houttuynia cordata* Thunb. (Fig. 11.79)
*Impatiens balsamina* Linn. (Fig. 11.80)
*Iphigenia indica* Kunth. (Fig. 11.81)
*Iris lactae* Pall. var *chinensis* (Fisch.) Kioidz (Fig. 11.82)
*Juglans regia* Linn. (Fig. 11.83)
*Lactarius hatsudake* Tanaka (Fig. 11.84)
*Lampteromyces japonicus* (Kawam. ) Sing. (Fig. 11.85)
*Lentinus edodes* (Berk.) Sing (Fig. 11.86)
*Lepista nuda* (Bull. ex Fr.) Cooke (Fig. 11.87)
*Ligustrum lucidum* Ait. (Fig. 11.88)
*Livistona chinensis* R. Br. (Fig. 11.89)
*Lloydella subpileata* (Berk. et Curt.) Hölm. & Litsch. (Fig. 11.90)
*Lobelia chinensis* Lour. (Fig. 11.91)
*Lonicera japonica* Thunb. (Fig. 11.92)
*Lycium barbarum* Linn. (Fig. 11.93)
*Lycoris radiata* (L. Hérit.) Herb. (Fig. 11.94)
*Lysurus mokusin* (Linn. ex Pers.) Fr. (Fig. 11.95)
*Mahonia bealei* (Fort.) Carr. (Fig. 11.96)
*Marsdenia tenacissima* (Roxb.) Wight et Arn. (Fig. 11.97)
*Morus alba* Linn. (Fig. 11.98)
*Oldenlandia diffusa* (Wild.) Roxb. (Fig. 11.99)
*Oudemansiella radicata* (Relh. ex Fr.) Sing (Fig. 11.100)
*Paeonia suffruticosa* Andrews (Fig. 11.101)
*Panax ginseng* C. A. Meyer (Fig. 11.102)
*Panellus stypticus* (Bull. ex Fr.) Karst. (Fig. 11.103)
*Panus conchatus* (Bull. ex Fr.) Karst. (Fig. 11.104)
*Paris polyphylla* Sm. (Fig. 11.105)
*Patrinia scabiosaefolia* Fisch. (Fig. 11.106)
*Phellinus igniarius* (Linn. ex Fr.) Quél. (Fig. 11.107)
*Pholiota lubrica* (Fr.) Sing. (Fig. 11.108)
*Physalis alkekengi* Linn. var. *franchetti* (Masters) Hort. (Fig. 11.109)
*Pinellia ternata* (Thunb.) (Fig. 11.110)
*Pleurotus ostreatus* (Jacq. ex Fr.) Quél. (Fig. 11.111)
*Pogostemon cablin* (Blanco) Benth. (Fig. 11.112)

*Polygonum cuspidatum* Sieb. et Zucc. (Fig. 11.113)
*Polyporus umbellatus* (Pers.) Fries. (Fig. 11.114)
*Poria cocos* (Schw.) Wolf (Fig. 11.115)
*Prunella vulgaris* Linn. (Fig. 11.116)
*Prunus armeniaca* Linn. (Fig. 11.117)
*Pseudostellaria heterophylla* (Miq.) Pax ex Pax et Hoffm. (Fig. 11.118)
*Psoralea corylifolia* Linn. (Fig. 11.119)
*Pyropolyporus fomentarius* (Linn. ex Fr.) Teng (Fig. 11.120)
*Ranunculus japonicus* Thunb. (Fig. 11.121)
*Rheum officinale* Baillon (Fig. 11.122)
*Rhodophyllus clypeatus* (Linn. ex Fr.) Quél (Fig. 11.123)
*Ricinus communis* Linn. (Fig. 11.124)
*Rozites caperata* (Pers. ex Fr.) Karst. (Fig. 11.125)
*Rumex japonica* Houtt. (Fig. 11.126)
*Russula delica* Fr. (Fig. 11.127)
*Salvia miltiorrhiza* Bge. (Fig. 11.128)
*Sarcandra glabra* (Thun.) Nakei (Fig. 11.129)
*Sarcodon fulgineo-albus* (Fr.) Quél (Fig. 11.130)
*Sargassum pallidum* (Turn.) C. Ag. (Fig. 11.131)
*Schizandra chinensis* (Turcz.) Baill. (Fig. 11.132)
*Schizophyllum commune* Fr. (Fig. 11.133)
*Sclerotinia sclerotiorum* (Lib.) de Bary (Fig. 11.134)
*Scutellaria barbata* Don (Fig. 11.135)
*Selaginella doederleinii* Hieron. (Fig. 11.136)
*Senecio scandens* Buch.-Hamil. (Fig. 11.137)
*Simblum gracile* Berk. (Fig. 11.138)
*Smilax china* Linn. (Fig. 11.139)
*Solanum nigrum* Linn. (Fig. 11.140)
*Sophora flavescens* Ait. (Fig. 11.141)
*Sparganium stoloniferum* Buch.-Hamil. (Fig. 11.142)
*Stephania tetrandra* S. Moore (Fig. 11.143)
*Strobilomyces floccopus* Karst. (Fig. 11.144)
*Strychnos nux-vomica* Linn. (Fig. 11.145)
*Suillus aeruginascens* (Secr.) Snell (Fig. 11.146)
*Taraxacum mongolicum* Hand.-Mazz. (Fig. 11.147)
*Terfezia leonis* Tul. (Fig. 11.148)
*Terminalia chebula* Retz. (Fig. 11.149)
*Trametes cinnabarina* (Jacq.) Fr. (Fig. 11.150)
*Trapa bispinosa* Roxb. (Fig. 11.151)
*Tremella fuciformis* Berk. (Fig. 11.152)
*Tricholoma matsuke* (S. Ito et Imai) Sing. (Fig. 11.153)

*Trichosanthes kirilowii* Maxim. (Fig. 11.154)
*Tripterygium wilfordii* Hook. (Fig. 11.155)
*Usnea longissima* Ach. (Fig. 11.156)
*Ustilago maydis* (DC. ) Corda (Fig. 11.157)
*Wikstroemia indica* C. A. Meyer (Fig. 11.158)
*Xanthium sibiricum* Patrin. (Fig. 11.159)
*Zanthoxylum nitidum* (Roxb. ) D.C. (Fig. 11.160)
*Ziziphus jujuba* Mill. (Fig. 11.161)

## Authors' Comments

The *Panax ginseng* used in the Tien Hsien formula lives in a mountainous region where germanium is available. When organic germanium is taken up in the plant it is available to the plant in the sesquioxide form. According to Asai (1980) germanium sesquioxide has been successfully used in the treatment of various types of cancer and leukemia.

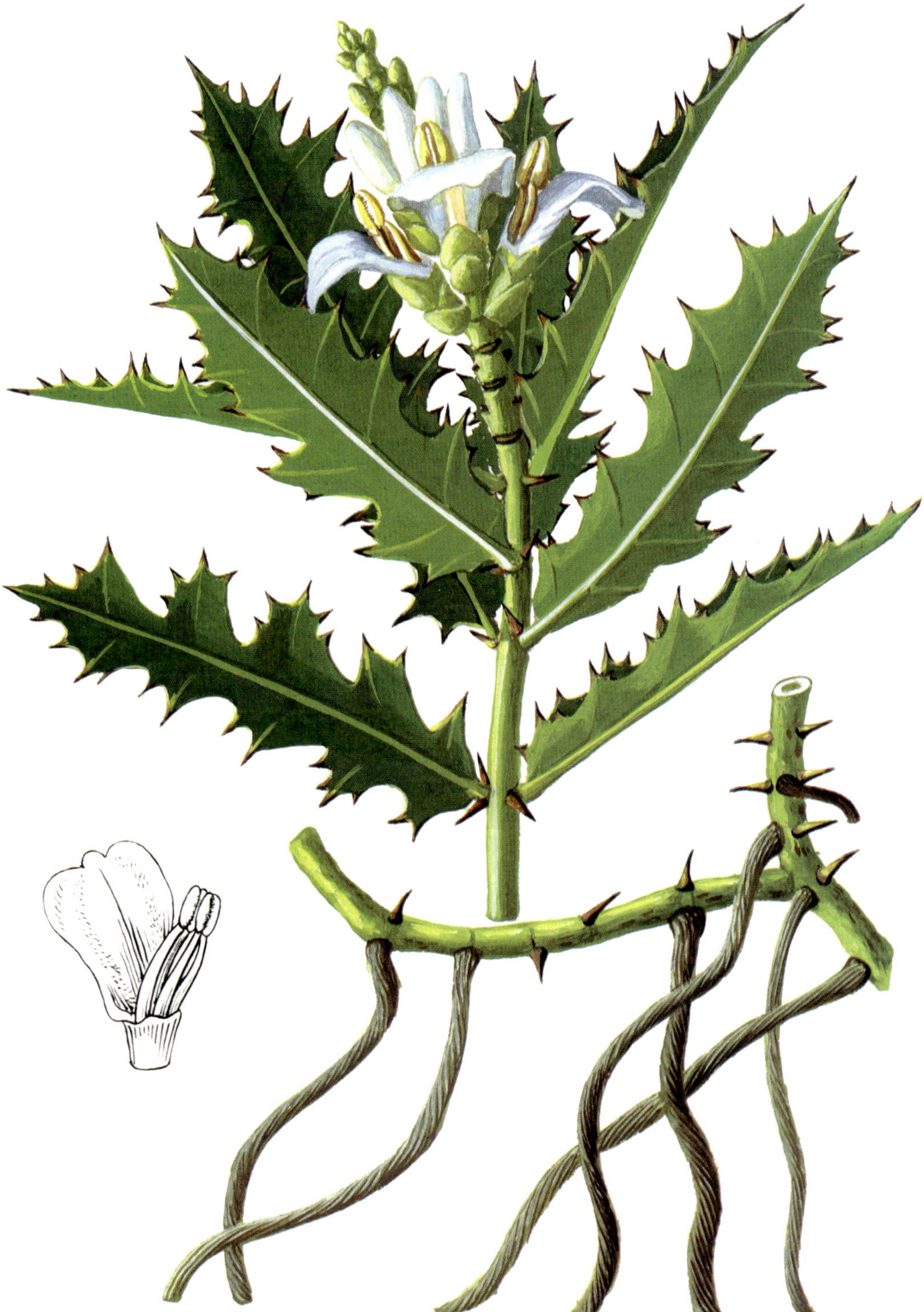

Fig. 11.1. ***Acanthus ilicifolius*** Linn. —This plant contains flavones and amino acids, which have anticancer properties, and is used to treat malignancy (Cheung, 1979; Duke & Ayensu, 1985; Hsu, et al, 1986).

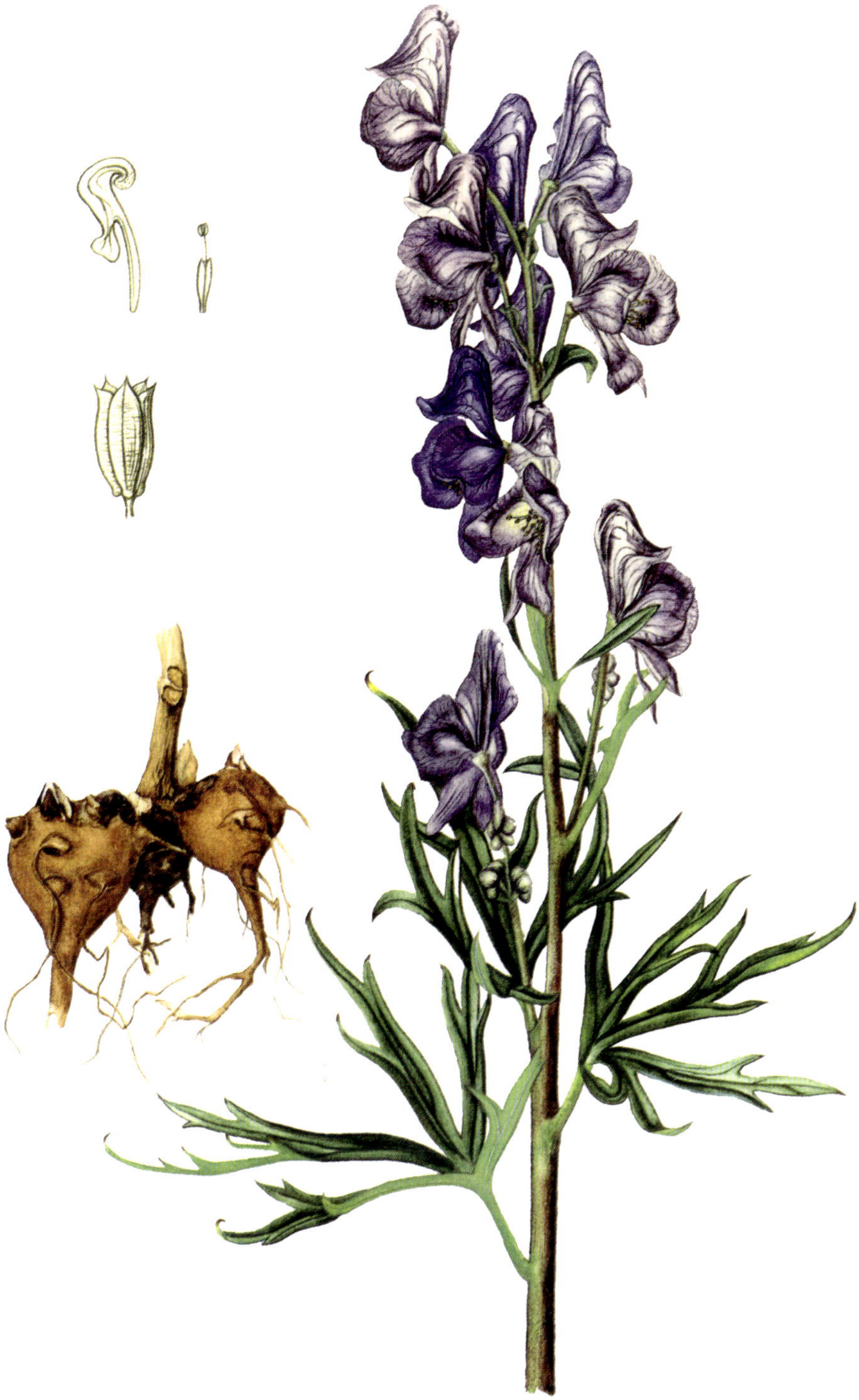

Fig. 11.2. ***Aconitium carmichaeli*** Debx. — The root contains aconitine, hypaconitine, and mesaconitine, which have been found to inhibit human lung, liver and stomach cancer cell lines, and sarcoma-180 in rats. It is used in the treatment of gastric carcinoma, lung cancer, and liver cancer. (Minyi, 1992; Lee, 1999)

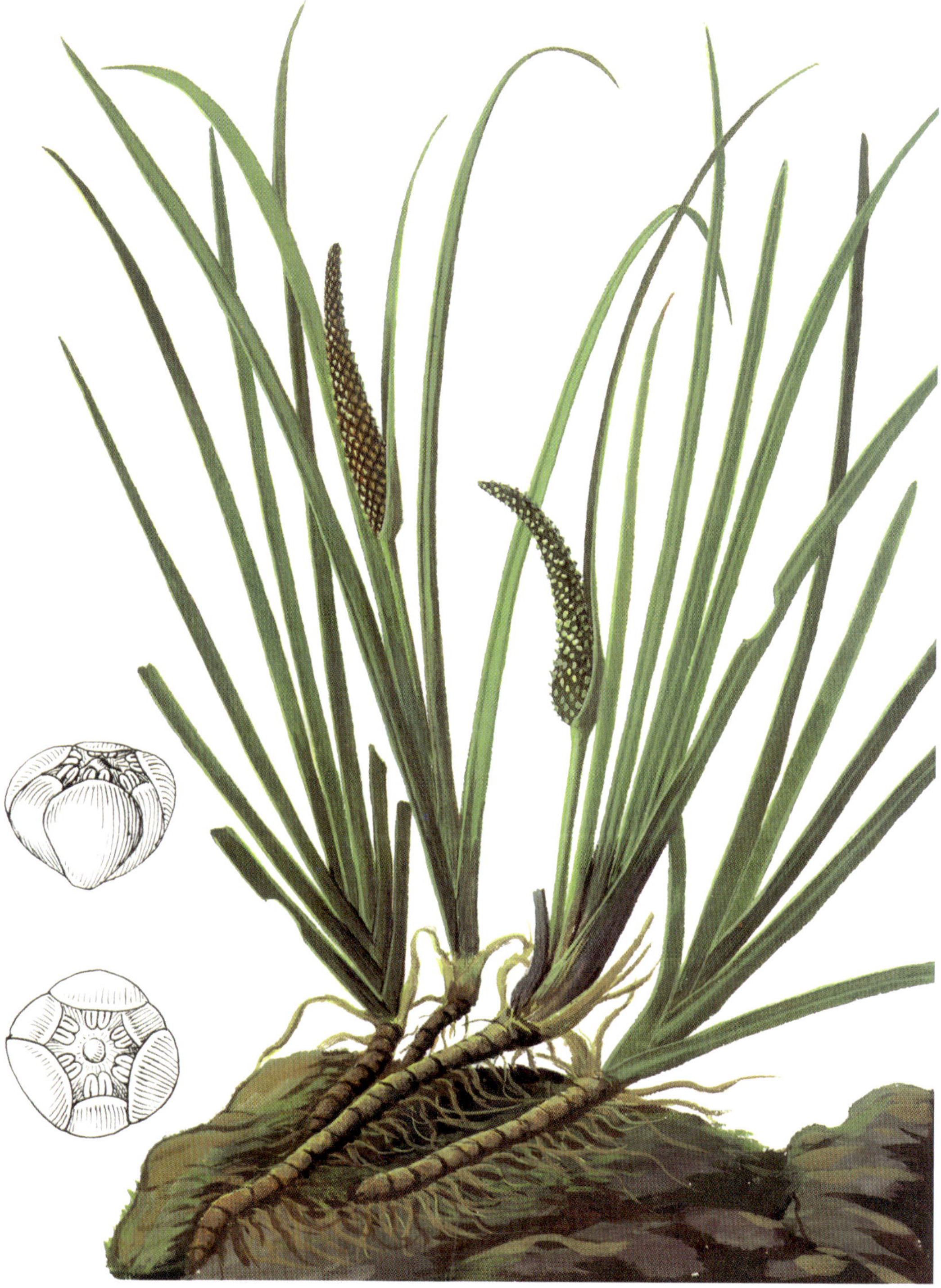

Fig. 11.3. ***Acorus gramineus*** Soland. — The rhizome contains asarone, palmitic acid, and a phenol compound. In vivo it inhibits sarcoma-180 and hepatoma in mice; in vitro it inhibits Hela cell, and strains of human lung and gastric carcinomas, and kills Erlich's ascites carcinoma cells of mice and HL-60 cells. It has been used in the treatment of cervical cancer, intracranial tumors, and various other forms of cancer. (Hsu, et al, 1986; Minyi, 1992; Lee, 1999)

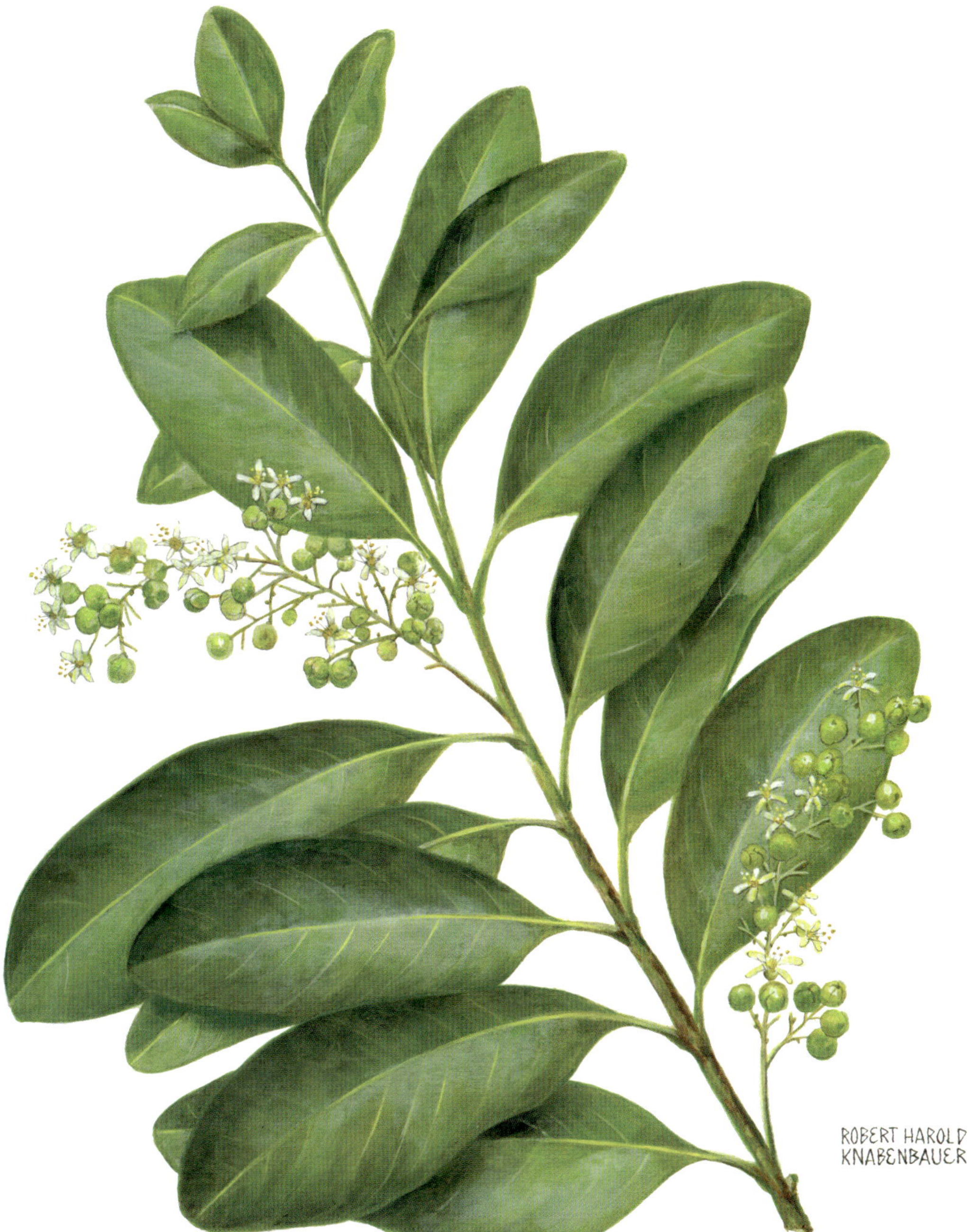


Fig. 11.4. ***Acronychia pedunculata*** (Linn.) Mig. — This plant contains β-sitosterol, bauerenol, acronycine, nitroacronycine, acrovestone, acronylin, 6-demethylacronylin, and essential oils. Acronycine is effective against reticulocytic leukemia-615 in mice and reticulohistiocytoma, and inhibits mouse liver cancer, cervical cancer-14 in mice, myeloid leukemia-1499, plasma cell myeloma, and adenocancer-755. It inhibits cancer cells, but does not affect normal cells. It has been used in the treatment of Hodgkin's disease, fibrosarcoma, liposarcoma, and various other cancers including esophageal, stomach, liver, and rectal cancer. (Duke & Ayensu, 1985; Hsu, et al, 1986; Minyi,1992; Duong, 1993; Lee, 1999)

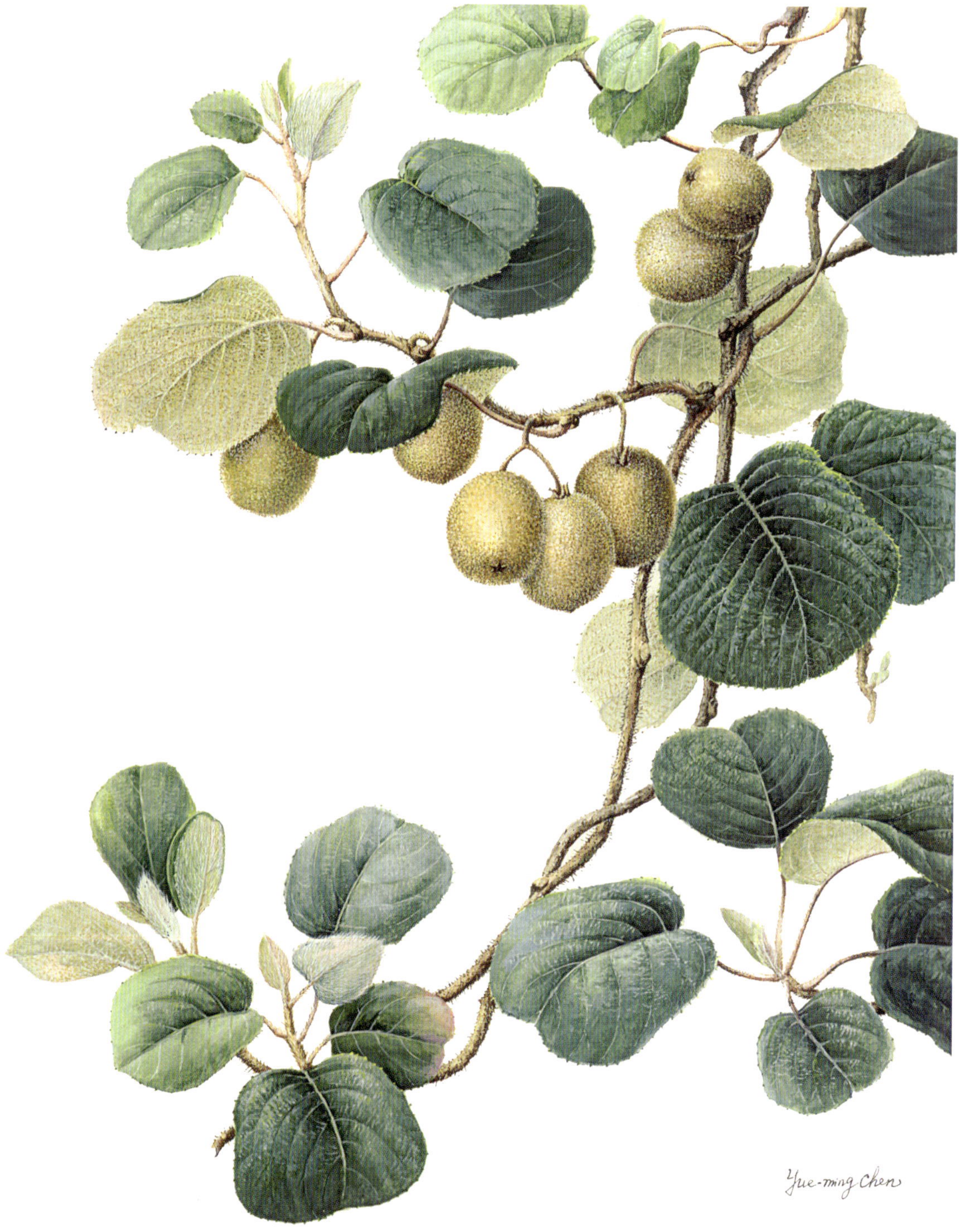


Fig. 11.5. ***Actinidia chinensis*** Planch. — This plant is rich in vitamin C and contains actinidine, quercetin, kaempterol, cumaric acid, leucodelphinidin, leucocyanidin, caffeine, and volatile oils. It inhibits Erlich's ascites carcinoma, sarcoma-180, and transplanted tumors in mice. It has been used in the treatment of esophageal, stomach, liver, lung, and mammary cancer. (Duke & Ayensu, 1985; Minyi, 1992; Huang, 1999; Lee, 1999)

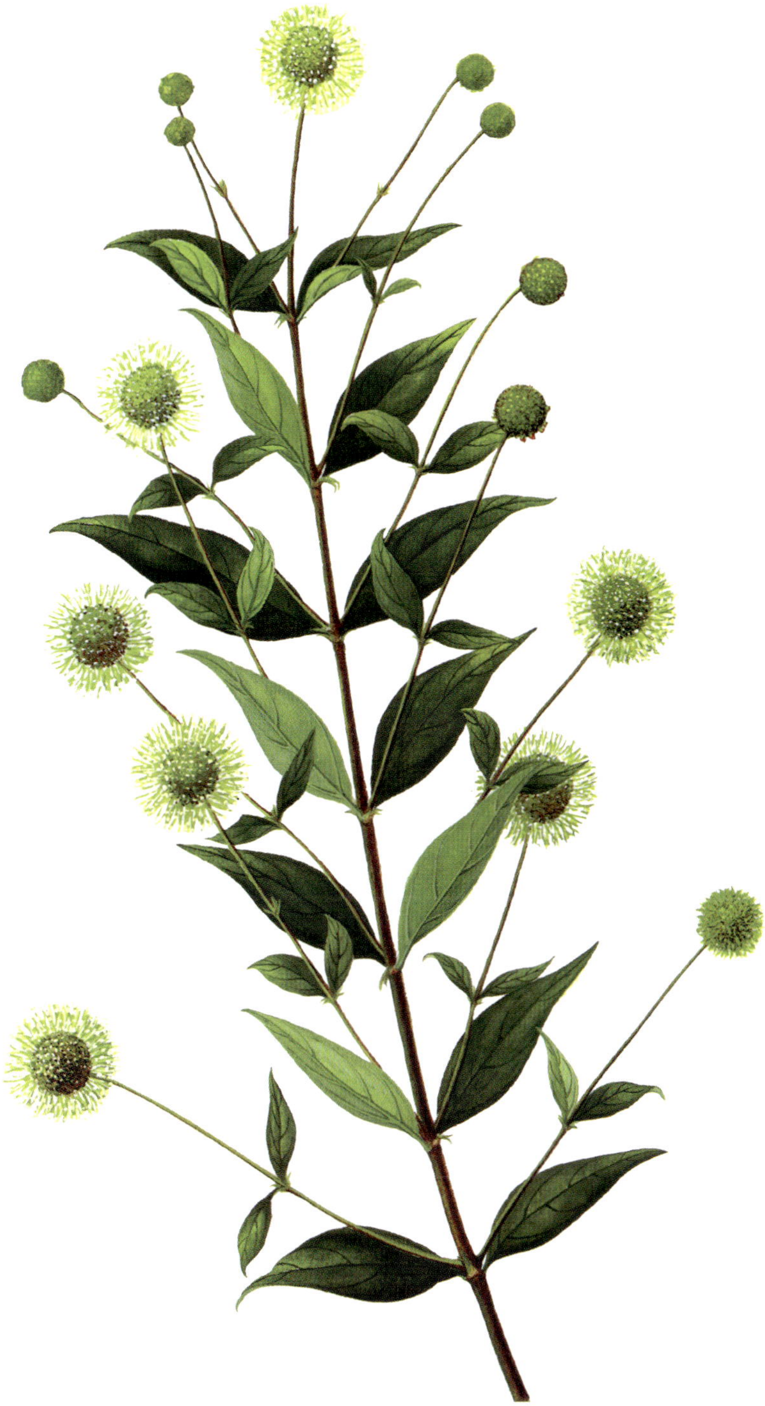

Fig. 11.6. ***Adina rubella*** (Sieb. & Zuc.) Hance — This plant contains triterpenoids, β-sitosterol, salicyclic acid, pectine, ursolic acid, tannin, and alkaloids. It inhibits sarcoma-180, cervical cancer cells, and Walker's cancer-256 in rats and JTC-26 in mice and has been used in the treatment of lymphoma, cancer of the esophagus, stomach, lungs, liver, colon, and cervix. (Hsu, et al, 1986; Minyi, 1992; Huang, 1999; Lee, 1999)

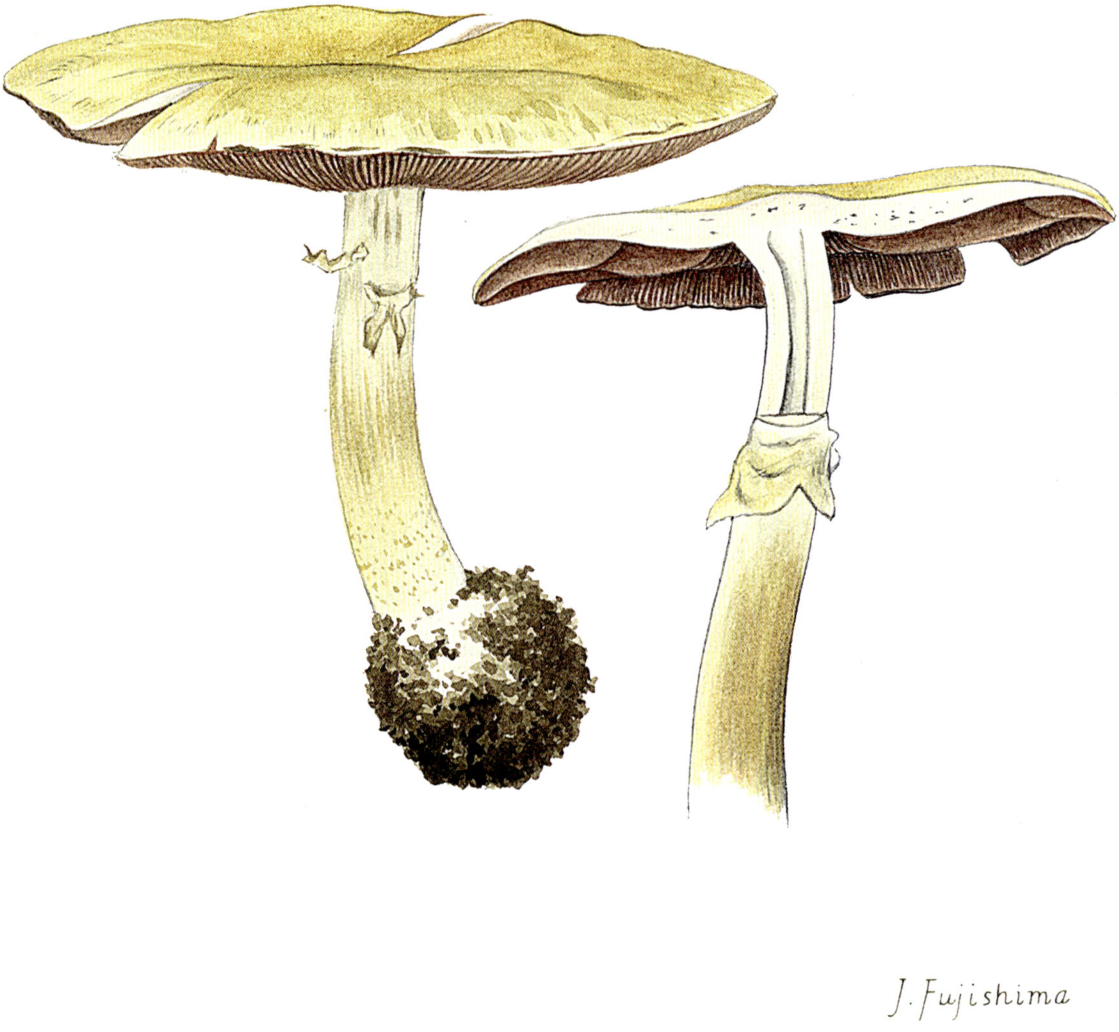


Fig. 11.7. ***Agaricus arvensis*** Schaeff. ex Fr. — This mushroom contains a variety of polysaccharides, which in laboratory mice inhibits sarcoma-180 and Ehrlich's carcinoma (Ying, et al, 1987).

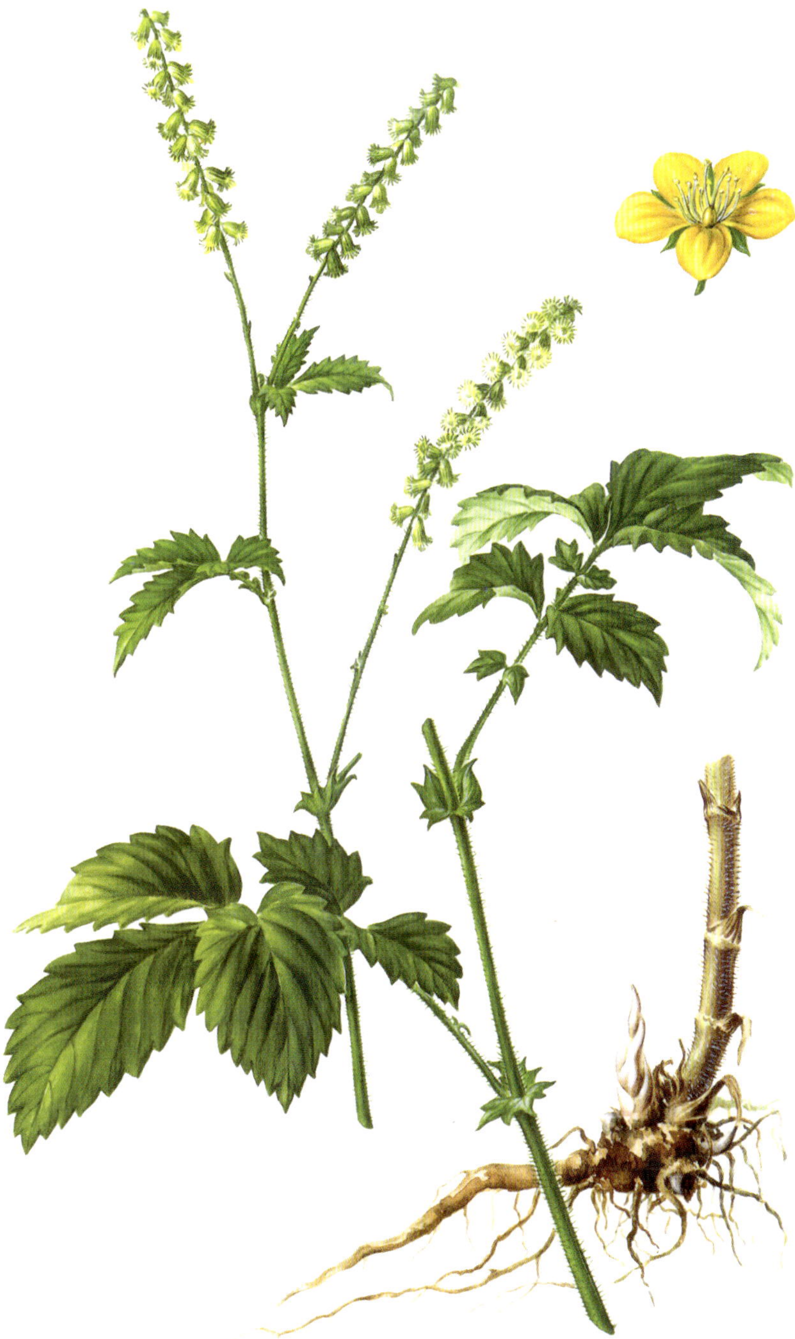

Fig. 11.8. ***Agrimonia pilosa*** Ledeb. — This plant contains agrimonins, agrimonol (= agrimonine), the derivatives of phloroglucinol agrimols A, B, C, D, and E, agrimonolide, agrimophol, phlobaphene, pyrogallic acid, pimic acid, and flavenoid glycosides, volatile oils, tannins, such as agrimoniin, and vitamins C and K. It inhibits human cancer cells JTC-26 in vitro, kills HL-60, and is effective against sarcoma-180 in rats; it also has been shown to increase the survival rat of mice implanted with Erlich's ascites carcinoma. It has been used in the treatment of esophageal and lung cancer and for tumors of the digestive system and bones. (Chang & But, 1986; Minyi, 1992; Huang, 1999; Lee, 1999)

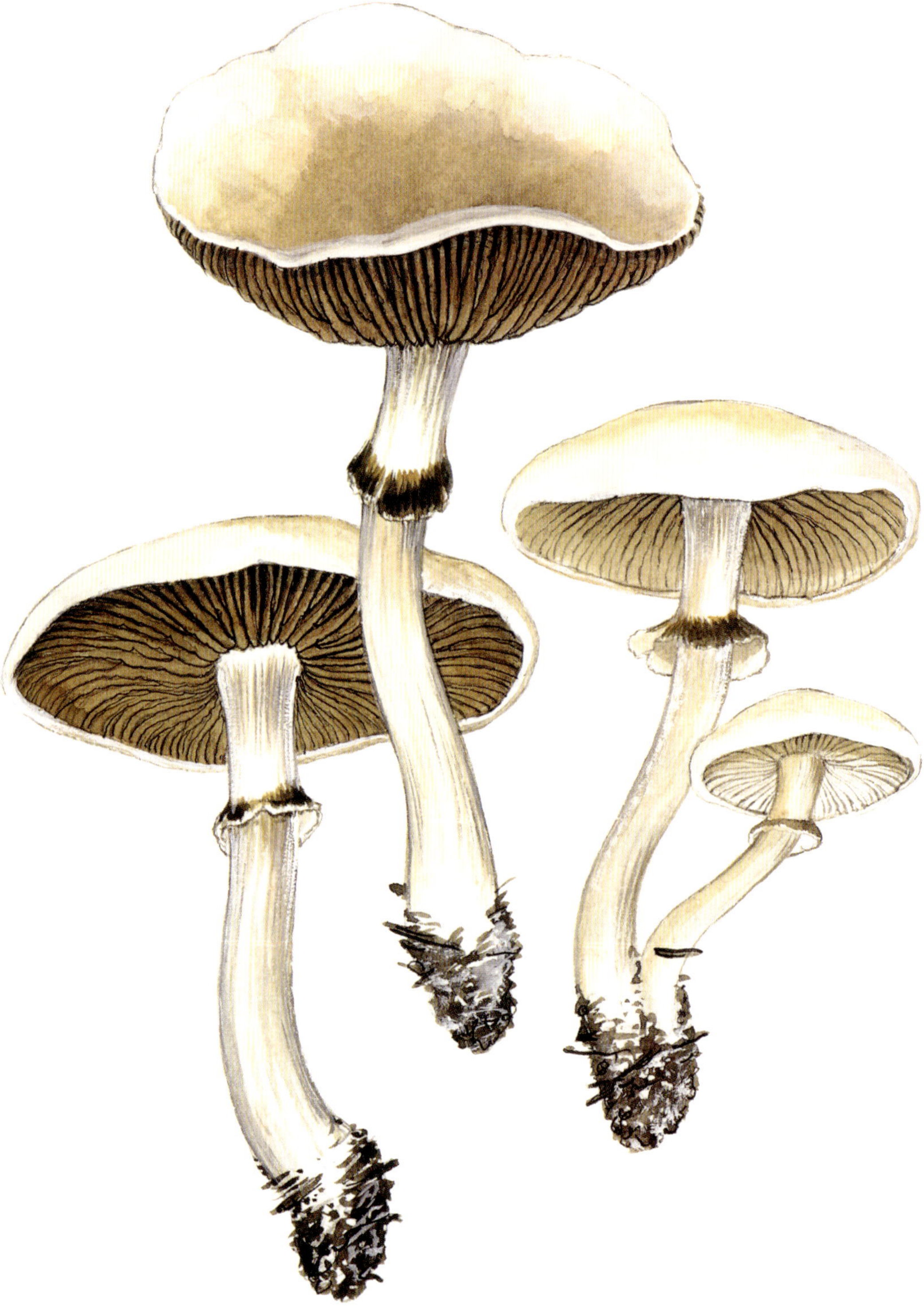

Fig. 11.9. ***Agrocybe praecox*** (Pers ex Fr.) Fayod. — This mushroom contains polysaccharides and other substances, which have been found to inhibit sarcoma-180 and Ehrlich's carcinoma (Ying, et al, 1987).

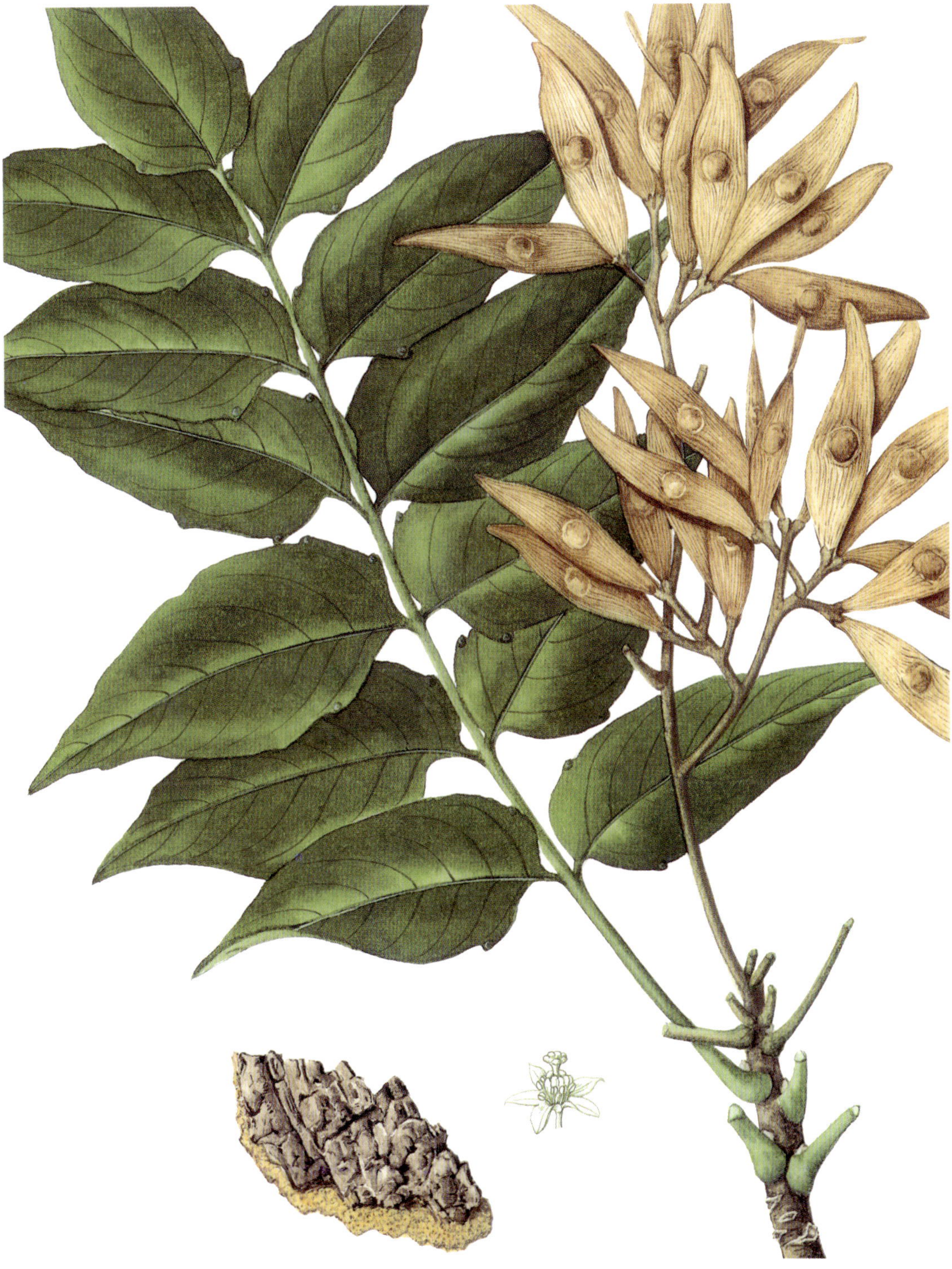

Fig. 11.10. ***Ailanthus altissima*** (Mill.) Swingle — This plant contains ailanthone, margoside, mersosin, tannin, and amarolide. It inhibits murine tumors sarcoma-37, sarcoma-180, HL-60 cells, and leukemia-16, and has been used in the treatment of cervical and stomach cancer. (Hsu, et al, 1986; Minyi, 1992; Lee, 1999)

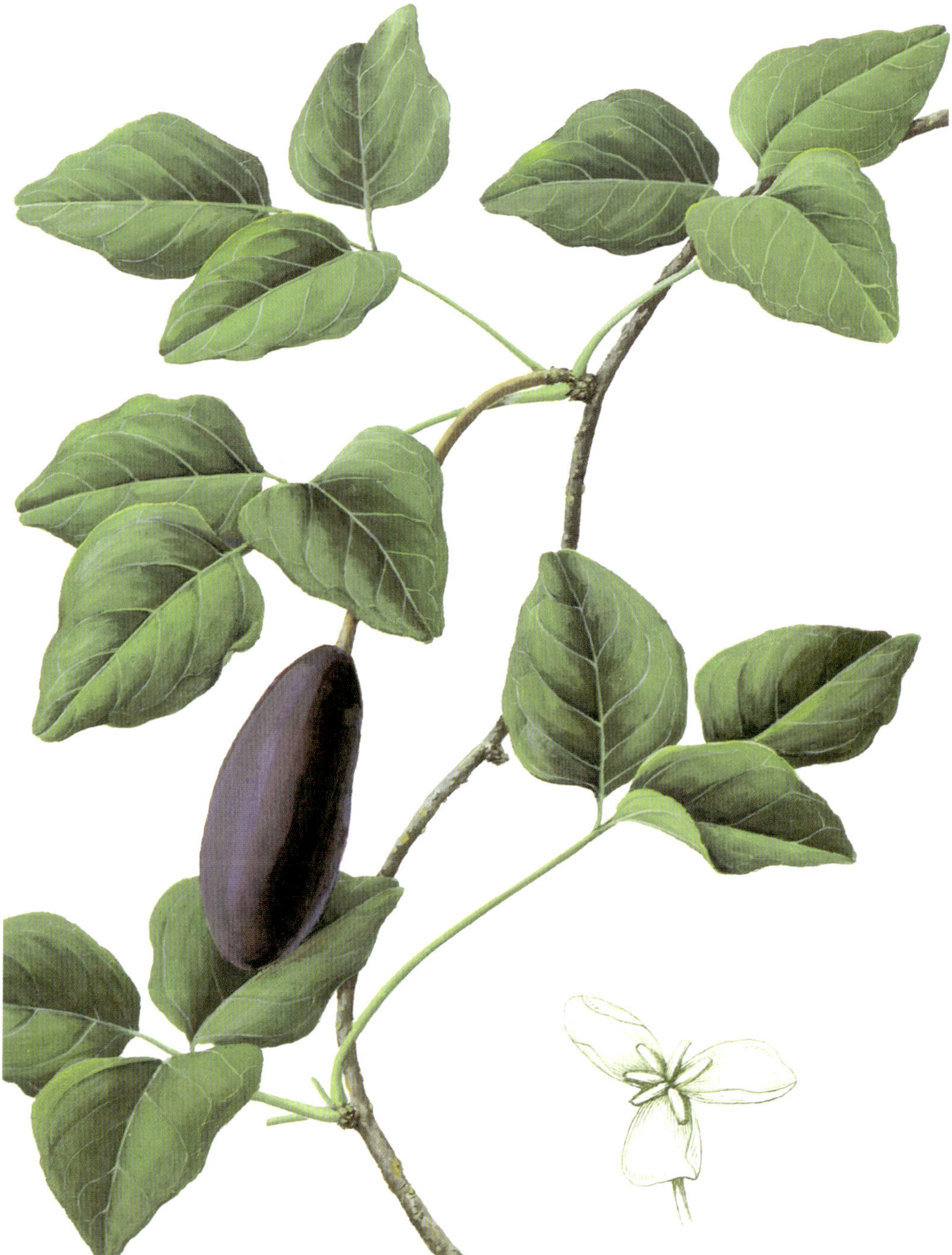

Fig. 11.11. ***Akebia trifoliata*** (Thunb.) Koidz — This plant contains akebin, hydrolyzed products of akebin (hederagenin, oleanolic acid, glucose, and rhamnose), palmitic acid, stearic acid, oleic acid, linoleic acid, acetic acid, and the triterpenoid saponins: akebia saponins A, B, C, D, E, F, and G. It inhibits sarcoma-37 and sarcoma-180 in rats, and JTC-26 in vitro. It has been used in the treatment of lymphosarcoma, and cancers of the mouth, stomach, and pancreas. (Hsu, et al, 1986; Minyi, 1992; Lee, 1999)

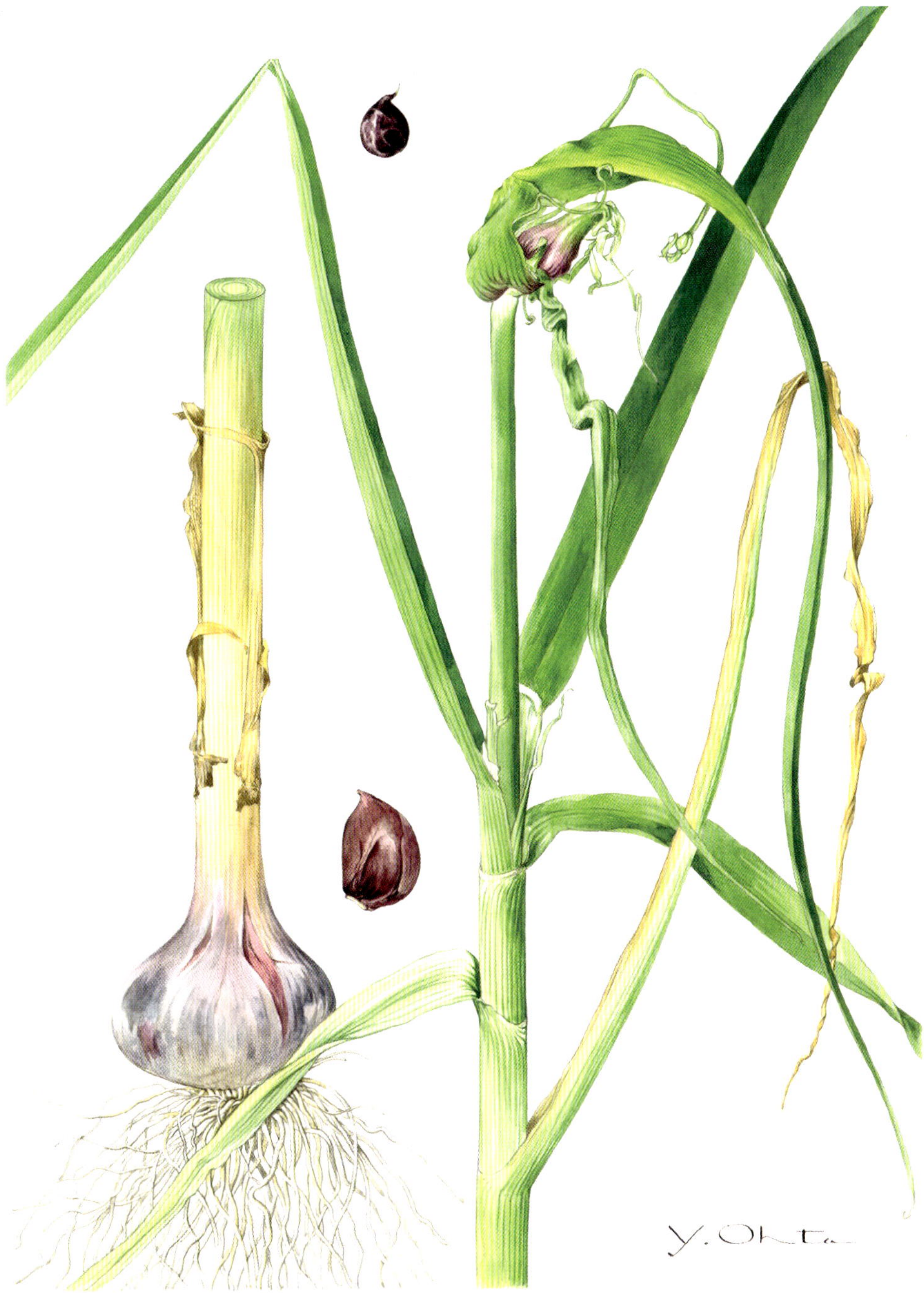


Fig. 11.12. ***Allium sativum*** Linn. — The bulb contains allitin, which when hydrolyzed by allinase produces allicin and diallyldisulfide, allistatin, glucominol, neo-allicin, diallylthiosulfonate, steroid saponins, and polysaccharides, and allisatin. It inhibits reticular cell tumors, sarcoma-180, parenchymal liver cancer, cervical cancer-14, JTC-26, transplanted human gastric cell line MGC80-3 in mice, and is effective against Erlich's ascites carcinoma and MTK-III in rats, and various other tumors in laboratory animals. It has been used to treat leukemia, nasopharyngeal carcinoma, lymphoepithelioma, carcinomas of the lung, stomach, and heart, and has preventative action against stomach cancer. (Chang & But, 1986; Minyi, 1992; Huang, 1999; Lee, 1999)

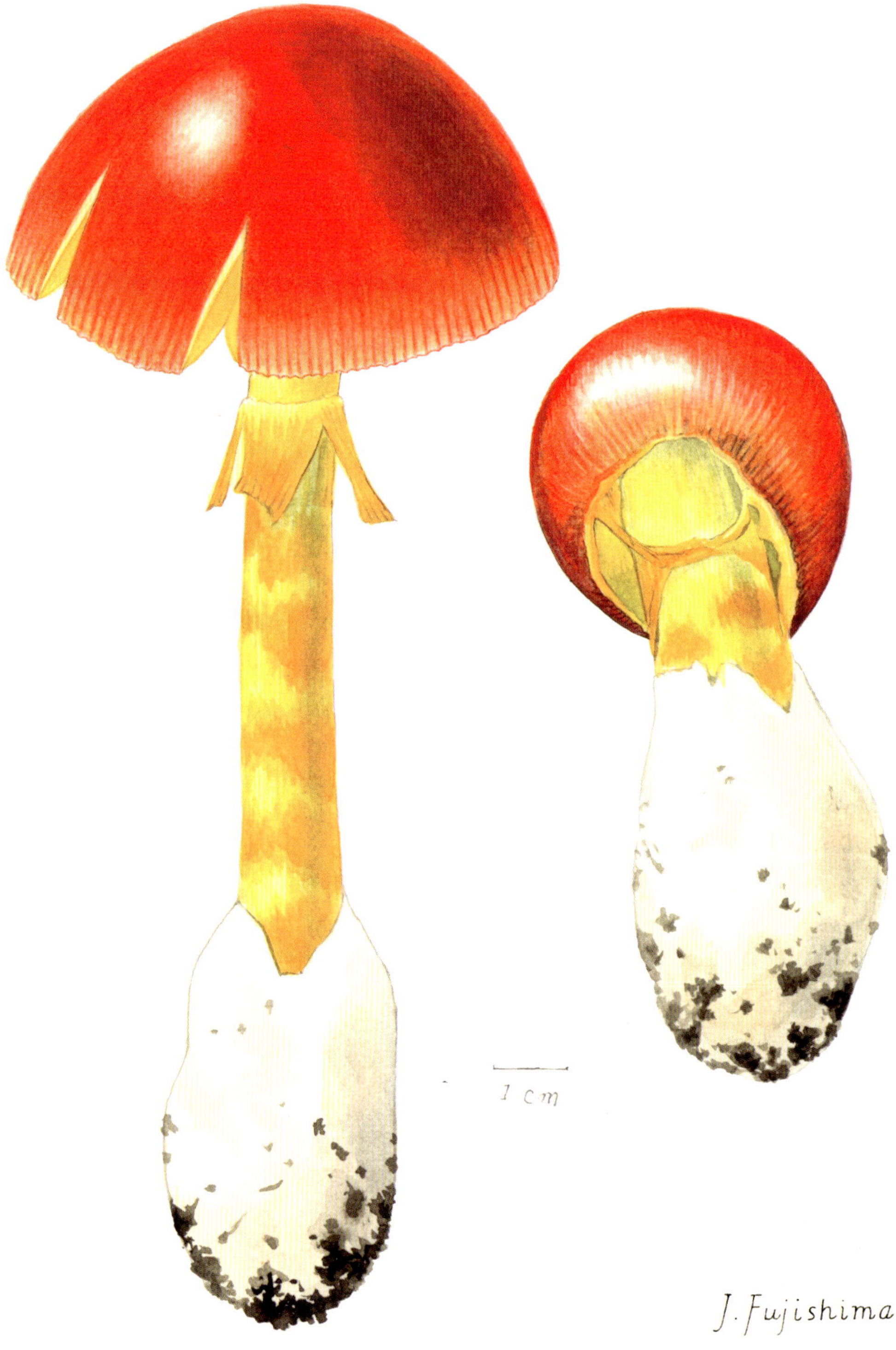


Fig. 11.13. ***Amanita caesaria*** (Scop. ex Fr.) Pers. ex Schw. — Extracts from the sporophore of this mushroom inhibit sarcoma-180 in laboratory mice (Jianzhe, et al, 1987).

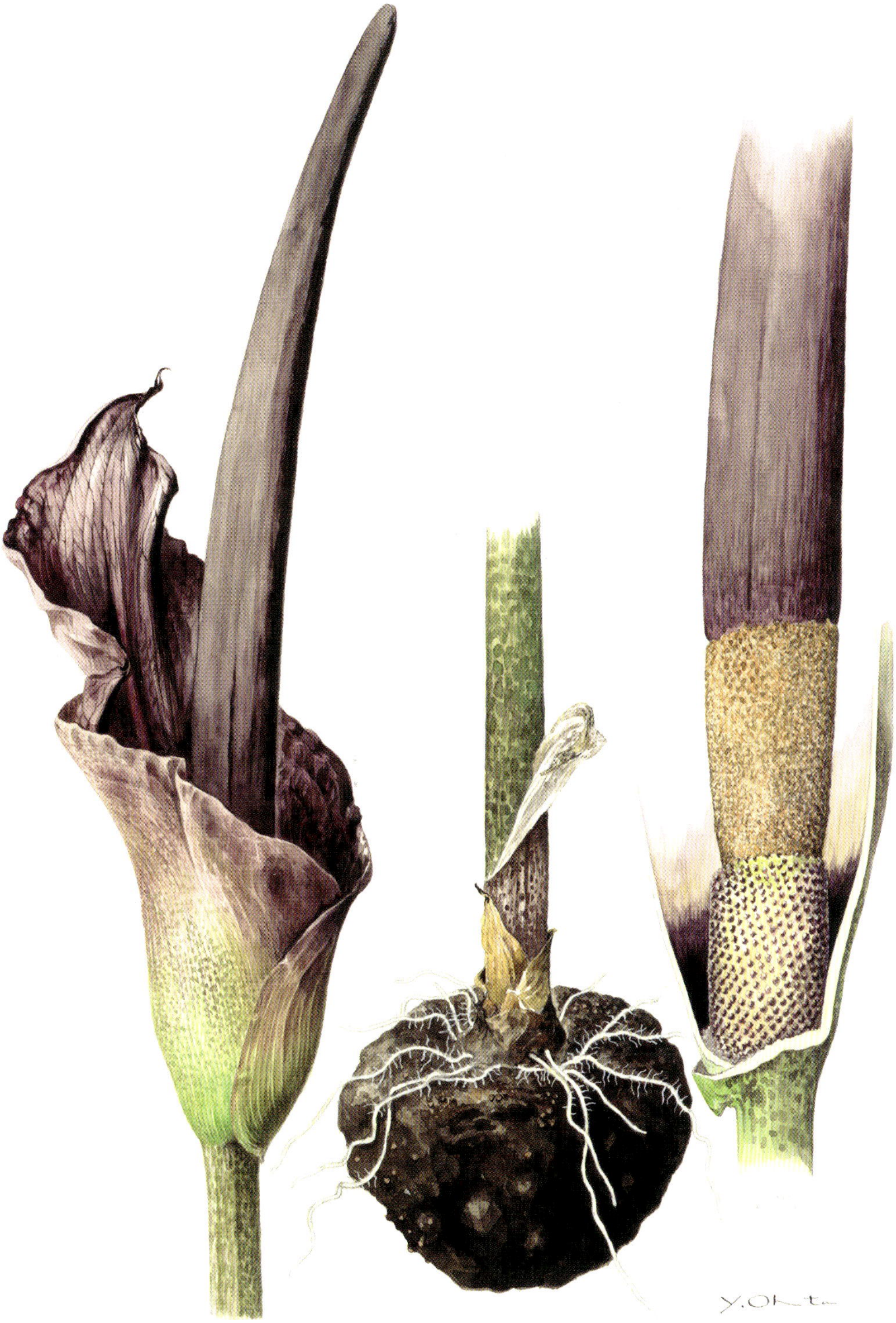

Fig. 11.14. ***Amorphophallus konjac*** Belval — The rhizome contains glucomannan, adenine, trigonelline, choline, and trimethylamine; the flower contains large quantities of vitamin $B_1$. It inhibits sarcoma-180, ESC, and HepS in laboratory animals. (Hsu, et al, 1986; Minyi, 1992; Lee, 1999)

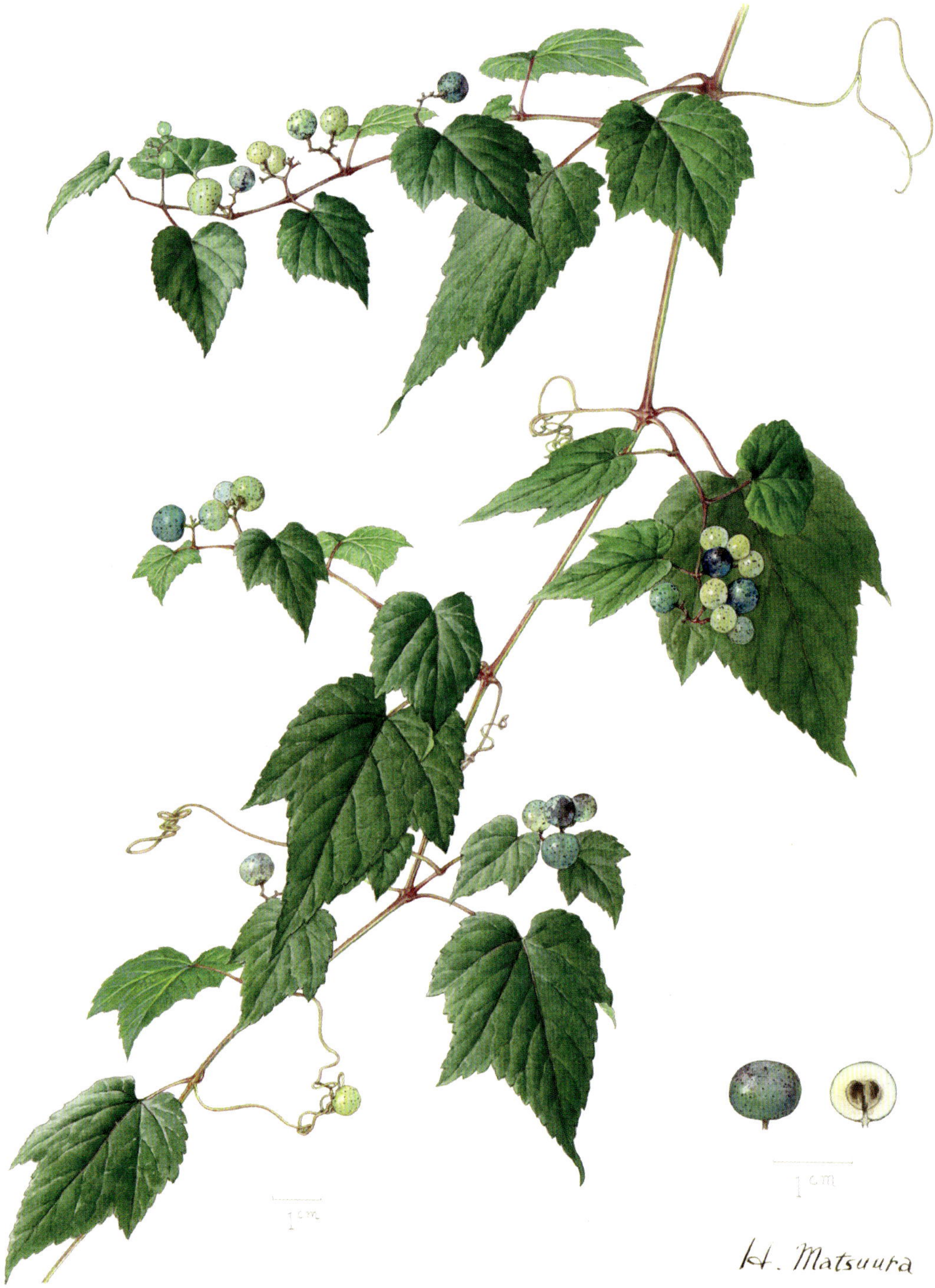


Fig. 11.15. ***Ampelopsis brevipedunculata*** Trautv. — This plant contains ampelopsin, myricetin, flavenoid glycosides, phenols, amino acids, and polysaccharides. It has been found to inhibit sarcoma-180 in mice, and is used in the treatment of carcinomas of the gastrointestinal tract, lymphoma, mammary cancer, and cancers of the lung, stomach, and kidney in humans. (Minyi, 1992; Huang, 1999; Lee, 1999)

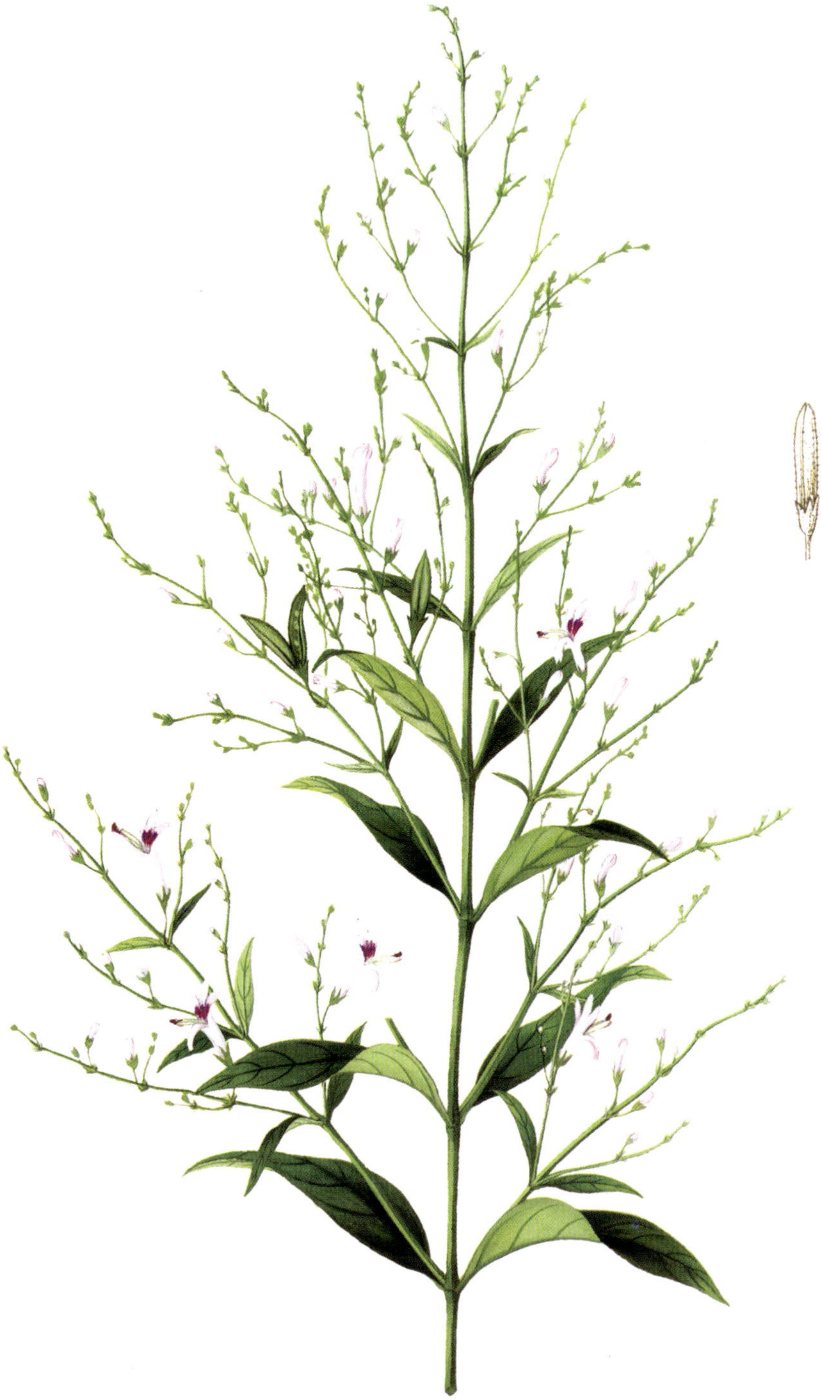

Fig. 11.16. ***Andrographis paniculata*** (Burm f.) Nees — This plant contains andrographolide, neoandrographolide, paniculide A, B, C, 14-deoxy-11-oxoandographolide, 14-deoxy-11-dehydroandrographolide, lactones, alkanes, ketones, aldehydes and the flavenoids andrographin, panicolin, mono-O-methylwightin, and apigenin-7,4′-dimethyl ethers. It has properties that enhance the immune system and inhibit Walker's carcinoma-256. (Hsu, et al, 1986; Huang, 1999)

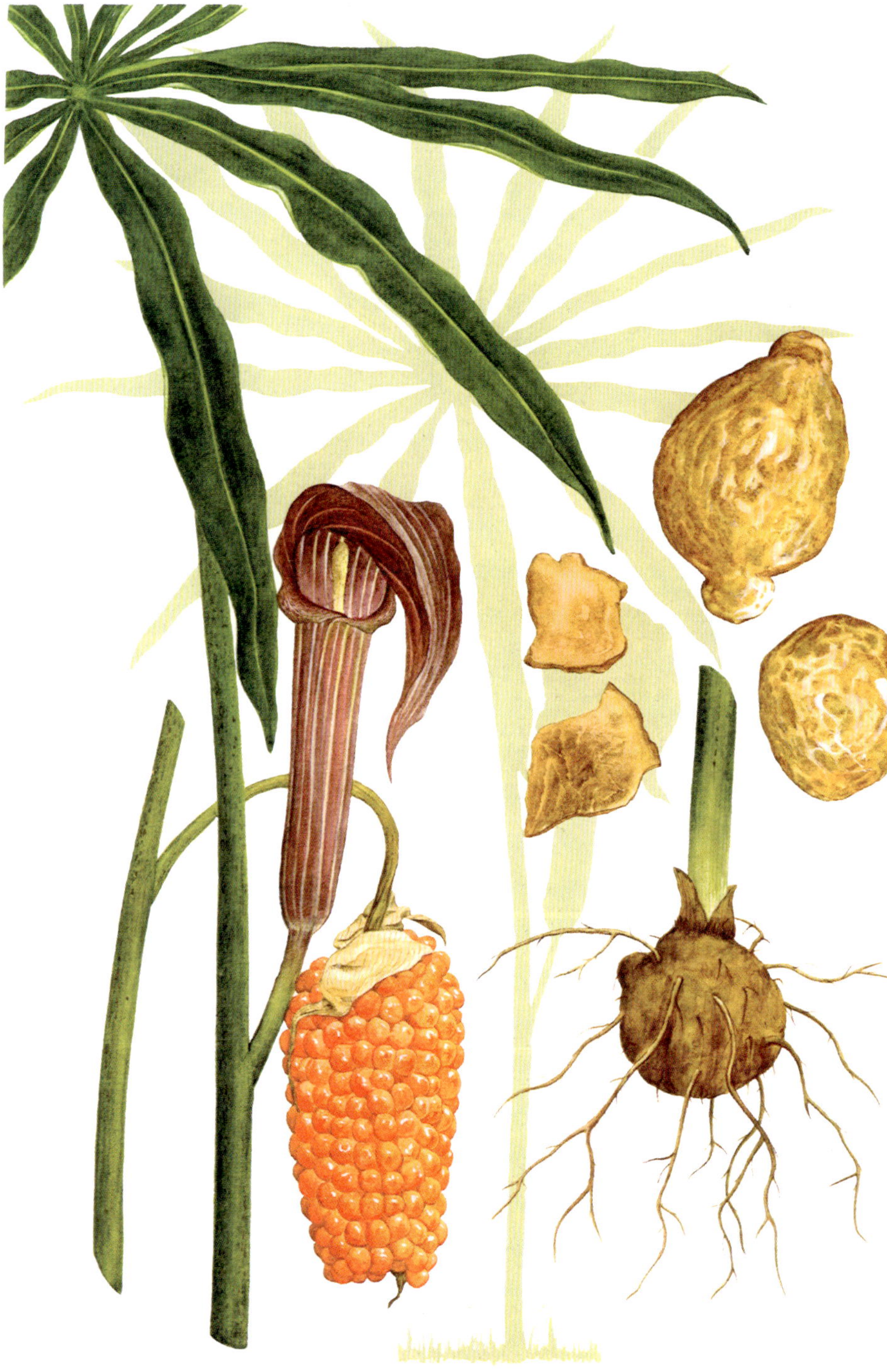

Fig. 11.17. ***Arisaema consanguineum*** Schott. — This plant contains saponins, d-mannitol, muscarine analogues, benzoic acid, β-sitosterol, trigonelline, and other alkaloids. It inhibits Hela cells in vitro, is effective against tumors in mice such as sarcoma-180 and $U_{14}$ cervical carcinoma, and has been found useful in the treatment cancer of the cervix and esophagus. The fresh herb is quite toxic. (Chang & But, 1986; Hsu, et al, 1986; Huang, 1999)

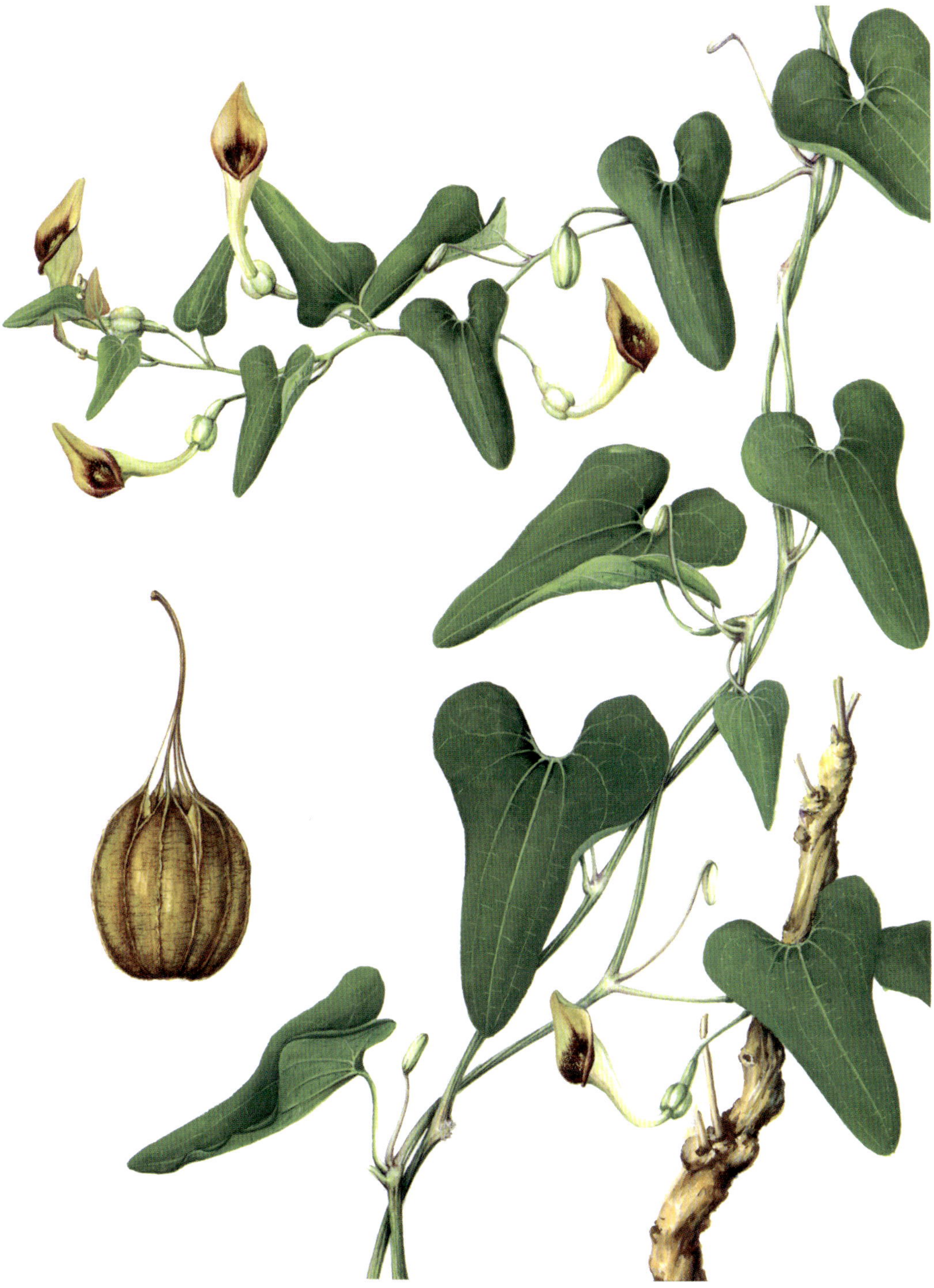

Fig. 11.18. ***Aristolochia debilis*** Sieb. et Zucc. — The root contains aristolochic acid, debilic acid, aristolone, aristoic acid, aristolo-lactum, magnoflorine, debilone, cyclanoline, and allantoin. It inhibits sarcoma-37, adenocarcinoma-775, and Erlich's ascites carcinoma in mice and has been found to reduce the toxic side effects of chemotherapy and radiation in humans. (Chang & But, 1986; Hsu, et al, 1986; Huang, 1999; Lee, 1999)

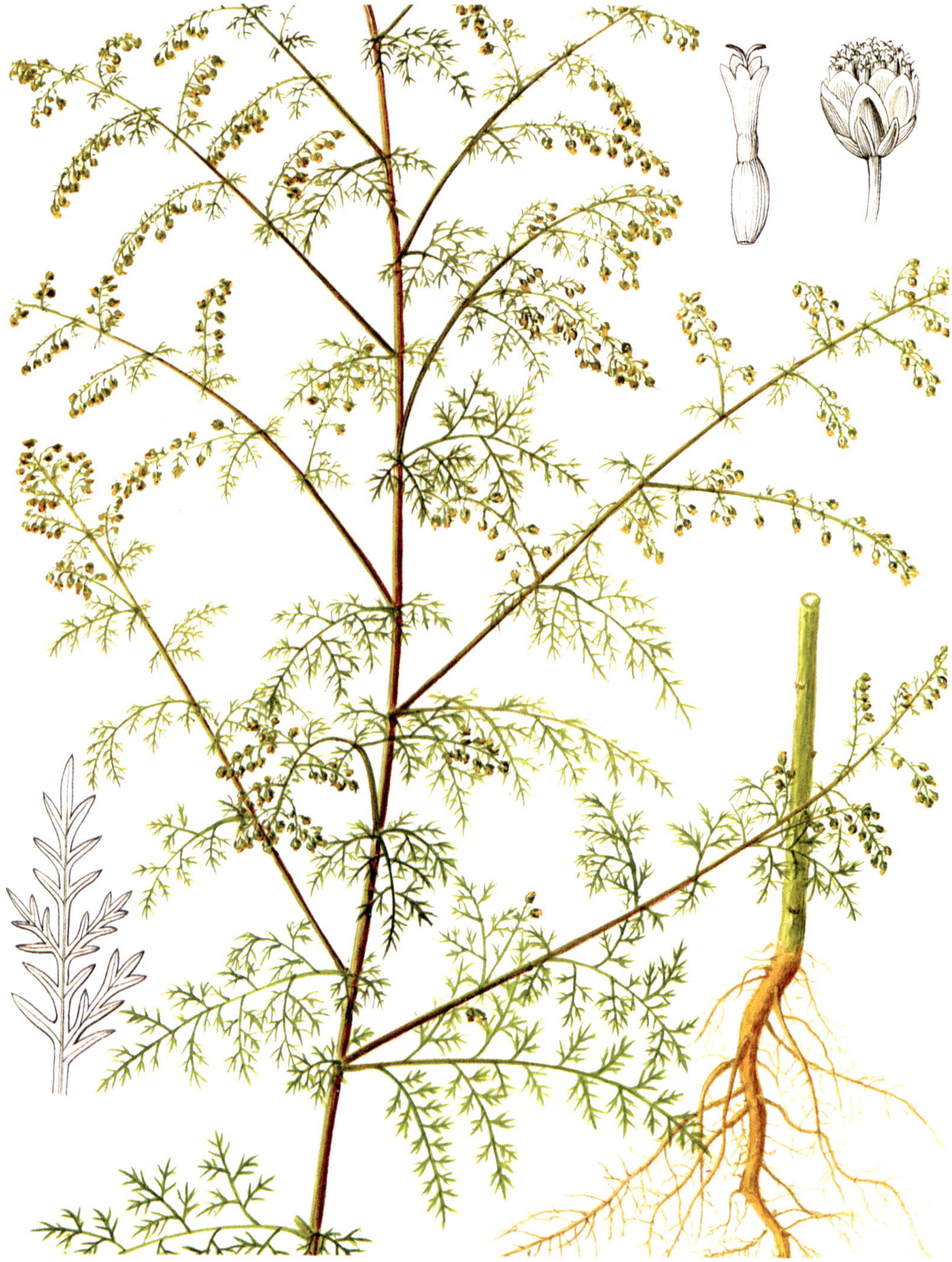

Fig. 11.19. ***Artemesia annua*** Linn. — This plant contains cineol (or eucalyptil), cuminal, artemesia alcohol, artemesia ketone, d-α-cadinene, α-, β-, γ-caryophyllene, caryophyllene oxide, arteannuin B, caumarin, thujone, sesquiterpene, and vitamin A. It inhibits JTC-26 and is effective against Hela, $CNE_2$, and SUNE-1 cell lines; in vivo it inhibits sarcoma-180, HepS, reticulosarcoma, $L_2$, $CNE_2$, and transplanted SUNE-1 in mice. It has been used to treat a variety of cancers including osteocarcinoma, and nasopharyngeal, gastrointestinal, breast, and liver cancer. (Chang & But, 1986; Hsu, et al, 1986; Minyi, 1992; Lee, 1999)

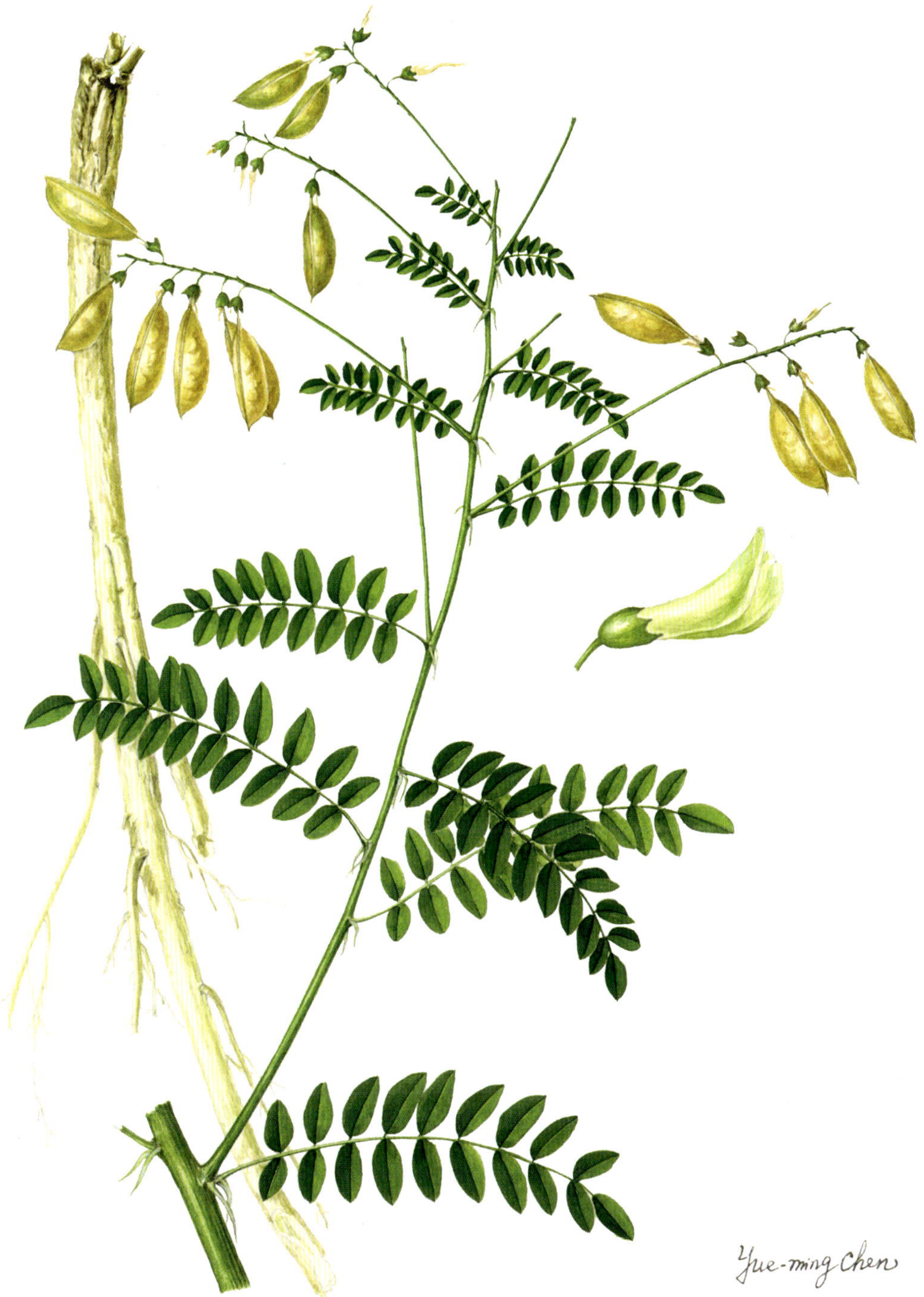


Fig. 11.20. ***Astragalus membranaceus*** (Fisch.) Bunge — The root contains glycoside astragaloside, coumarin, flavenoids, rhamnocitrin, betaine, saponins, glucoronic acid, choline, folic acid, β-sitosterol, and polysaccharides. It has antitumor properties, inhibits sarcoma-180 in mice, inhibits the formation of lipid peroxidation resulting from free radical damage, and is an immune enhancer. (Chang & But, 1986; Minyi, 1992; Harborne, 1994; Huang, 1999; Ebadi, 2002)

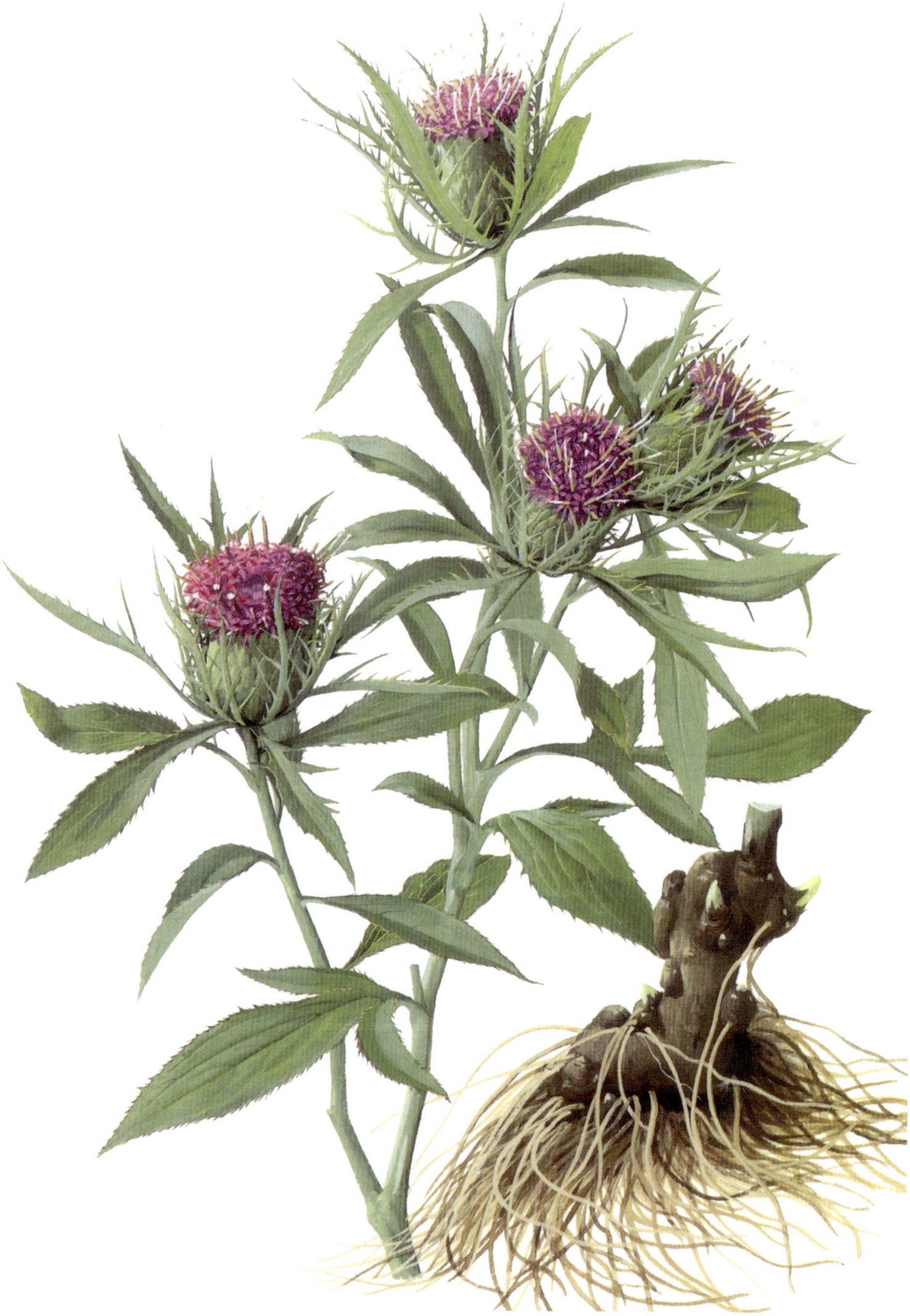

Fig. 11.21. ***Atractylodes macrocephalus*** Koidz. Baizu. — The root contains a volatile oil containing atractylol and atractylone, atractylenolide, sesquiterpene, furfural, hinesol, butenelolides A and B, and vitamin A. It has anticancer activity, inhibits sarcoma-180 and Erlich's ascites carcinoma in mice, is effective against EAC cells, sarcoma-180, and human esophageal cancer cells in vitro, and enhances the immune system. It has been used to treat cancers of the esophagus, stomach, thymus, liver, kidney, and lung. (Chang & But, 1986; Hsu, et al, 1986; Minyi, 1992; Lee, 1999)

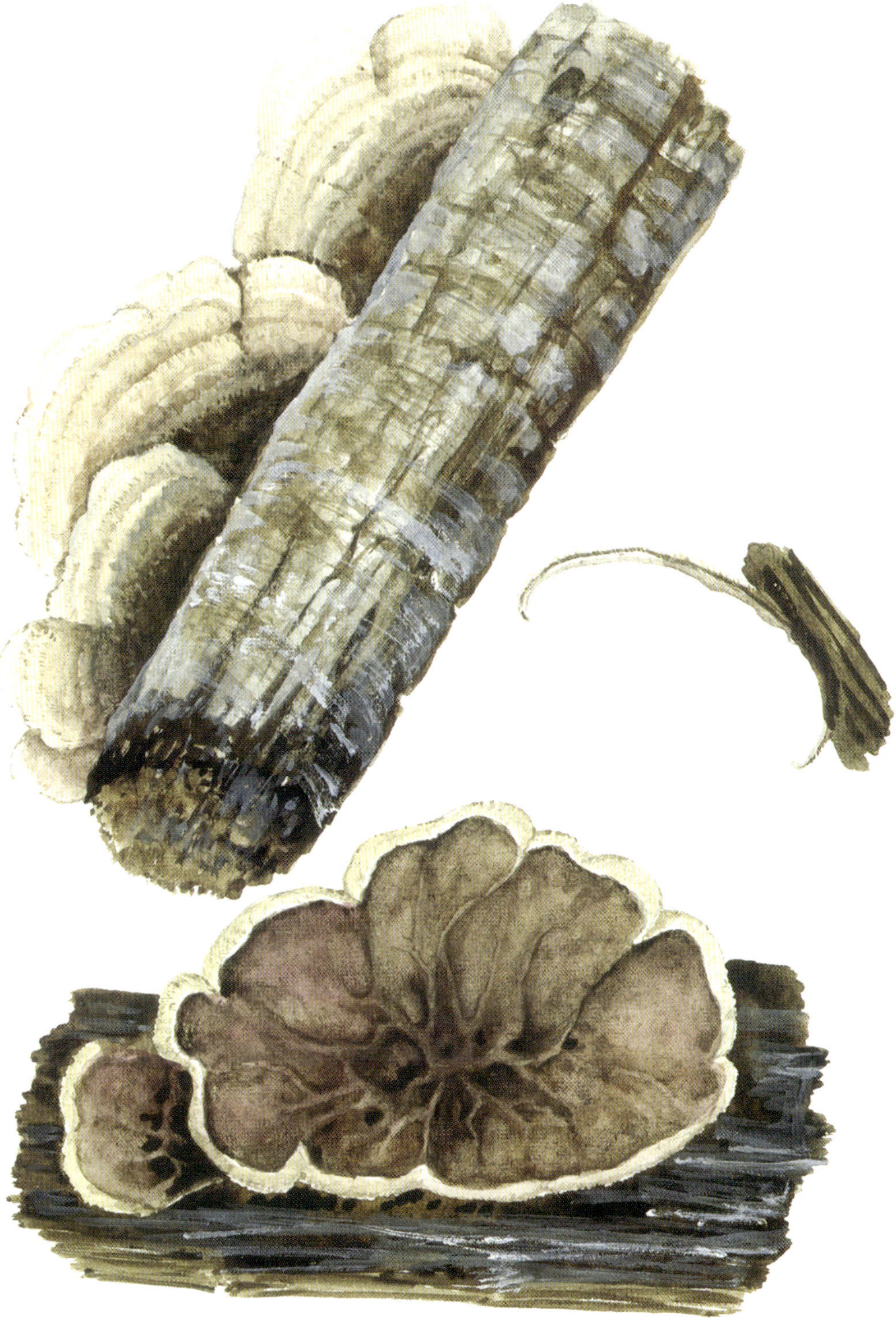

Fig. 11.22. ***Auricularia mesenterica*** (Dicks) Pers. — Extracts of the sporophore of this mushroom contain polysaccharides that inhibit sarcoma-180 and Ehrlich's carcinoma in laboratory mice (Ying, et al, 1987).

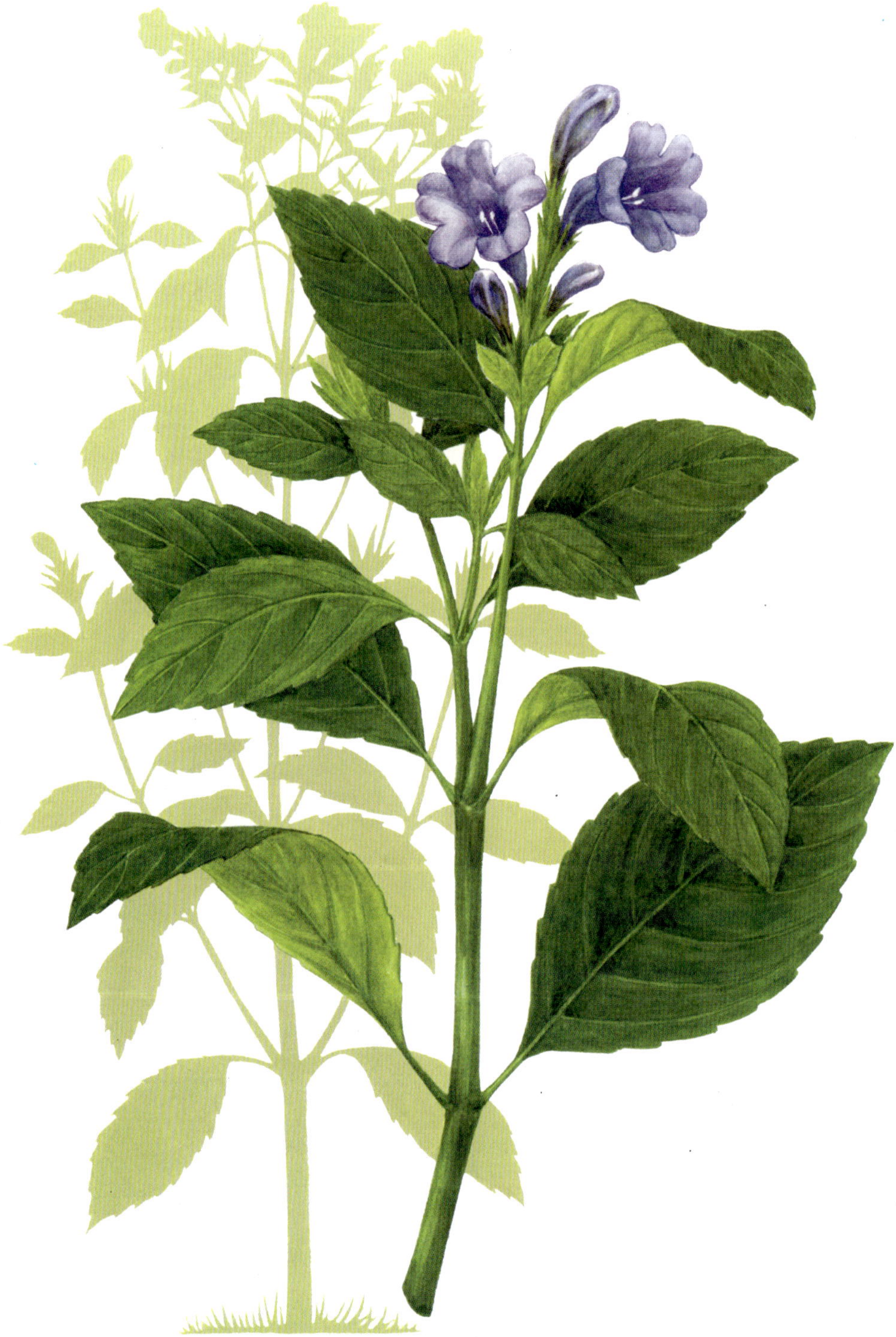

Fig. 11.23. ***Baphicacanthus cusia*** (Nees) Bremek. — This plant is used to make the dye indigo. It contains indican, sinirin, indigotin, indirubin, isoindigo, β-sitosterol, tannic acid, inorganic salts, and proteins. It has antineoplastic effects and has been used to treat myeloma and leukemias. (Chang & But, 1986; Lee, 1999)

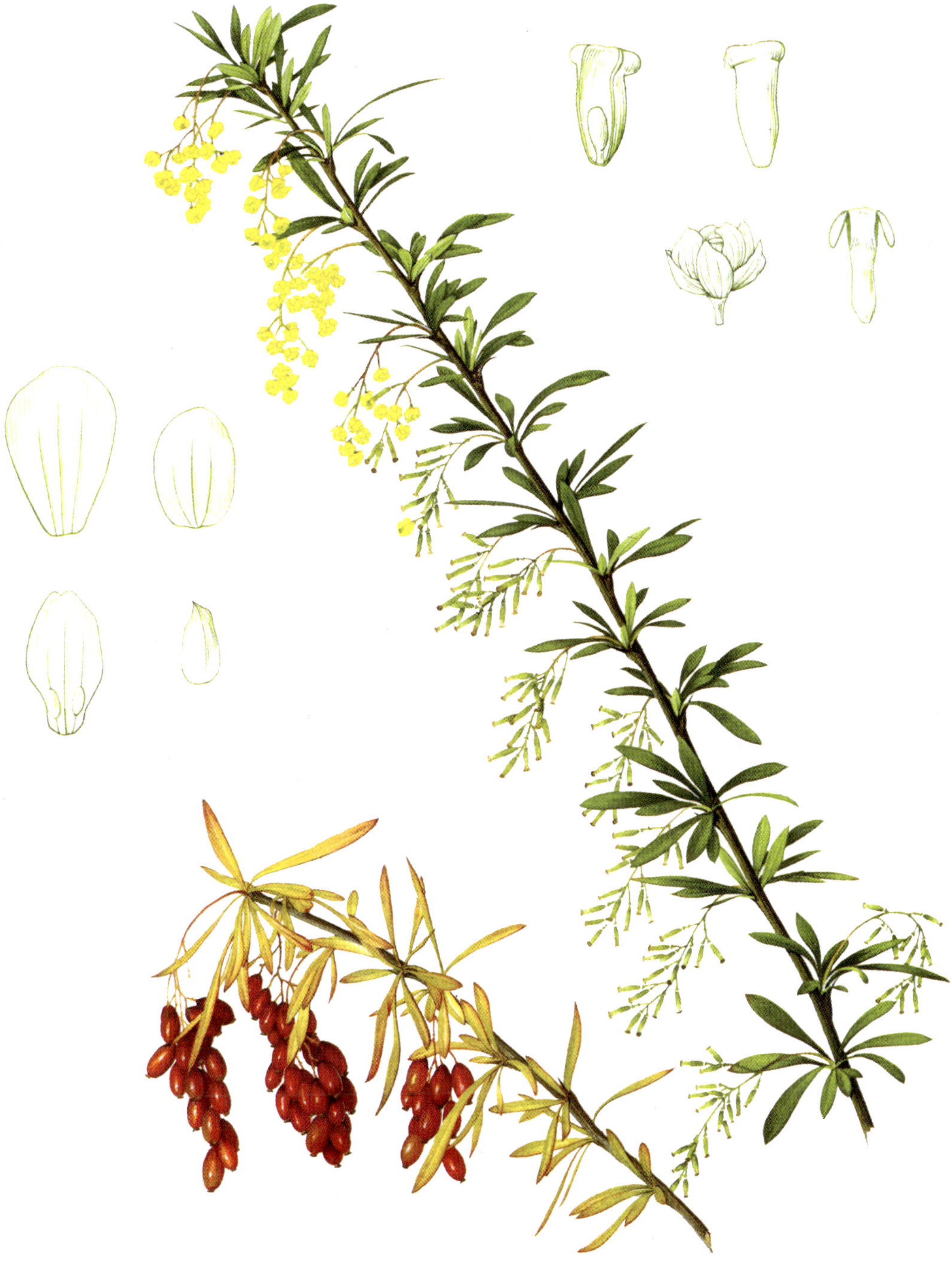

Fig. 11.24. ***Berberis poiretii*** Schneid. — The main ingredient in this plant is berberine; it also contains berbamine, beringamine, isotetramdrine, palmatine, jatrorhizzine, oxycanthine, columbamine, isotetrandrine, and magnoflorine. It inhibits Walker's carcinoma-256 in rats, Erlich's ascites carcinoma, sarcoma-180, and HepA, inhibits the cancer cell lines lymphocytic leukemia P-388, leukemia-1210, and cerebroma-16, is effective against ascitic cancer cells in mice, inhibits lipid peroxidation, and is used in the treatment of leukopenic complications of cancer. (Chang & But, 1986; Huang, 1999; Lee, 1999)

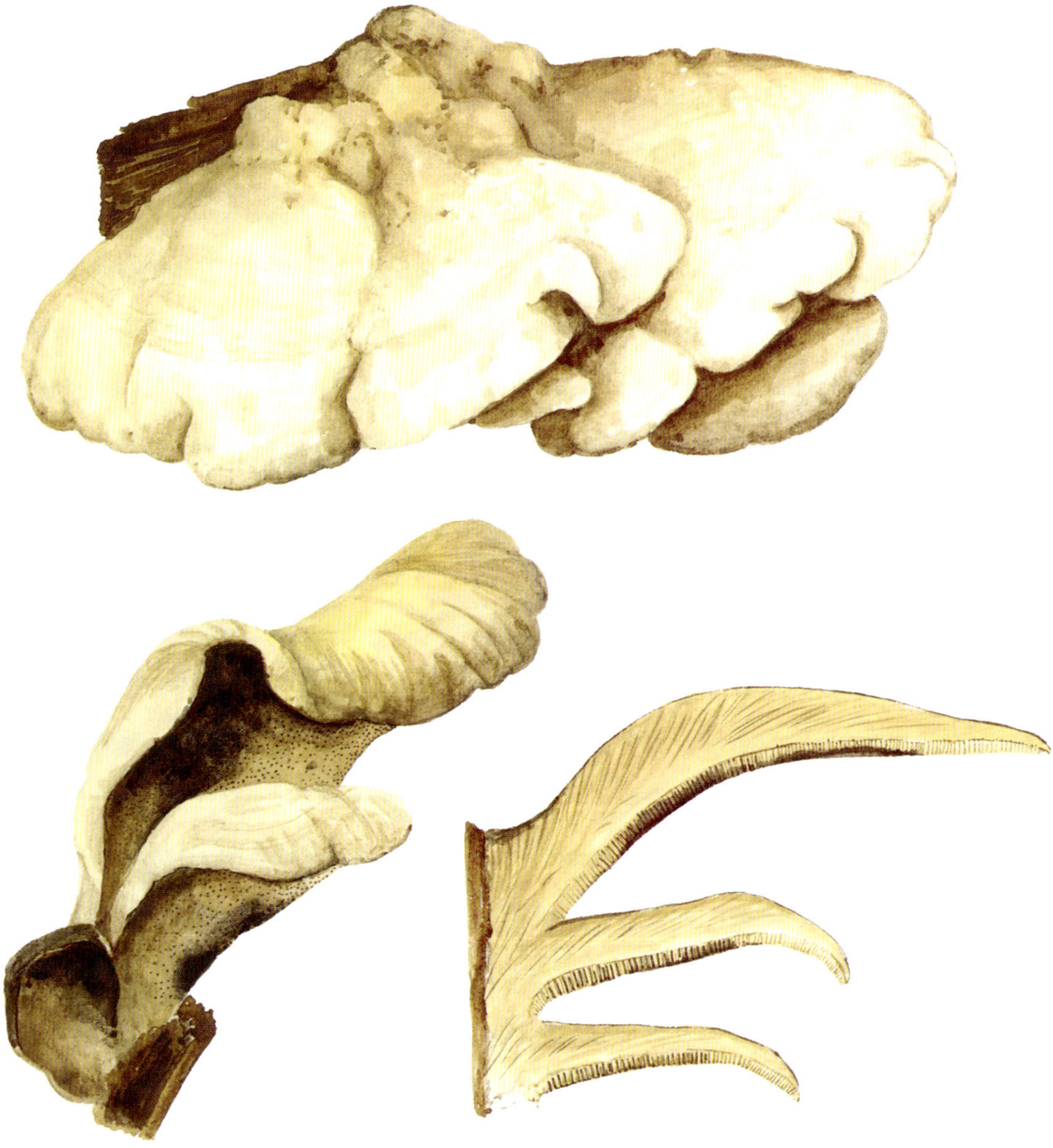

Fig. 11.25. ***Bjerkandera fumosa*** (Pers. ex Fr.) — This mushroom contains polysaccharides, which are used in the treatment of uterine cancer (Ying, et al, 1987).

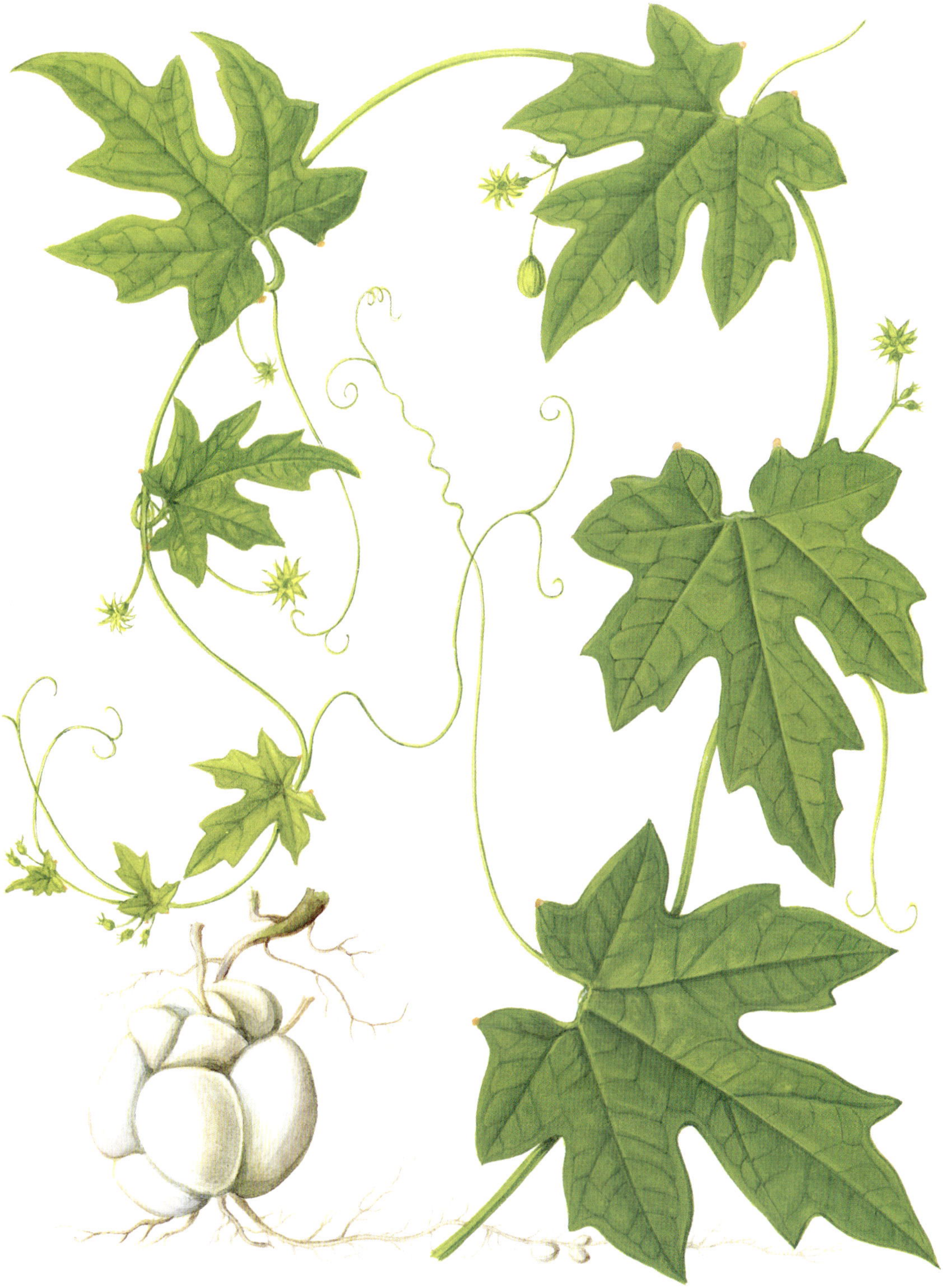

Fig. 11.26. ***Bolbostemma paniculatum*** (Maxim.) Franquet — This plant contains mannose, sucrose, and the triterpenoid saponins tubeioside I, II, and III, which have antitumor and antitumor-promoting effects. It has been used in the treatment of breast cancer. (Minyi, 1992; Yu, et al, 2001)

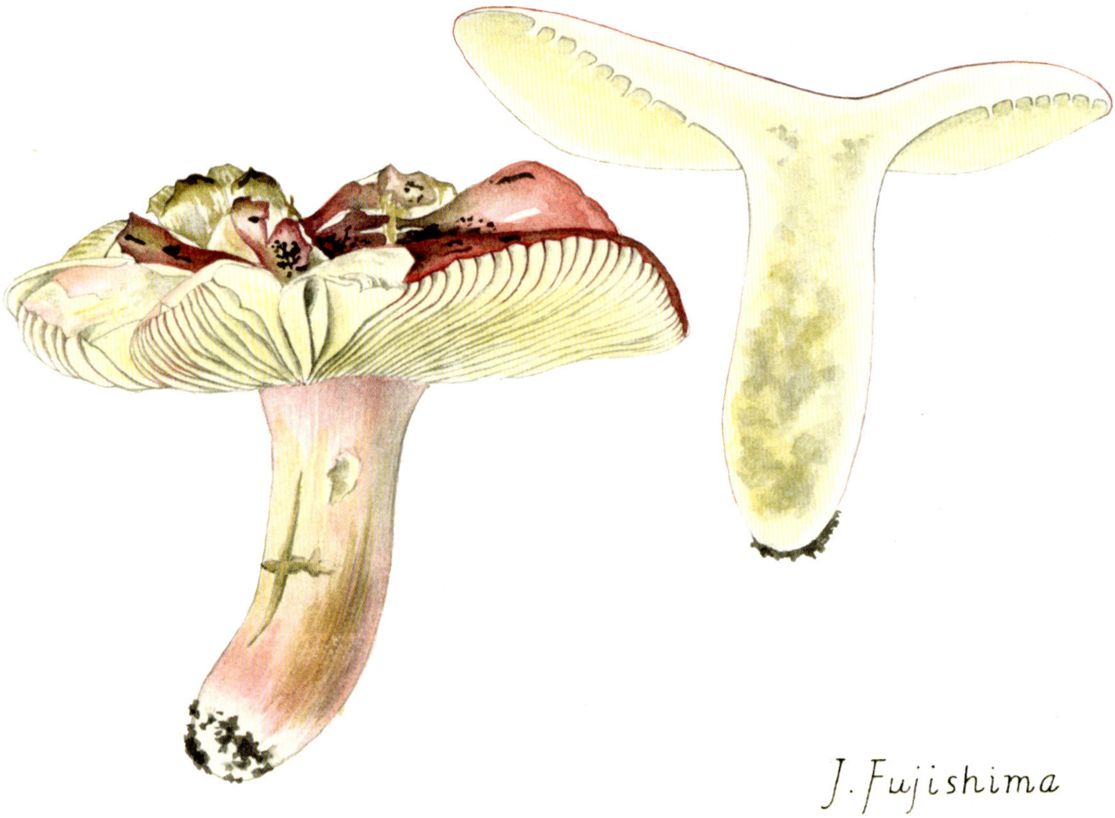


Fig. 11.27. ***Boletus erythropus*** Pers. ex Fr. — This mushroom contains polysaccharides that inhibit sarcoma-180 and Ehrlich's carcinoma in laboratory mice (Jianzhe, et al, 1987).

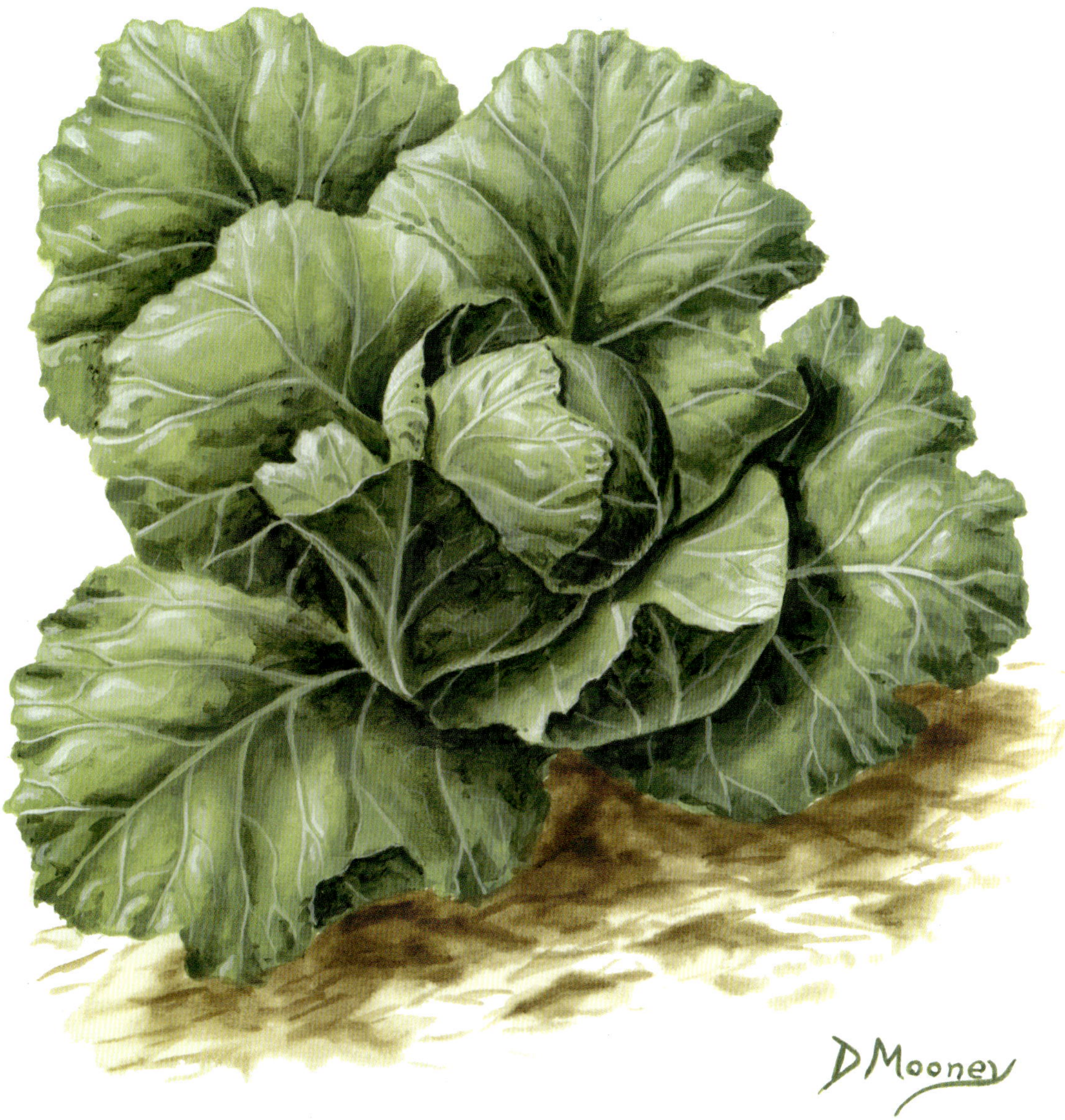


Fig. 11.28. ***Brassica oleracea*** Linn. — This plant, which is commonly known as cabbage, contains sulfhydryl dithiolthiones that are protective against cancer and radiation sickness (Bueding, Ansher & Dolan, 1985).

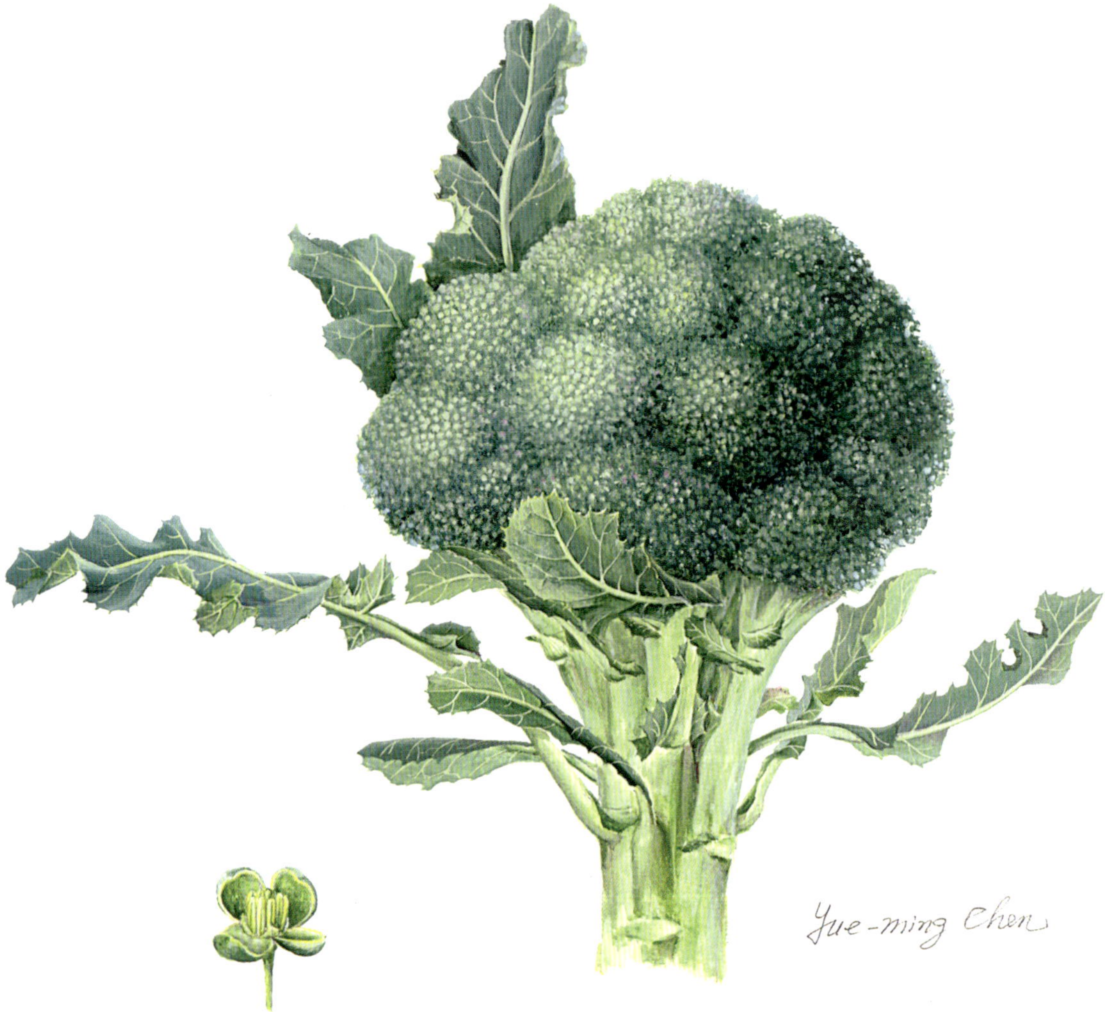


Fig. 11.29. ***Brassica oleracea*** var ***italica*** Plenck. — This plant, which is commonly known as broccoli, and its cruciferous relatives contain sulfhydryl dithiolthiones and sulforaphane, which are highly protective against cancer and radiation sickness (Bueding, Ansher & Dolan, 1985; Zhang, et al, 1992).

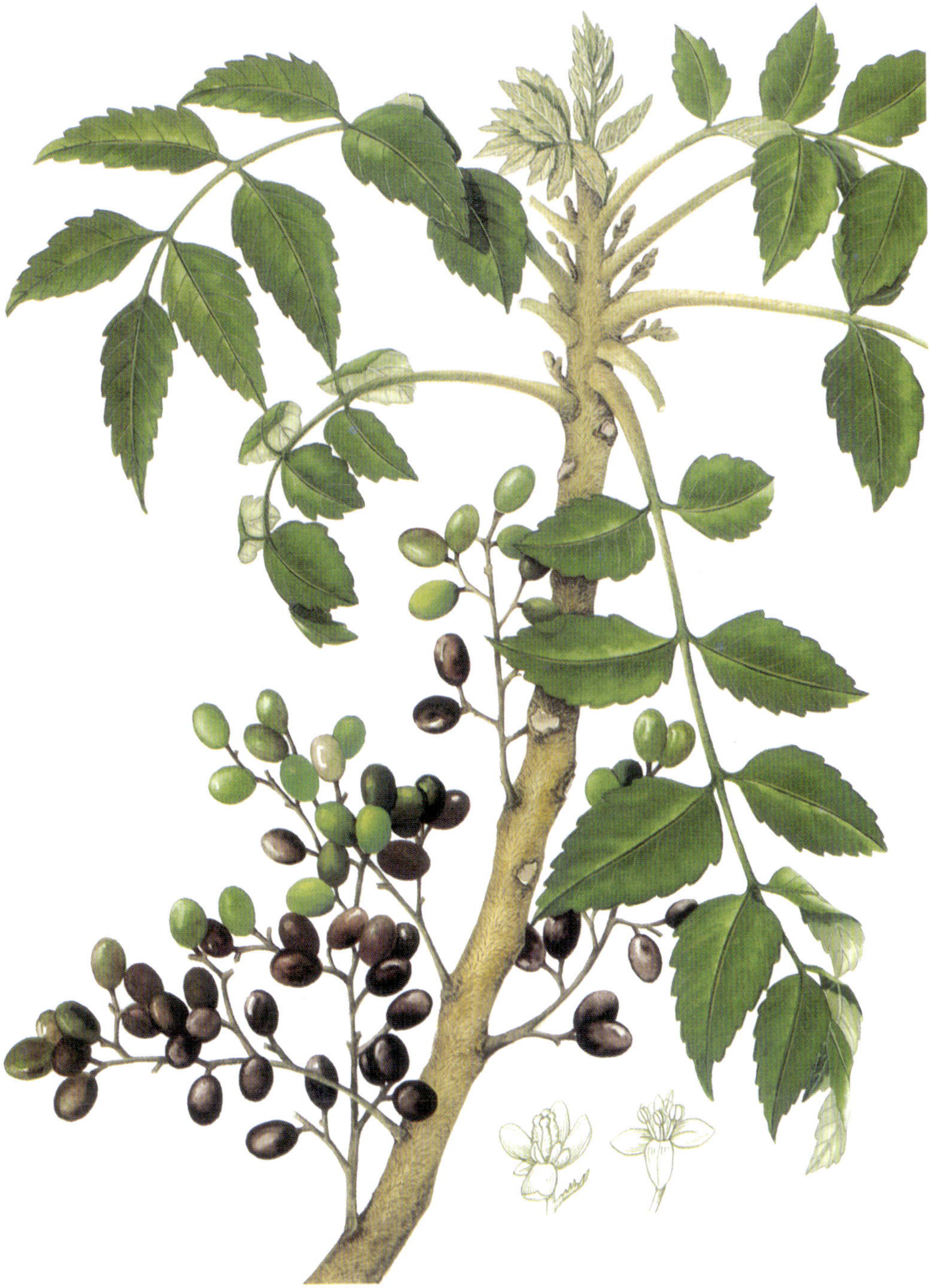

Fig. 11.30. ***Brucea javanica*** (Linn.) Merr. — This plant contains brusatol, brucenol, yatanin bruceolide, bruceine A, B, C, D, E, F, G, and H, bruceosides A and B (the glucosides of bruceines), yatanoside, brucealin, yatanin, kosamine, brucamarine, yatanine, oleic acid, bruceolic acid, linoleic acid, stearic acid, and palmitoleic acid. It exhibits antineoplastic activity, inhibits Erlich's ascites carcinoma, Walker's carcinoma-256, and lymphocytic leukemia P-388, and has been used to treat cervical and esophageal cancer. (Chang and But, 1986; Hsu, et al, 1986)

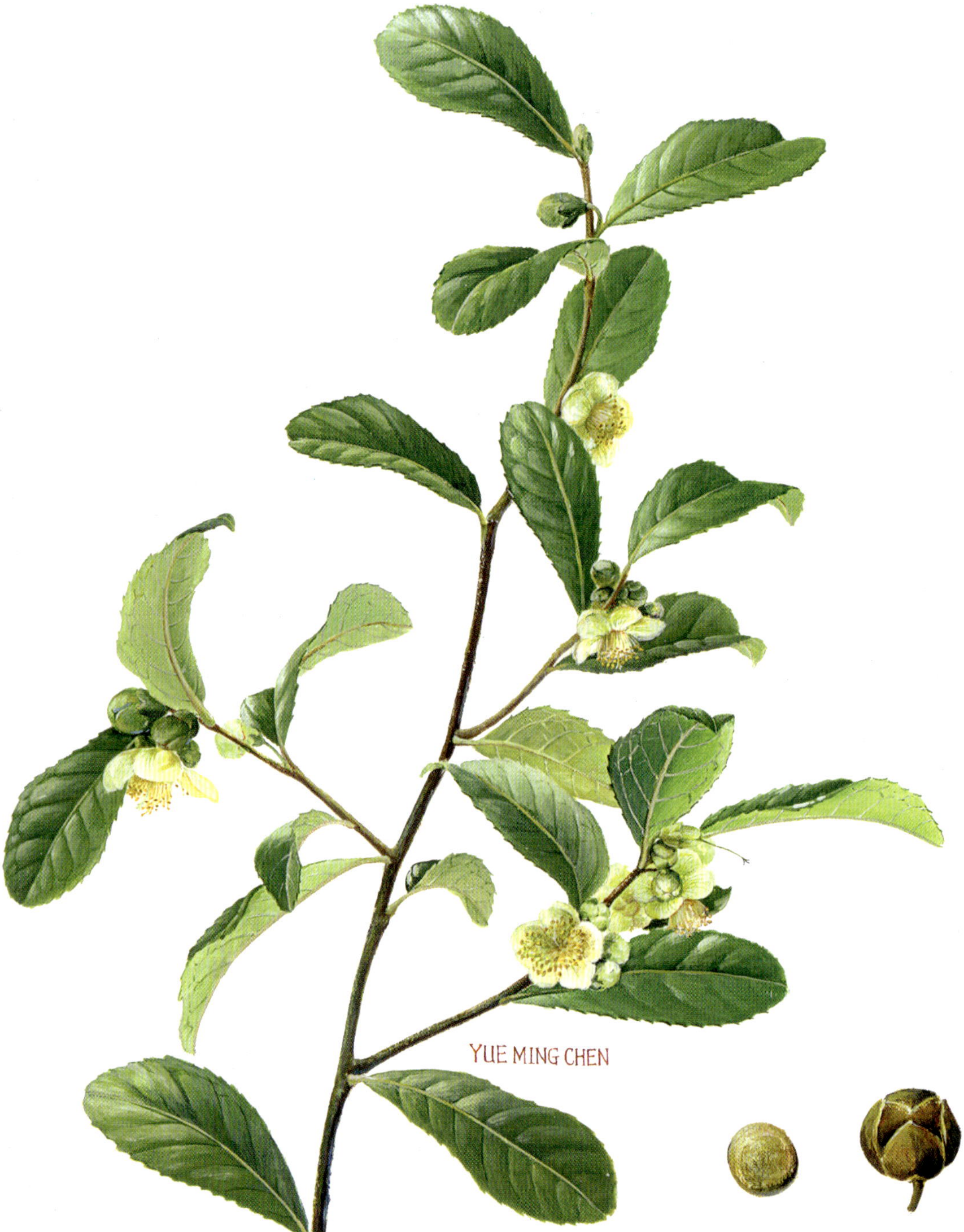


Fig. 11.31. ***Camellia sinensis*** (Linn.) Kuntze — The tea leaf contains quercetin, naringenin, heptenol, theaspirone, jasmone, chlorogenic acid, tannin, various alkaloids including caffeine, theophylline, theobromine, and xanthine, and polyphenols including(–)-epigallocatechin gallate (EGCG). There is an abundance of data that supports the fact that green tea prevents and is useful in the treatment of cancer. (Hsu, et al, 1986; Huang, 1999)

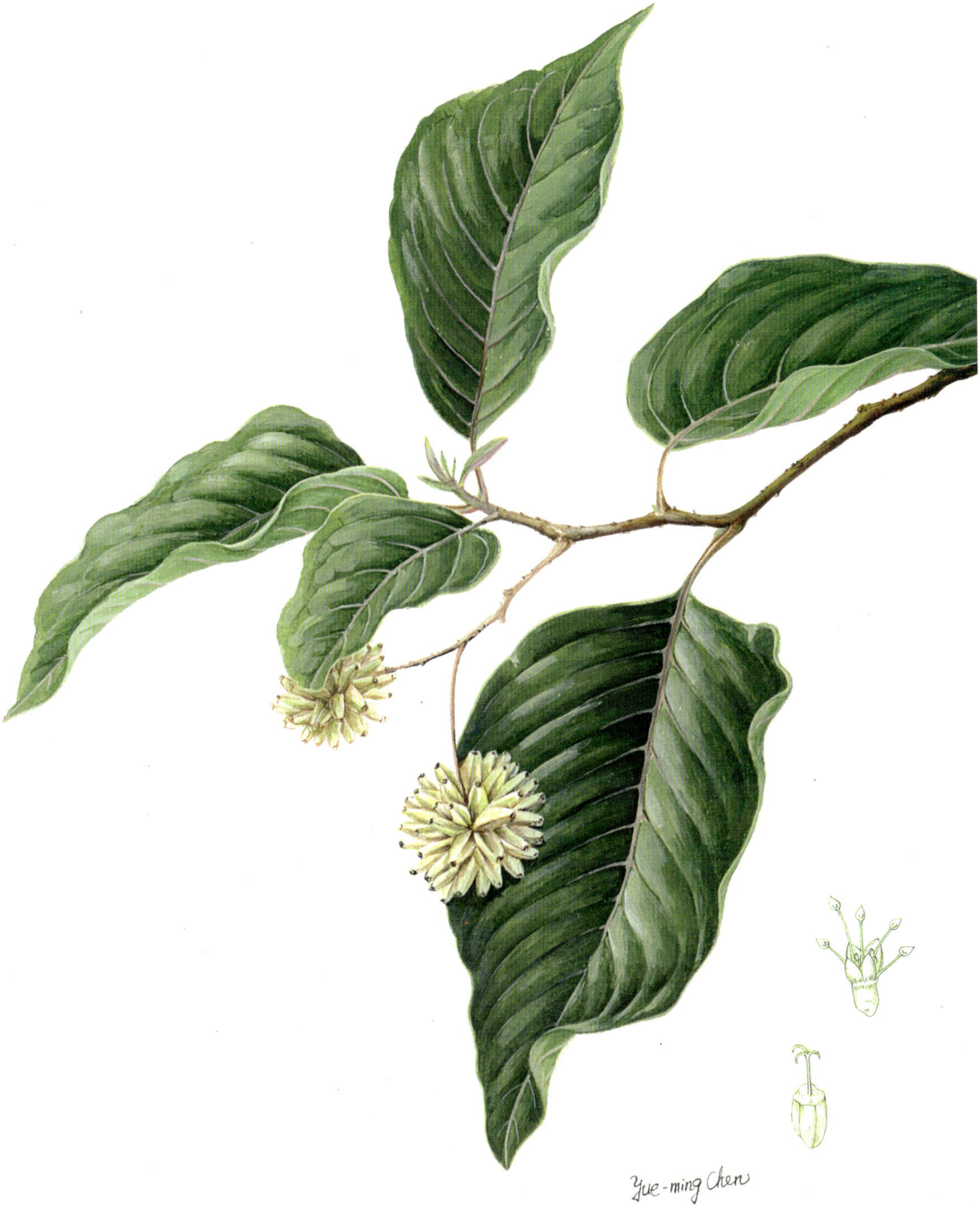


Fig. 11.32. ***Camptotheca acuminata*** Decne. — This plant contains camptothecine, chlorocamptothecine, venoterpine, deoxycamptothecine, hydroxycamptothecine, methoxycamptothecine, trimethylellagic acid, betulic acid, vincoside-lactam, and camptoglucoside. Studies have shown that it has strong anticancer activity against a variety of animal tumors. It has been used to treat a variety of cancers including leukemia, skin cancers, and cancers of the head, neck, alimentary tract, heart, liver, breast, ovaries, and lung. (Chang & But, 1986; Minyi, 1992; Huang, 1999; Lee, 1999)

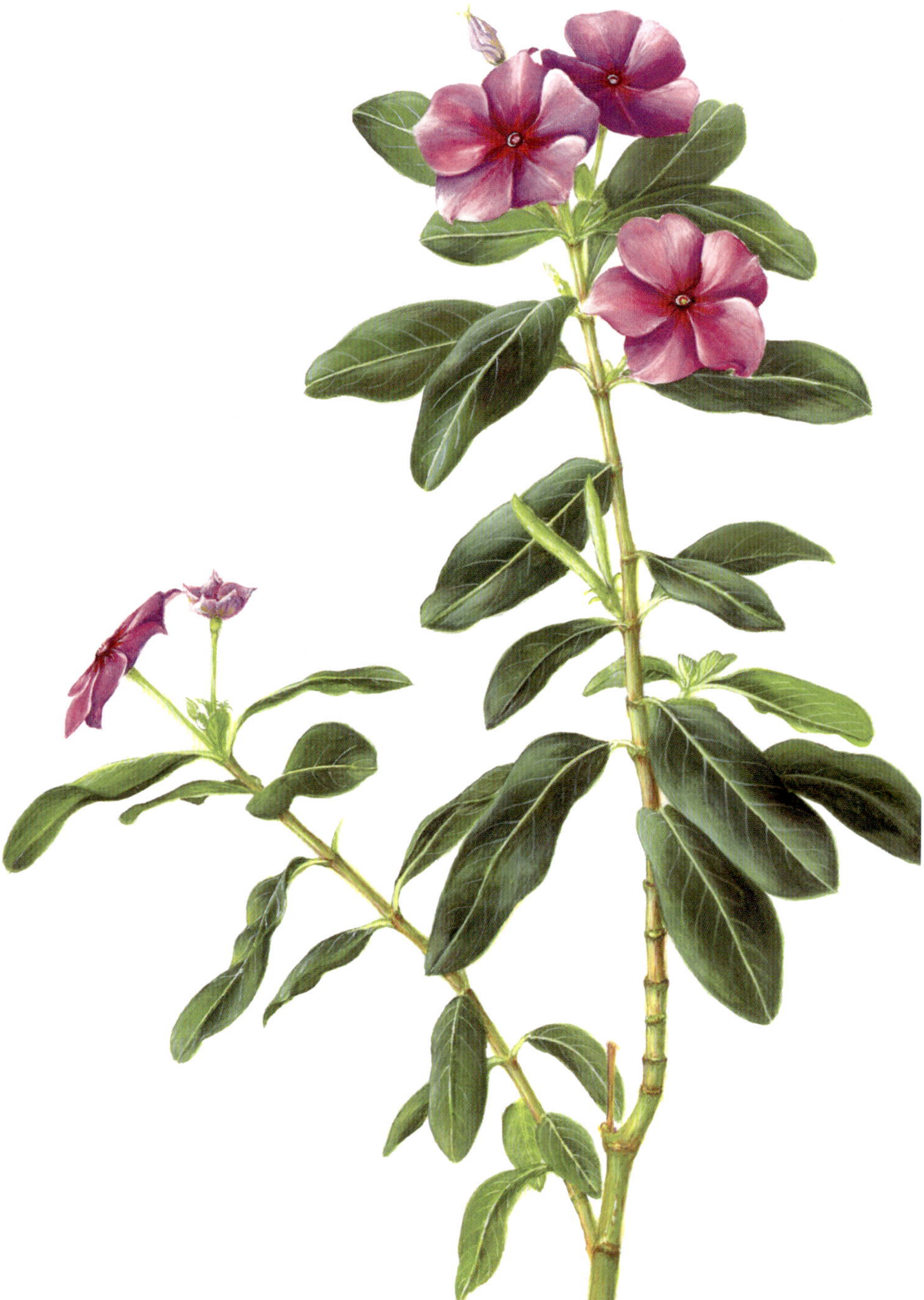

Fig. 11.33. ***Cantharanthus roseus*** (Linn.) G. Don. — There are 70 different alkaloids that have been extracted from this plant, several of which have been found to have anticancer activity. They are vinblastine, vincristine, leurosine, leurosidine, isoleusosine, lochneridine, vinrosidine, rovidine, carosine, perivine, perividine, vindolinine, and pericalline. It has been used in the treatment of Hodgkin's disease, chorioepithelioma, leukemia, lymphoma, and cancers of the breast ovaries, testes, liver, and lung. (Chang & But, 1986; Minyi, 1992; Huang, 1999)

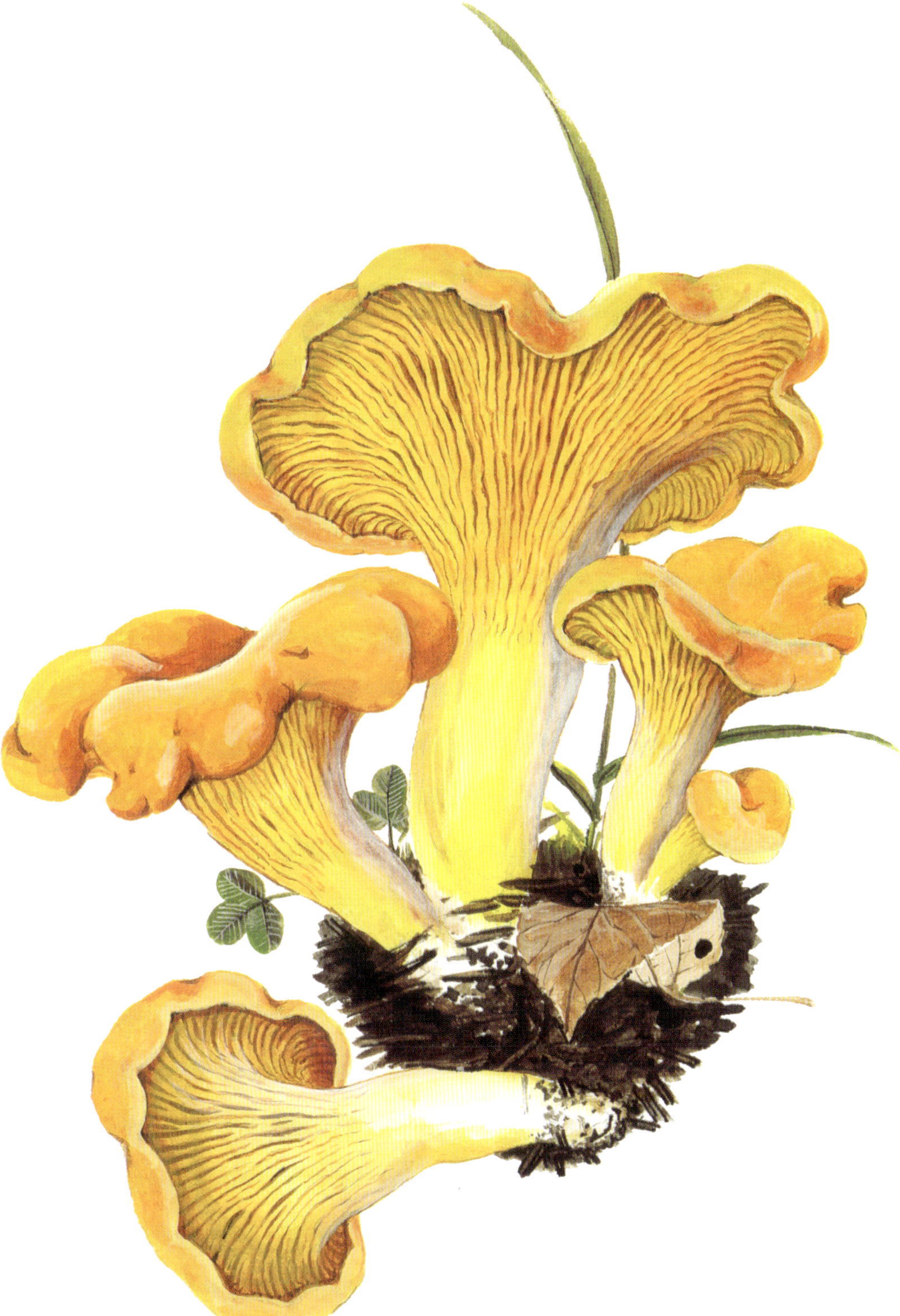

Fig. 11.34. ***Cantharellus cibarius*** Fr. — This fungus contains amino acids, vitamin A, and polysaccharides and has an inhibitory effect on sarcoma-180 in laboratory mice (Ying, et al, 1987).

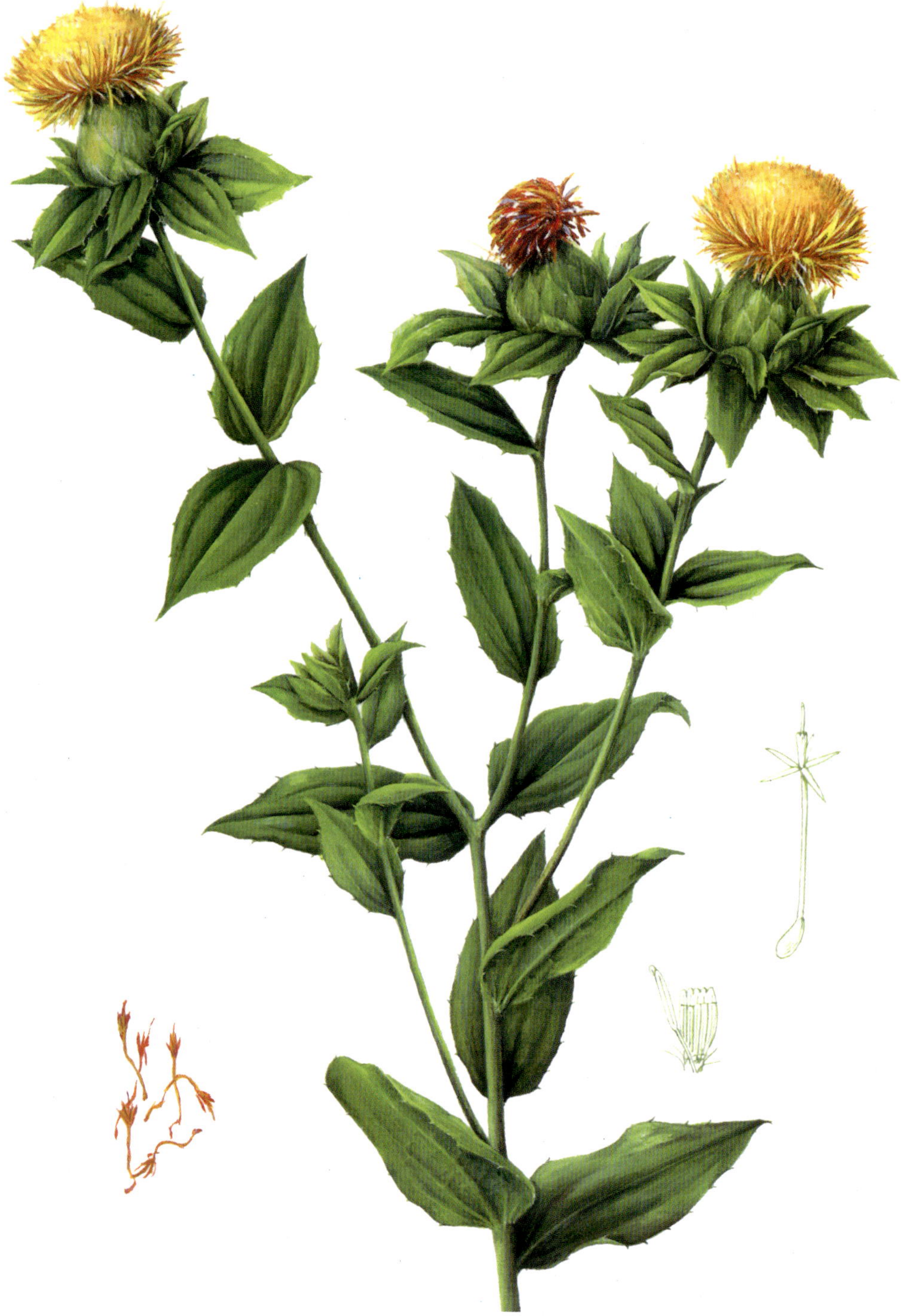

Fig. 11.35. ***Carthamus tinctorius*** Linn. — This plant contains carthamin, carthamone, neocarthamin, luteolin-7-glucoside, linoleic acid, matairesinol-4-*o*-β-glucopyranoside, and tracheloside. In vivo it inhibits JTC-26 and mouse sarcoma-180; in vitro it inhibits leukemia cells. It has been used in the treatment of leukemia, myeloma, and cervical, esophageal, and pancreatic cancer. (Hsu, et al, 1986; Minyi, 1992; Lee, 1999)

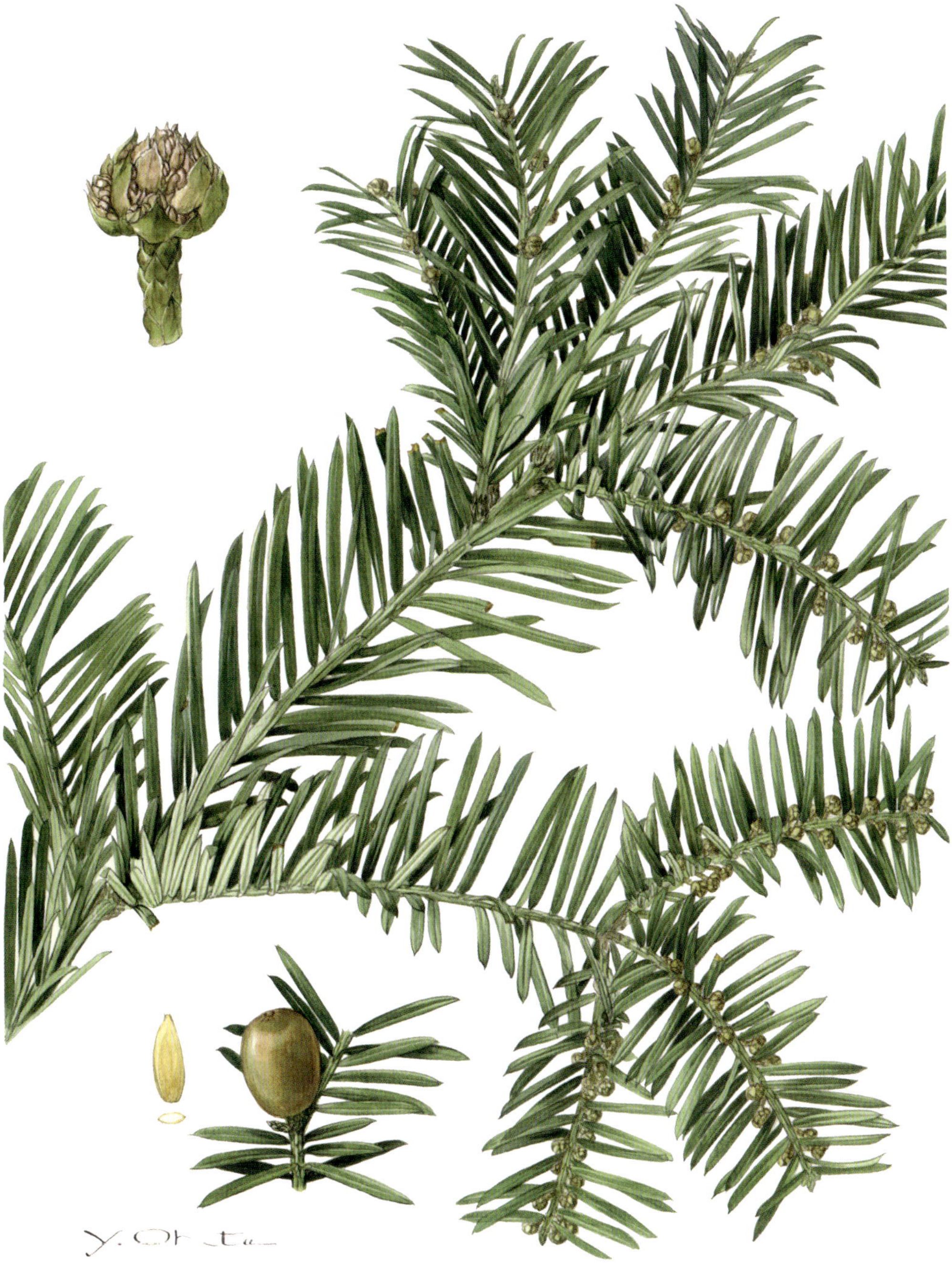

Fig. 11.36. ***Cephalotaxus harringtonia*** K. Koch — This plant contains 20 different alkaloids, including cephalotaxine, demethylcephalotaxine, epicephalotaxine, acetylcephalotaxine, cephalotaxinone, demethylcephalotaxinone, harringtonine, homoharringtonine, wilsonine, and epiwilsonine. It inhibits sarcoma-180, cerebroma-22, and lymphocytic leukemia P-388 in mice, and Walker's carcinoma-256 in rats, increases the survival rate of mice with leukemia-615 and leukemia-7212, is effective against reticulosarcoma, Erlich's ascites carcinoma, and uterine cervix carcinoma murine tumors. It has been used in the treatment of leukemia and malignant tumors including cancers of the lung, breast, and colon. (Chang & But, 1986; Minyi, 1992; Huang, 1999; Lee, 1999)

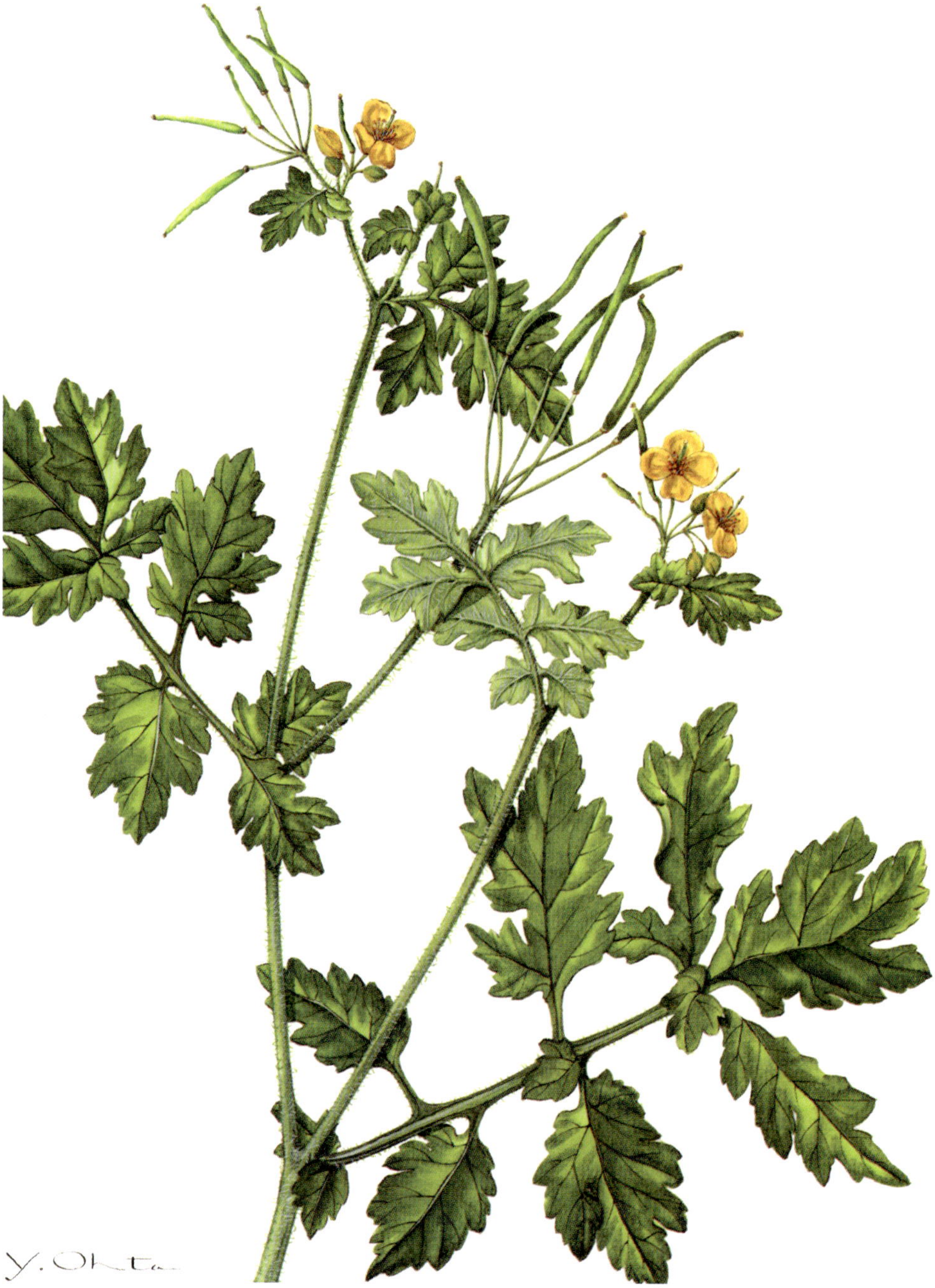


Fig. 11.37. ***Chelidonium majus*** Linn. — This plant contains chelidonine, chilidone, chelerythrine, crytopine, protopine, α-, β-, γ-homochelidonines, chelidonic acid, berberine, sanguinarine, sparteine, choline, histamine, tyramine, saponins, flavonol, chelidoniol, vitamin C, and carotene. It has immunomodulatory effects, inhibits sarcoma-180, and Erlich's ascites carcinoma in mice, inhibits mitosis of cancer cells in vitro, and prevents the growth of malignant tumors. It has been used to treat malignant tumors, including cancers of the digestive tract, stomach, pancreas, lung, respiratory tract, and bone. (Chang & But, 1986; Hsu, et al, 1986; Minyi, 1992; Lee, 1999; Gansauge, et al, 2002; Song, et al, 2002)

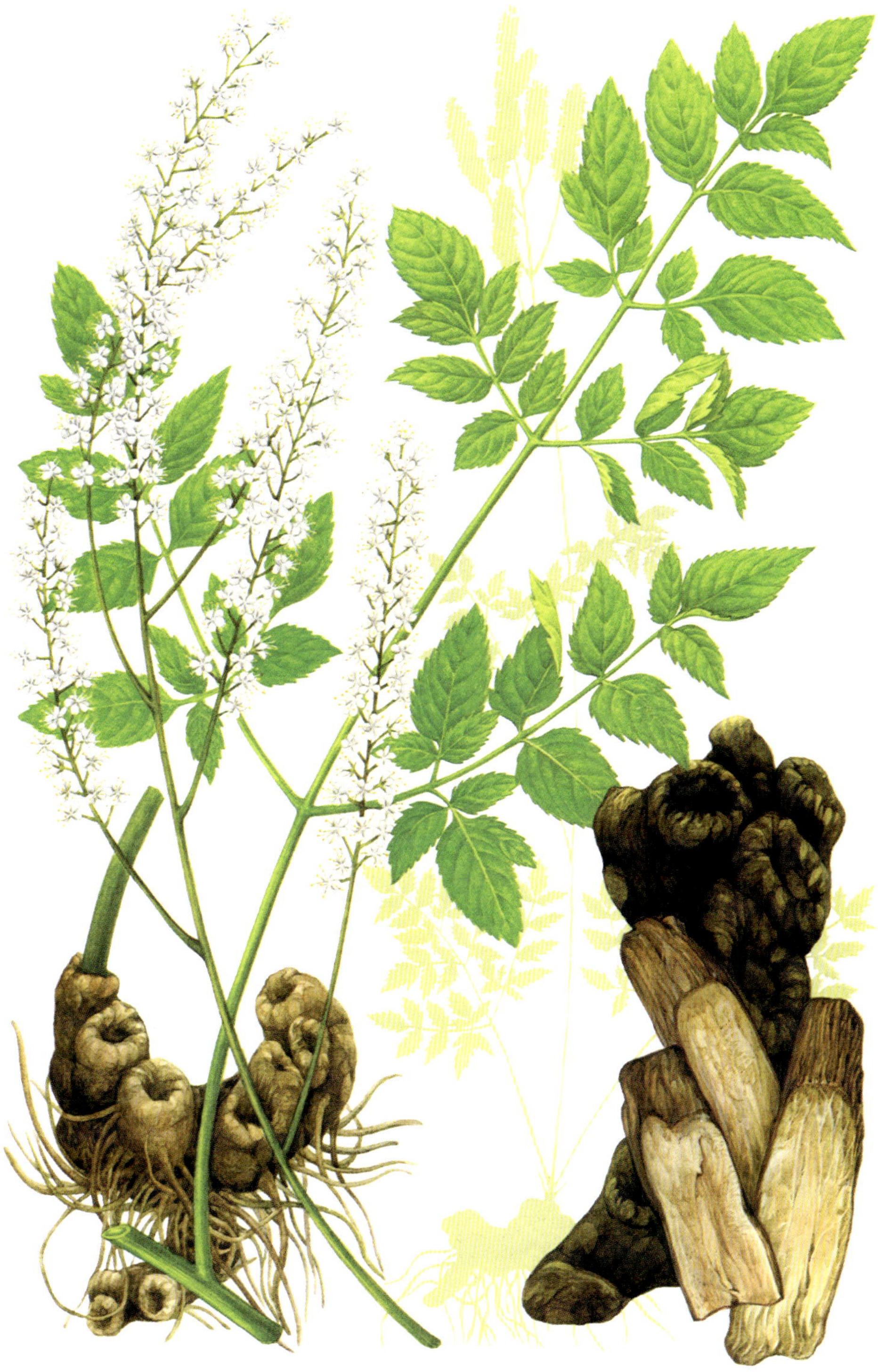

Fig. 11.38. ***Cimicifuga heracleifolia*** Kom. — This plant contains cimicfugine, salicylic acid, caffeic acid, ferulic acid, isoferulic acid, cemigenol, khellol, aminol, cimifugenol, cimitin, tannin, and fatty acids. It inhibits human cervix carcinoma JTC-26 cells in vitro and has been used to treat cancers of the tongue, larynx, and breast. (Minyi, 1992; Huang, 1999)

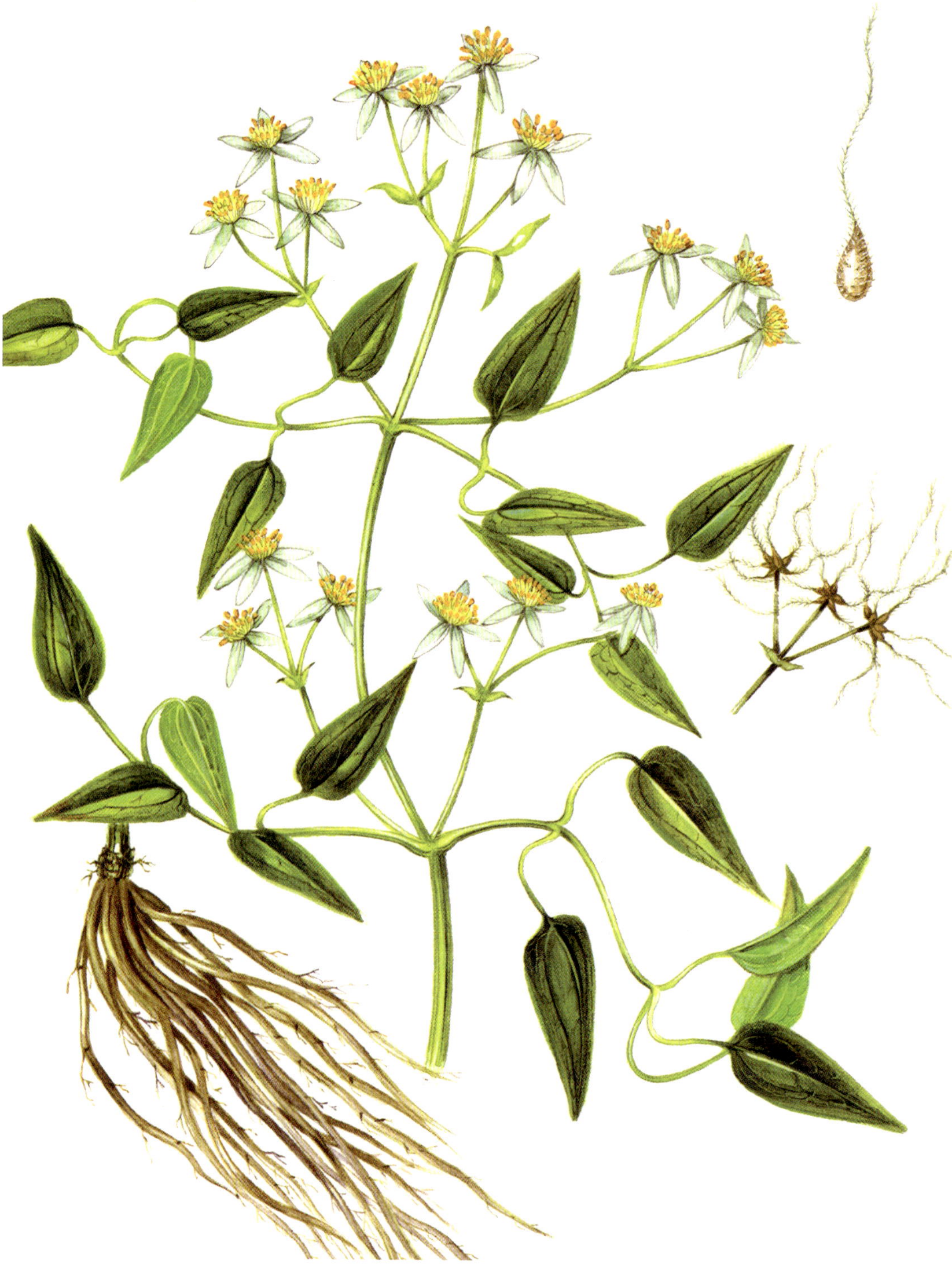

Fig. 11.39. ***Clematis chinensis*** Osbeck — The root contains ranunculin, anemonin, anemonol, and other saponins, steroids, amino acids, and phenols. It inhibits uterine cervix carinoma U-26 cells in vitro, is effective against sarcoma-180 in mice and Hela and Hep2 cell lines in vitro, and has been used to treat esophageal, parotid, and colon cancer. (Lee, 1992; Hsu, et al, 1986; Huang, 1999)

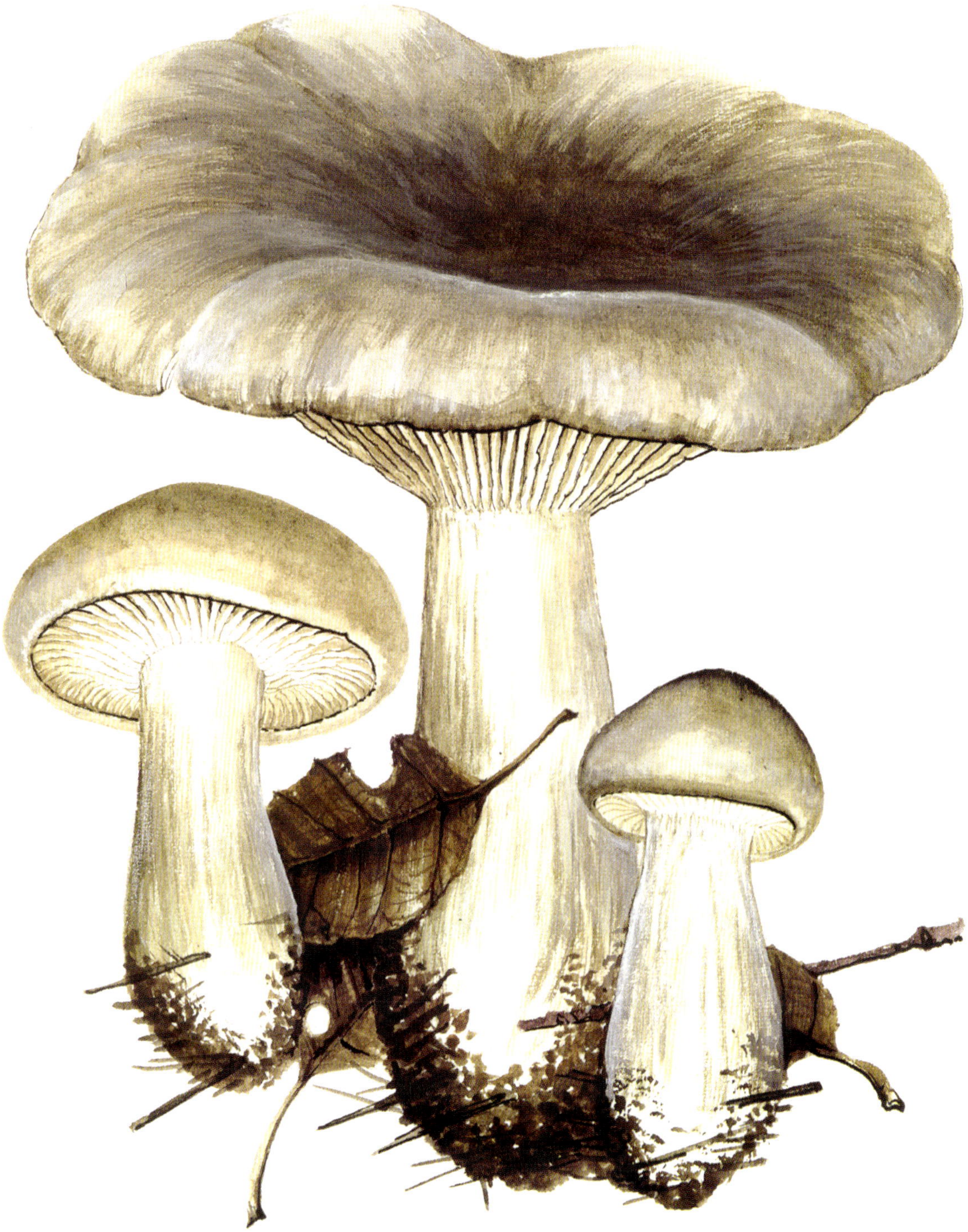

Fig. 11.40. ***Clitocybe nebularis*** (Batsch. ex Fr.) Qué — This mushroom contains nebularin and polysaccharides and has been shown to inhibit sarcoma-180 in laboratory mice (Ying, et al, 1987).

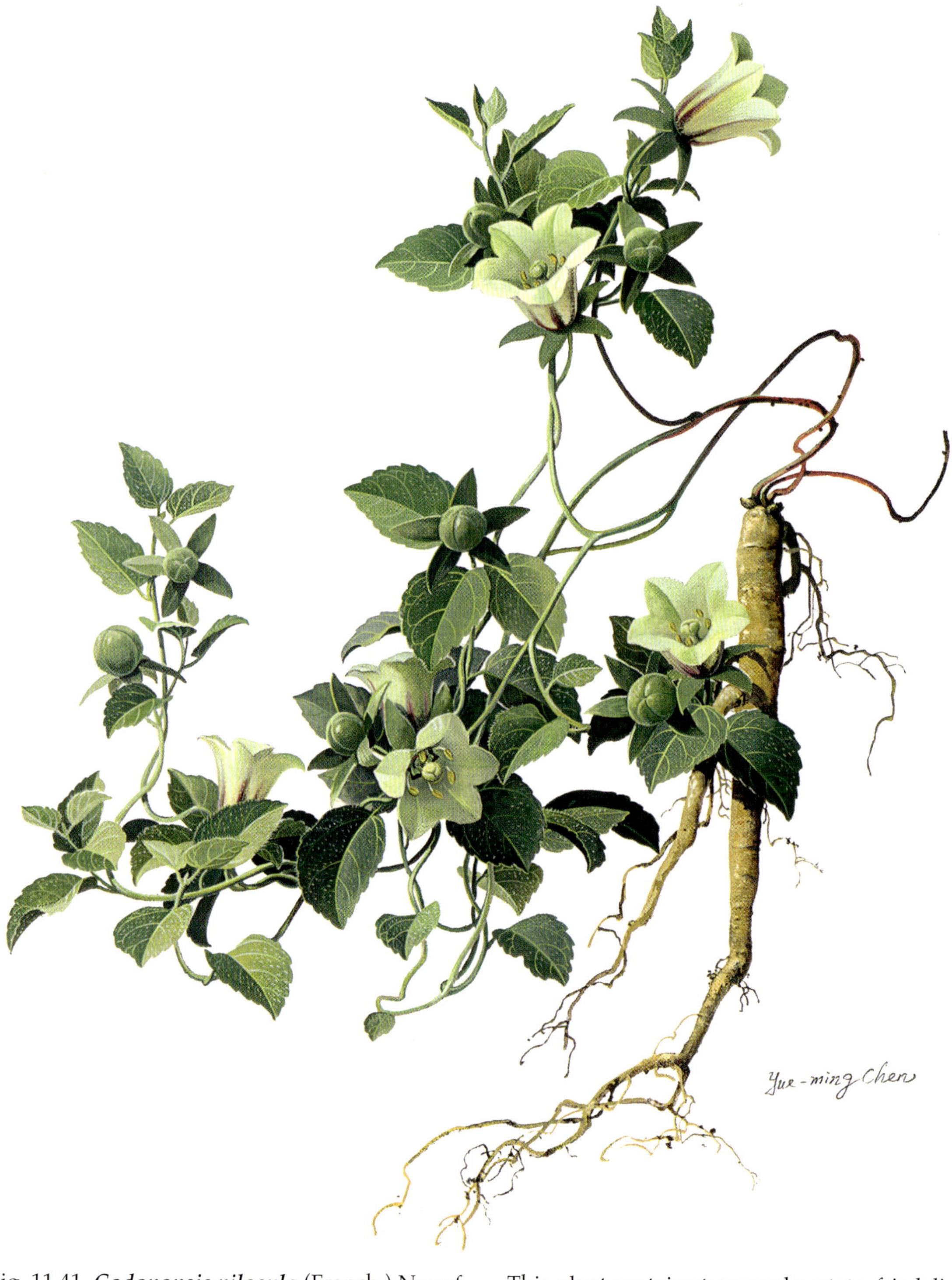


Fig. 11.41. ***Codonopsis pilosula*** (Franch.) Nannf. — This plant contains taraxeryl acetate, friedelin, saponin, inulin, alkaloids, saccharides, proteins, starches, vitamin $B_1$ and $B_2$. It inhibits transplanted sarcoma-180 in mice and exhibits immune-enhancing properties. It has been used to treat thyroid, stomach, and lung cancer. (Hsu, et al, 1986; Minyi, 1992; Lee, 1999)

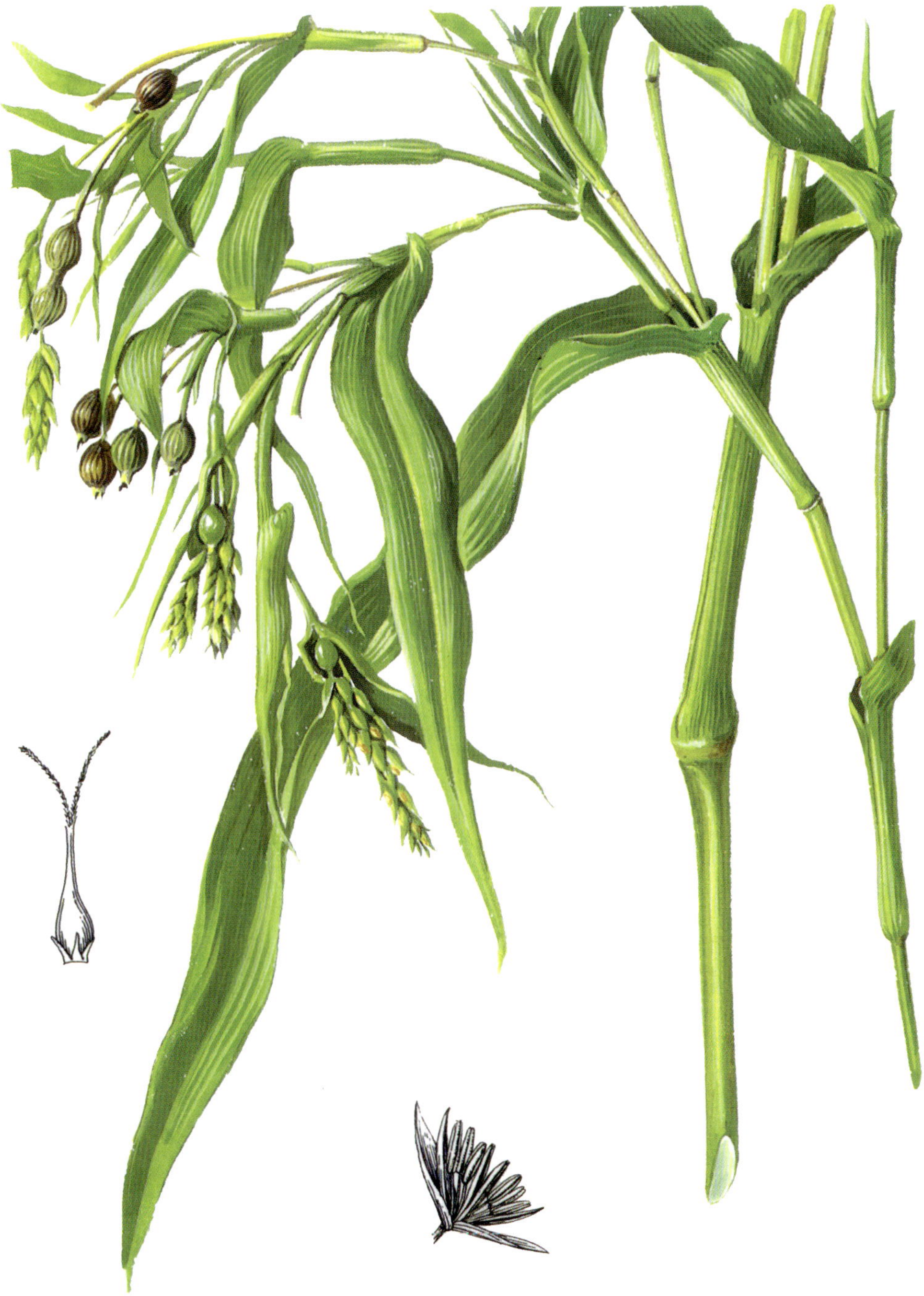

Fig. 11.42. ***Coix lacryma*** Linn. — The kernels of the seeds of this plant contain coixenolide, coixol, stigmasterol, amino acids, saccharides, α-, β-, and γ-sitosterol, glycerides of palmitic acid, myristic acid, 8-octadecenoid acid, proteins, starch, phytin, alkaloids, and vitamin $B_1$. It inhibits Erlich's ascites carcinoma, cervical cancer U-14, and HCA solid tumor of mice, and has been used to treat Yoshida's sarcoma, chorioepithelioma, malignant reticular cellular hyperplasia, and cancers of the larynx, lung, stomach, breast, and uterus. (Chang & But, 1986; Hsu, et al, 1986; Minyi, 1992; Huang, 1999)

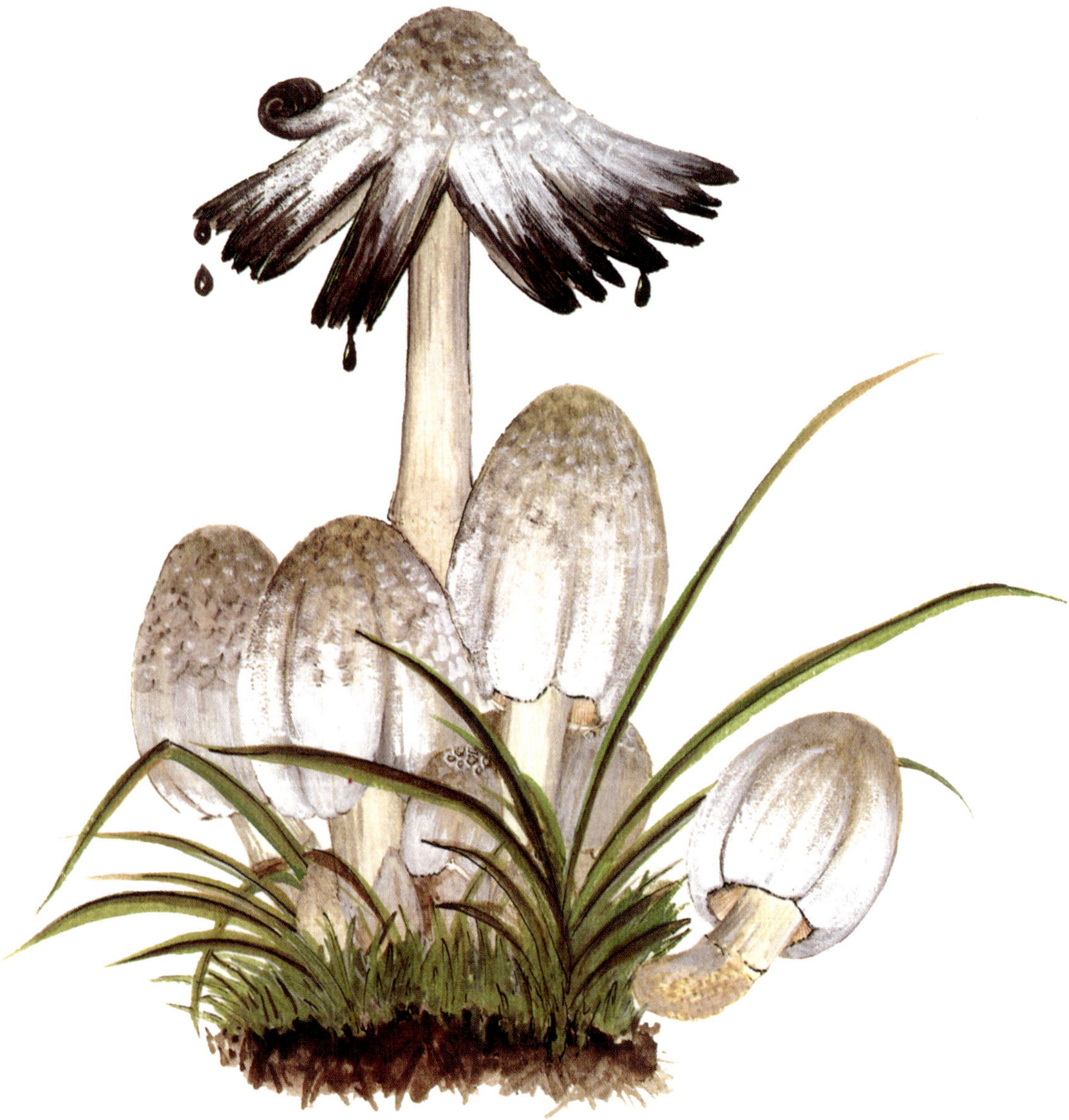

Fig. 11.43. ***Coprinus atramentarius*** (Bull.) Fr. — This mushroom contains polysaccharides that inhibit sarcoma-180 and Ehrilch's carcinoma (Jianzhe, et al, 1987).

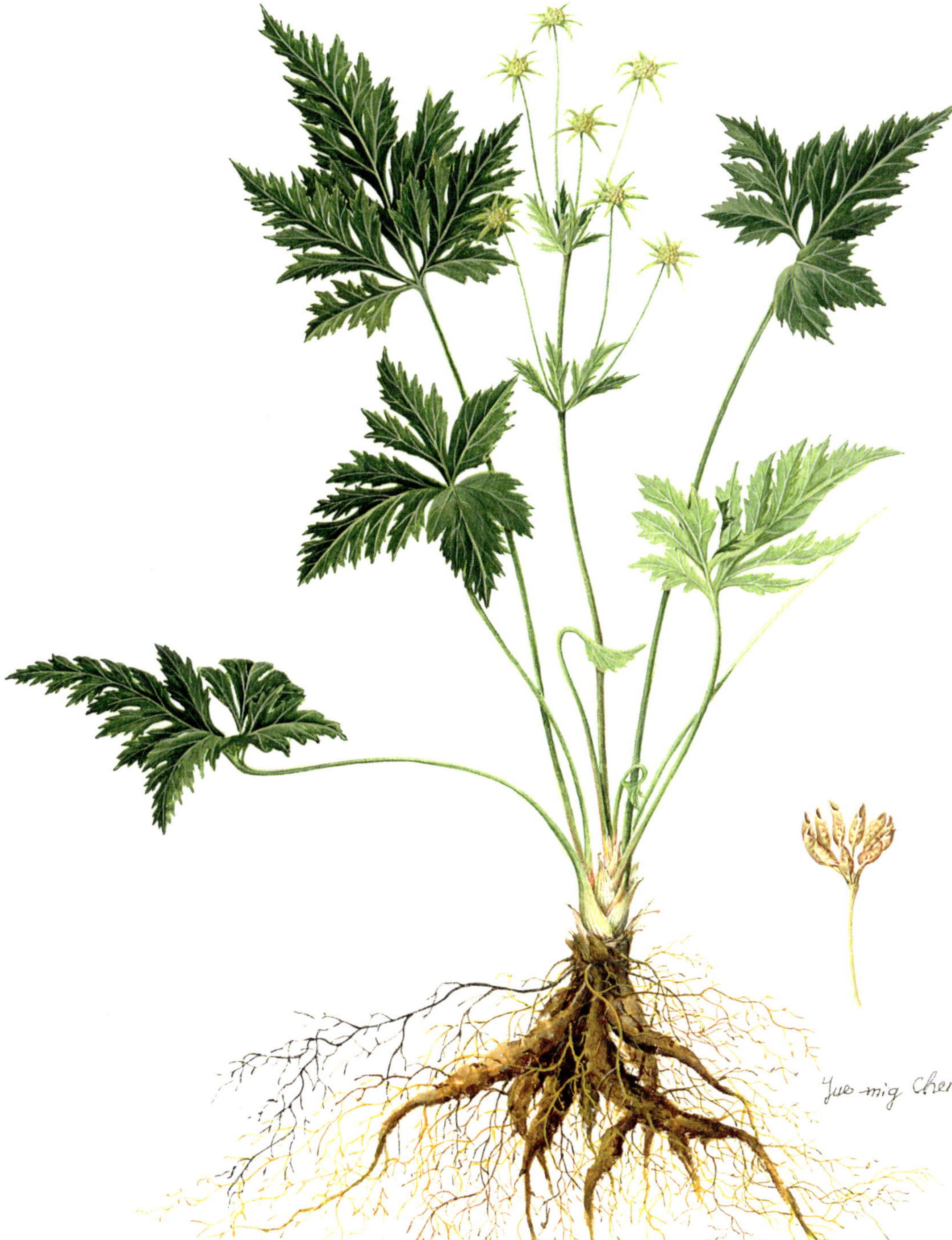


Fig. 11.44. ***Coptis chinensis*** Franch. This plant contains alkaloids including berberine, coptisine, methyl-coptisine, worenine, palmatine, columbine, jateorrhizine, and magnoflorine, and ferulic acid, obakunone, and obakulactone. It has antineoplastic effects, inhibits Erlich's ascites carcinoma, lymphoma NK/LY cells, and JTC-26 cells in vitro, and has been used to treat cancers of the ear, esophagus, rectum, and cervix. (Chang & But, 1986; Hsu, et al, 1986; Minyi, 1992; Lee, 1999)

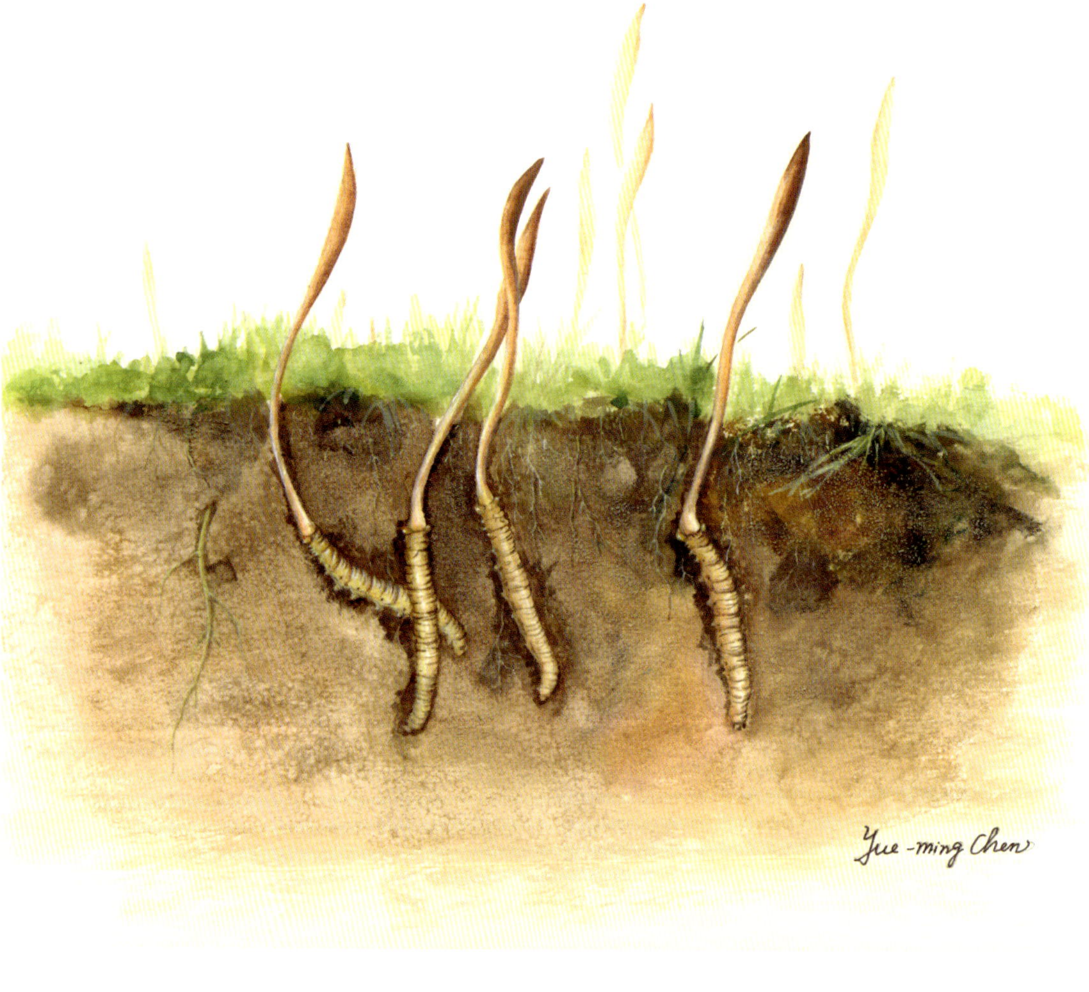


Fig. 11.45. ***Cordyceps sinensis*** (Berk.) Saccardo — This fungus, which grows on the head of the larvae of *Hepialus armori* Oberthuer, contains cordycepin 3'-deoxyadenosine, glutamic acid, phenylalanine, proline, histidine, alanine, lysine, arginine, and mannitol. It inhibits human nasopharyngeal carcinoma, HFp-2, and HL-60 cell lines, inhibits Erlich's ascites carcinoma in mice, and is effective against P-388, hepatoma tumors, and the metastasis of LC tumor in mice. It is widely used in China because of its anticancer and immune enhancing effects and has been used to treat leukemias and cancers of the nasopharynx, lymphocytes, and lung. (Chang & But, 1986; Huang, 1999; Lee, 1999)

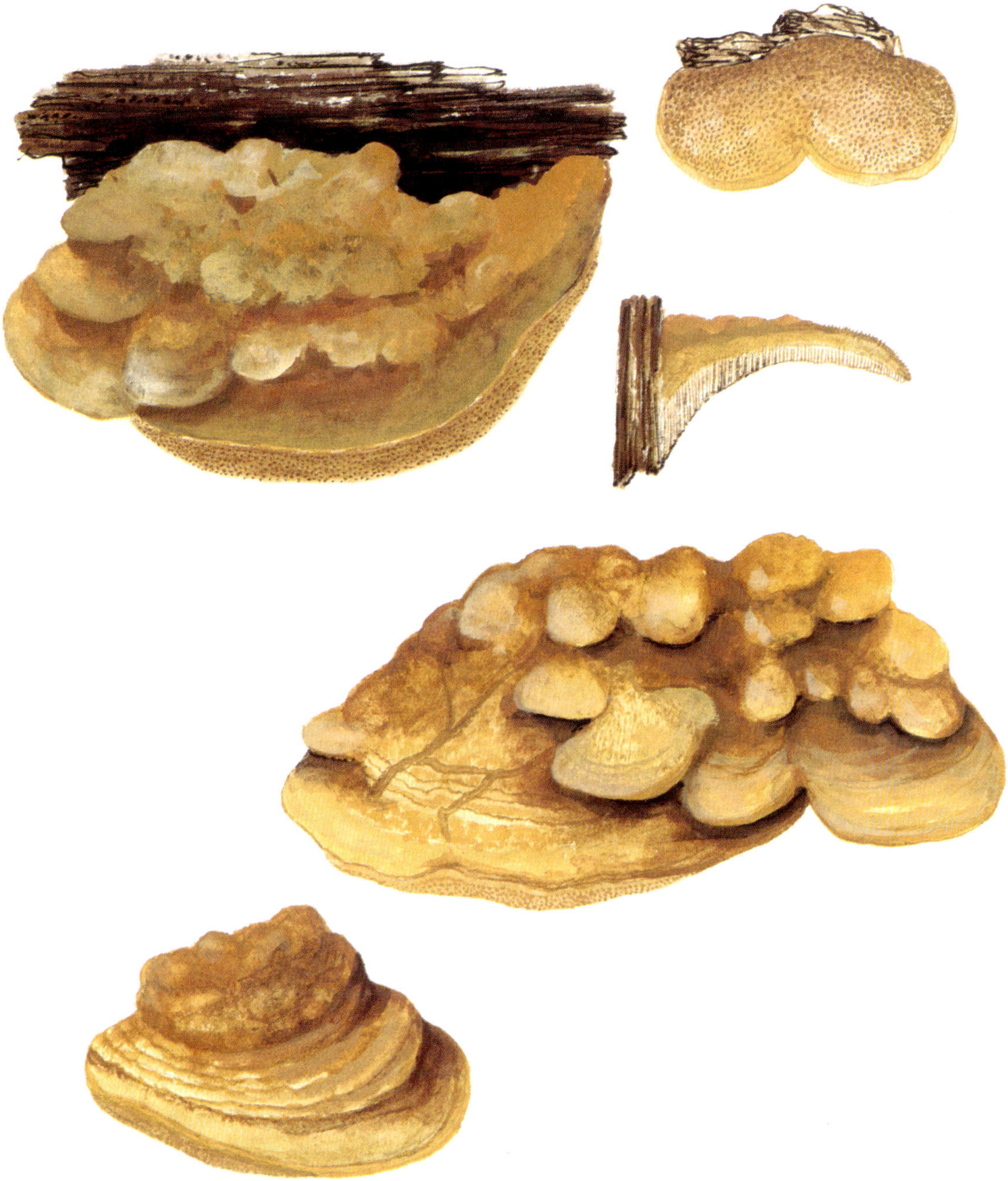

Fig. 11.46. ***Coriolopsis occidentalis*** (Kl.) Murr. — The extracts of the sporophore of this mushroom contain polysaccharides that inhibit sarcoma-180 and adenoma-755 in laboratory mice (Ying, et al, 1987).

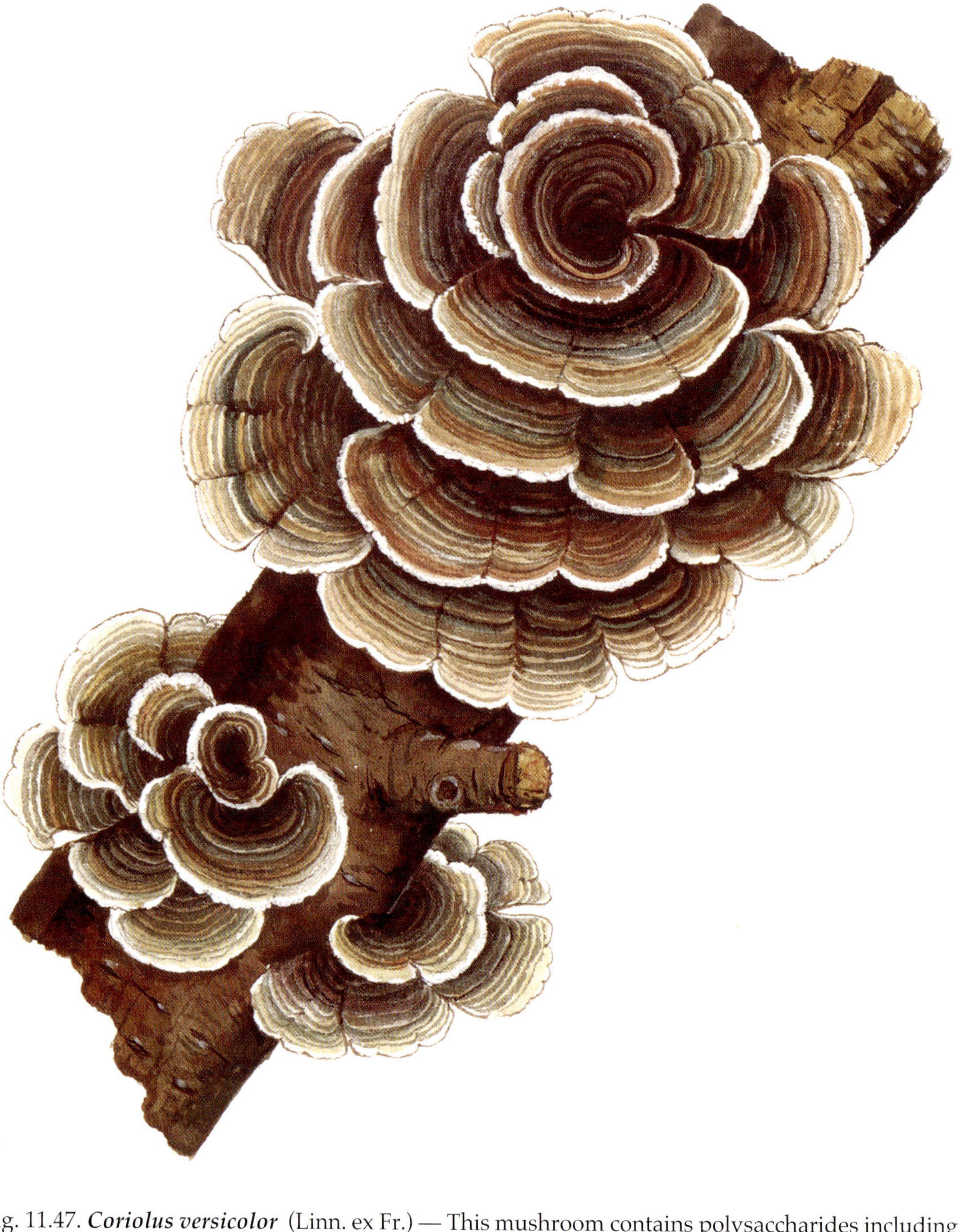

Fig. 11.47. ***Coriolus versicolor*** (Linn. ex Fr.) — This mushroom contains polysaccharides including dextran, PS-K, and coriolan, which inhibit many tumors, such as sarcoma-180, adenocancer-755, cervical cancer-14, lympholeukemic cell-7212, and lympholeukemic cell-388 in laboratory animals. It has been used to treat malignant tumors and to treat and prevent liver cancer. (Ying, et al, 1987; Minyi, 1992)

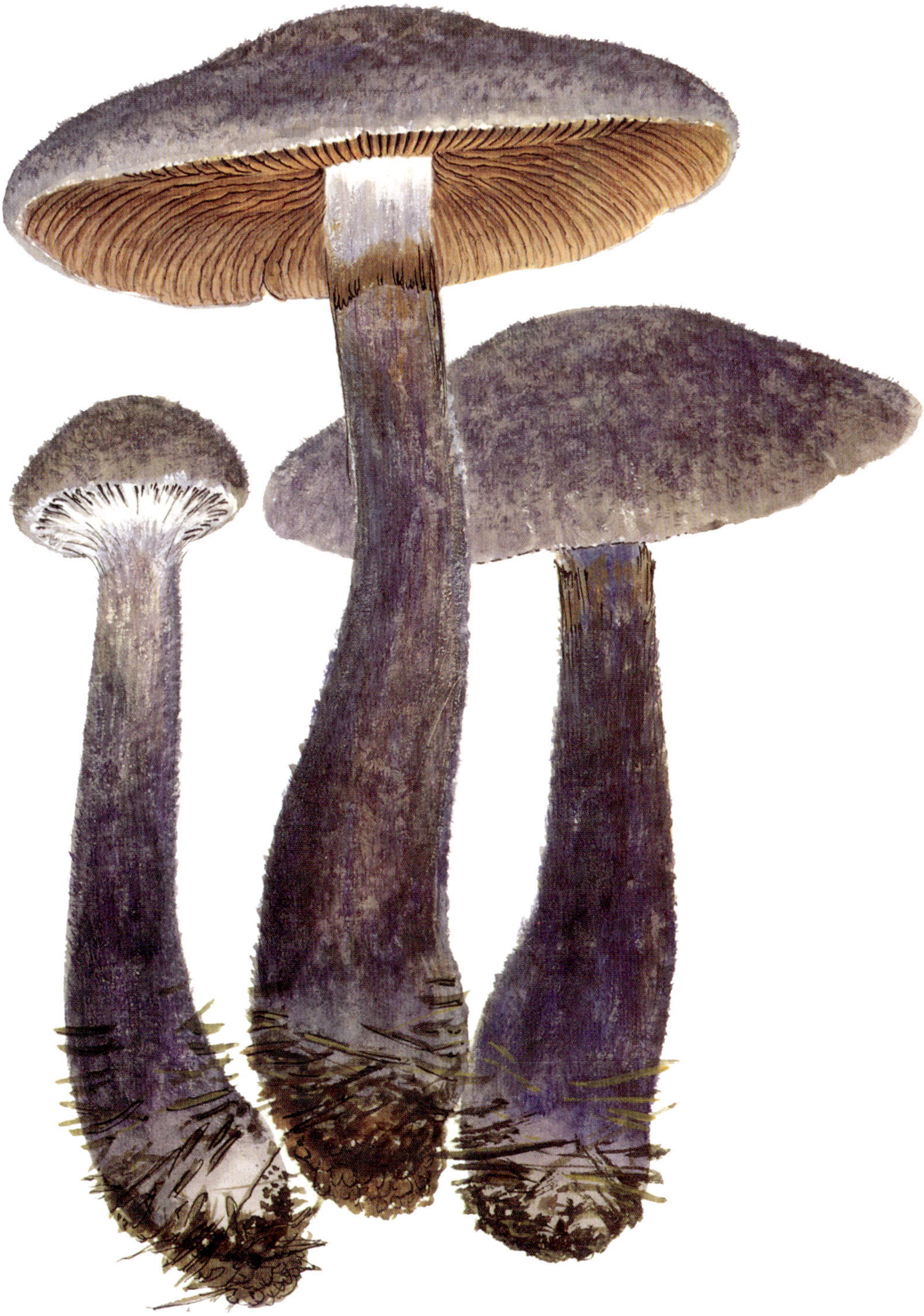

Fig. 11.48. ***Cortinarius violaceus*** (Linn.) Fr. — This mushroom contains polysaccharides that inhibit sarcoma-180 and Ehrlich's carcinoma (Ying, et al, 1987).

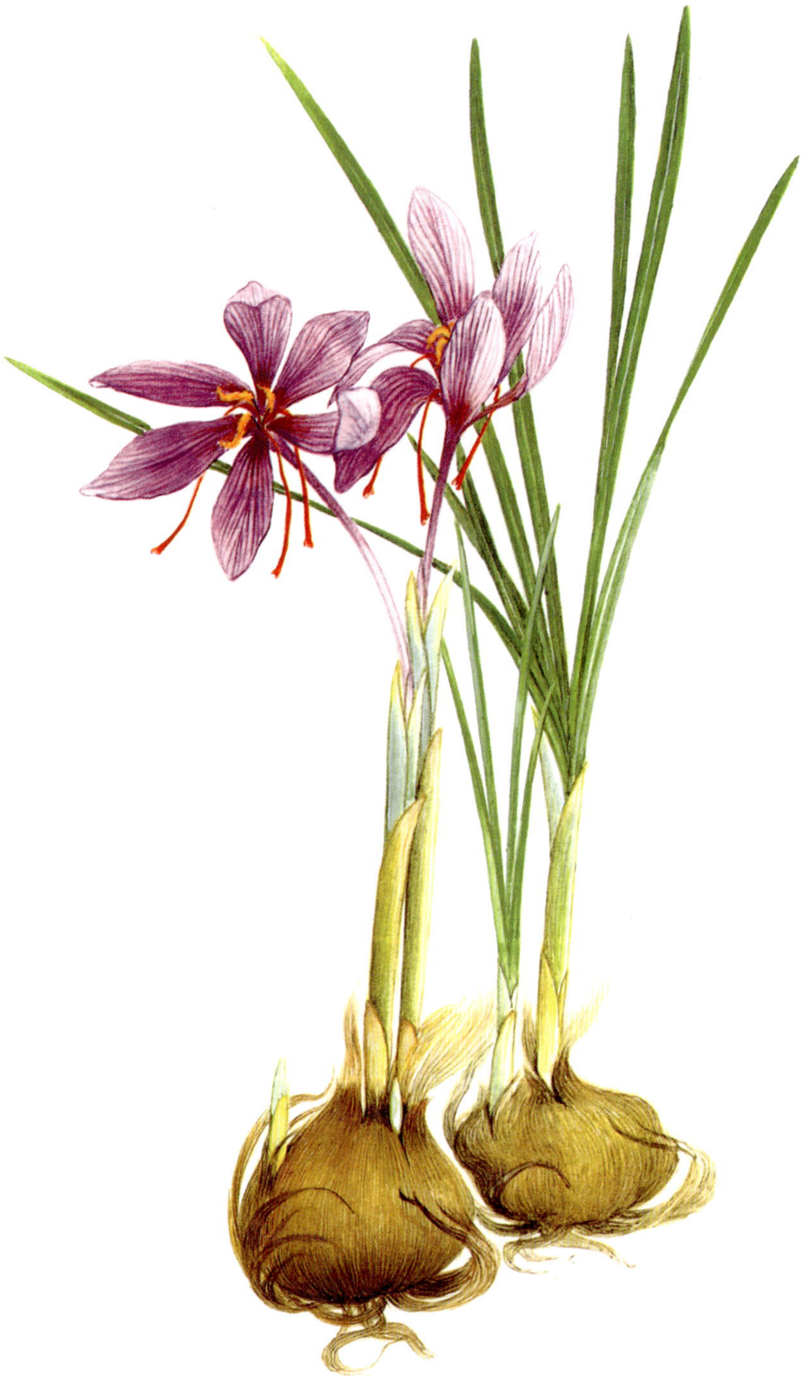

Fig. 11.49. ***Crocus sativas*** Linn. — This plant contains carotene derivatives, glycosides including crocin (crocetin digentibiose ester) and picrocrocin, α-, β-, γ-carotenes, lycopene, and the essential oil safranal. Crocin and dimethyl-crocetin exhibit a potent cytotoxic effect on human cancer cells by disrupting DNA protein interaction, which is vital to the synthesis of cancer cells. It shows protective properties against carcinogenic and hepatotoxic agents. (Hsu, et al, 1986; Chang, et al, 1996; Huang, 1999)

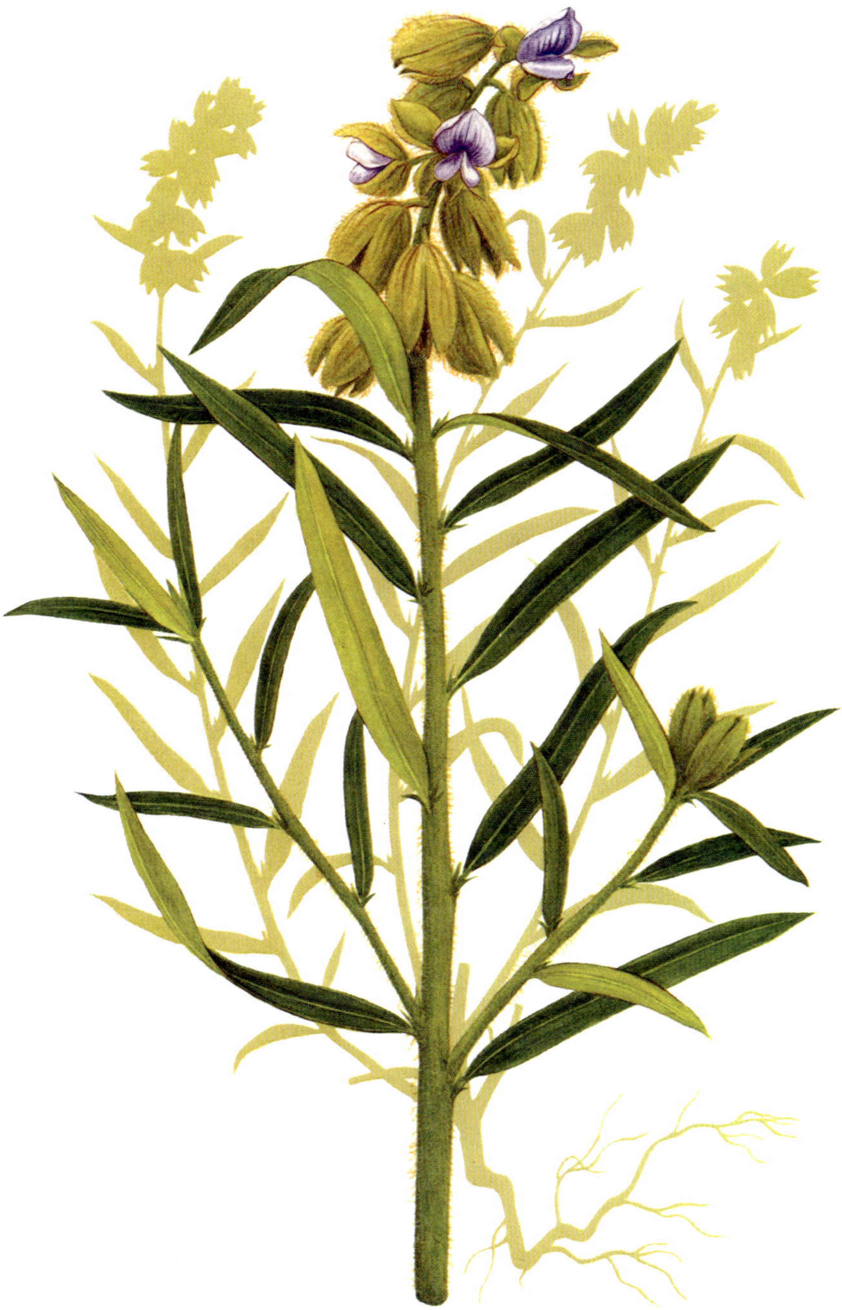

Fig. 11.50. ***Crotalaria sessilflora*** Linn. — This plant contains alkaloids, including monocrotaline A, B, C, which are credited for the anticancer activity of the plant. Laboratory studies show it inhibits sarcoma-37, sarcoma-180, lymphocytic leukemia-1210, leukemia-615, Ehrlich's ascites carcinoma, Walker's carcinoma-256, lymphosarcoma ascitic type $L_1$, metastatic Lewis lung cancer, melanoma B-16, plasma cell tumor, and adenoma-755 in laboratory animals, and in vitro inhibits human hepatoma BEL-7402 cells, and KB cells. It has been used in the treatment of leukemia and cancers of the esophagus, skin, cervix, and rectum. (Chang & But, 1986; Hsu, et al, 1986; Huang, 1999; Lee, 1999)

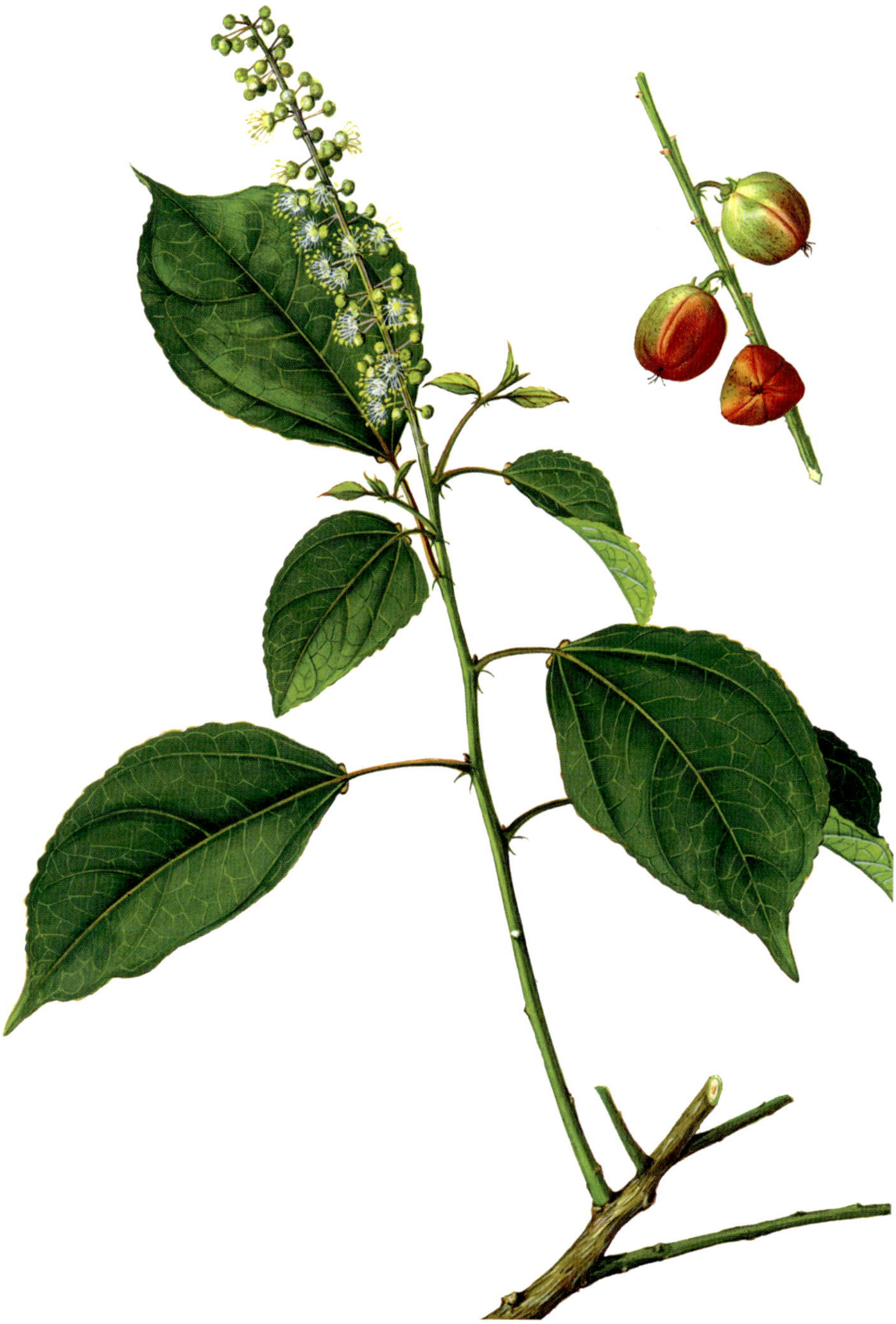

Fig. 11.51. ***Croton tiglium*** Linn. — This plant contains crotonoside, arginine, crotin, β-sitosterol, isoguanosine, and croton oil, which is made up of oleic acid, linolic acid, arachic acid, stearic acid, palmitic acid, lauric acid, tiglic acid, crotonic acid, and croton resin, which includes phorbol esters. It inhibits solid and ascitic sarcoma-180, solid and ascitic cervical carcinoma-14, lymphocytic leukemia P-388, solid hepatoma, transplanted cutaneous carcinoma, and Erlich's ascites carcinoma in mice, inhibits JTC-26 in vitro, kills EAC cells and ascitic liver carcinoma, and has been used in the treatment of stomach and cervical cancer. (Chang & But, 1986; Hsu, et al, 1986; Minyi, 1992; Kim, et al, 1994; Lee, 1999)

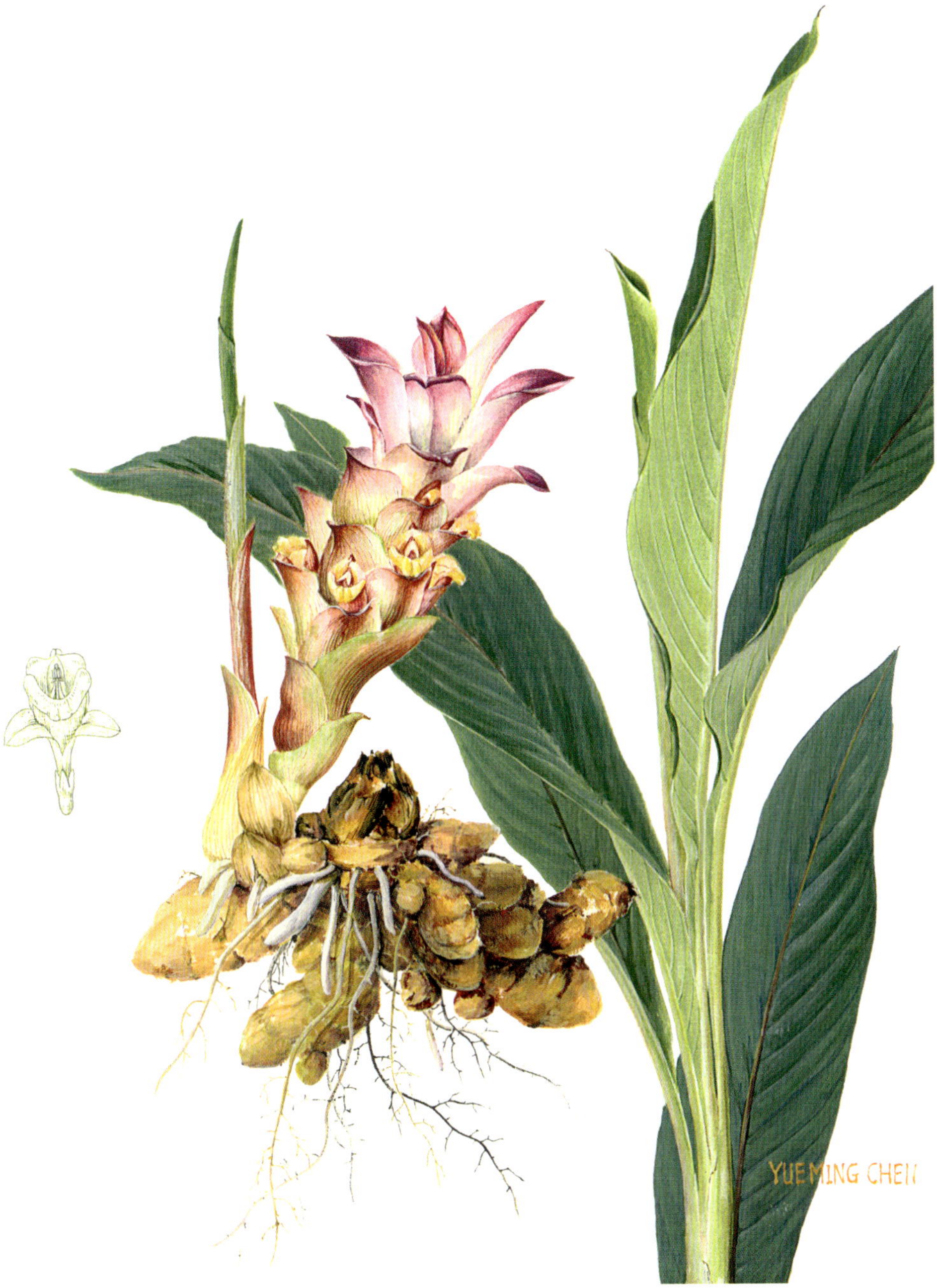


Fig. 11.52. ***Curcuma aromatica*** Salisb. — This plant contains curzerenone, pyrocurcuzerenone, dehydrocurdione, zederone, curidone, curzerene, curcolone, furanodienone, isofuranodienone, furanodiene, curcumin, isocurcumenol, epicurcumenol, procurcumenol, and curcumol (curcumenol), tumerone, (+)-ar-tumerone, zingiberene, (+)-α-phellandrene, l-curcamene, camphor, camphene, curcumin, p-coumaroylferuoyl methane, di-p-coumaroyl methane. It has antitumor and anticancer promoting properties. It inhibits sarcoma-180 in mice, ascites cells, and mouse cervical cancer-14 cells, kills Erlich's ascites carcinoma cells in vitro, and has antimutagenic and antitumor properties. It has been used in the treatment of cervical cancer, cystocarcinoma, spermatocytoma, and celiac tumor. (Chang & But, 1986; Hsu, et al, 1986; Huang, 1999)

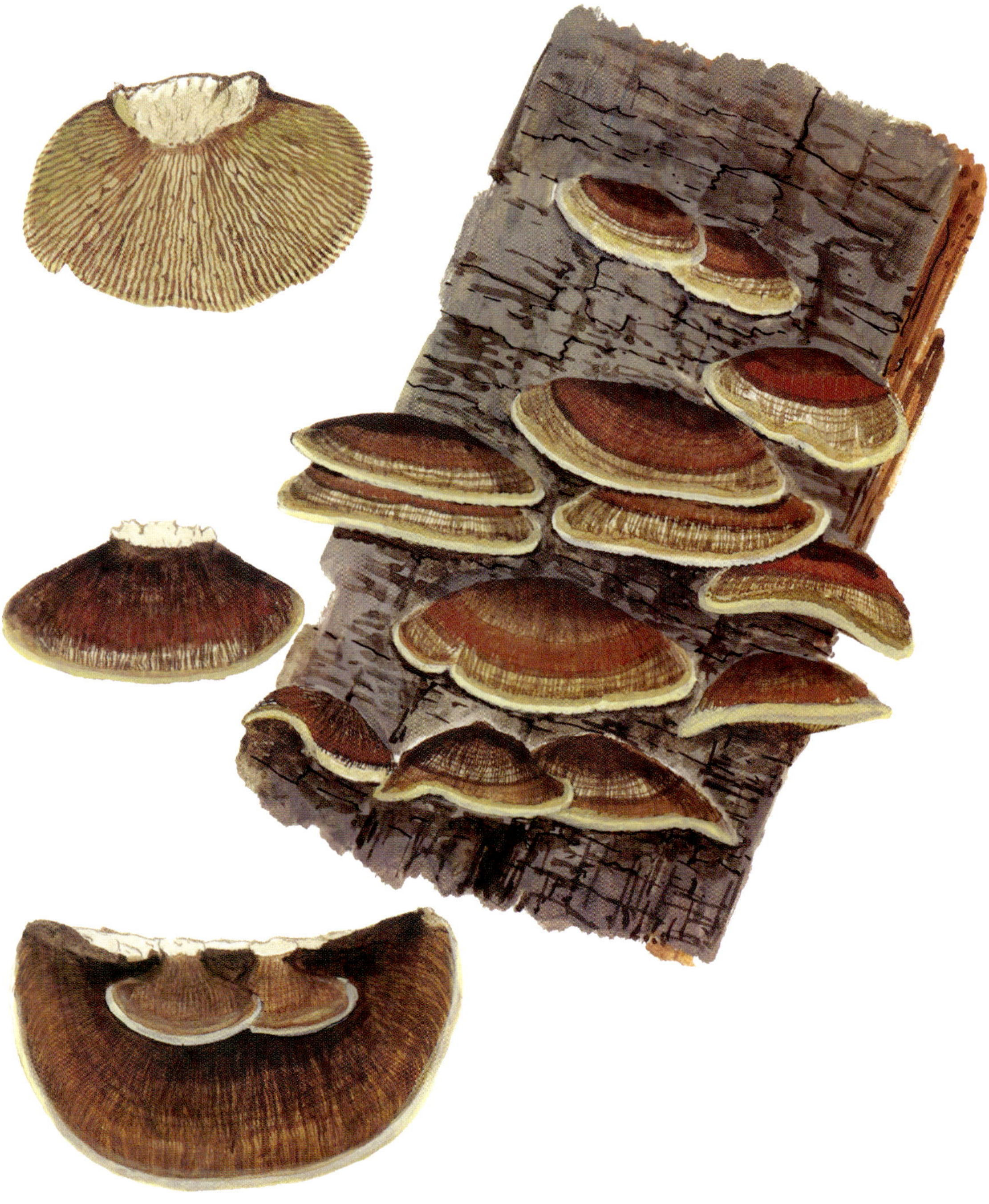

Fig. 11.53. ***Daedaleopsis tricolor*** (Fr.) Band. et Sing. — This mushroom contains polysaccharides that inhibit sarcoma-180 in mice (Ying, et al, 1987).

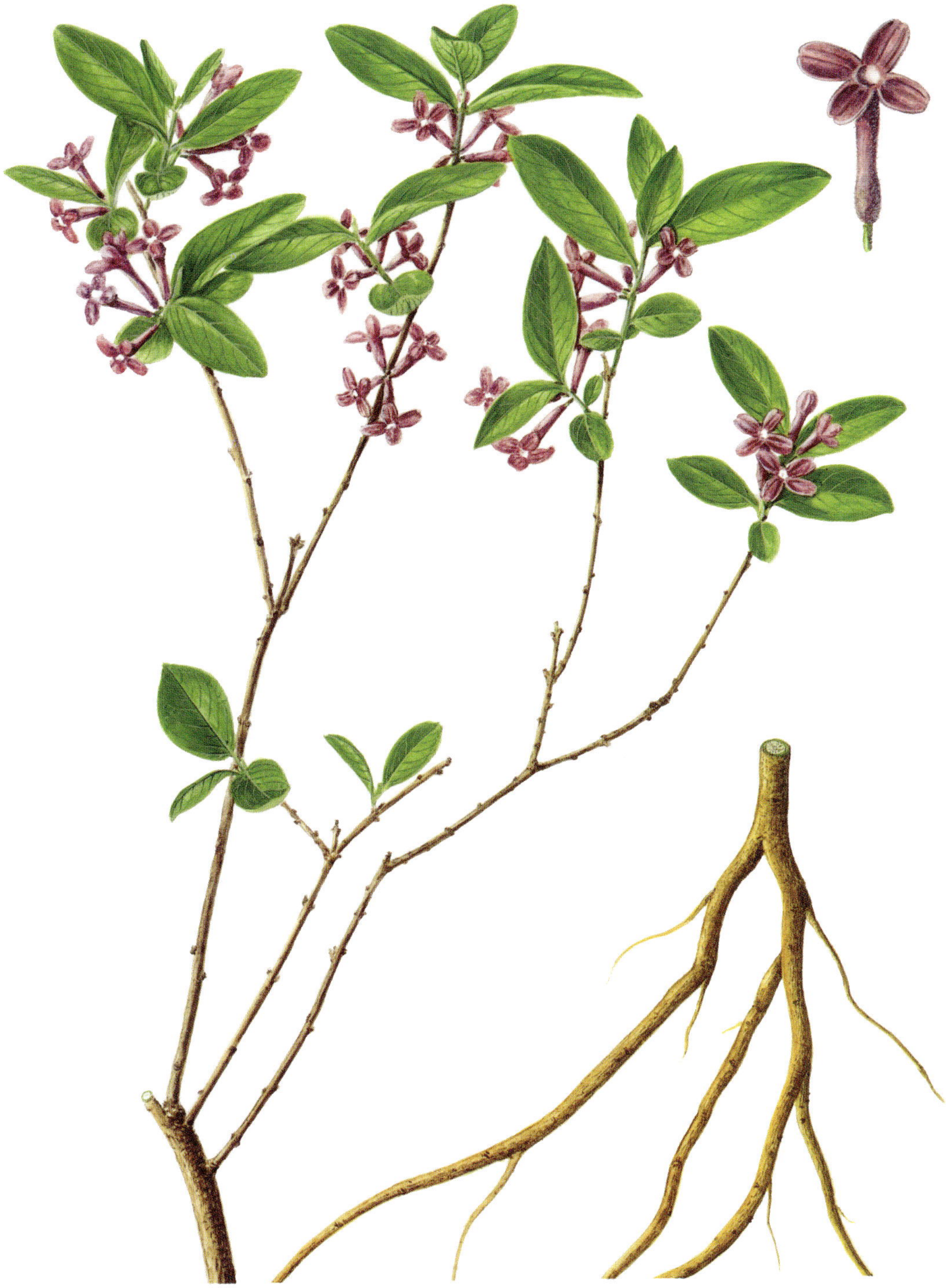

Fig. 11.54. ***Daphne genkwa*** Sieb. et Zucc. — This plant contains flavenoids, apigenin, genkwanin, and hydroxygenkwanin, bezoic acid, sitosterol, guidilatichin, yuankanin, and fatty oils. It has anticancer activity on rectal cancer, and inhibits lymphatic leukemia-388 in laboratory animals. It has been used in the treatment of skin cancer, lymphosarcoma, and lymphadenoma. (Hsu, et al, 1986; Minyi, 1992; Huang, 1999)

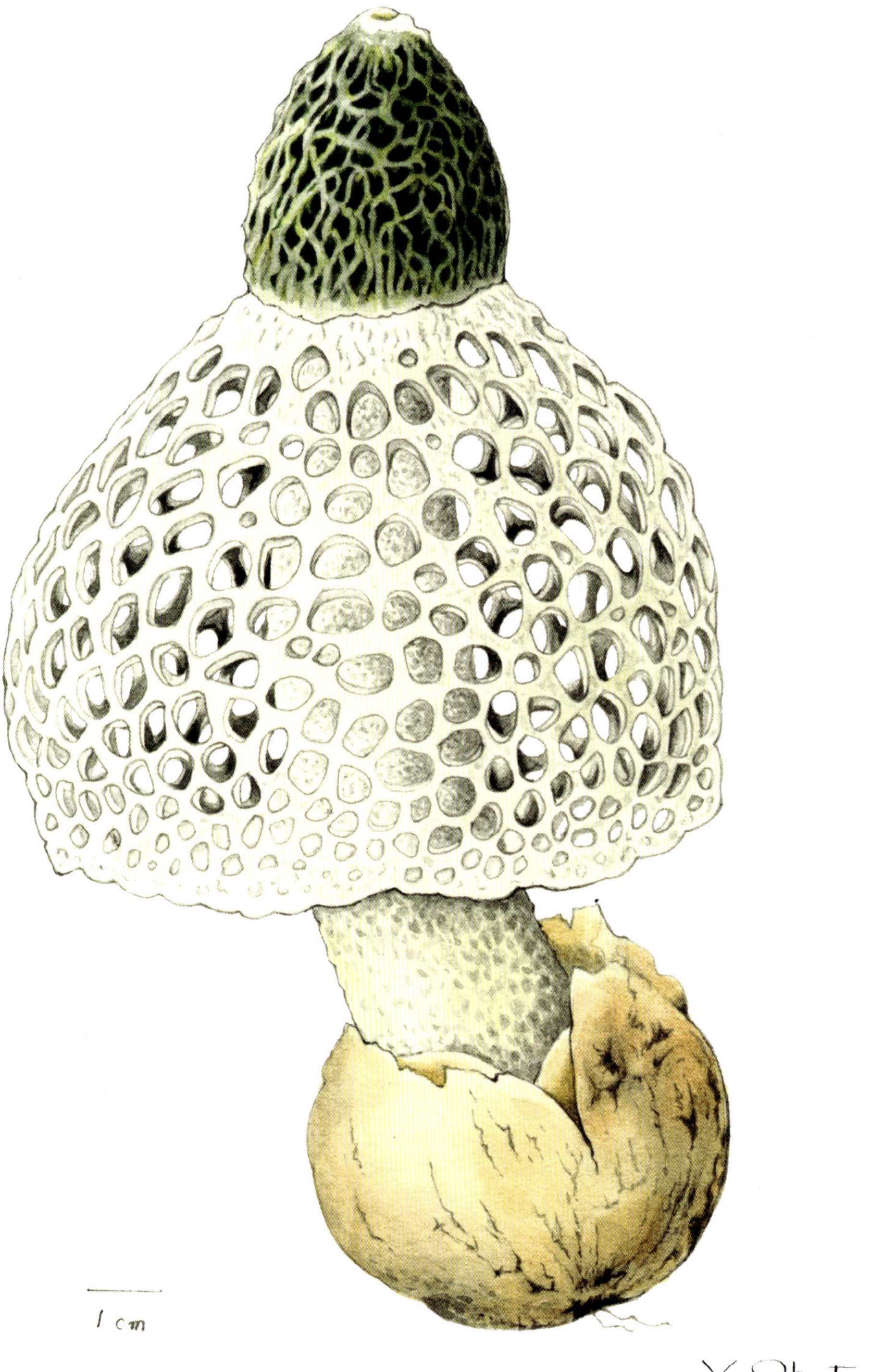


Fig. 11.55. ***Dictyophora indusiata*** (Vent. ex Pers.) Fischer — This mushroom contains polysaccharides that inhibit sarcoma-180 and Ehrlich's carcinoma (Ying, et al, 1987).

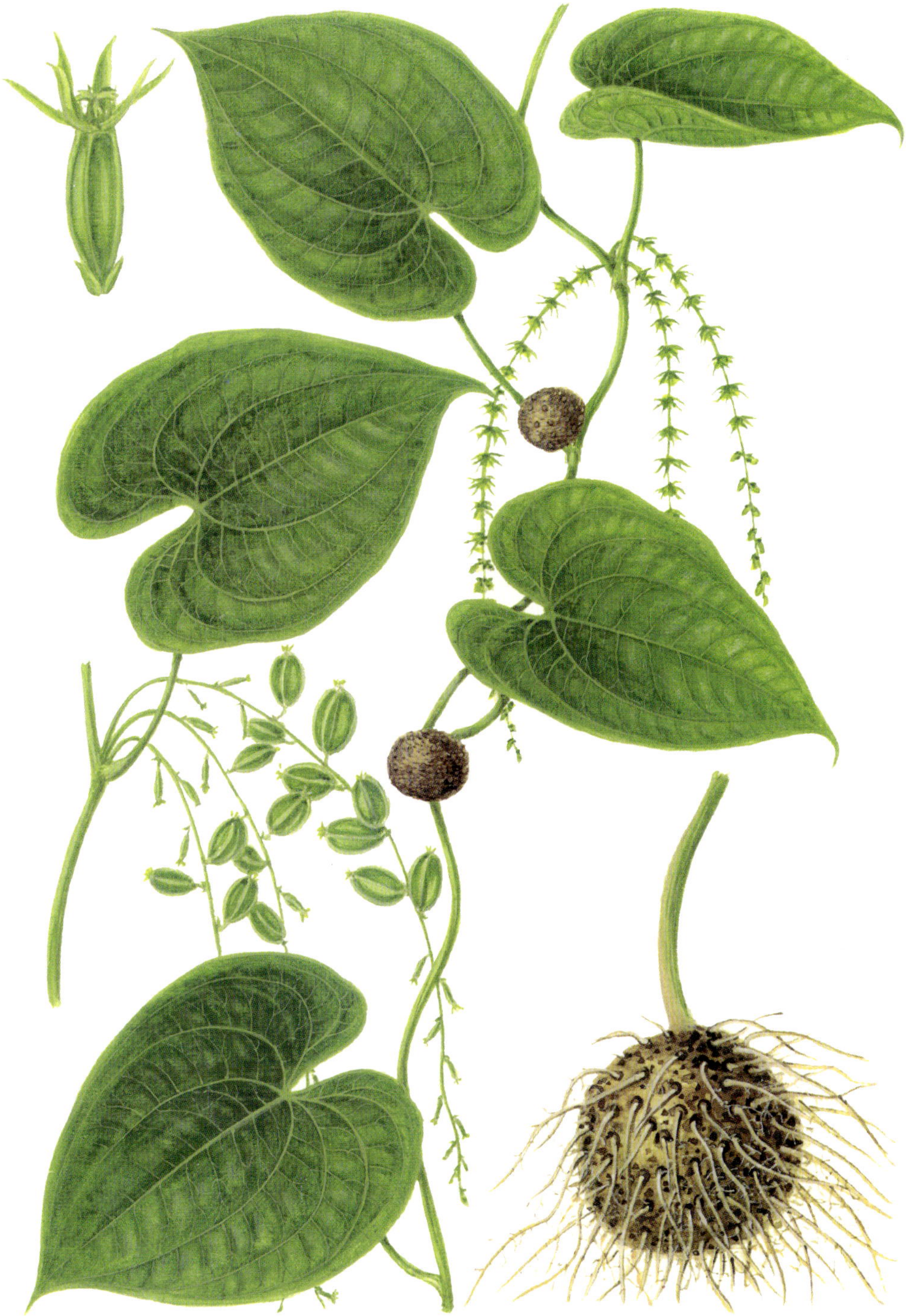

Fig. 11.56. ***Dioscorea bulbifera*** Linn. — This plant contains the terpenes diosbulbin A, B, C, and D, 2,4,6,7-tetrahydroxy-9,10-dihydrophenanthrene, 2,4,5,6-tetrahydroxy-phenanthrene, and tannin. It inhibits mouse sarcoma-180 and cervical cancer-14, is effective against leukemia-615, and has been used to treat cancer of the esophagus, heart, and rectum. (Hsu, et al, 1986; Minyi, 1992; Huang, 1999; Lee, 1999)

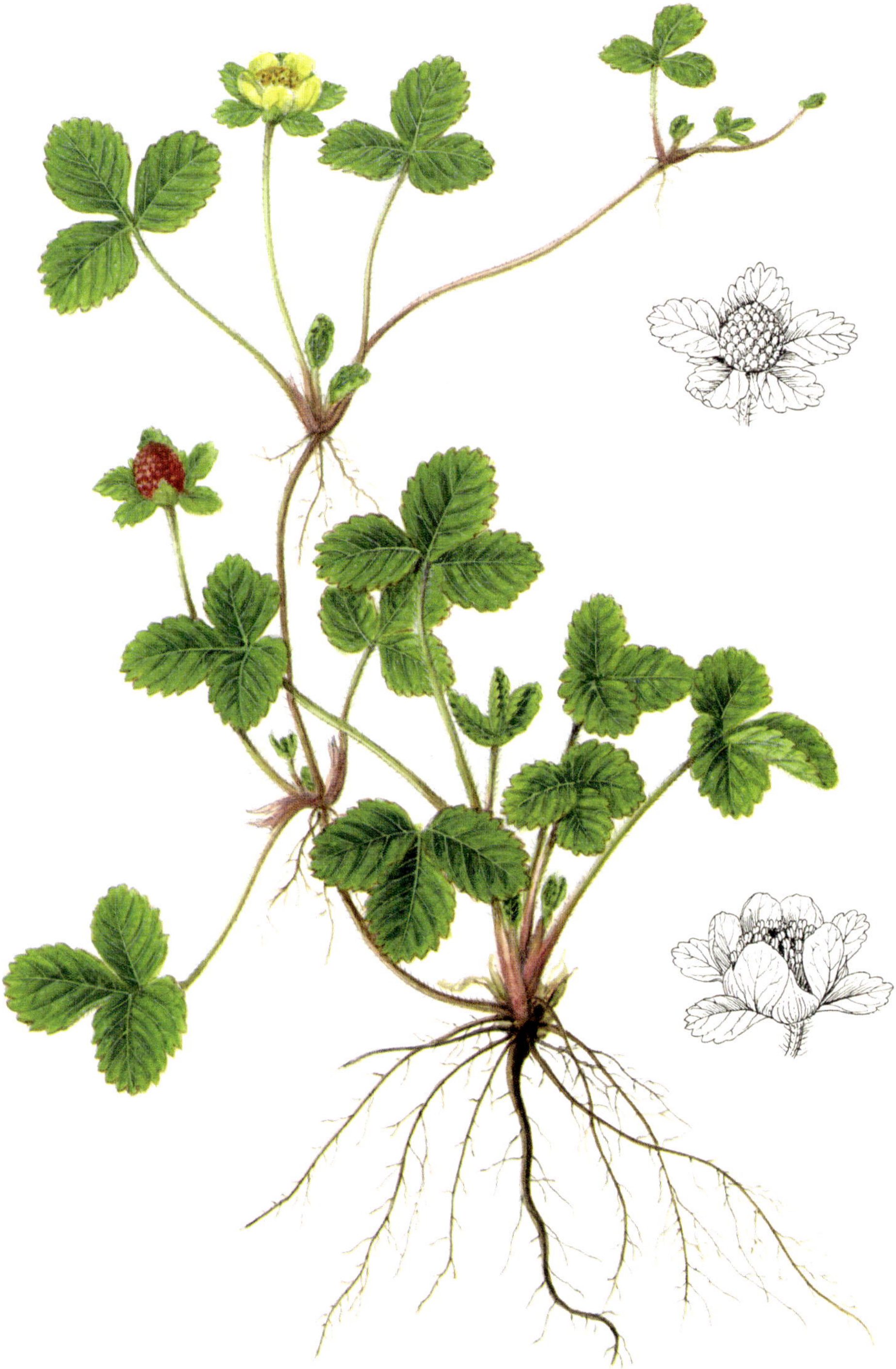

Fig. 11.57. ***Duchesnea indica*** (Andr.) Focke — This plant contains saponins, oleic acid, and β-sitosterol. It inhibits sarcoma-180 in mice, JTC-26, and Erlich's ascites cancer, and has been used to treat cystoma, thoracic cancer, carcinoma of the urinary bladder, rectal cancer, cervical cancer, thyroid cancer, hepatoma, leukemia, and various other cancers. (Hsu, et al, 1986; Minyi, 1992; Huang, 1999; Lee, 1999)

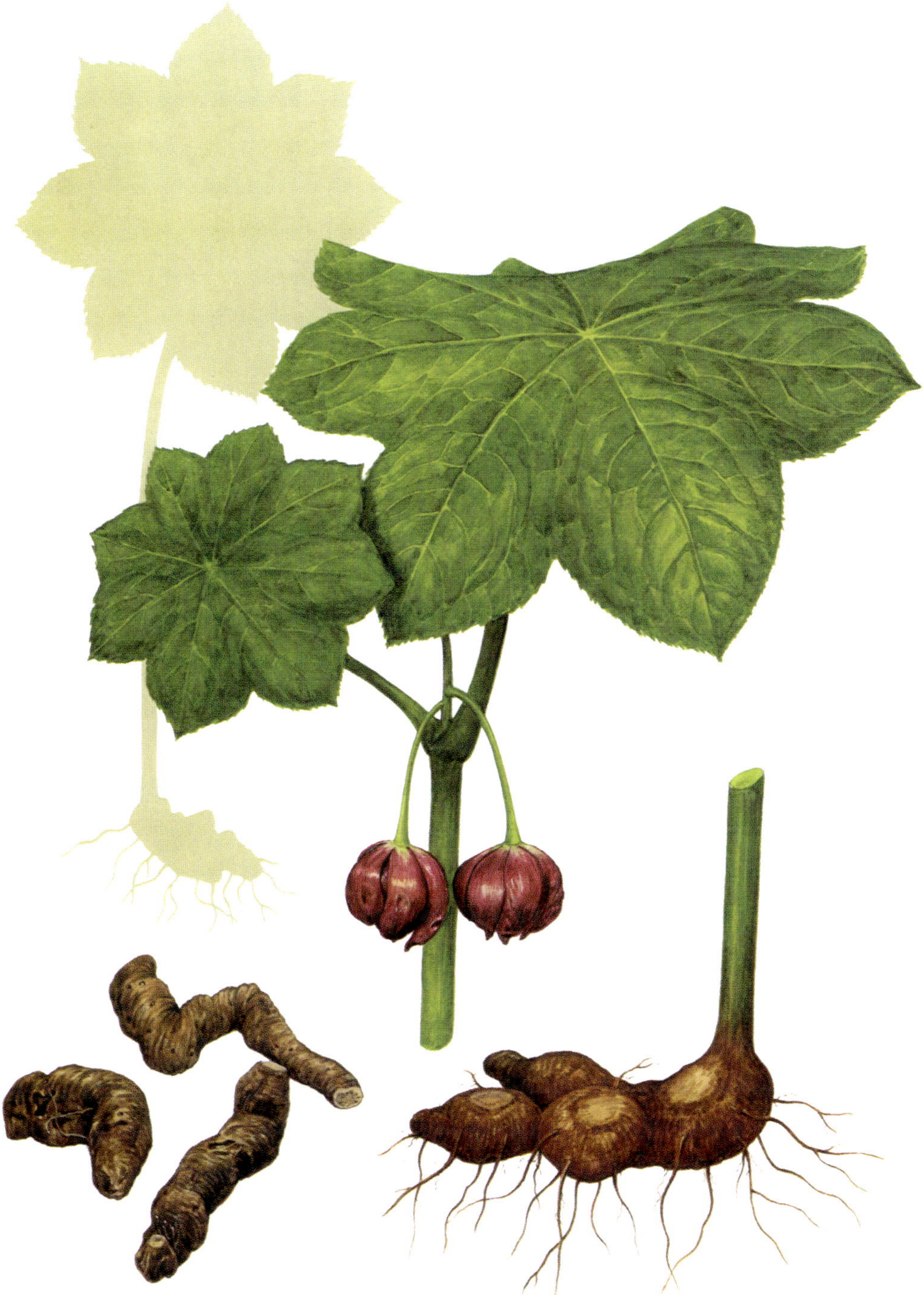

Fig. 11.58. ***Dysosma pleiantha*** (Hance) Woodson — This plant contains podophyllotoxin, desoxypodophyllotoxin, isopicropodophyllone, quercetin, kaempferol, astragalin, pellatin, and hyperin. It has an antineoplastic action that is active against several types of cancer, and has been used to treat cancers of the skin, nasopharynx, esophagus, lung, cervix, and uterus. (Hsu, et al, 1986; Minyi, 1992; Huang, 1999)

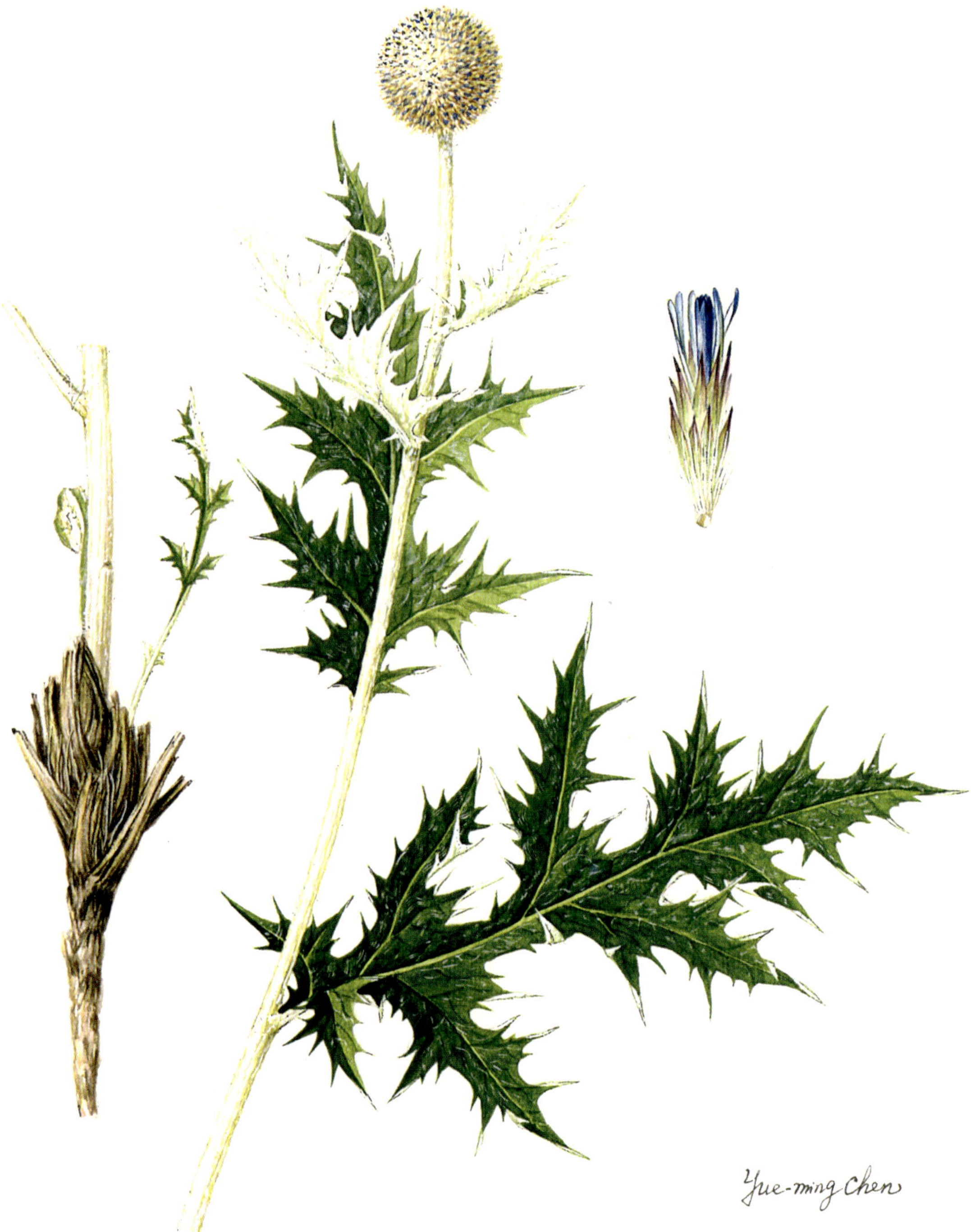


Fig. 11.59. ***Echinops latifolius*** Tausch. — This plant contains volatile oils, phenols, echinopsine, and β-sitosterol. It enhances the immune system, inhibits carcinogenesis, and has been used to treat glossocancer and breast cancer. (Minyi, 1992)

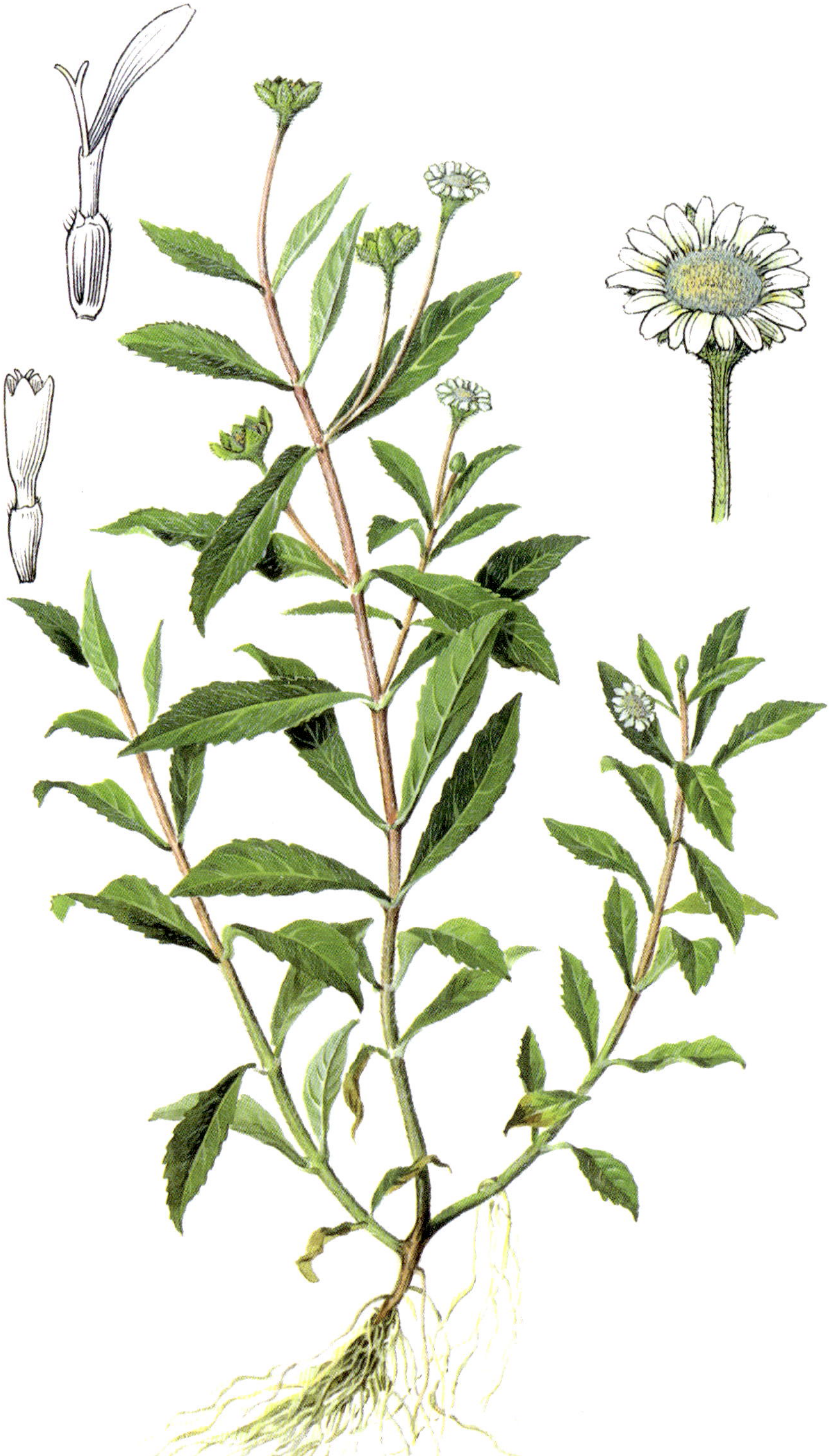

Fig. 11.60. ***Eclipta prostrata*** Linn. — This plant contains saponins, nicotine, ecliptine, wedelolactone, tannins, and vitamin A. It inhibits oncocytoplasia and has been used to treat esophageal and uterine cancer. (Minyi, 1992)

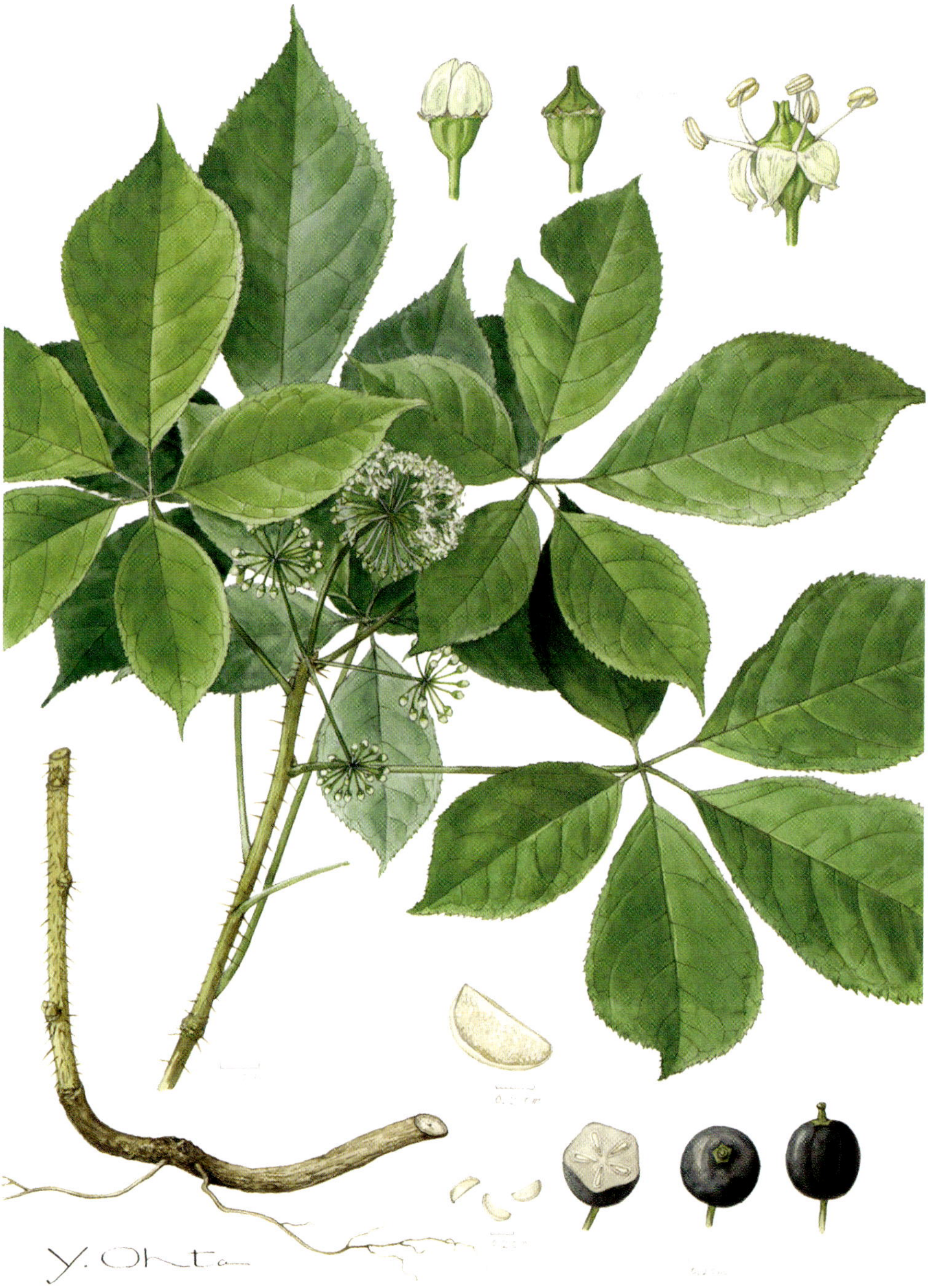

Fig. 11.61. ***Eleutherococcus senticosus*** (Rupr. et Maxim.) Maxim. — This plant contains the following glycosides, β-sitosterol, eleutherosides, daucosterol, syringin, 7-hydroxy-6,8-dimethoxycoumarin glycoside, ethylgalactoside, syringaresinol, and a number of sugars. It inhibits induced tumors, metastasis of SSK sarcoma, and Walker's carcinoma in rats, and is effective against transplanted tumors, has adaptogenic properties, enhances the immune system, and has been used in patients suffering from leukopenia resulting from cancer radiotherapy and chemotherapy. (Halstead & Hood, 1984a; Chang & But, 1986; Huang, 1999)

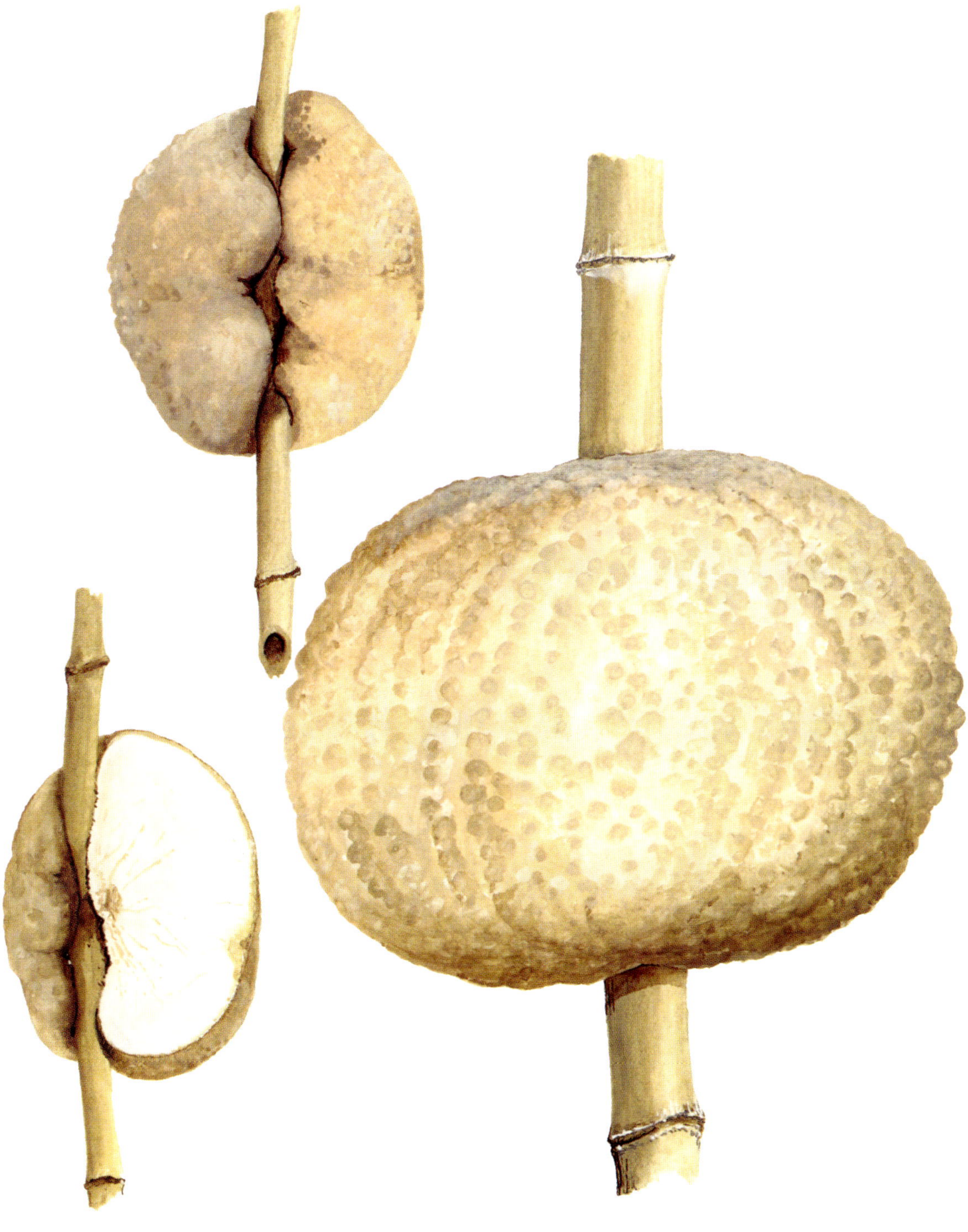

Fig. 11.62 *Engleromyces goetzi* P. Henn. — This mushrrom contains polysaccharides that have been effective in treating human cancers (Ying, et al, 1997).

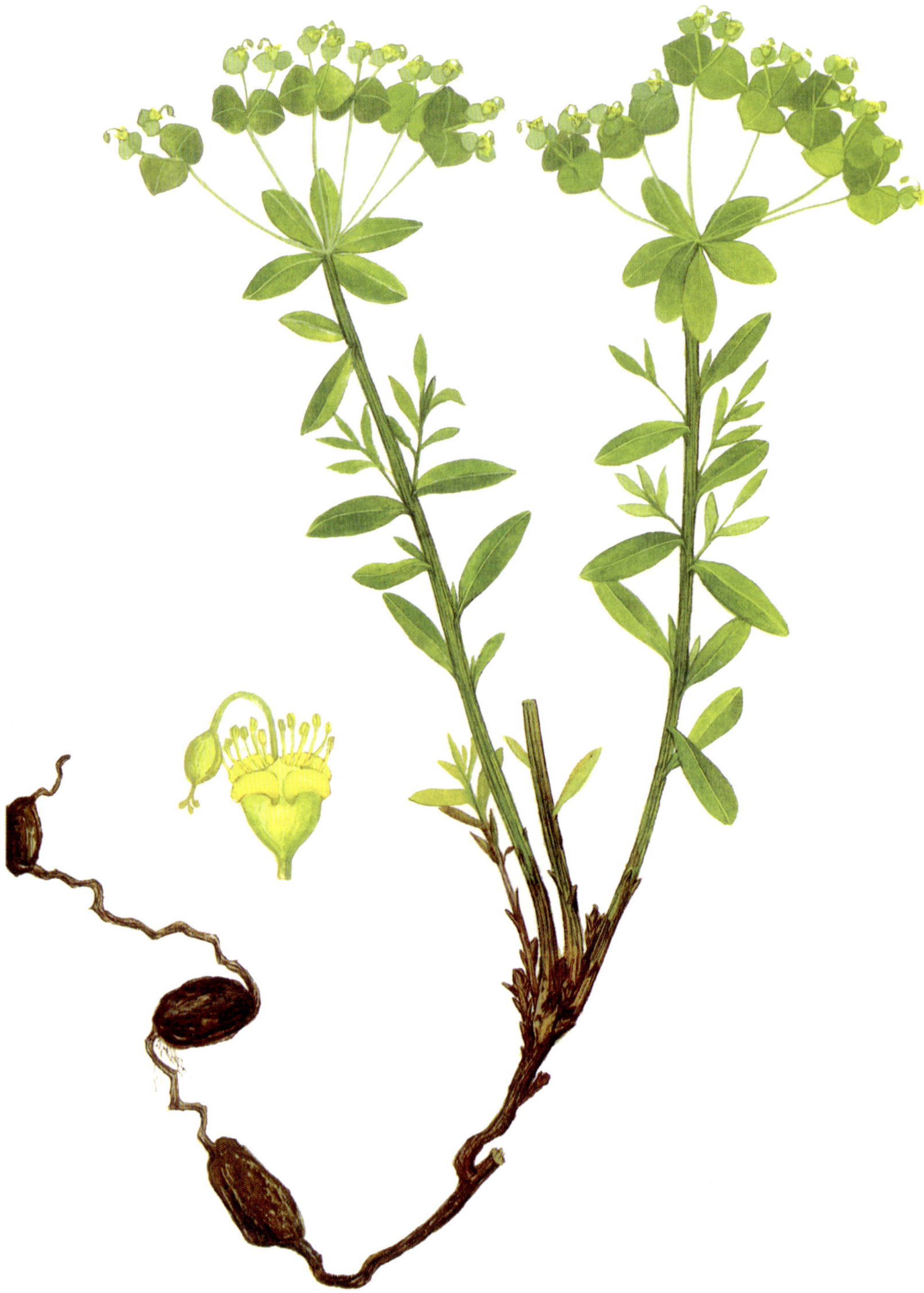

Fig. 11.63. ***Euphorbia kansui*** T. N. Lion ex T. P. Wang — This plant contains diterpenoids, triterpenoids, α-euphorbol, tirucallol, ingenol, and euphadienol. It is effective against squamous carcinoma and lung carcinoma, causes necrosis of cancer cells, and has been used to treat esophageal and liver cancer. (Lee, 1999)

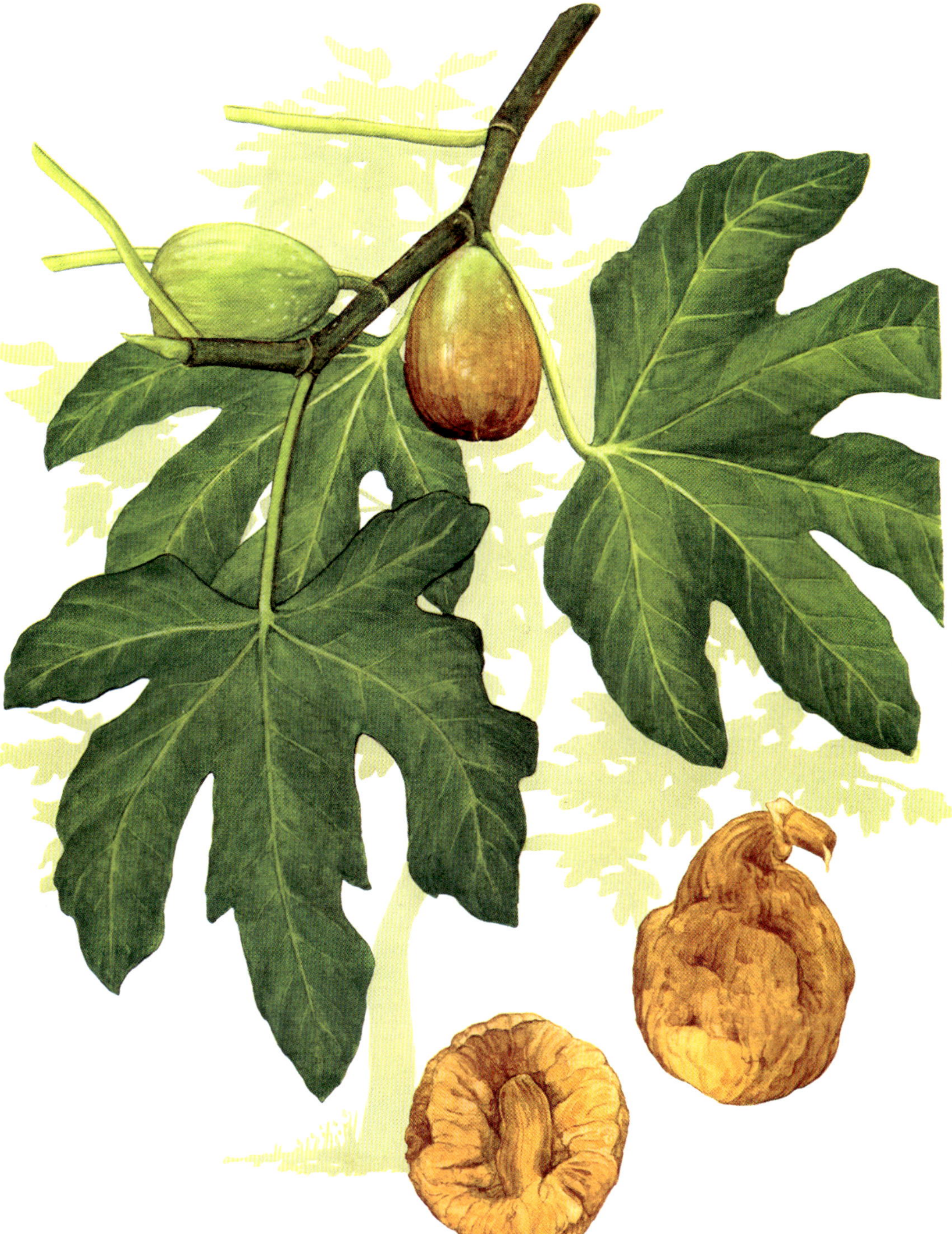

Fig. 11.64. ***Ficus carica*** Linn. — The fruit of this plant contains glucose, fructose, citric acid, quinic acid, and shikimic acid, which show an anticancer effect on Ehrlich's sarcoma, and inhibits transplanted sarcoma in rats and mastocarcinoma of mice. It has been used in the treatment of esophageal, stomach, bowel, and urinary bladder cancer. (Hsu, et al, 1986; Minyi, 1992)

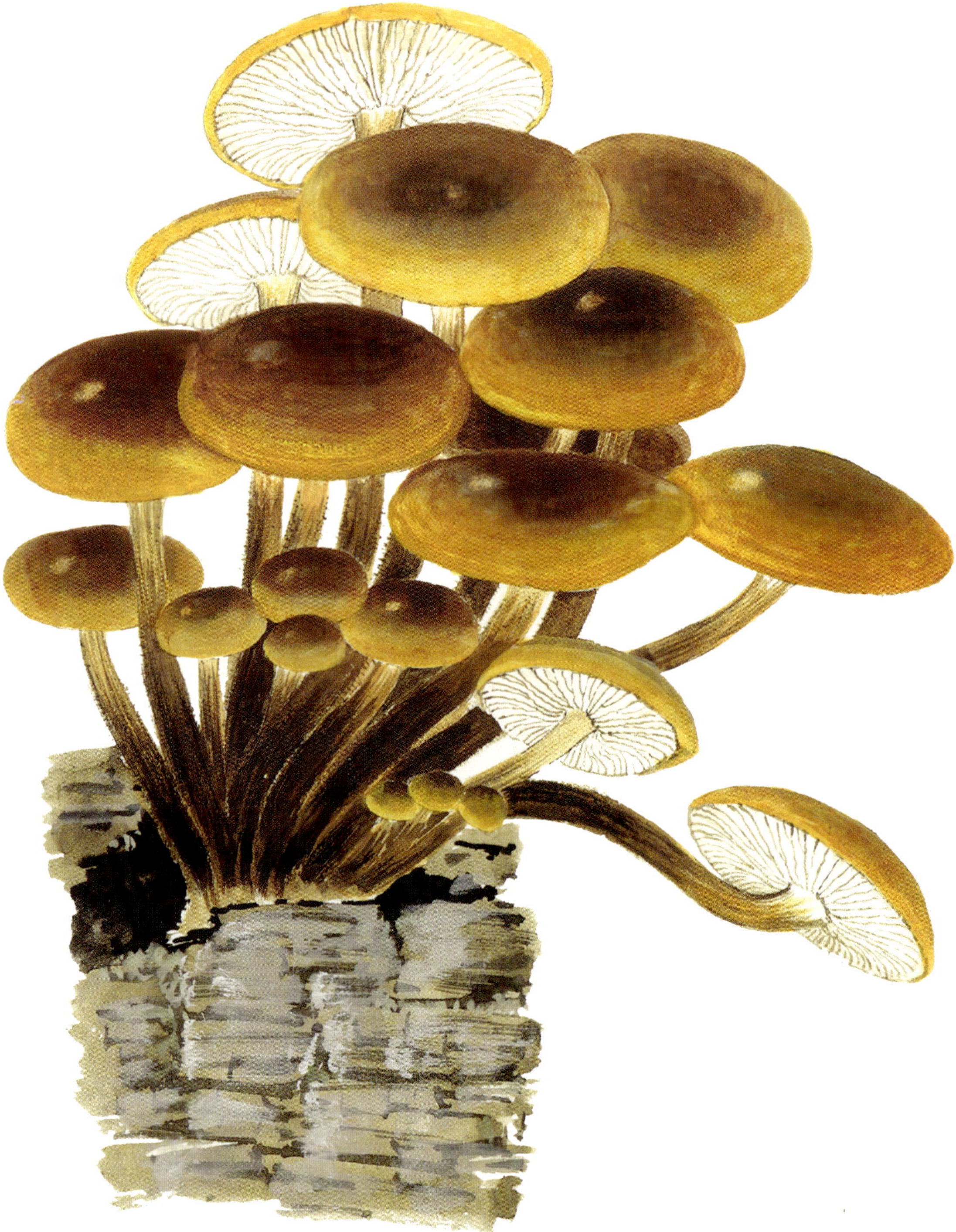

Fig. 11.65. ***Flamulina velutipes*** (Curt. ex Fr.) Sing. — This mushroom contains proflamin, flammulinin (a sporophore extract), arginine, methionine, lysine, polysaccharides, and vitamins. It inhibits sarcoma-180 and Ehrlich's carcinoma in white mice. (Ikekawa, et al, 1985; Ying, et al, 1987; Leung, et al, 1997)

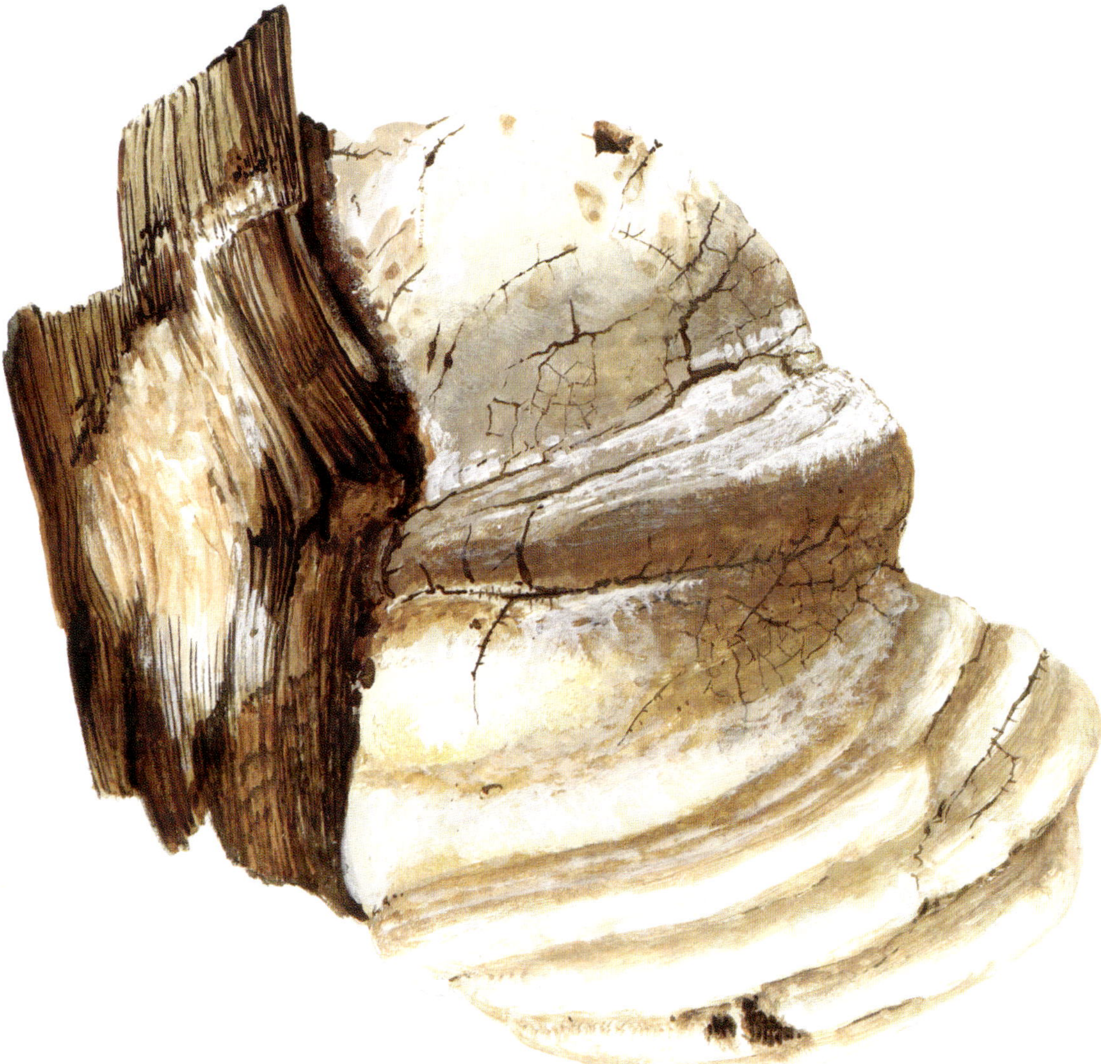

Fig. 11.66. ***Fomitopsis officinalis*** (Vill. ex Fr.) Bond et Sing. — This mushroom contains agaric acid and polysaccharides that inhibit sarcoma-180 and Ehrlich's carcinoma in mice (Ying, et al, 1987)

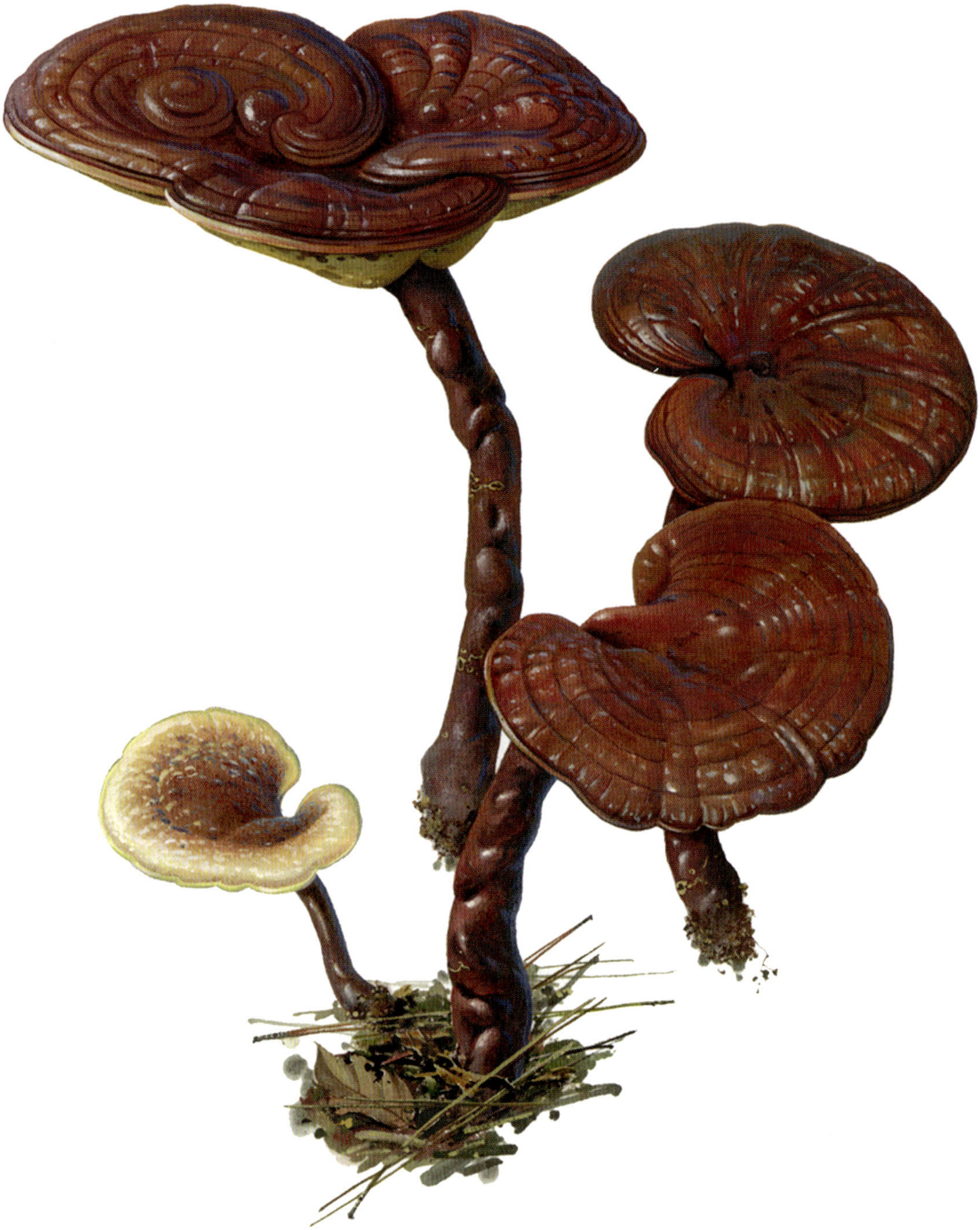

Fig. 11.67. ***Ganoderma lucidum*** (Leys. ex Fr.) Karst. — This mushroom contains ergosterol, fumaric acid, polysaccharides, aminoglucose, coumarins, mannitol, lactones, steroid, triterpene, glucoside, riboflavin, alkaloids, organic acids, ascorbic acid, and a variety of enzymes. It has antitumor effects, inhibits sarcoma-180 in mice, enhances the immune system, and has been used to treat various types of cancers including stomach cancer. (Hsu, et al, 1986; Ying, et al, 1987; Minyi, 1992; Huang, 1999)

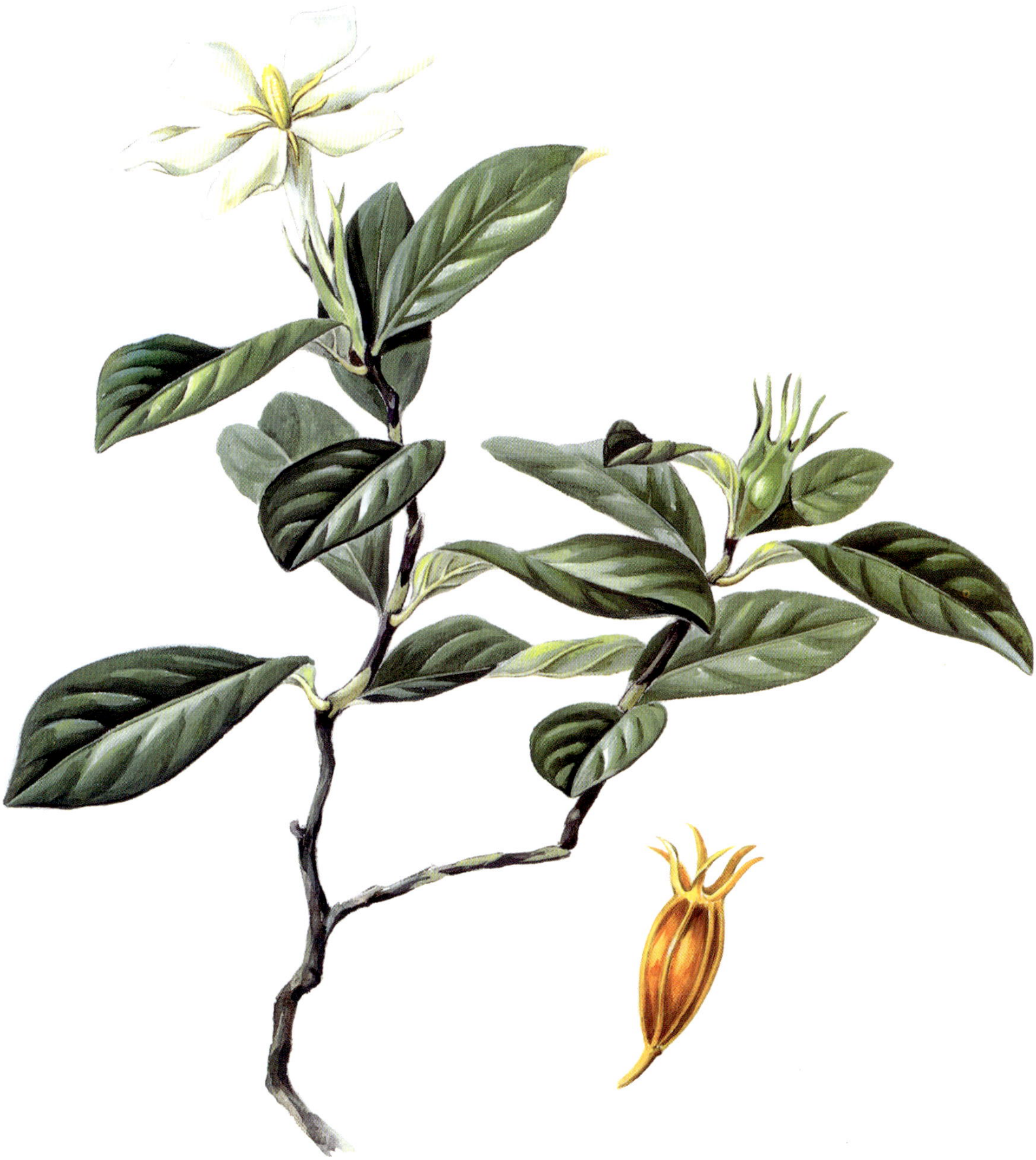

Fig. 11.68. ***Gardenia jasminoides*** Ellis — This plant contains flavones, gardenoside, shanzhiside, geniposide, genipin, gentiobioside, crocin (crocetin, digentiobiose ester), gardenin, β-sistosterol, mannitol, nonacosane, fatty oil, tannin, and pectin. It has antitumor effects, inhibits sarcoma-180 in mice, and has been used to treat lymphocytic leukemia, cheilocarcinoma, and other cancers. (Hsu, et al, 1986; Minyi, 1992; Lee, 1999)

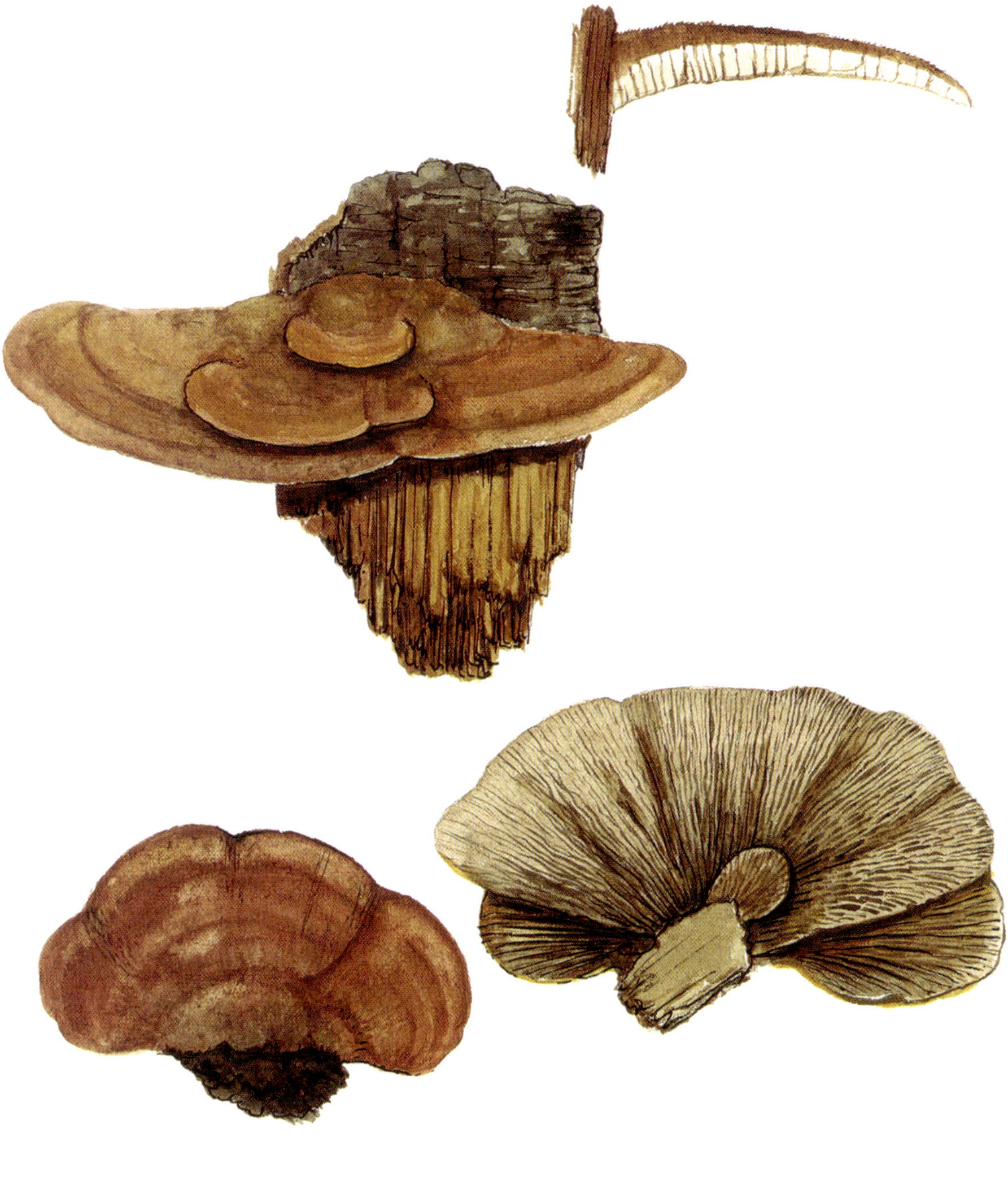

Fig. 11.69. ***Gloeophyllum trabeum*** (Pers. ex Fr.) Murr. — This mushroom contains polysaccharides that inhibit sarcoma-180 in white mice (Ying, et al, 1987).

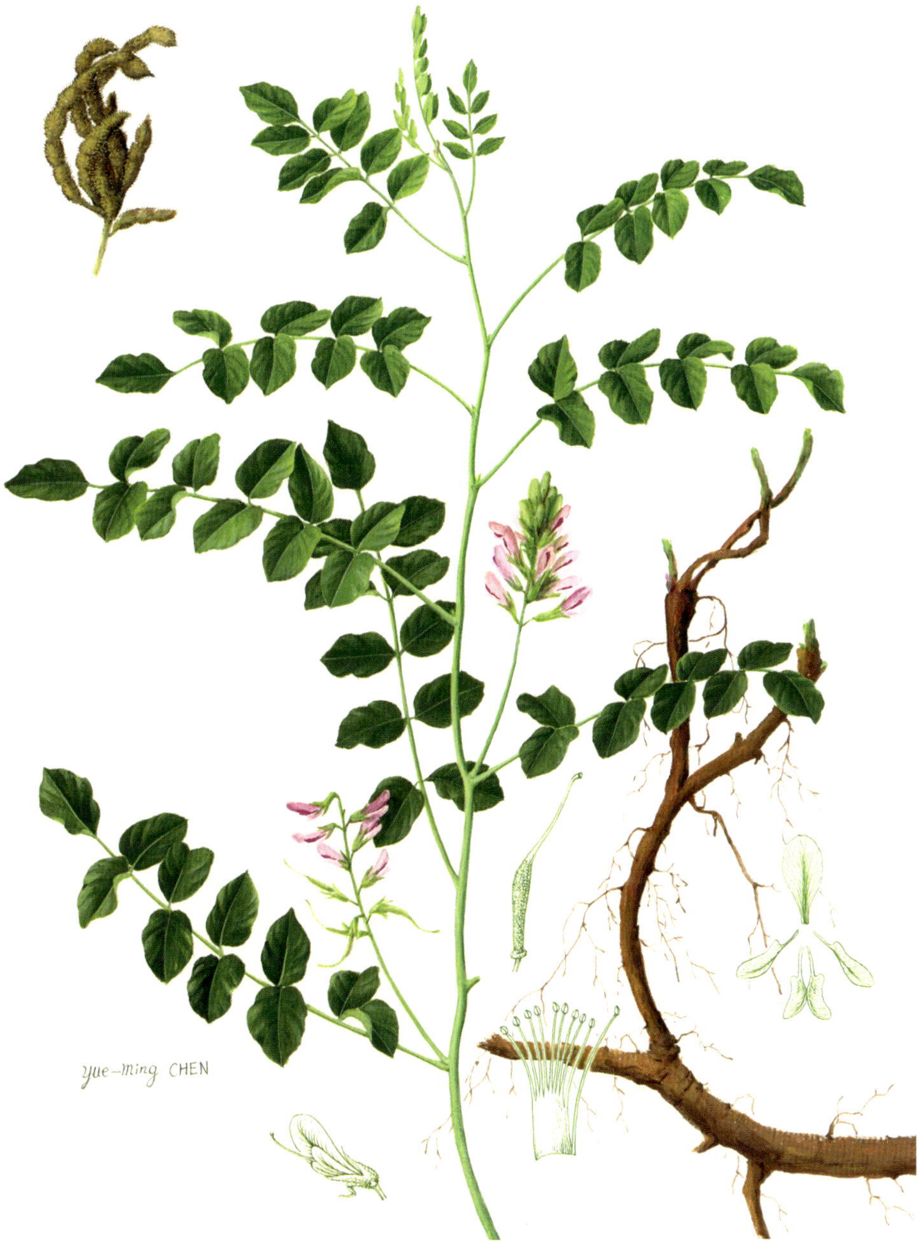


Fig. 11.70. ***Glycyrrhiza uralensis*** Fisch. et DC. — The plant contains the saponin glyccyrrhrizin, which when hydrolyzed produces glycyrrhetic acid and glucoronic acid, flavenoids, such as liquiritin, liquiritigenin, isoliquiritin, isoliquiritigenin, licoflavone, licoricone, 2-methyl-7-hydroxyisoflavone, and licoricidin, berniarin, umbelliferone, ferulic acid, sinapic acid, amino acids, glucoses, sucroses, mannitol, asparanic acids, glycyrols, isoglycyrols, biotin, and β-sitosterol. It inhibits transplanted Oberling-Guerin myeloma, Hep A, and Yoshida's sarcoma in rats and transplanted Jitian sarcomas and Erlich's ascites carcinoma in mice, and in vitro inhibits JTC-26 cells, exhibits antileukemic activity in mice and antitumor effects in rats with ascitic hepatocarcinoma, prevents hepatocarcinoma induced by polyoxybenzidine in mice, and acts as a detoxification agent. It has been used in the treatment of chorioepithelioma and stomach cancer. (Chang & But, 1986; Lee, 1999)

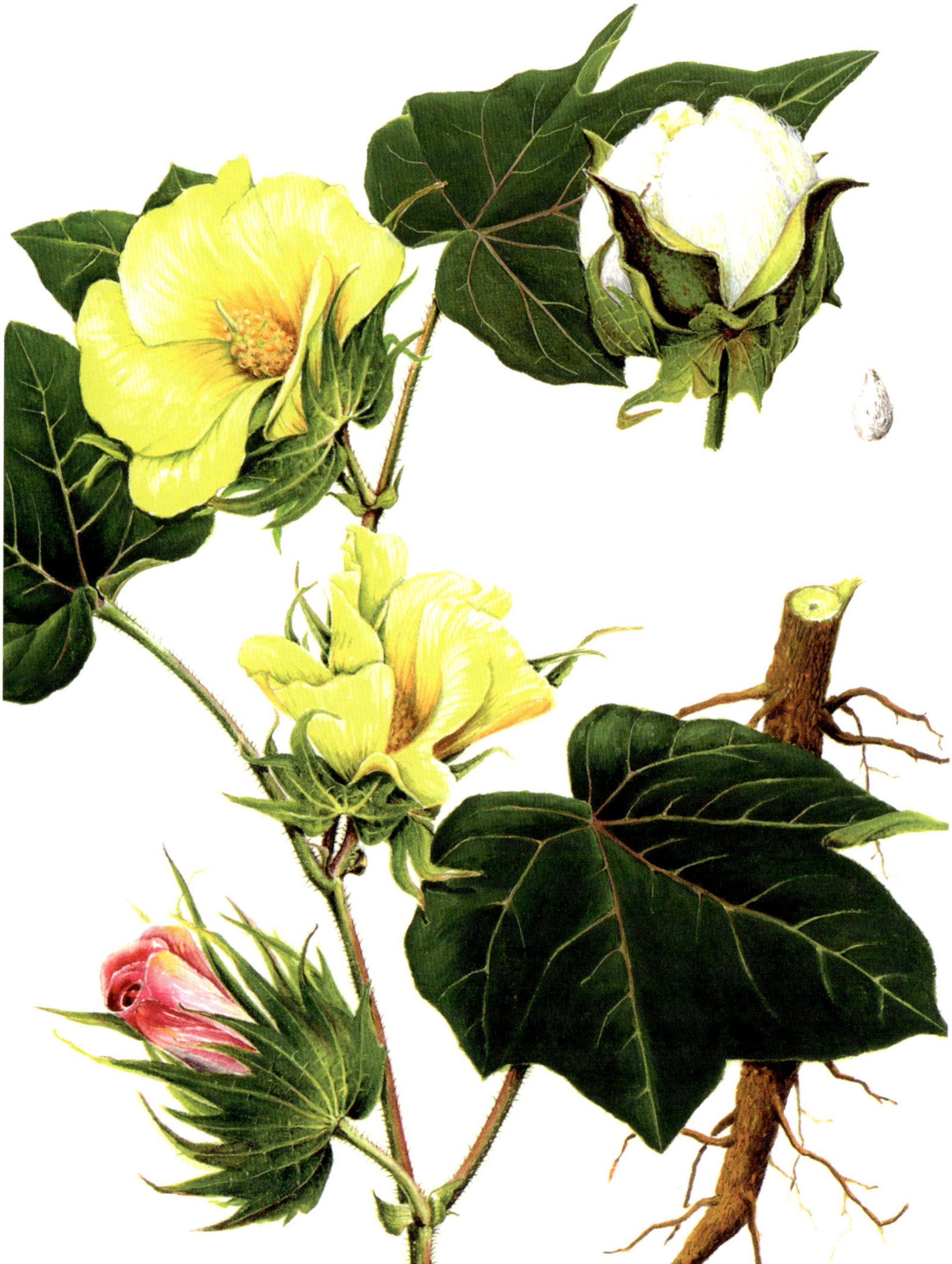

Fig. 11.71. ***Gossypium hirsutum*** Linn. — This plant contains gossypol, asparagine, arginine, quercimeritrin, and resins. In vitro it inhibits Yoshida's sarcoma, Erlich's ascites carcinoma, Walker's carcinoma-256, lymphocytic leukemia-388, and melanoma. It is effective against sarcoma-37, sarcoma-180, Walker's carcinoma, and breast cancer in mice. It has been used to treat spermatocytoma, malignant lymphoma, and cancers of the esophagus, stomach, lung, liver, and urinary bladder. (Chang & But, 1986; Minyi, 1992; Lee, 1999)

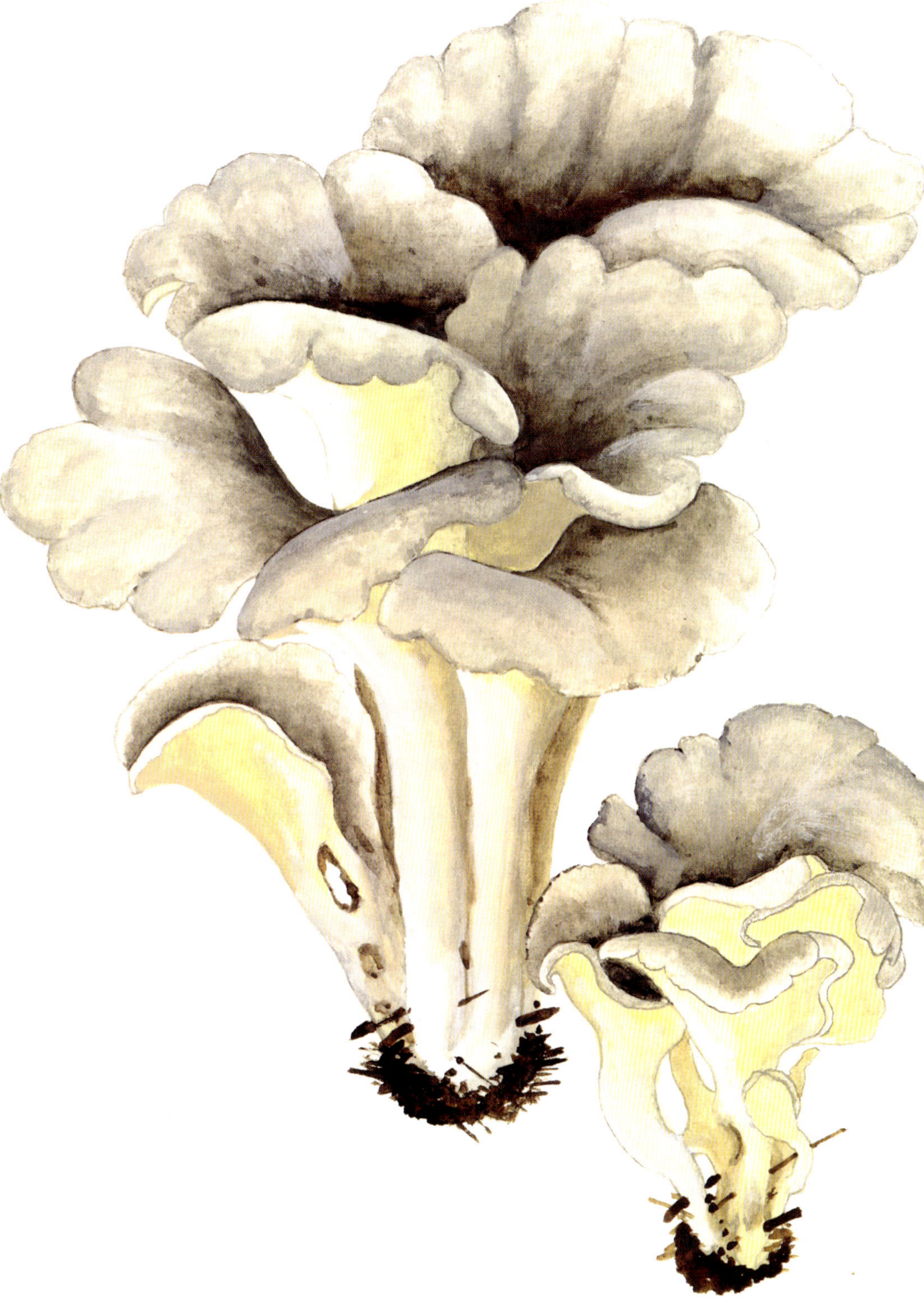

Fig. 11.72. ***Grifola frondosus*** (Dicks. ex Fr. ) S. F. Gray — Extracts from the sporophore of this mushroom contain polysaccharides that inhibit Ehrlich's carcinoma in mice (Ying, et al, 1987).

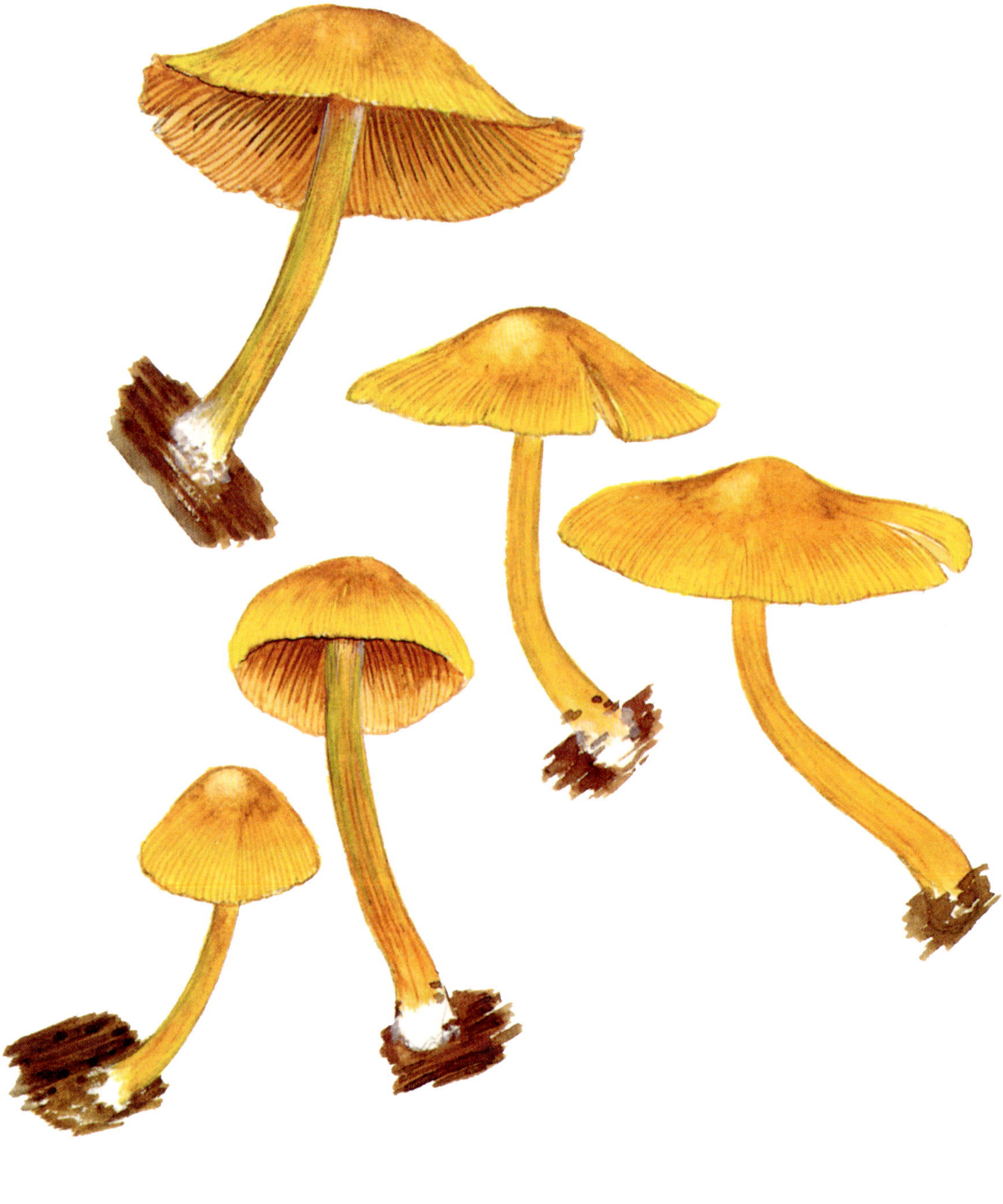

Fig. 11.73. ***Gymnopilus liquiritae*** (Pers. ex Fr.) Karst. — This mushroom contains polysaccharides, has anticarcinogenic properties, and inhibits sarcoma-180 and Ehrlich's carcinoma in white mice (Ying, et al, 1987).

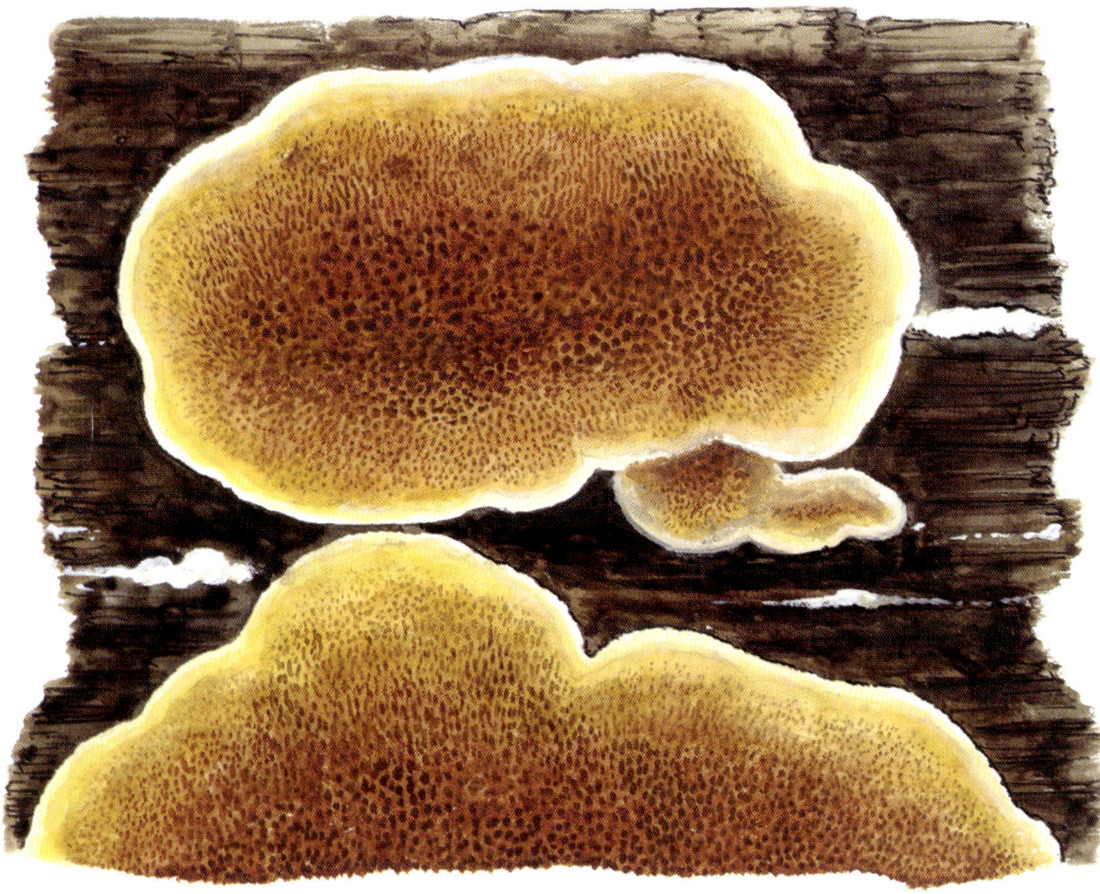

Fig. 11.74. ***Gyrophana lacrymans*** (Wulf.) Pat. — This mushroom contains polysaccharides that inhibit sarcoma-180 in mice and Ehrlich's carcinoma (Ying, et al, 1987).

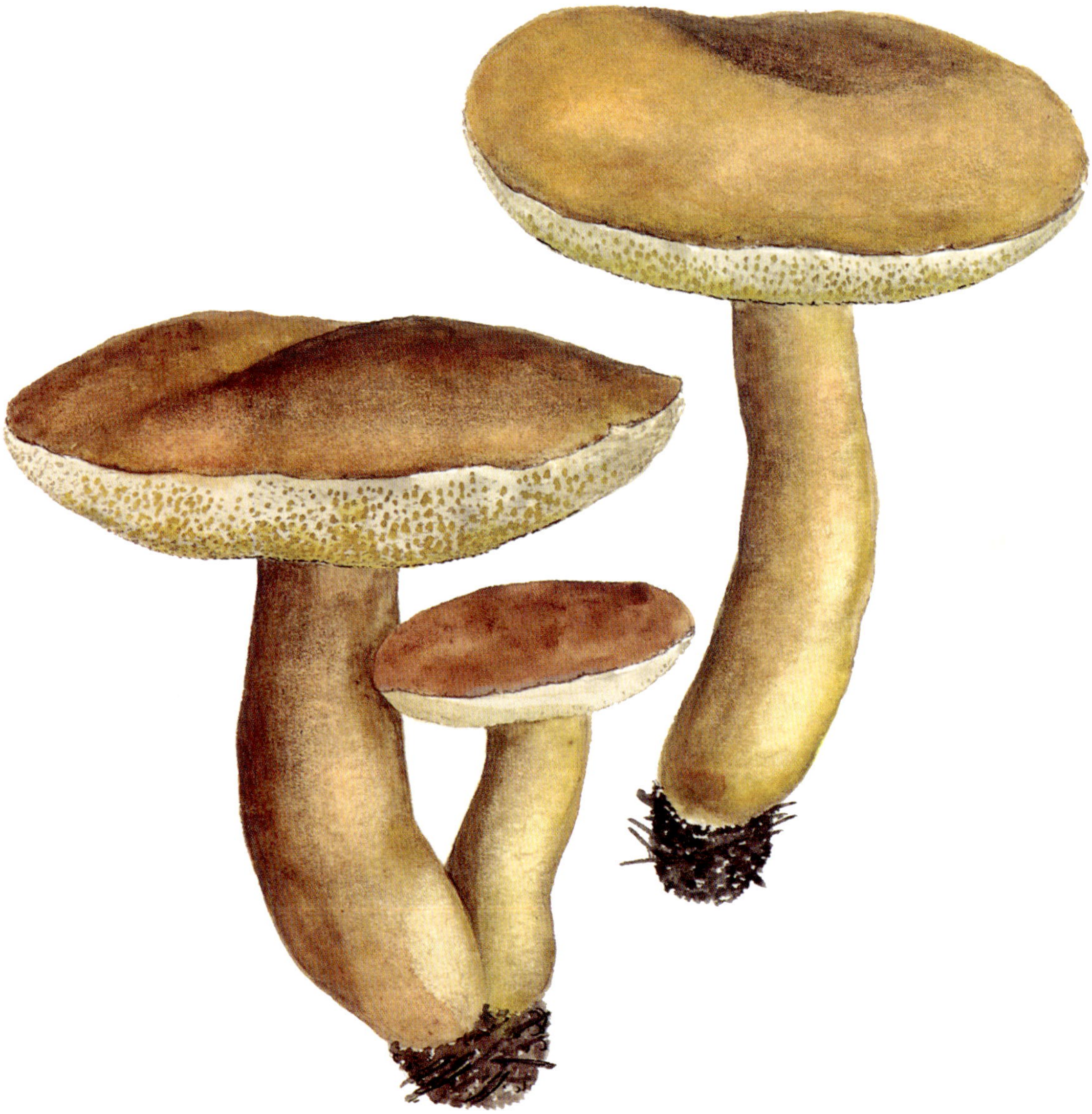

Fig. 11.75. ***Gyroporus castaneus*** (Bull. ex Fr.) Quél. — This mushroom contains polysaccharides that inhibit sarcoma-180 and Ehrlich's carcinoma (Ying, et al, 1987).

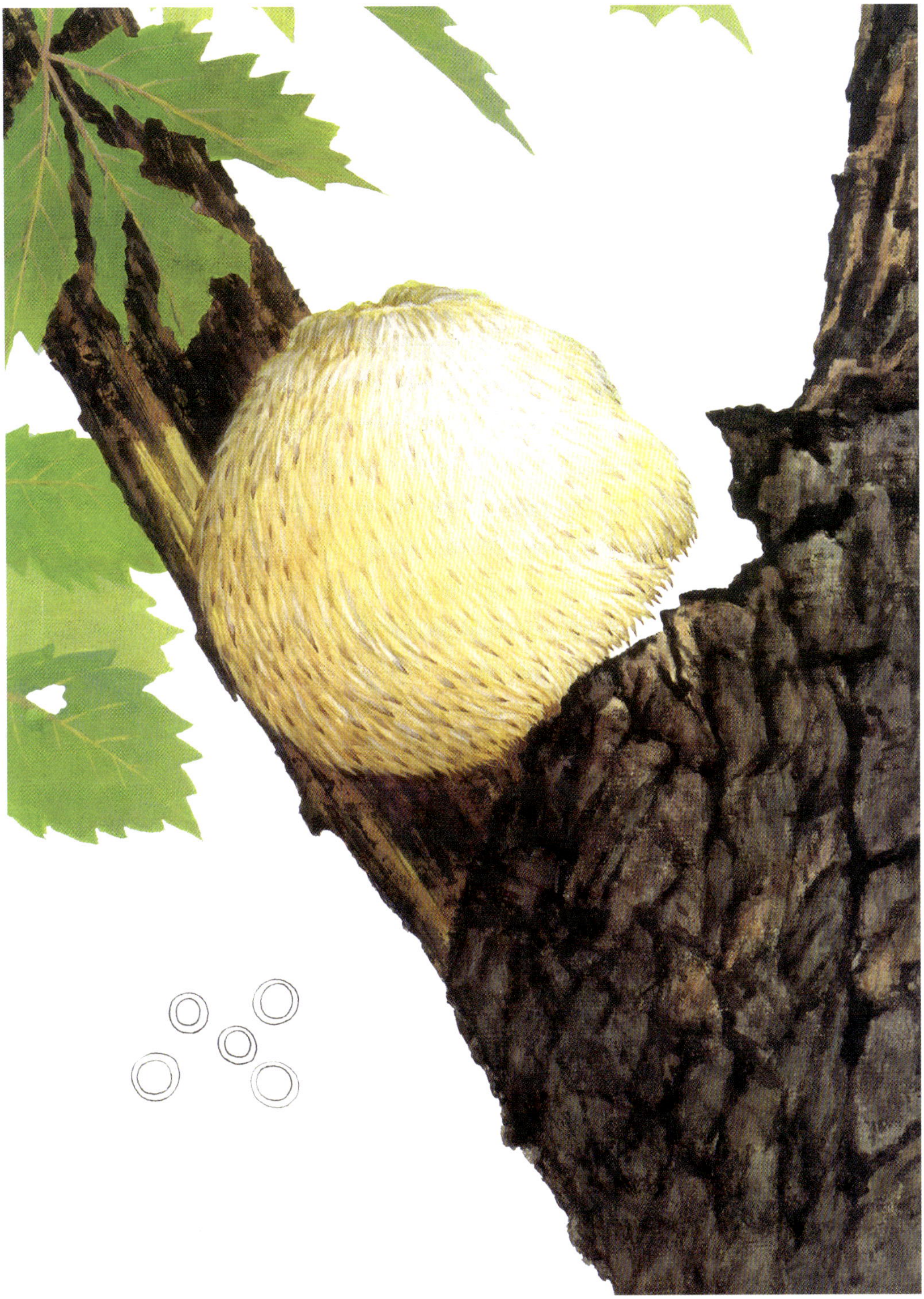

Fig. 11.76. ***Hericeum erinaceus*** (Bull. ex Fr.) Pers. — This fungus contains polysaccharides and polypeptides. It inhibits sarcoma-180 in mice, inhibits the synthesis of DNA and RNA in ascites carcinoma in vitro, and enhances the immune system. It has been used to treat esophageal, stomach, intestine, and cardiac cancers. (Ying, et al, 1987; Minyi, 1992; Lee, 1999)

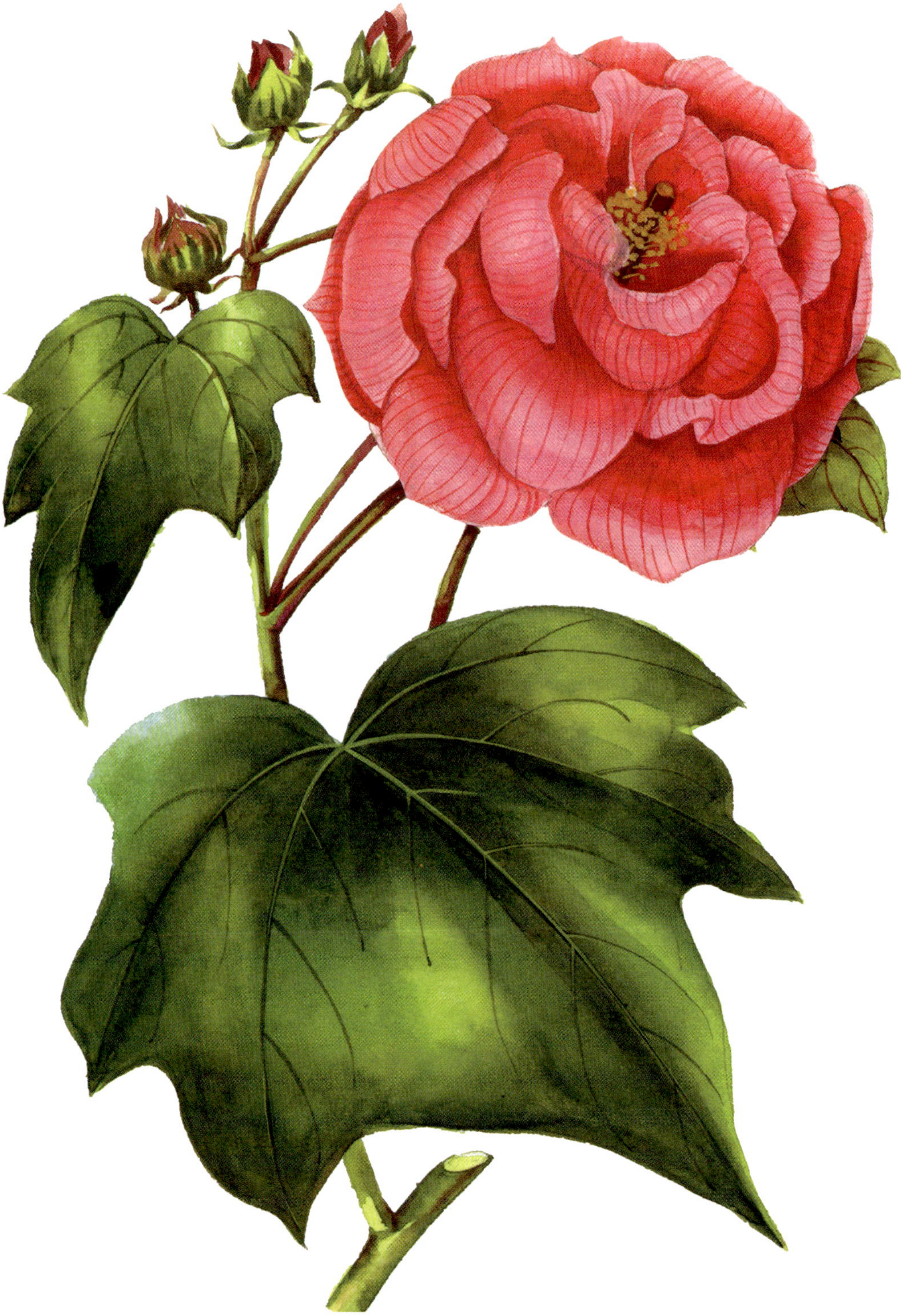

Fig. 11.77. ***Hibiscus mutabilis*** Linn. — This plant contains flavenoid glycosides, amino acids, tannins, hyperoside, rutin, and anthocyanin. It shows activity to stomach cancer cells and has been used to treat cancers of the digestive system, breast, and lung. (Minyi, 1992; Huang, 1999)

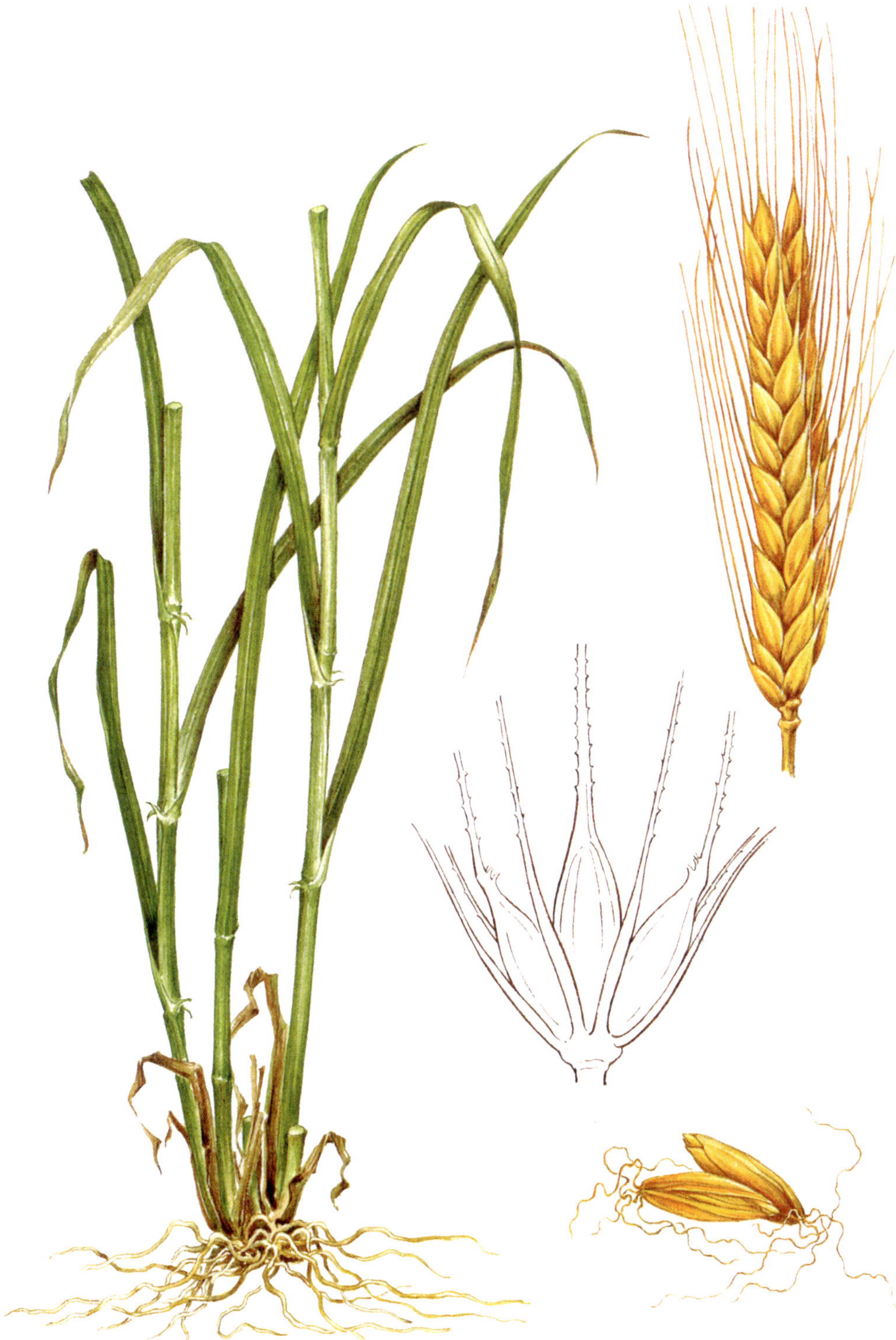

Fig. 11.78. ***Hordeum vulgare*** Linn. — This plant contains α-amylase, β-amylase, maltose, dextrin, proteins, hordenine, vitamins B and C, and maltoxin. It inhibits sarcoma-180 in mice (Chang & But, 1986).

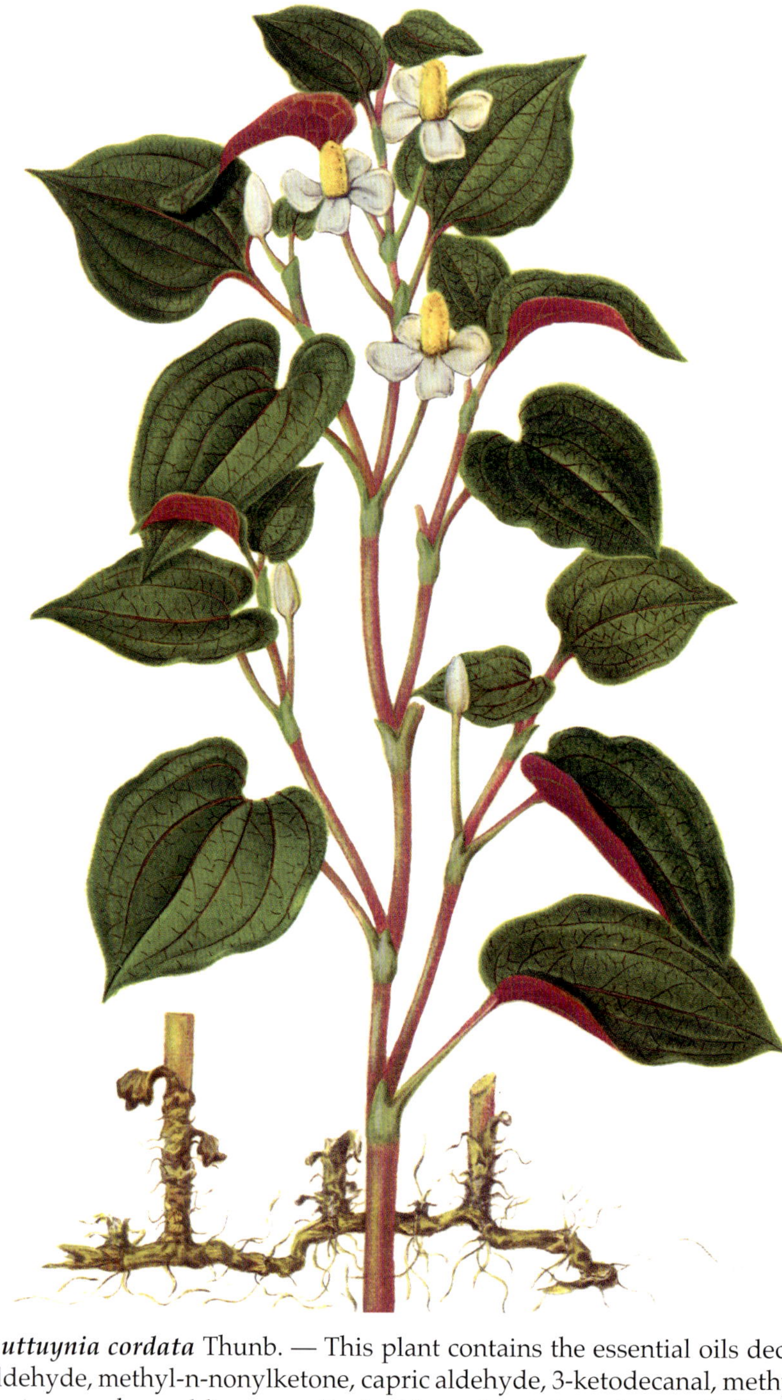

Fig. 11.79. ***Houttuynia cordata*** Thunb. — This plant contains the essential oils decanoyl acetaldehyde, lauric aldehyde, methyl-n-nonylketone, capric aldehyde, 3-ketodecanal, methyllaural sulfide, myrcene α-pinene, camphene, d-limonene, linalool, bornyl acetate, and caryophyllene, the flavenoids quercitrin, isoquercitrin, quercetin, reynoutrin, hyperin, and rutin, the alkaloids aristolactum, peperolactum, norcepharadione, cepharadione, and splendidine, potassium chloride, potassium sulfate, and cordarine. It shows cytotoxicity against leukemic cell lines and several other human cell lines, and has been used to treat cervical carcinoma. (Chang & But, 1986; Hsu, et al, 1986; Minyi, 1992; Chang, et al, 2001; Kim, et al, 2001)

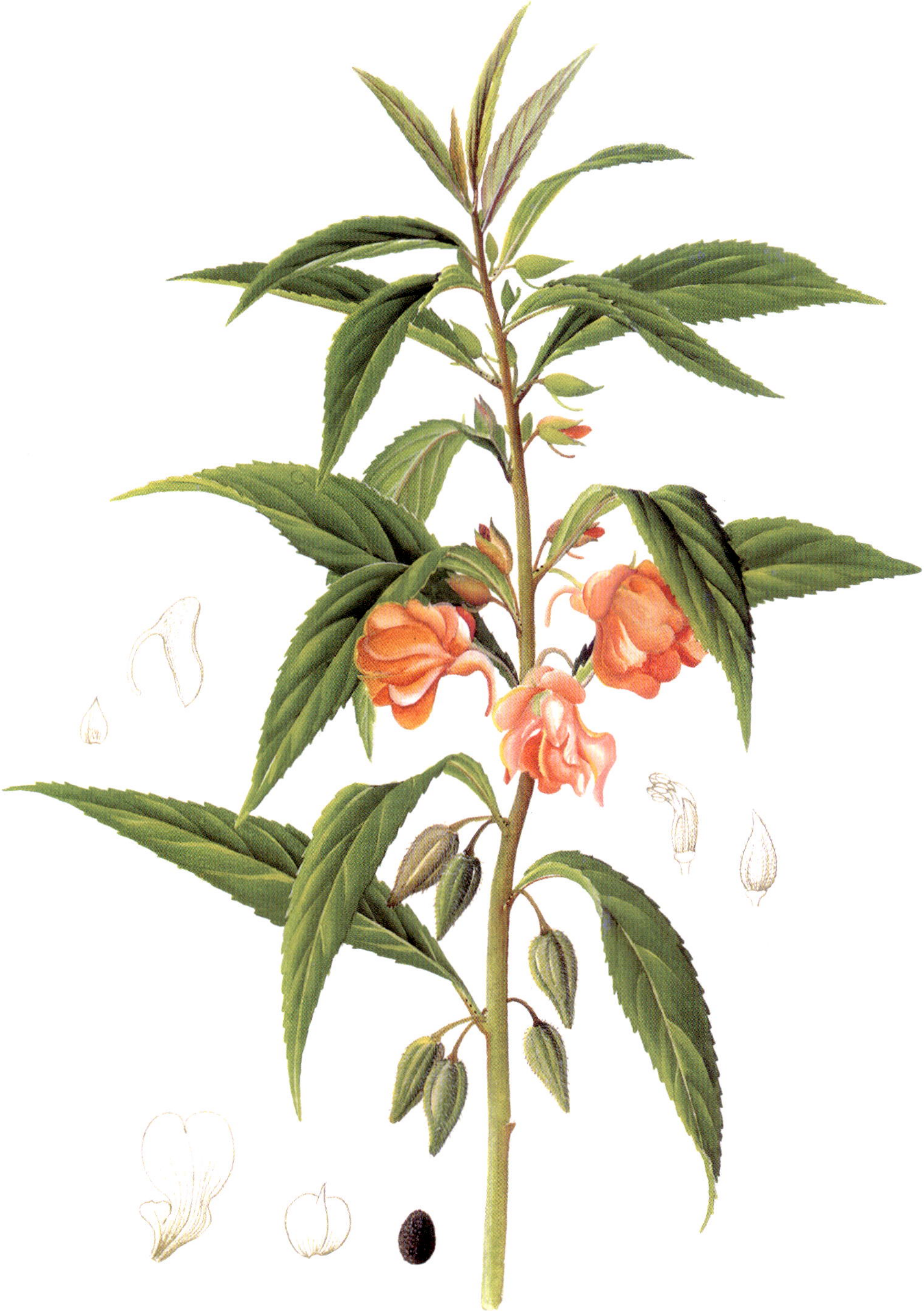

Fig. 11.80. ***Impatiens balsamina*** Linn. — This plant contains balsaminasterol, parinaric acid, γ-spinasterol, b-ergosterol, kaempferol-3-glucoside, quercetin-3-glucoside, pelargonidin-3-glucoside, cyanidin-3-glucoside, 1,2,4-trihydroxy napthalene-4-glucoside, kaempferol, kaempferol-3-arabinose, β-sitosterol, and saponins. It inhibits transplanted sarcoma-37 in mice, is sensitive to gastrolymphosarcoma, and has been used to treat esophageal and cardiac cancer. (Hsu, et al, 1986; Minyi, 1992; Lee, 1999)

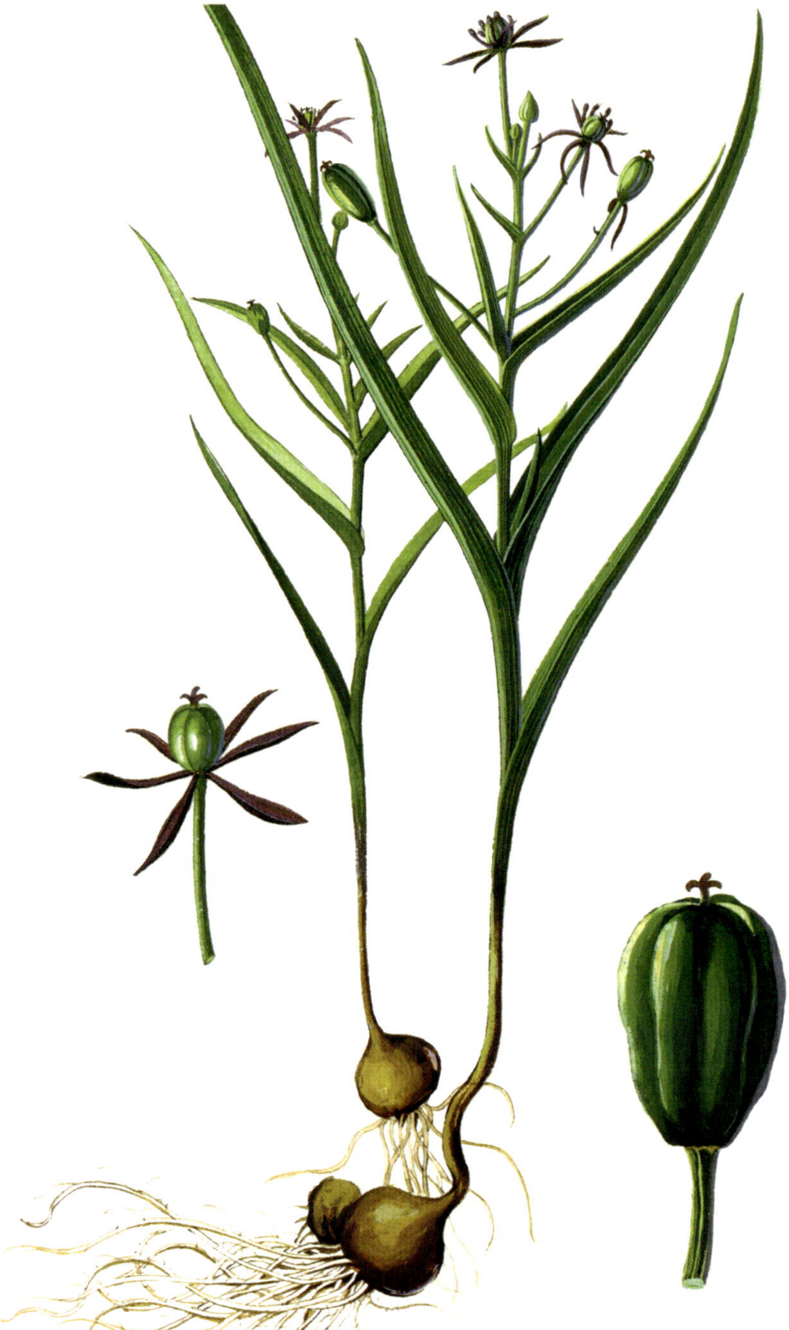

Fig. 11.81. ***Iphigenia indica*** Kunth. — This plant contains many alkaloids, including colchicine, its derivative colchinamide, β-lumicolchine, isocolchicine, cornigerine, and N-formyl-N-deacetylcolchicine. It inhibits transplanted tumors, Walker's carcinoma-256, sarcoma-180, sarcoma-37, lymphosarcoma, and hepatoma in laboratory animals. Its antineoplastic activity works by blocking the metaphase of mitosis in cell division. This plant is used widely throughout China in the treatment of cancer and has been used to treat epithelioma, leukemia, cancers of the esophagus, thyroid, stomach, breast, cervix, lung, and skin. (Chang & But, 1986; Huang, 1999; Minyi, 1999)

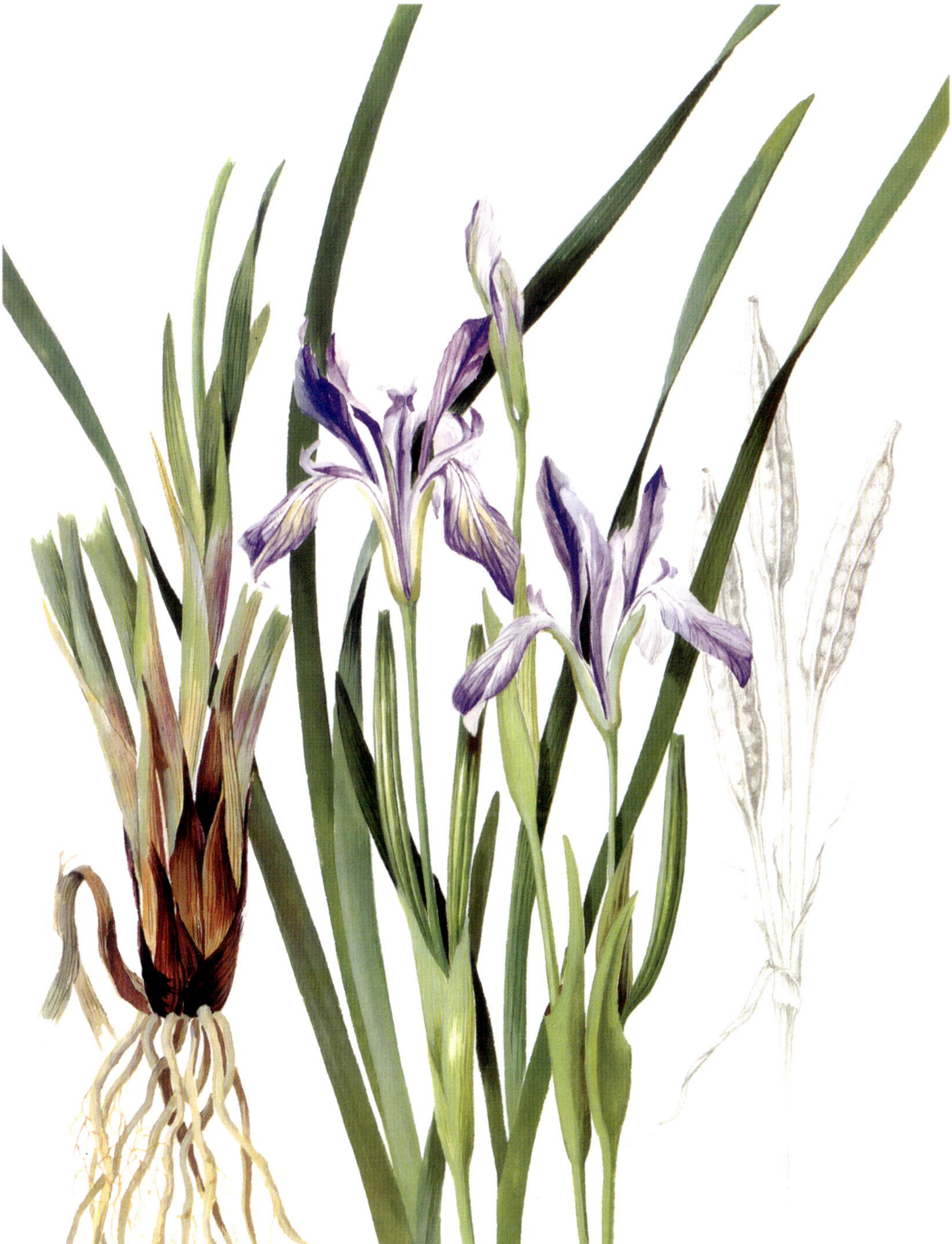

Fig. 11.82. ***Iris lactae*** Pall. **var *chinensis*** (Fisch.) Koidz — This plant contains irisquinone, dihydroirisquinone, and pallason A. It inhibits leukemia and some solid tumors, exhibits anticancer effects against lymphosarcoma, cervical cancer-14, sarcoma-180, Erlich's ascites carcinoma, LA-795, and B-16 tumors in laboratory animals, and inhibits DNA synthesis of cancer cells. It has been used to treat leukemias and various other cancers including head, neck, esophageal, gastric, liver, lung, and cervical cancer. (Minyi, 1992; Lee, 1999)

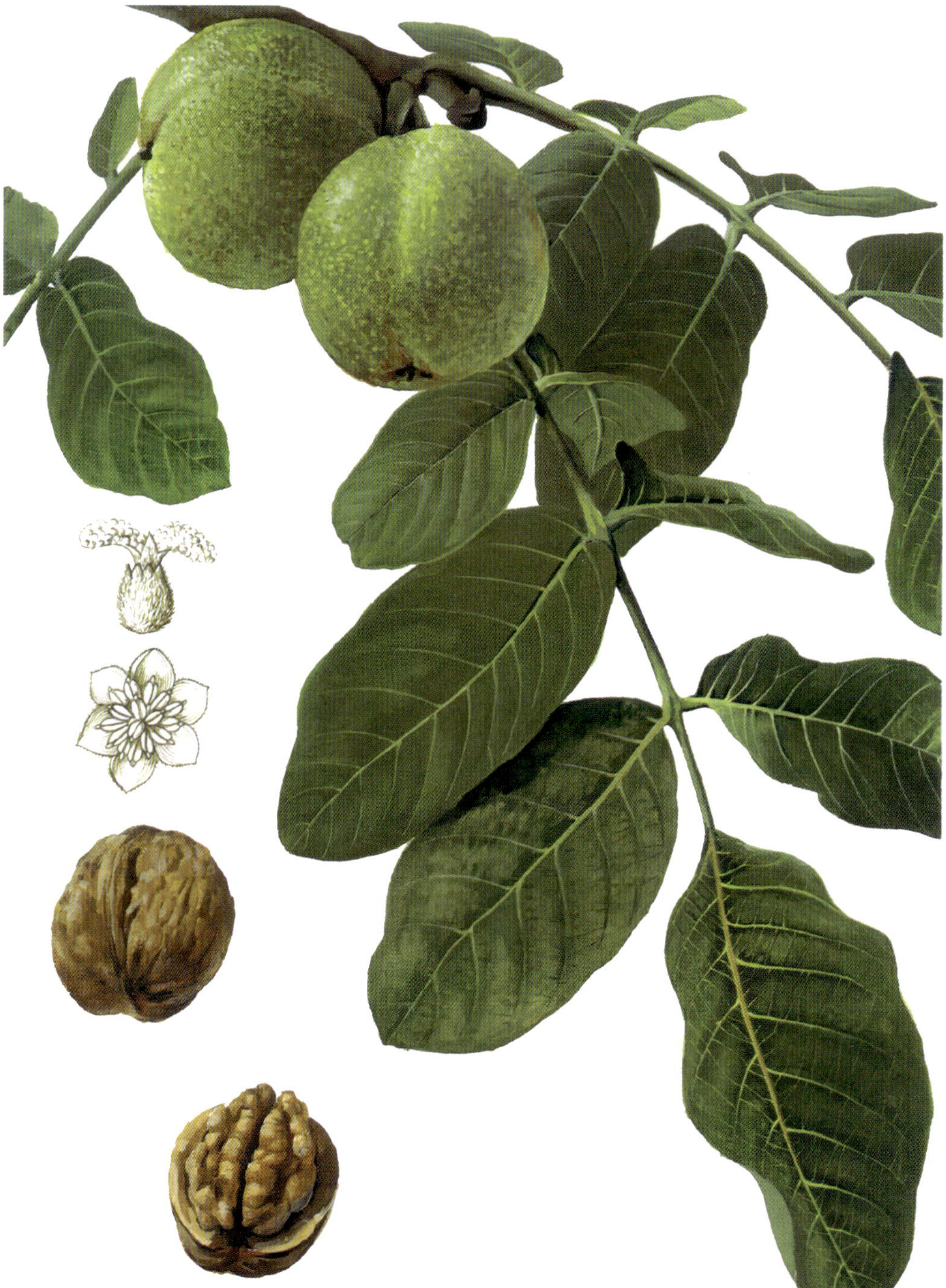

Fig. 11.83. ***Juglans regia*** Linn. — This plant contains juglanin, juglone, α-hydrojuglone-β-D-glucoside, napthoquinone, anthraquinone, caffeic acid, gallic acid, flavone, alkaloids, saccharides, proteins, vitamin C, tannins, and glucosides. It inhibits sarcoma-37, sarcoma-180, mammocancer, and Erlich's ascites carcinoma in mice, and has been used to treat leukemias and cancers of the esophagus, stomach, liver, and breast. (Minyi, 1992; Huang, 1999; Lee, 1999)

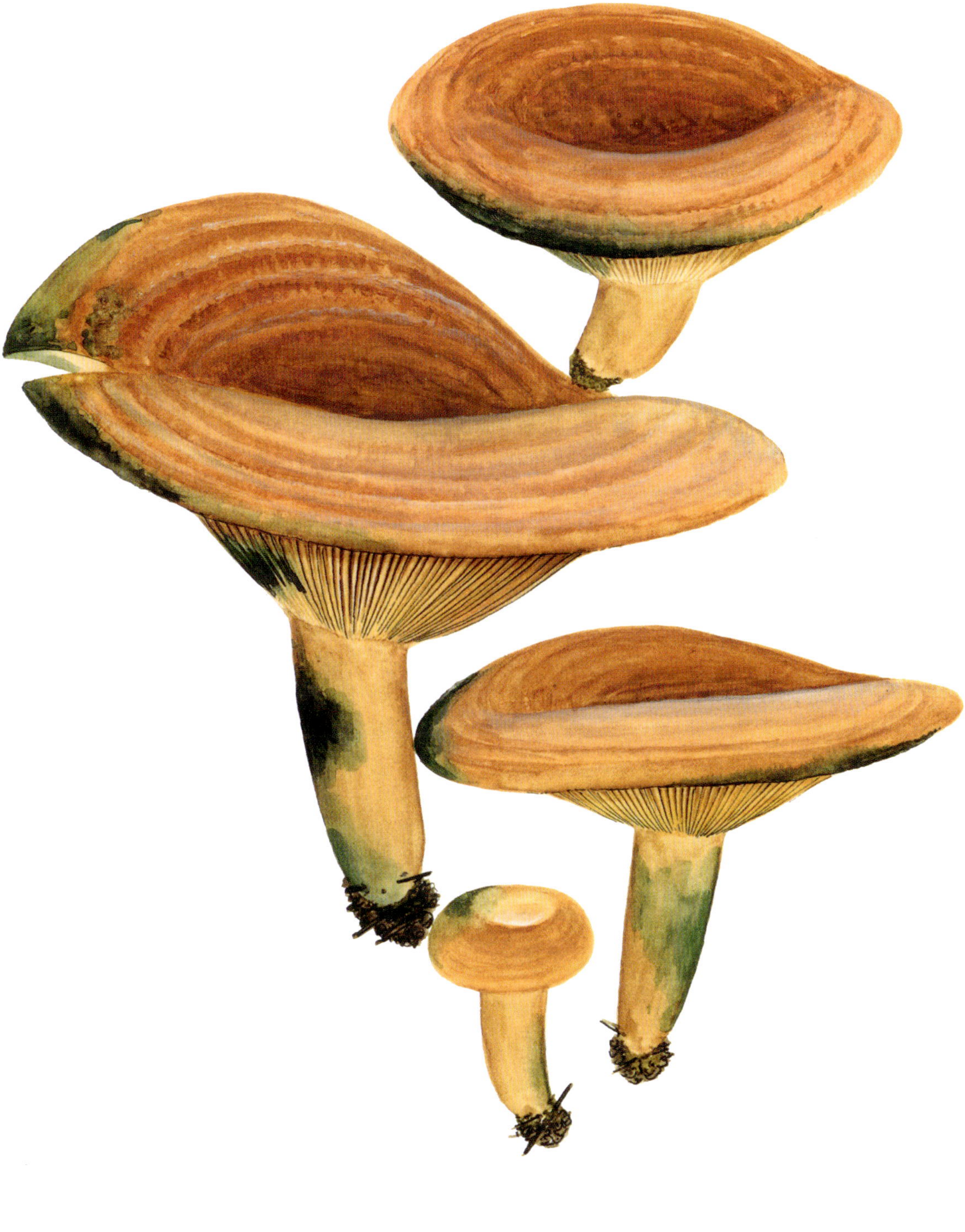

Fig. 11.84. ***Lactarius hatsudake*** Tanaka — This fungus contains polysaccharides that inhibit sarcoma-180 and Ehrlich's carcinoma (Ying, et al, 1987).

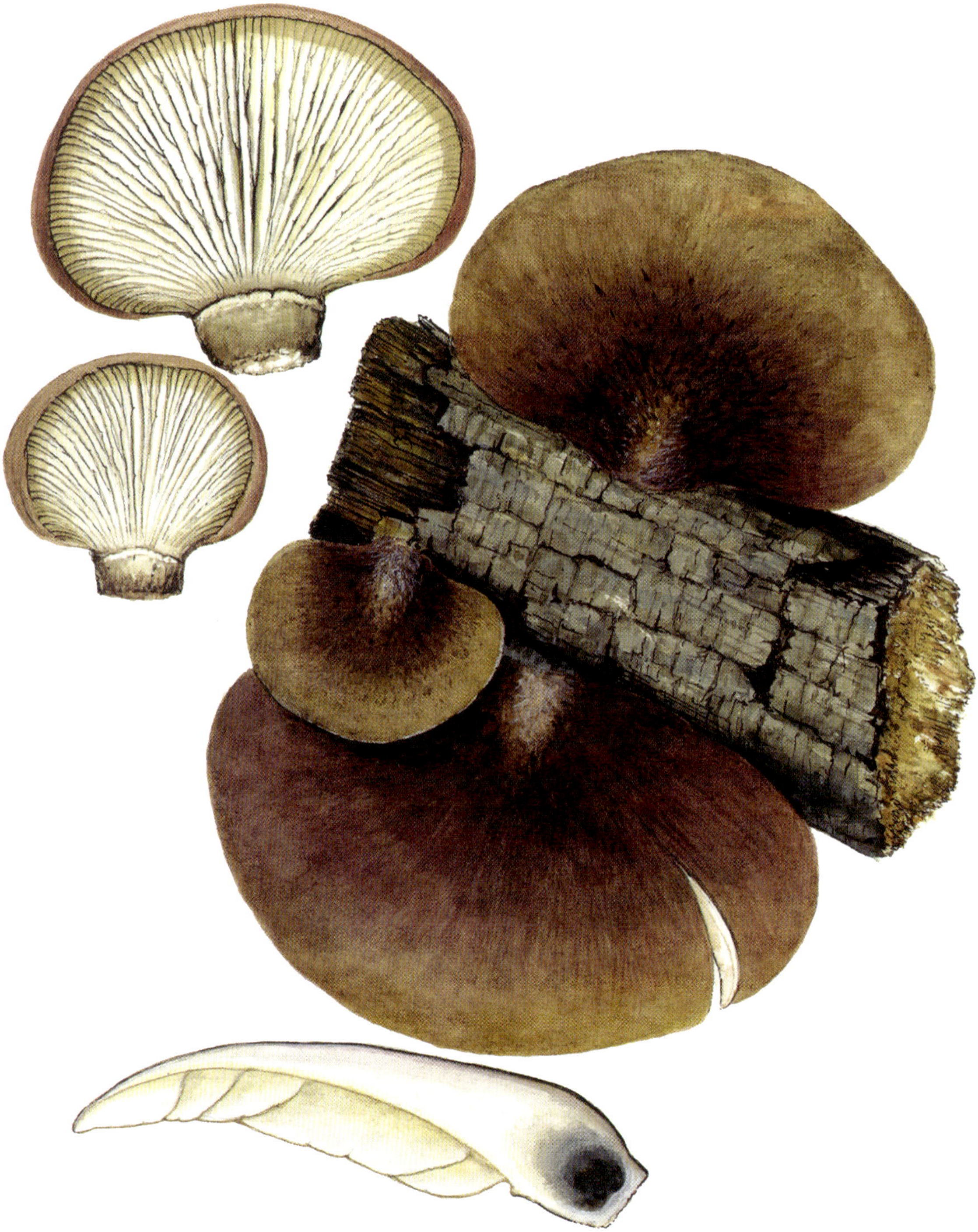

Fig. 11.85. ***Lampteromyces japonicus*** (Kawam.) Sing. — This mushroom contains lunaycin, which inhibits sarcoma-180 and Ehrlich's carcinoma (Ying, et al, 1987).

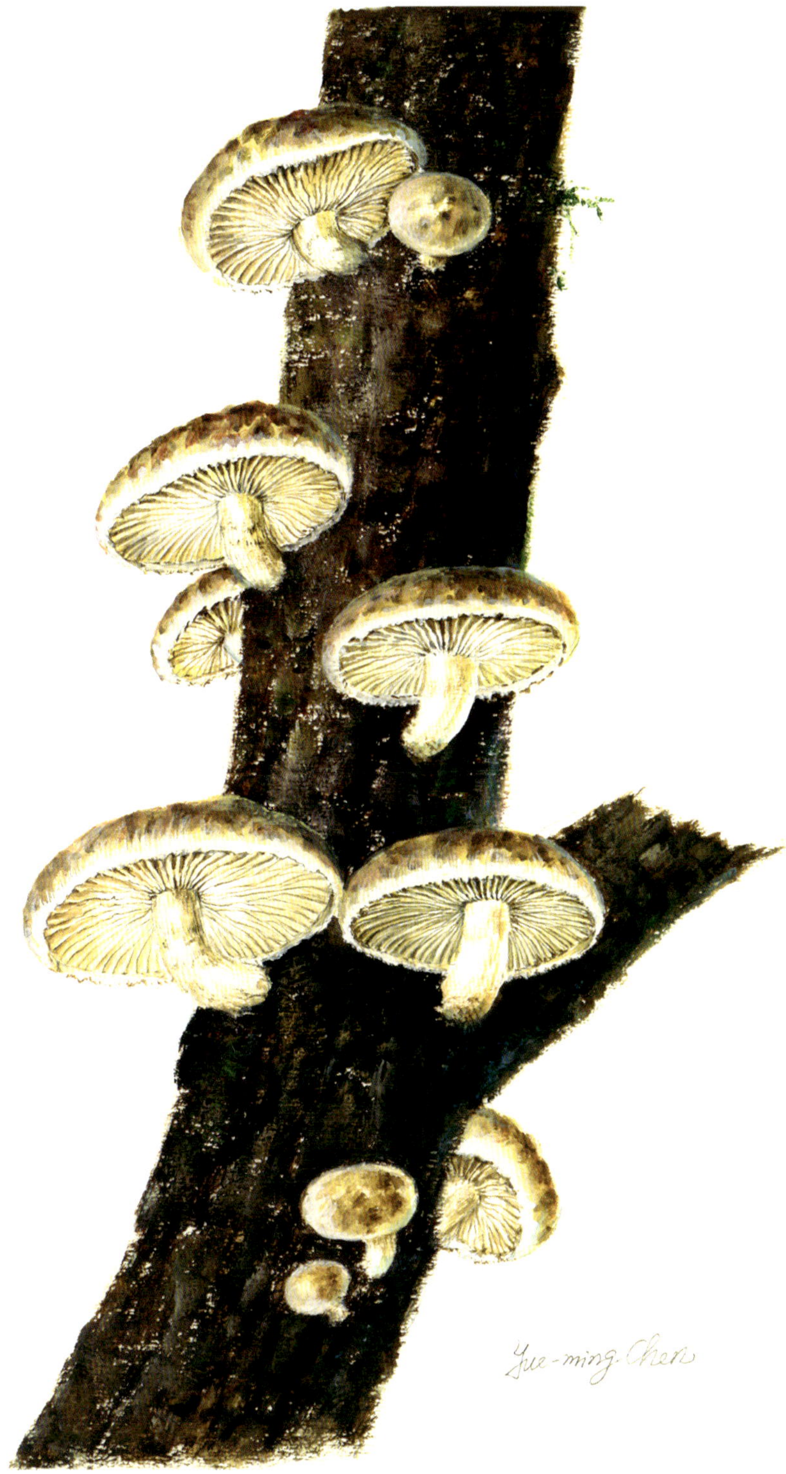

Fig. 11.86. ***Lentinus edodes*** (Berk.) Sing. — This mushroom contains ergosterol (which becomes vitamin D when exposed to ultra-violet light), vitamins A and B, butyric acid, and lentinan. It inhibits sarcoma-180 in mice and Erlich's carcinoma. (Ying, et al, 1987; Minyi, 1992)

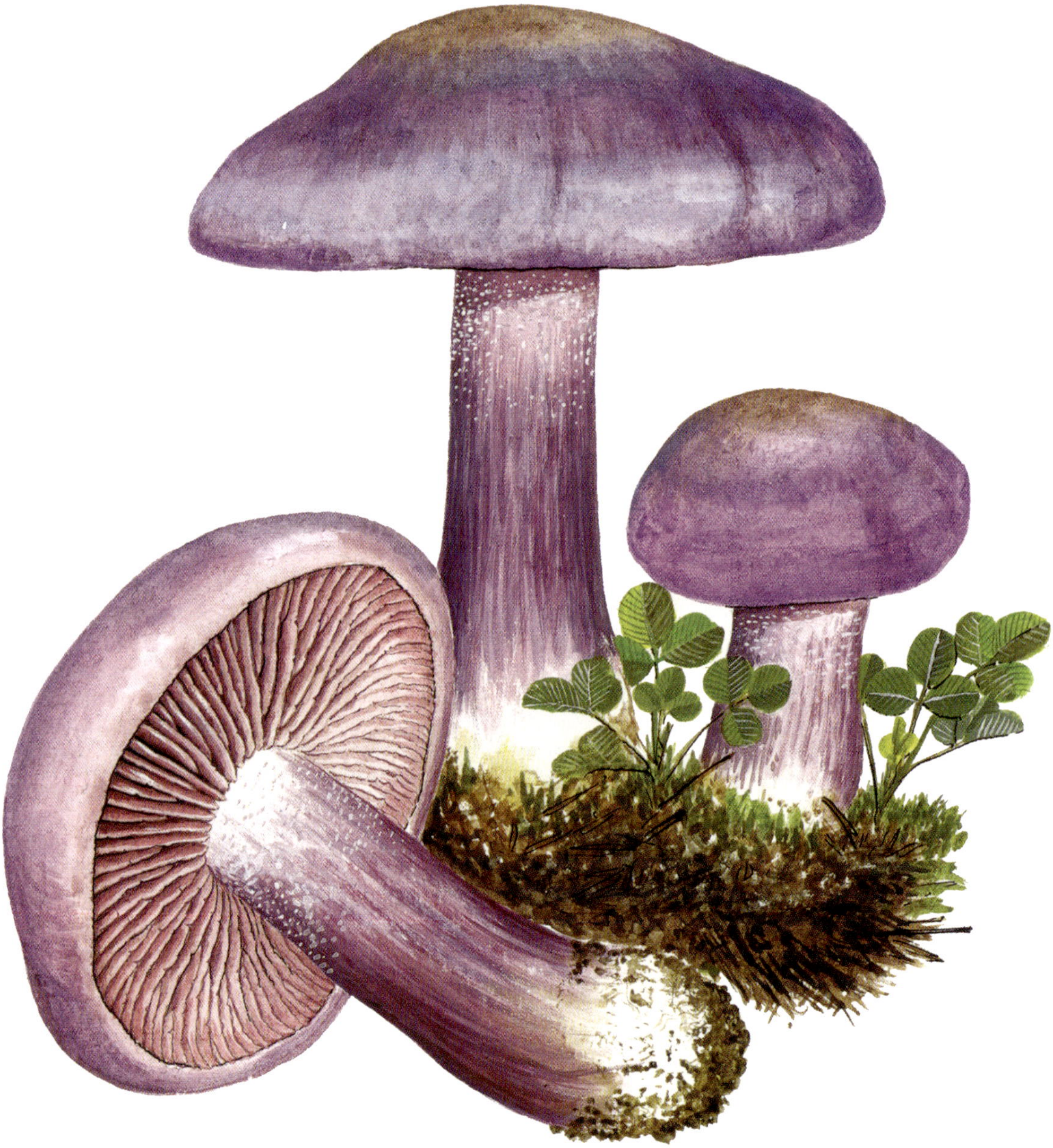

Fig. 11.87. ***Lepista nuda*** (Bull. ex Fr.) Cooke — This mushroom contains polysaccharides, vitamins A and $B_1$ and inhibits sarcoma-180 and Erlich's carcinoma (Ying, et al, 1987).

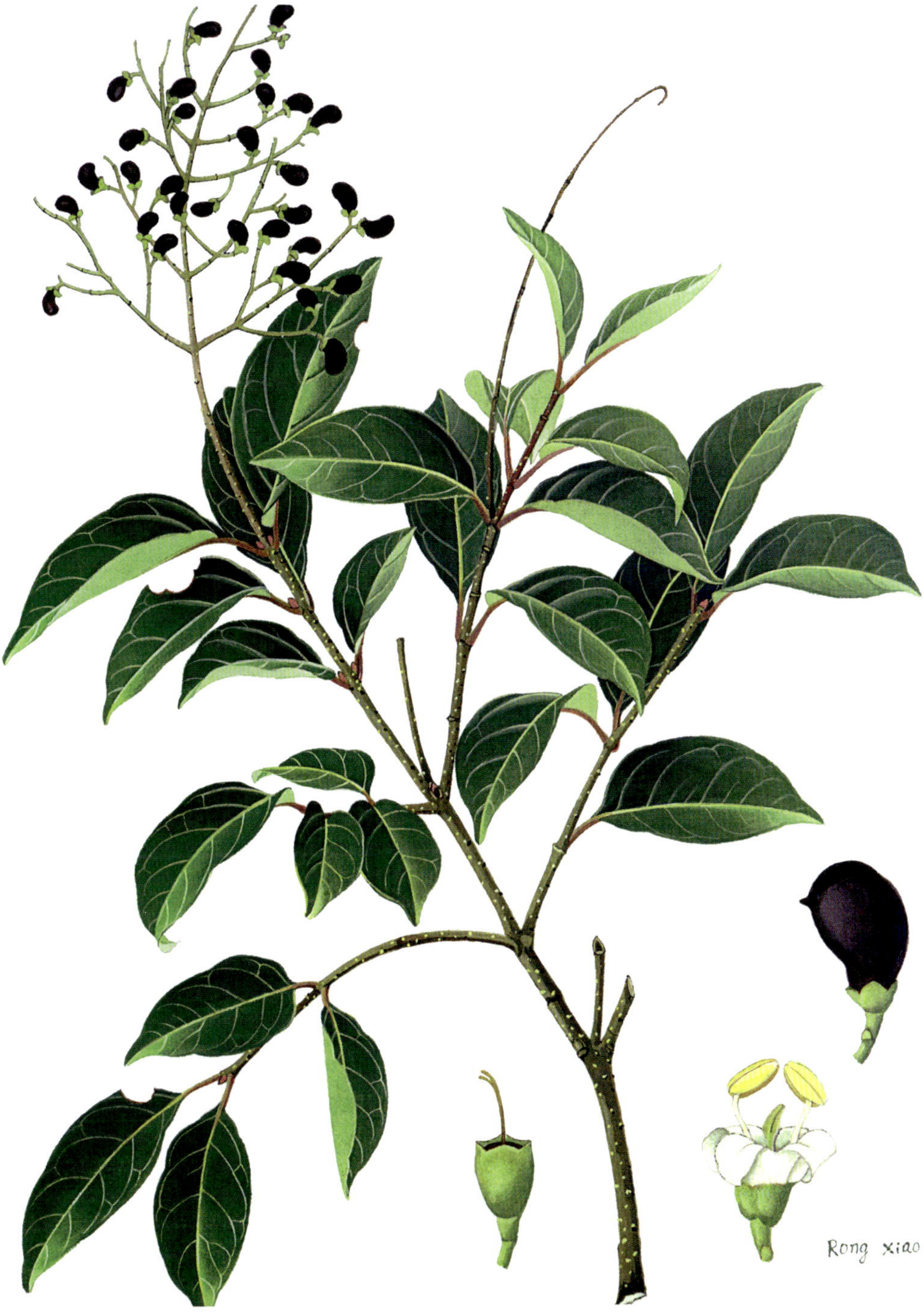


Fig. 11.88. ***Ligustrum lucidum*** Ait. — The fruit contains oleanolic acid, 10-hydroxy oleanolic acid, betulin, lupeol, mannitol, oleic acid, linoleic acid, ursolic acid, palmitic acid, nuzhenide, and hydroxy-nuzhenide. It inhibits U-14 in mice and is effective against HL-60 cells, and has liver protective, anticancer and immune enhancement action. It is one of the key ingredients of an anticancer drug known as "Shengbai" which is used for patients suffering from leukopenia resulting from cancer chemotherapy. (Chang and But, 1986; Lee, 1999)

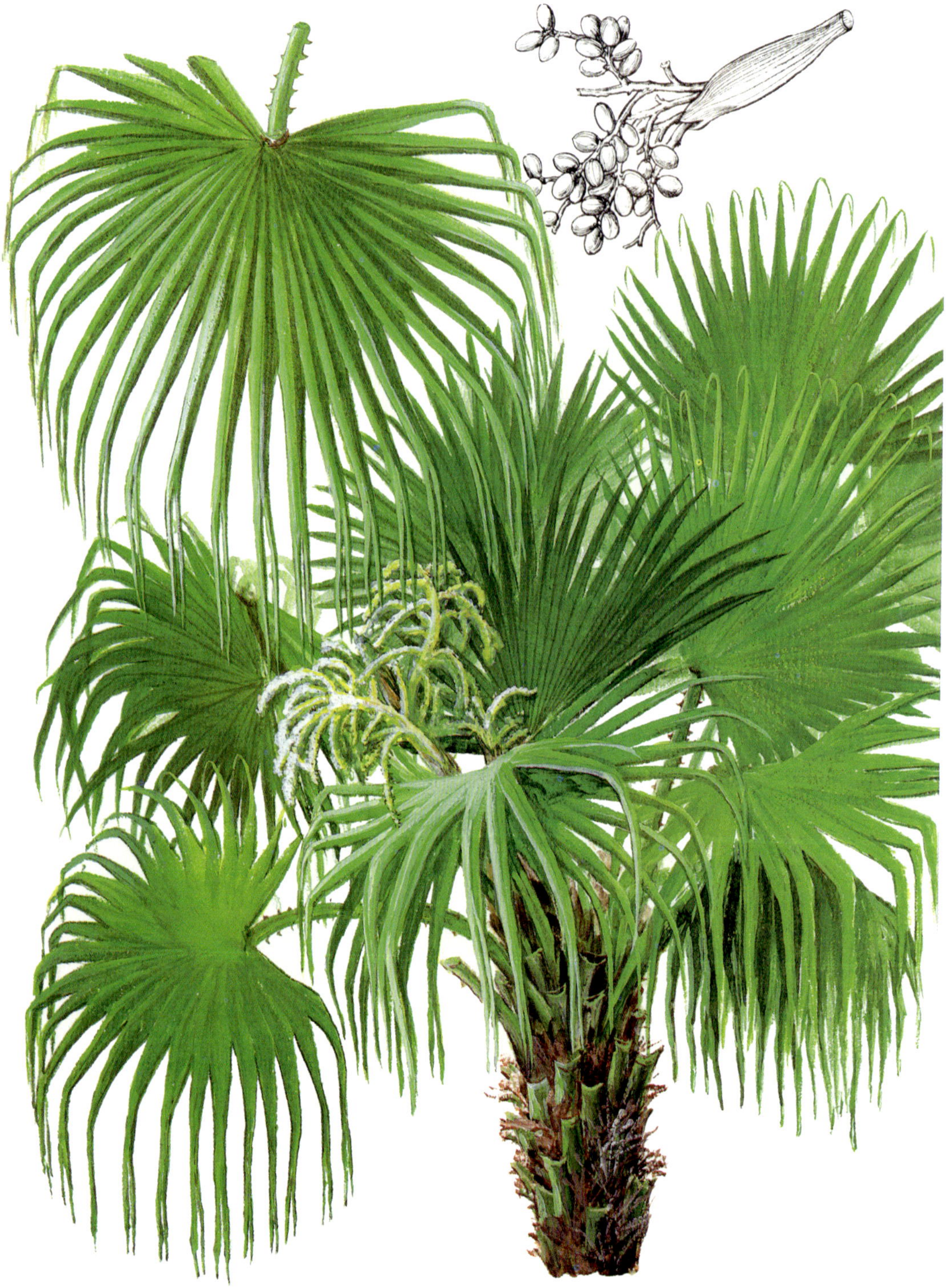

Fig. 11.89. ***Livistona chinensis*** R. Br. — This plant contains phenols, reduced saccharides, triglyceride, and tannins. It inhibits encephaloma-22 tumor cell lines in vitro and has been used to treat chorioepithelioma, choriocarcinoma, malignant moles, leukemia, nasopharyngeal, esophageal, and lung cancer. (Huang, 1999; Lee, 1999; Sartippour, et al, 2001)

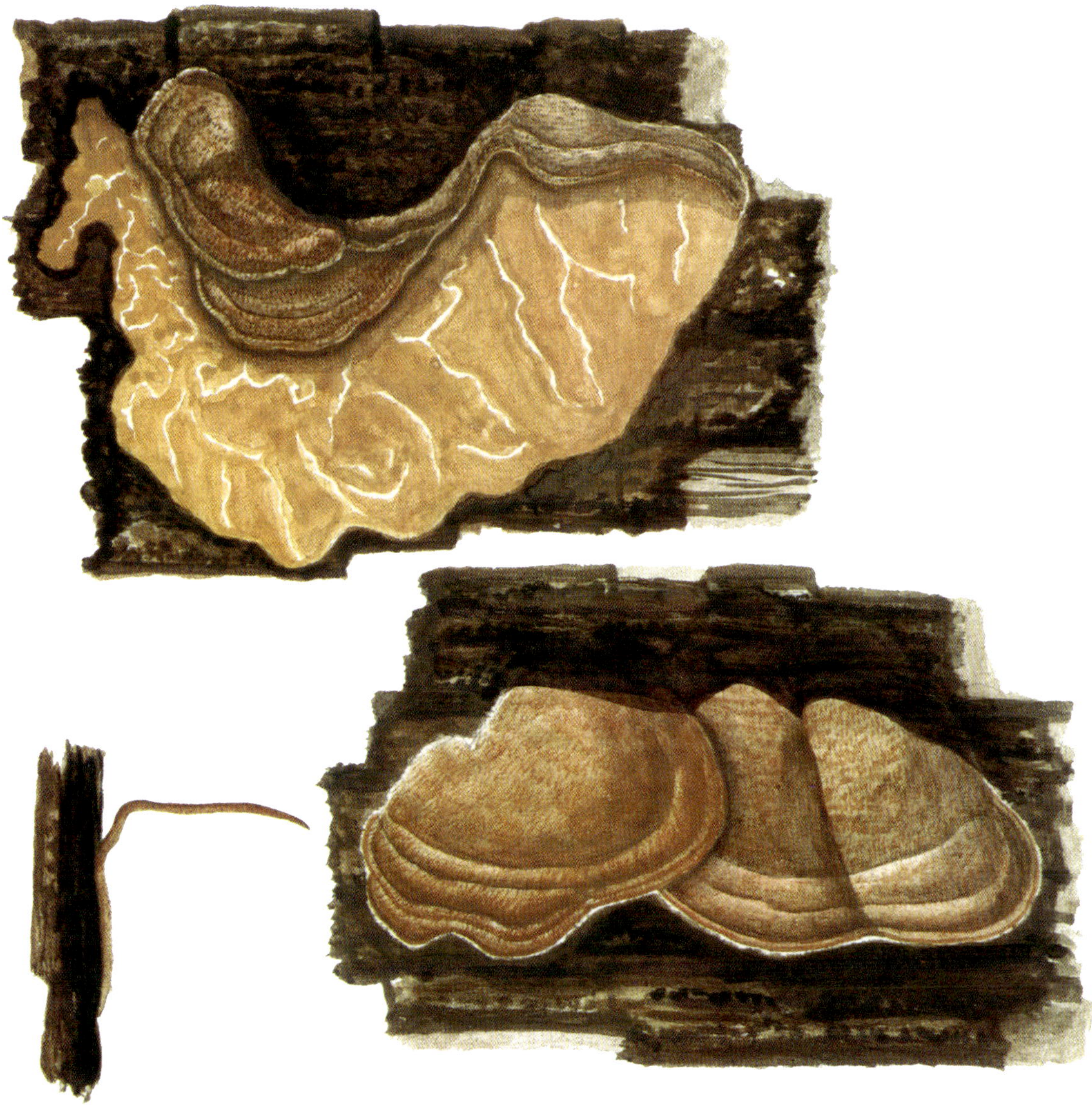

Fig. 11.90. ***Lloydella subpileata*** (Berk. et Curt.) Hölm. & Litsch. — This mushroom contains polysaccharides that inhibit sarcoma-180 in white mice (Ying, et al, 1987).

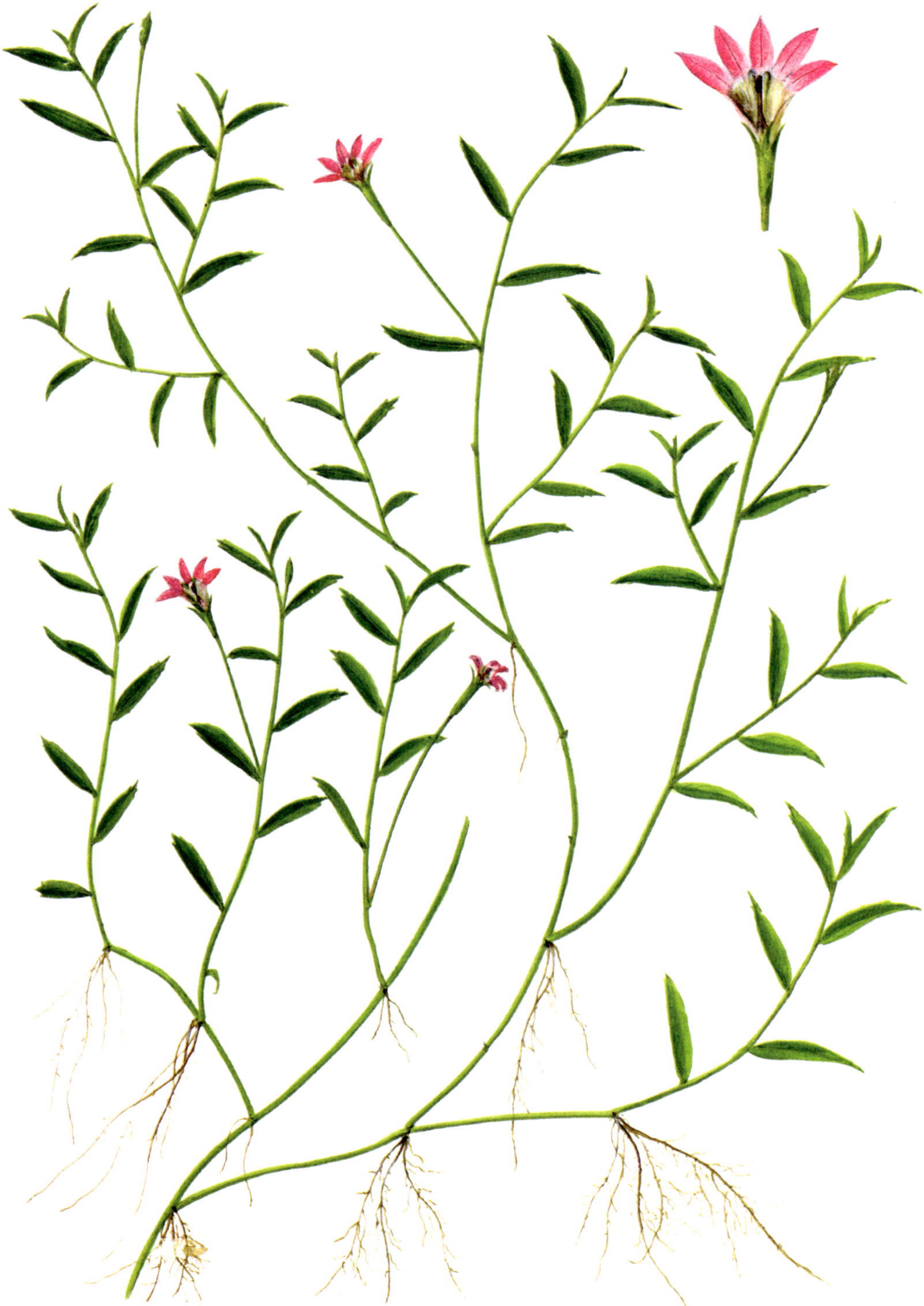

Fig. 11.91. ***Lobelia chinensis*** Lour. — This plant contains the alkaloids lobeline, lobelanine, lobelanidine, and isolobelanine, glucosides, and saponins. It is effective against Hela cells in vitro, inhibits sarcoma-37 and sarcoma-180 in mice, and has been used to treat cancers of the nasal cavity, and gastrointestinal, liver, kidney, and rectal cancers. (Hsu, et al, 1986; Minyi, 1992; Huang, 1999)

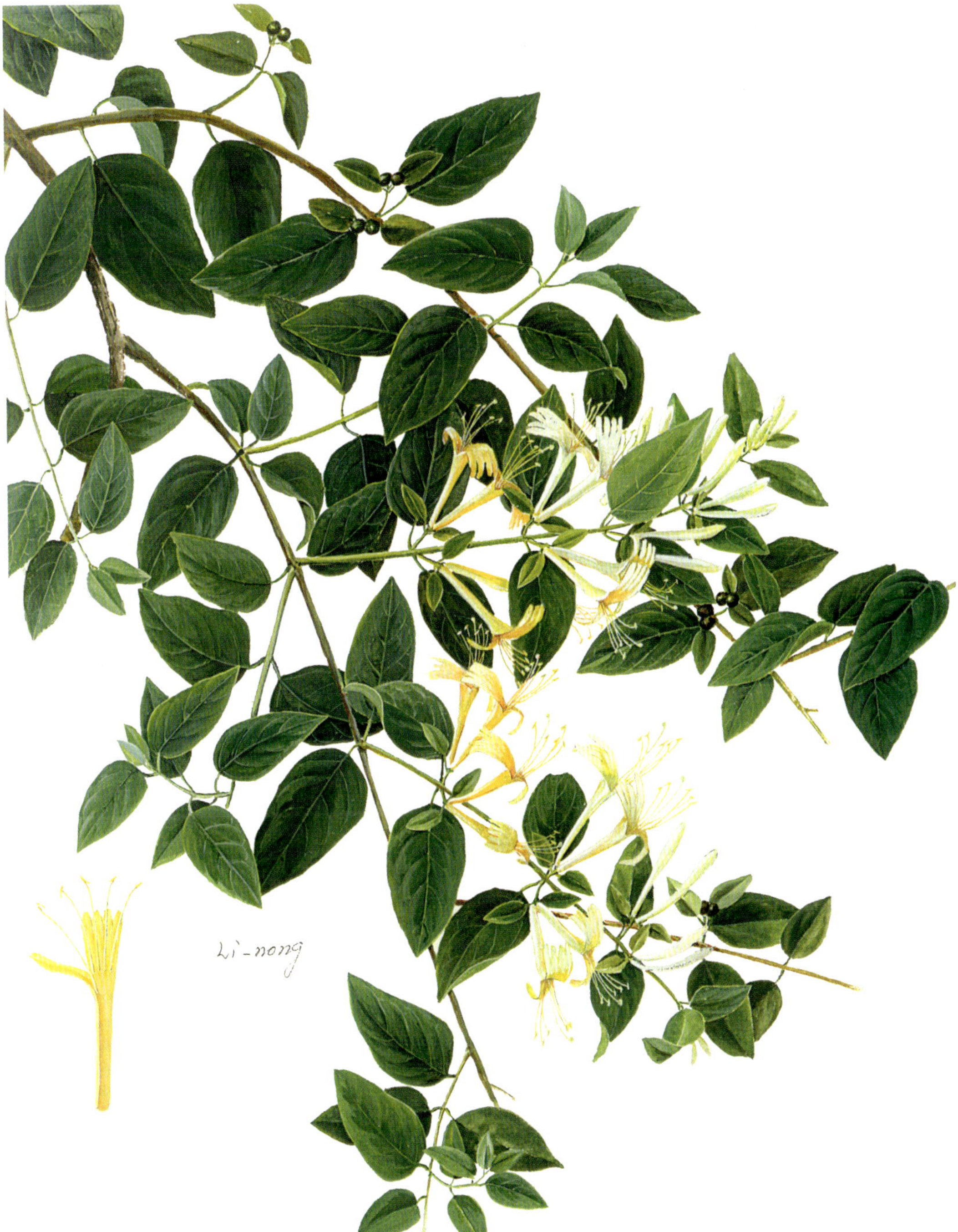


Fig. 11.92. ***Lonicera japonica*** Thunb. — This plant contains chlorogenic acid, isochlorogenic acid, neochlorogenic acid, 4-o-caffeoylquinic acid, 4,5-dicaffeoylquinic acid, 3,5-dicaffeoylquinic acid, 3,4-dicaffeoylquinic acid, flavenoids (including luteolin), lonicerin, inositol, and saponins. Laboratory tests have shown it is effective against Hela-60 cells and inhibits sarcoma-180 and ascites carcinoma. It has been used to treat leukemia and nasopharyngeal, breast, and cervical cancer. (Chang & But, 1986; Hsu, et al, 1986; Minyi, 1992; Lee, 1999)

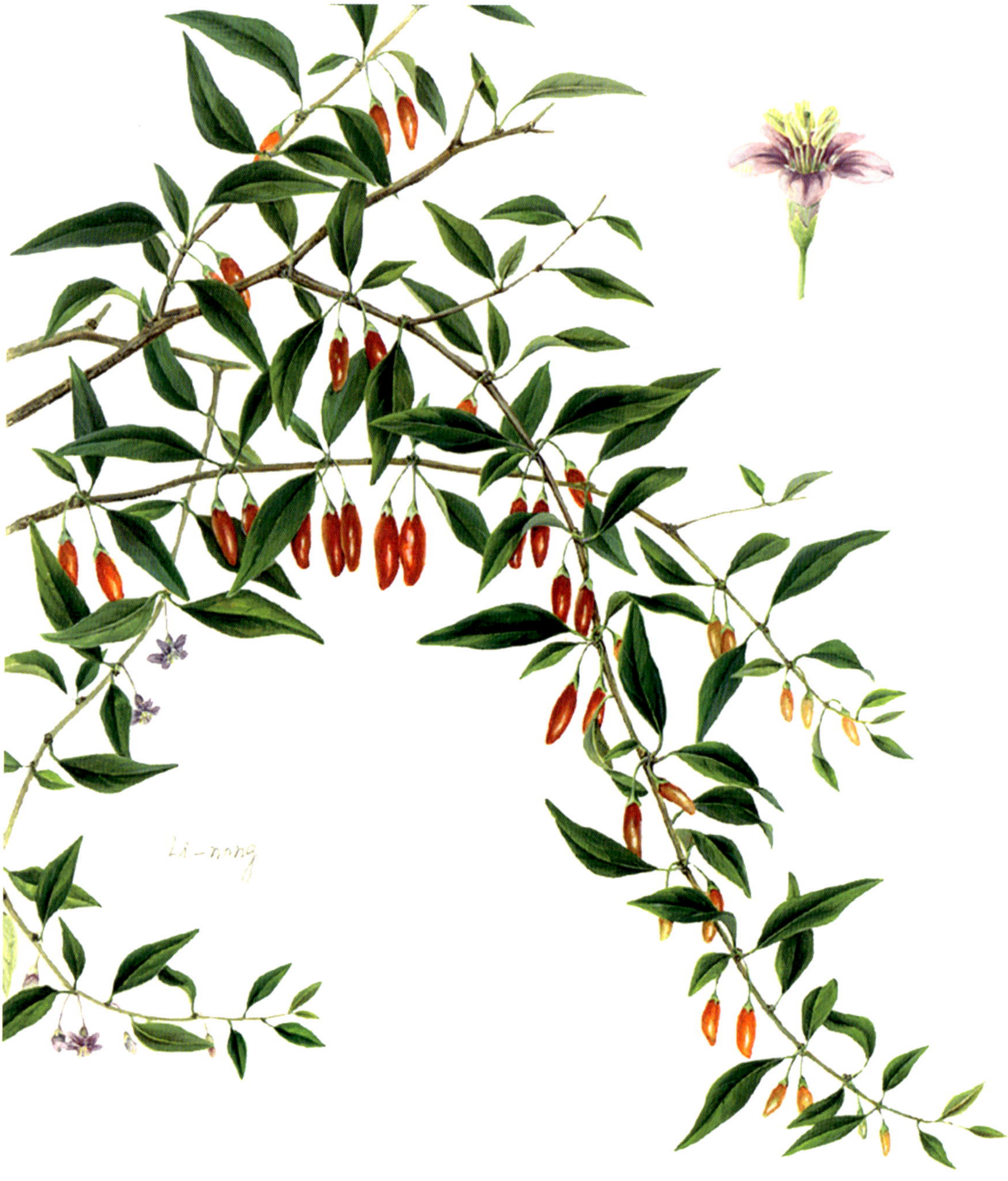

Fig. 11.93. ***Lycium barbarum*** Linn. — This plant contains amino acids, betaine, physalien, cinnamic acid, linolein acid, polysaccharides, zeaxanthin, vitamin A, $B_1$, $B_2$, and C, calcium, phosphorus, and iron. It is a potent immune enhancer, has anticancer activity, inhibits JTC-26 in vitro and sarcoma-180 in vivo, and has radiosensitizing effects on mice with transplanted Lewis lung cancer. It has been used to treat osteoma, leukemia, and cancers of the intestine, stomach, and pancreas, and is used extensively by the Chinese military. (Hsu, et al, 1986; Lu & Cheng, 1991; Lee, 1999; Halstead, 2002 - unpublished data)

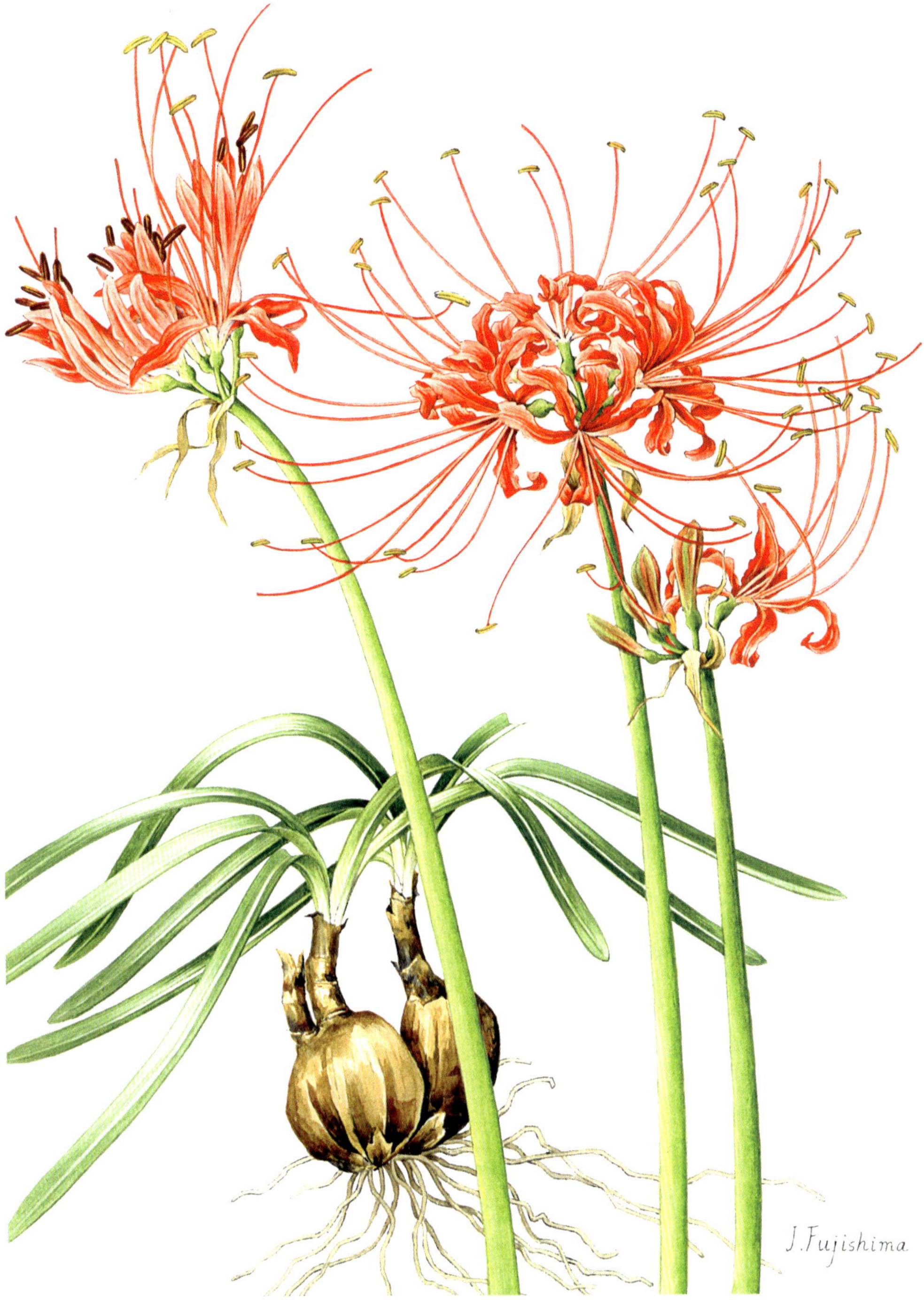


Fig. 11.94. ***Lycoris radiata*** (L. Hérit.) Herb. — This plant contains the alkaloids lycorine, lycoreine, lycoramine, lycorenine, lycoricidine, lycoricidinol, dihydrolycorine, homolycorine, pseudolycorine, galanthamine, tazettine, and haementhidine. It inhibits Ehrlich's ascites carcinoma, ascitic hepatocarcinoma-AH130, Yoshida's sarcoma, and sarcoma-180 in mice, and Walker's sarcoma-256 in rats, and has been used to treat gastrointestinal tract and cervical cancer. (Chang & But, 1986; Minyi, 1992; Huang, 1999; Lee, 1999)

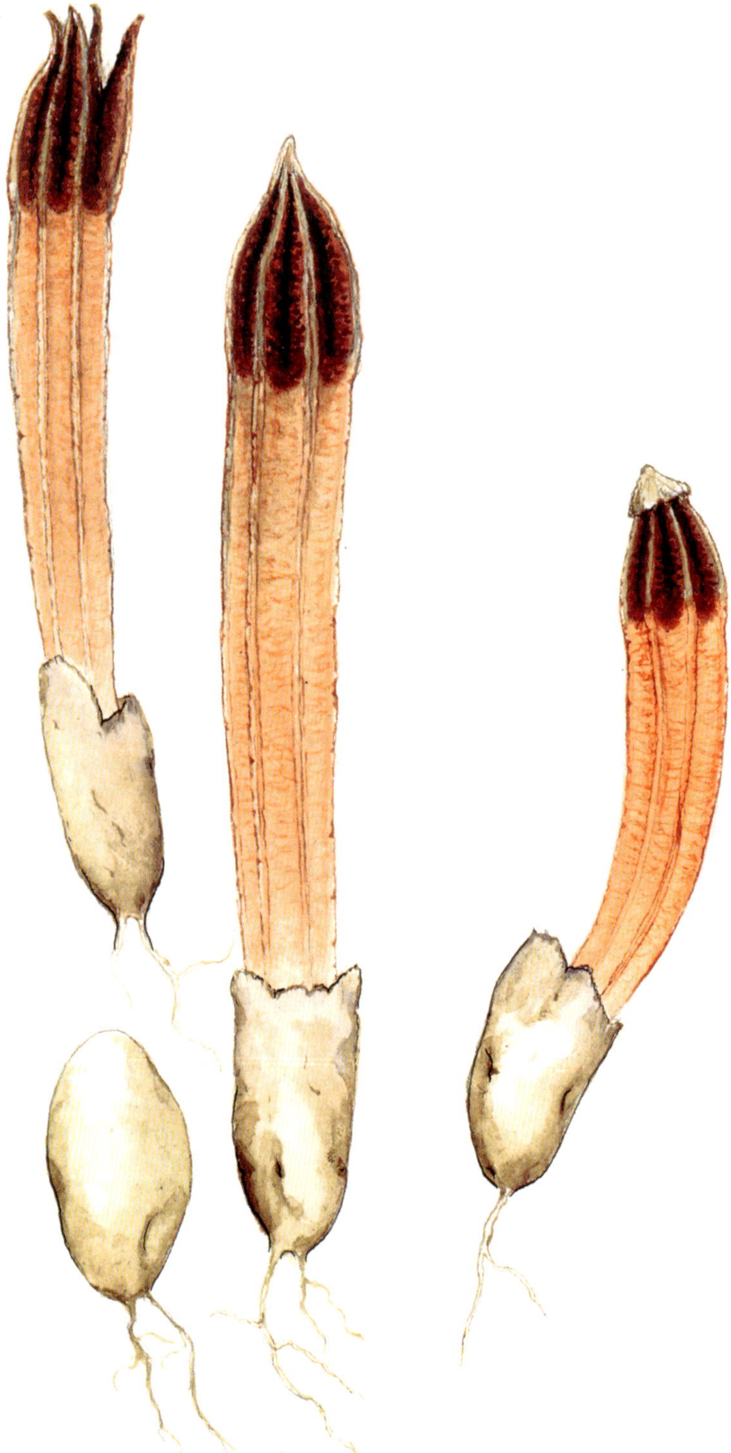

Fig. 11.95. ***Lysurus mokusin*** (Linn. ex Pers.) Fr. — This fungus contains polysaccharides that have anticarcinogenic properties and inhibit sarcoma-180 in mice and Ehrlich's carcinoma (Ying, et al, 1987).

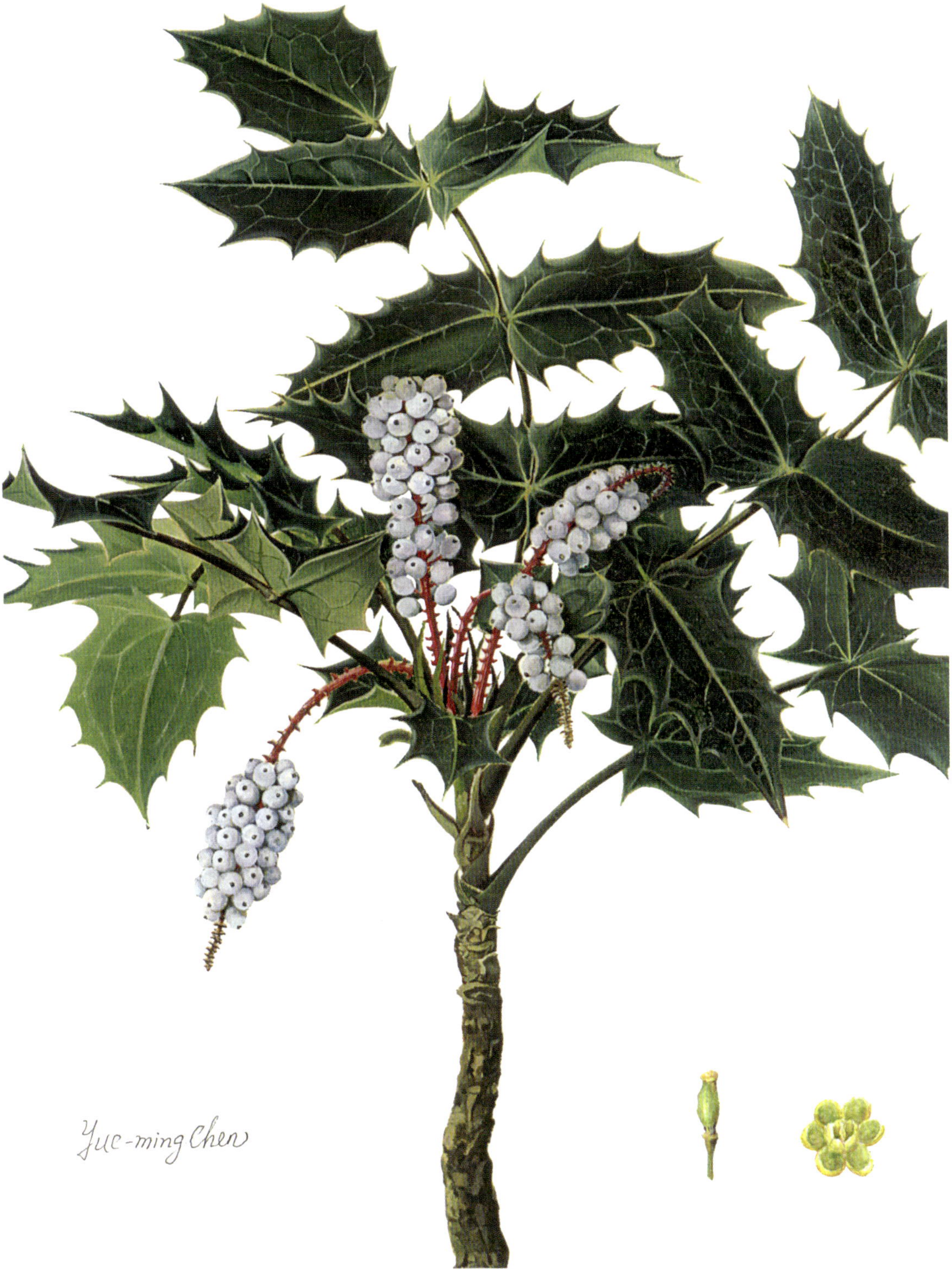


Fig. 11.96. ***Mahonia bealei*** (Fort.) Carr. — This plant contains berberine, which is found to have antineoplastic properties, and has been used in the treatment of pulmonary and liver cancer. (Duke & Ayensu, 1985; Zhicen, et al, 1987; Minyi, 1992)

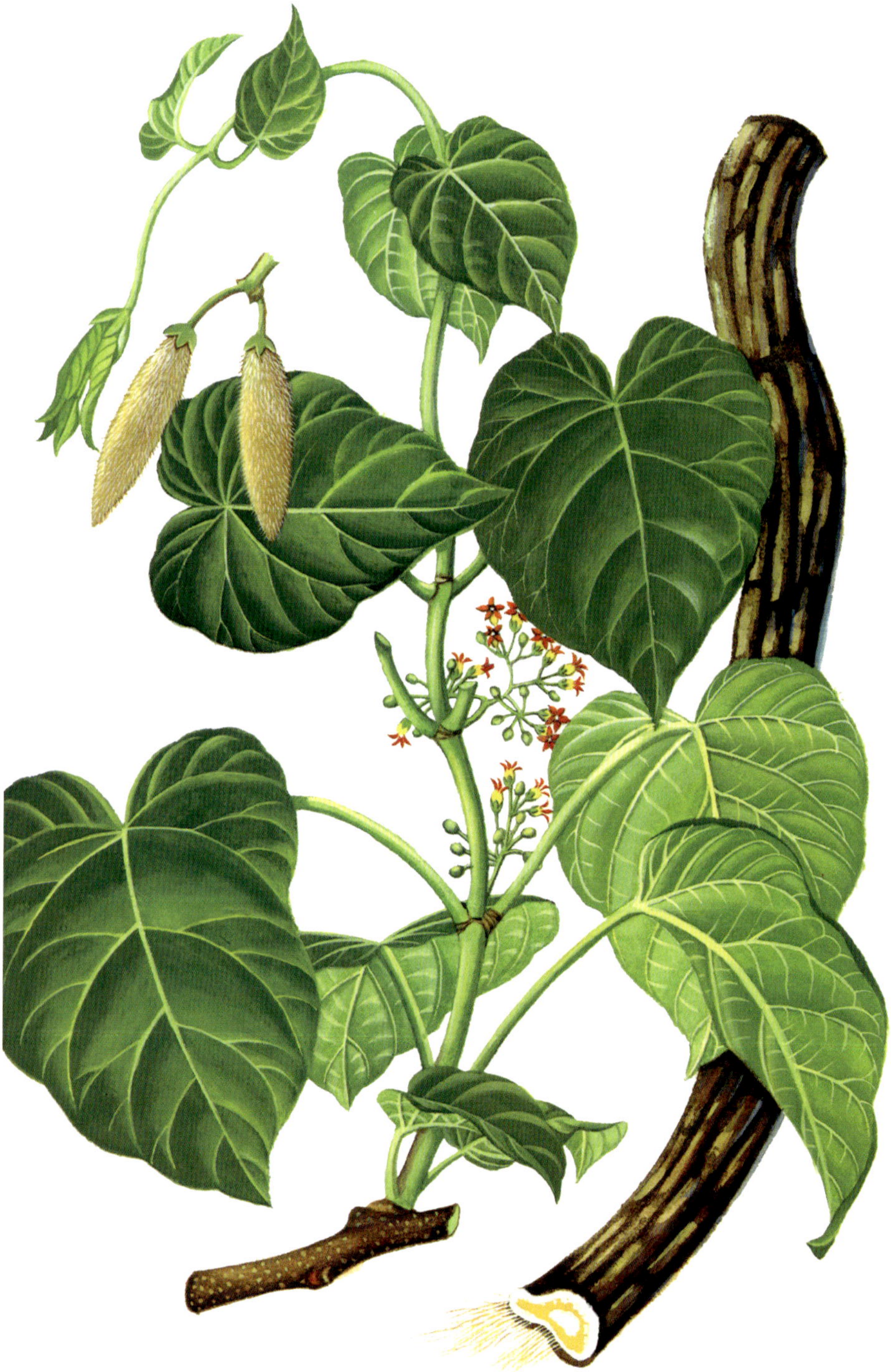

Fig. 11.97. ***Marsdenia tenacissima*** (Roxb.) Wight et Arn. — This plant contains sarcostin, steroidal saponins, polysaccharides, alkaloids, resins, and phytochromes, which inhibit cancer and enhance the immune system. It has been used in the treatment of Hodgkin's disease, lymphosarcoma, osteosarcoma, lingual and mandibular squamous epithelial carcinoma, and esophageal, gastrointestinal, heart, and cervical cancer. (Hsu, et al, 1986; Minyi, 1992; Huang, 1999)

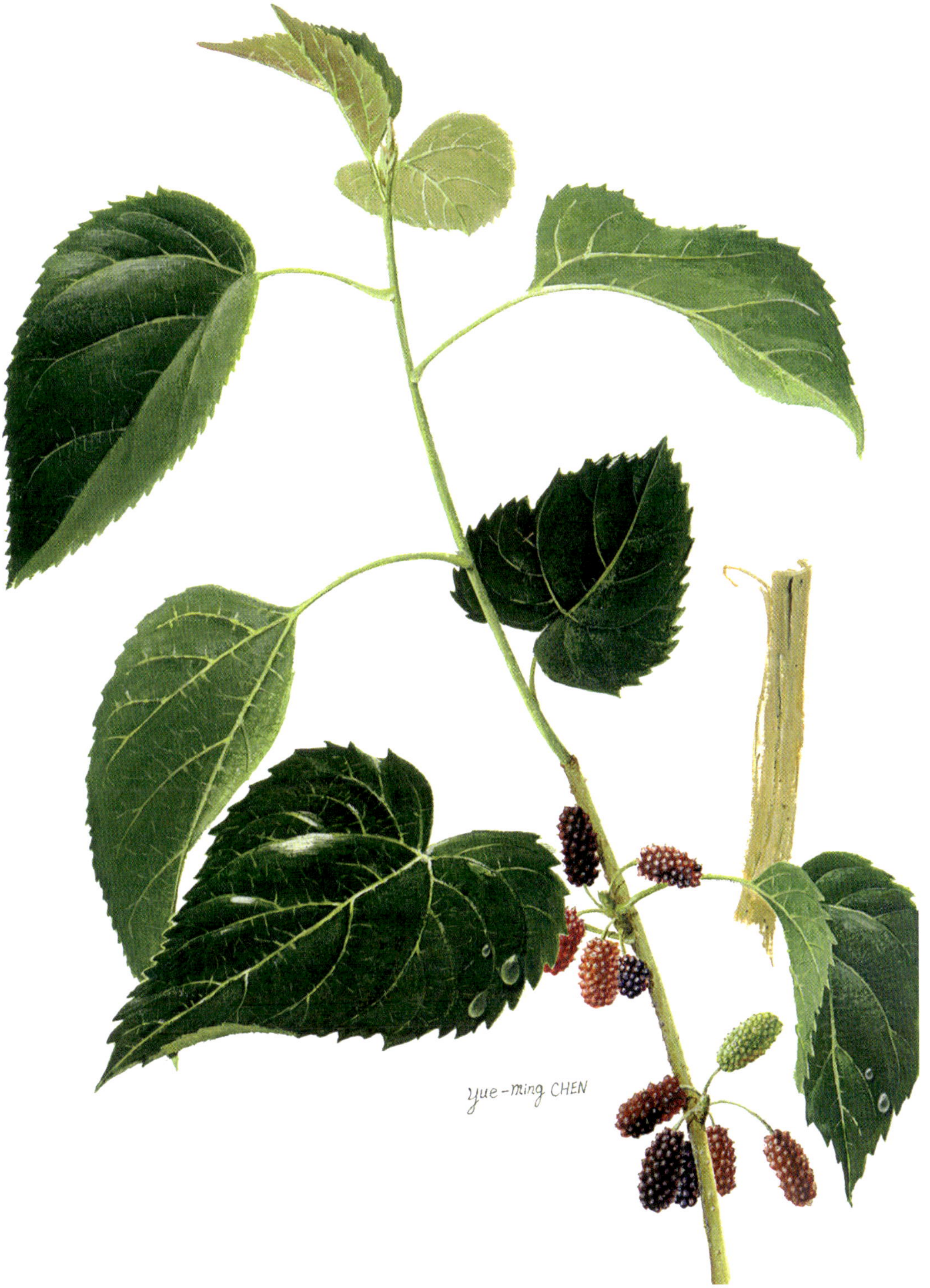


Fig. 11.98. ***Morus alba*** Linn. — This plant contains umbelliferone, scopoletine, mulberrin, flavenoids, and tannins. It inhibits sarcoma-180 in mice and JTC-26 and HL-60 in vitro, and has been used in the treatment of esophageal and gastrointestinal cancer. (Minyi, 1992)

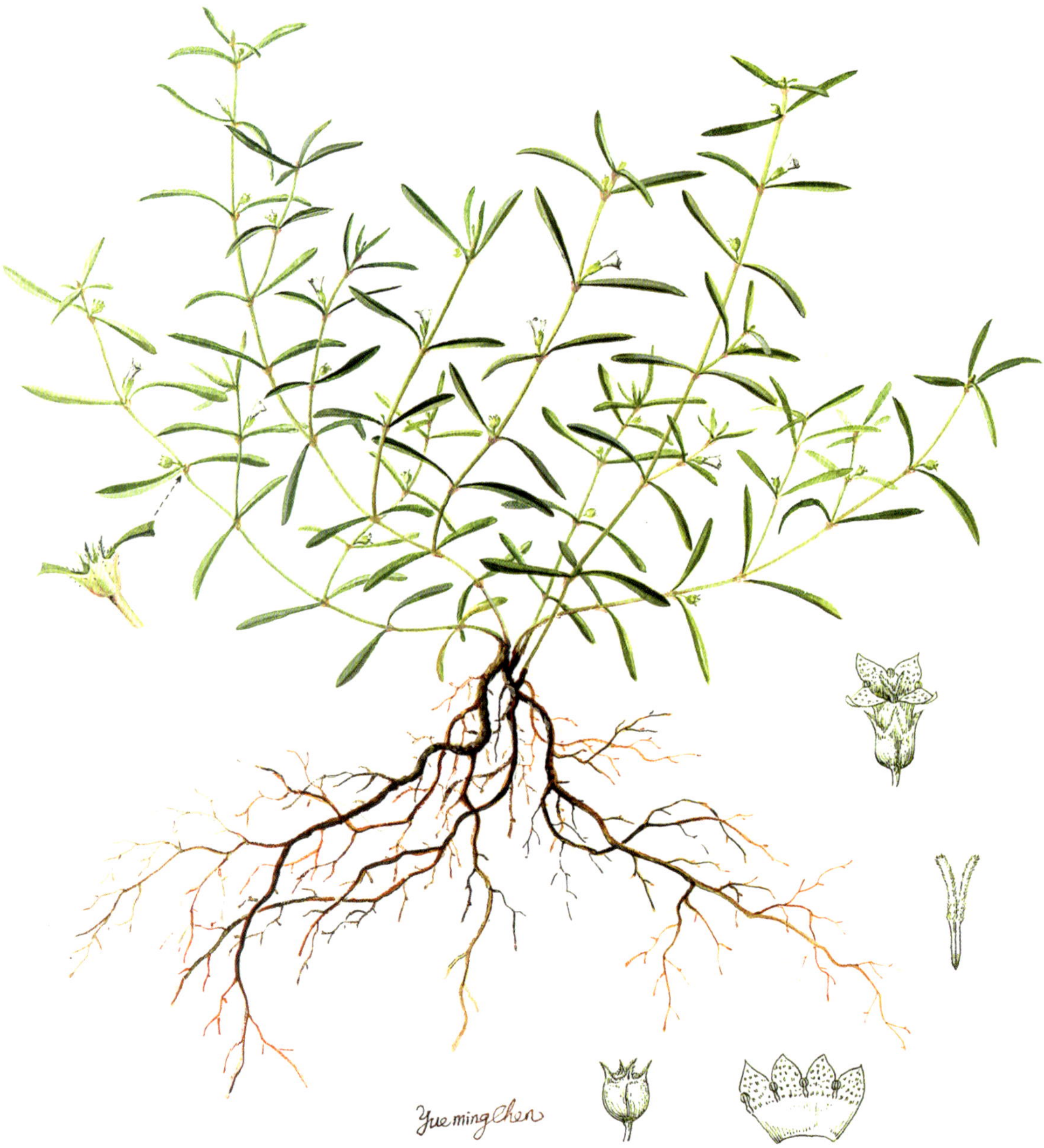


Fig. 11.99. ***Oldenlandia diffusa*** (Wild.) Roxb. — This plant contains hentriacontane, stigmasterol, ursolic acid, oleanolic acid, β-sitosterol, sitosterol-D-glucoside, coumaric acid, coumeic acid, and flavenoid glycosides, asperuloside, palderoside, desacetylasperuloside, and oldenlandoside. Laboratory studies have shown that it inhibits Erlich's carcinoma, Yoshida's sarcoma, Jitian sarcoma, and multiple kinds of leukemia in vitro. It has been used in the treatment of a variety of cancers including esophageal, stomach, liver, breast, and cervical cancer, fibrosarcoma, and lymphosarcoma. (Chang & But, 1986; Minyi, 1992; Huang, 1999)

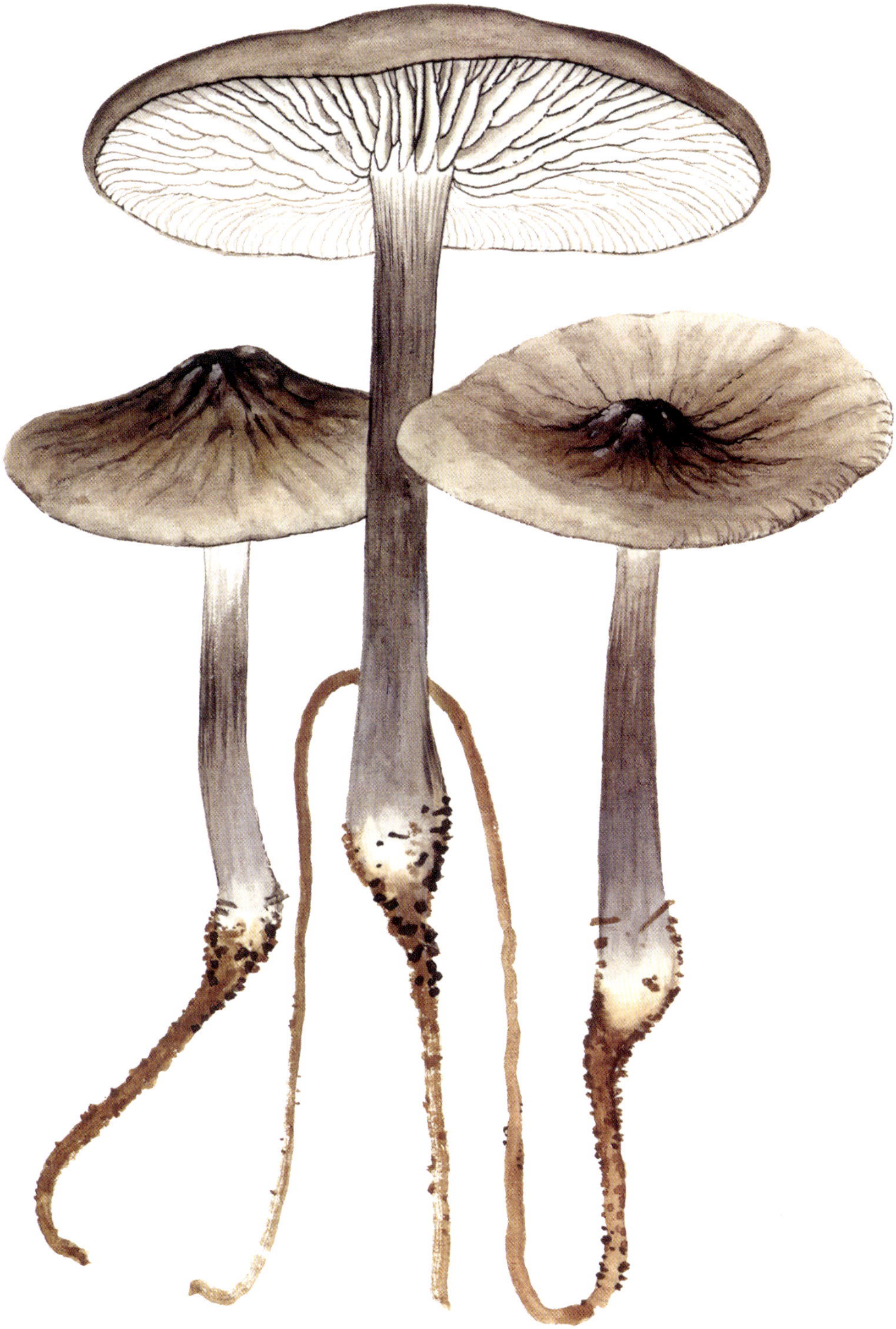

Fig. 11.100. ***Oudemansiella radicata*** (Relh. ex Fr.) Sing — This mushroom contains oudenone, which is made from its fermented liquid, and polysaccharides that inhibit sarcoma-180 in mice and Ehrlich's carcinoma (Ying, et al, 1987).

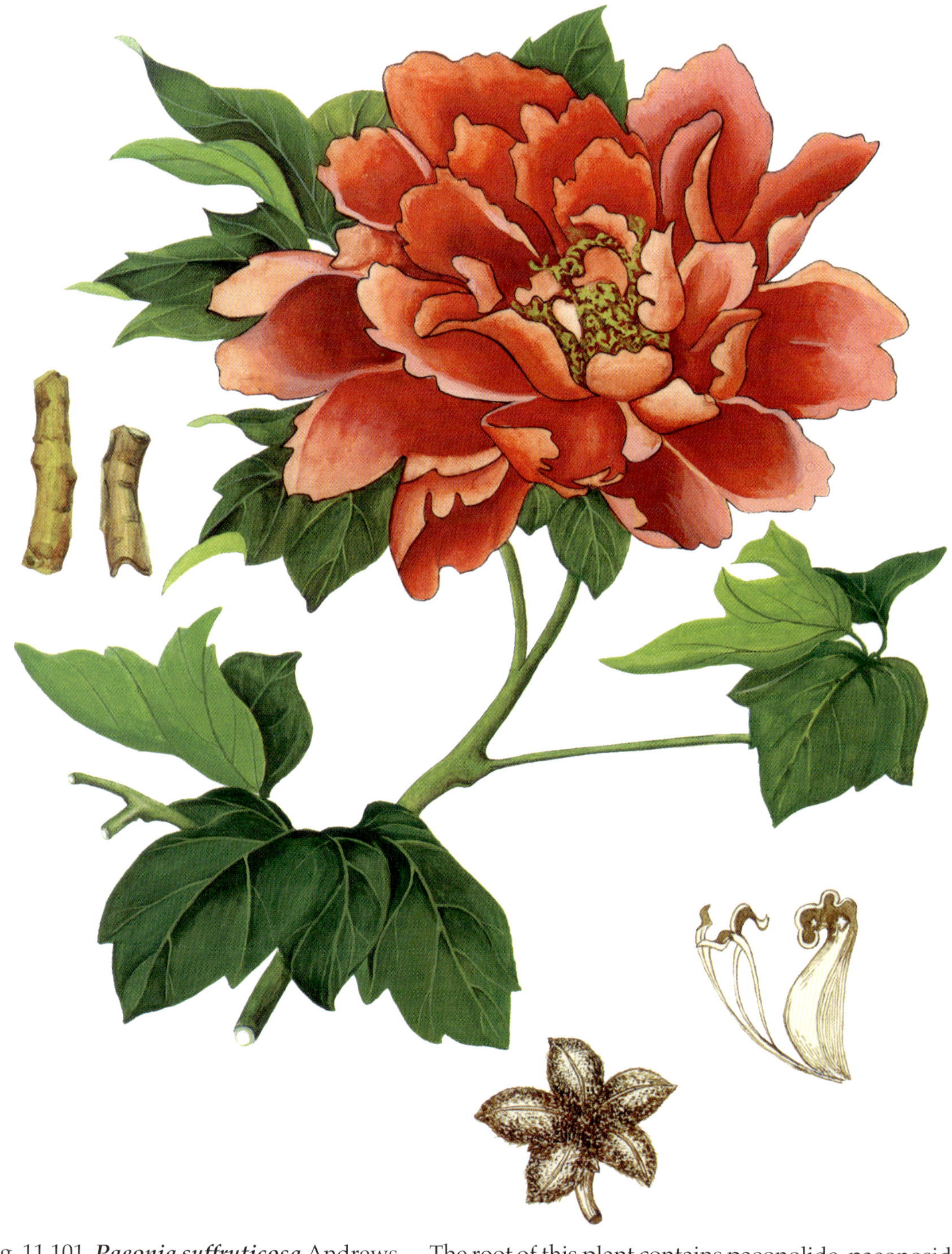

Fig. 11.101. ***Paeonia suffruticosa*** Andrews — The root of this plant contains paeonolide, paeonoside, paeonol, paeoniflorin, oxypaeoniflorin, benzoylpaeoniflorin, benzoyloxypaeoniflorin, benzoic acid, campesterol, and β-sitosterol. It inhibits human cervical carcinoma (JTC-26) and human hepatocellular carcinoma (SK-HEP-1) cell lines in vitro and sarcoma-180 in vivo, and has been used in the treatment of esophageal, lung, and cervical carcinoma, uterine myoma, and leukemia. (Hsu, et al, 1986; Sakamoto, et al, 1992; Lee, 1999; Oh, et al, 2001)

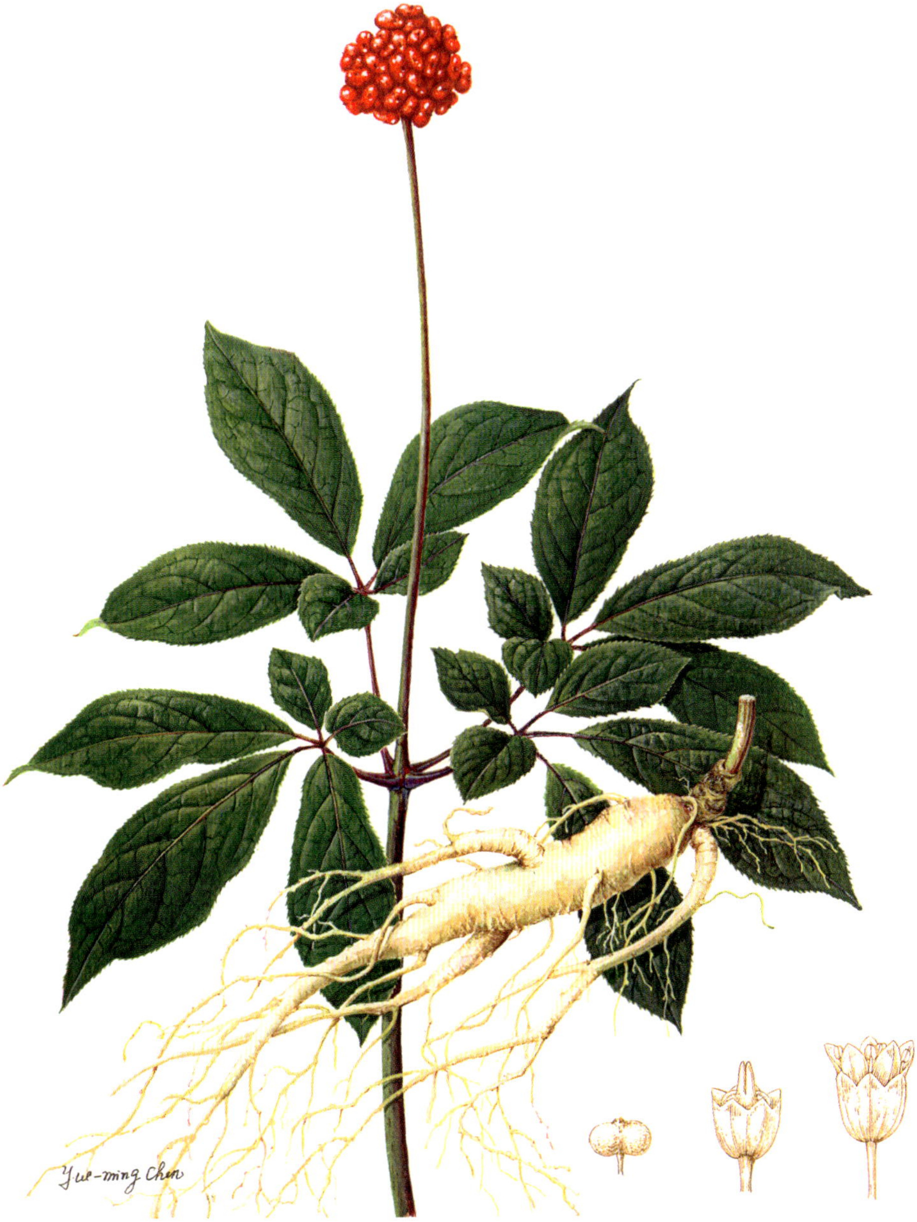


Fig. 11.102. ***Panax ginseng*** C. A. Meyer — This plant contains several pharmacologically active saponins such as ginsenosides and panaxosides A, B, C, D, E, and F, flavenoids, volatile oils including panacene, panaxin, β-elemene, and panaxynol, saccharides, panose, prostisol, vitamins, amino acids, antioxidants, peptides, fatty acids, alcohols, cholesteryl ester transfer protein inhibitors, β-sitosterol, β-sitosterol glucoside, kaempferol, trifolin, panasenoside, luteolin-7-glucoside, panaxadiol, panaxtriol, and oleanolic acid. These compounds have a broad range of pharmacological effects on the body. Ginseng is an adaptogen and tends to normalize the pathophysiology of the body, shows antineoplastic effects, enhances the immune system, and inhibits murine tumors sarcoma-180, adenocarcinoma-755, Erlich's ascites carcinoma, and U-14, and in vitro inhibits human uterine cervix-26 cancer cells. It has been used to treat cancers of the esophagus, lung, stomach, breast, and uterus. Ginseng has a low level of toxicity. (Chang & But, 1986; Hsu, et al, 1986; Minyi, 1992; Huang, 1999; Lee, 1999)

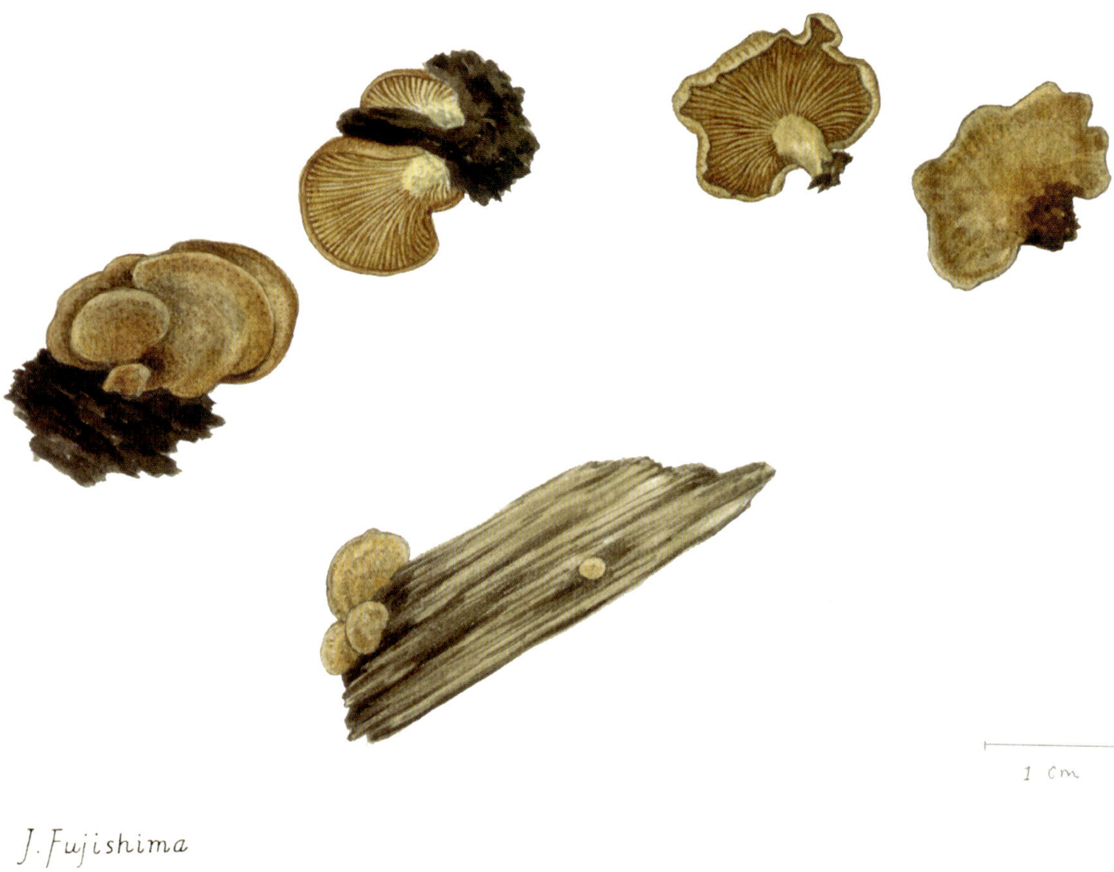


Fig. 11.103. ***Panellus stypticus*** (Bull. ex Fr.) Karst. — This fungus contains polysaccharides that inhibit sarcoma-180 and Ehrlich's carcinoma (Ying, et al, 1987).

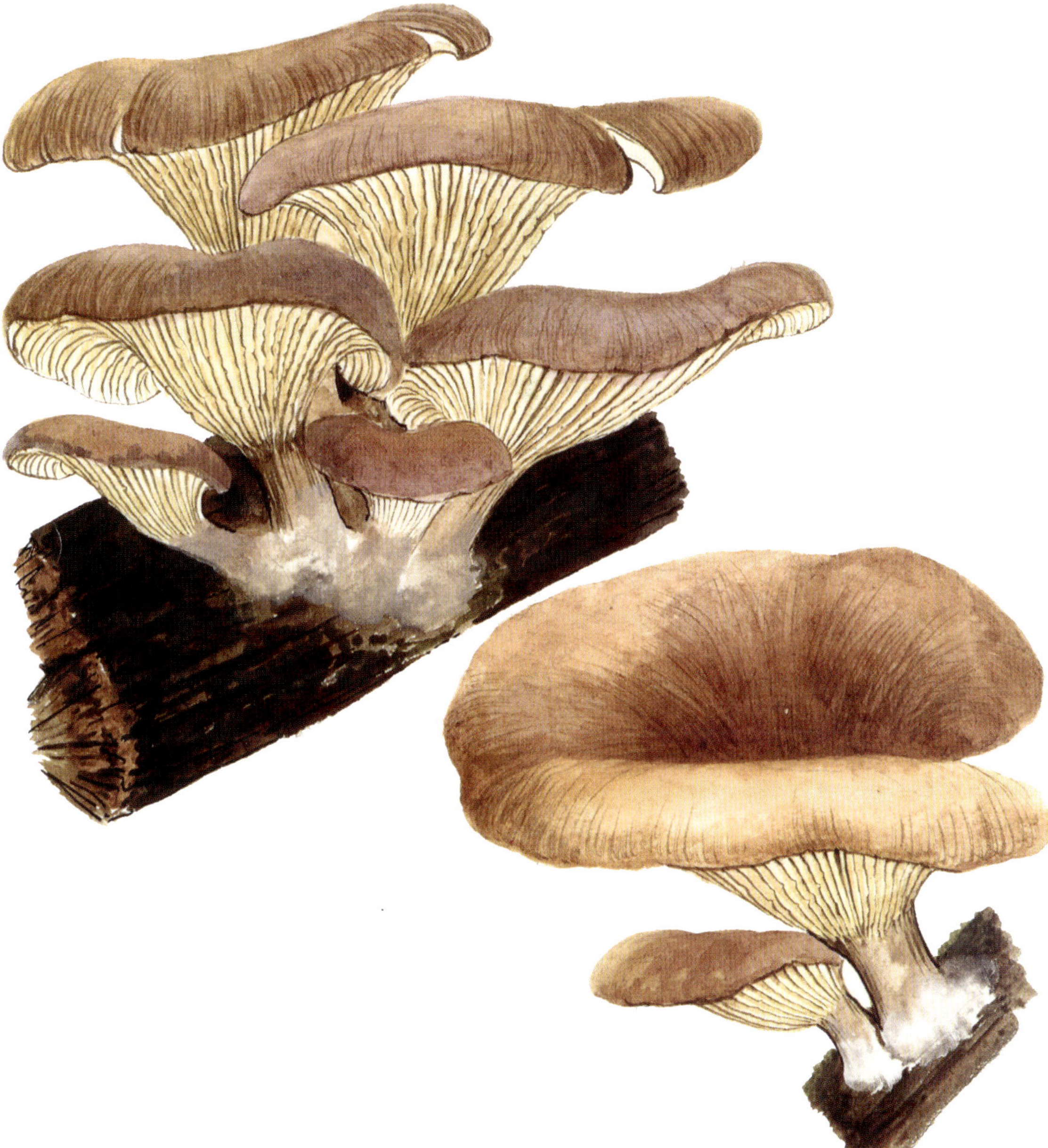

Fig. 11.104. ***Panus conchatus*** (Bull. ex Fr.) Karst. — This fungus contains polysaccharides that inhibit sarcoma-180 and Ehrlich's carcinoma in white mice (Ying, et al, 1987).

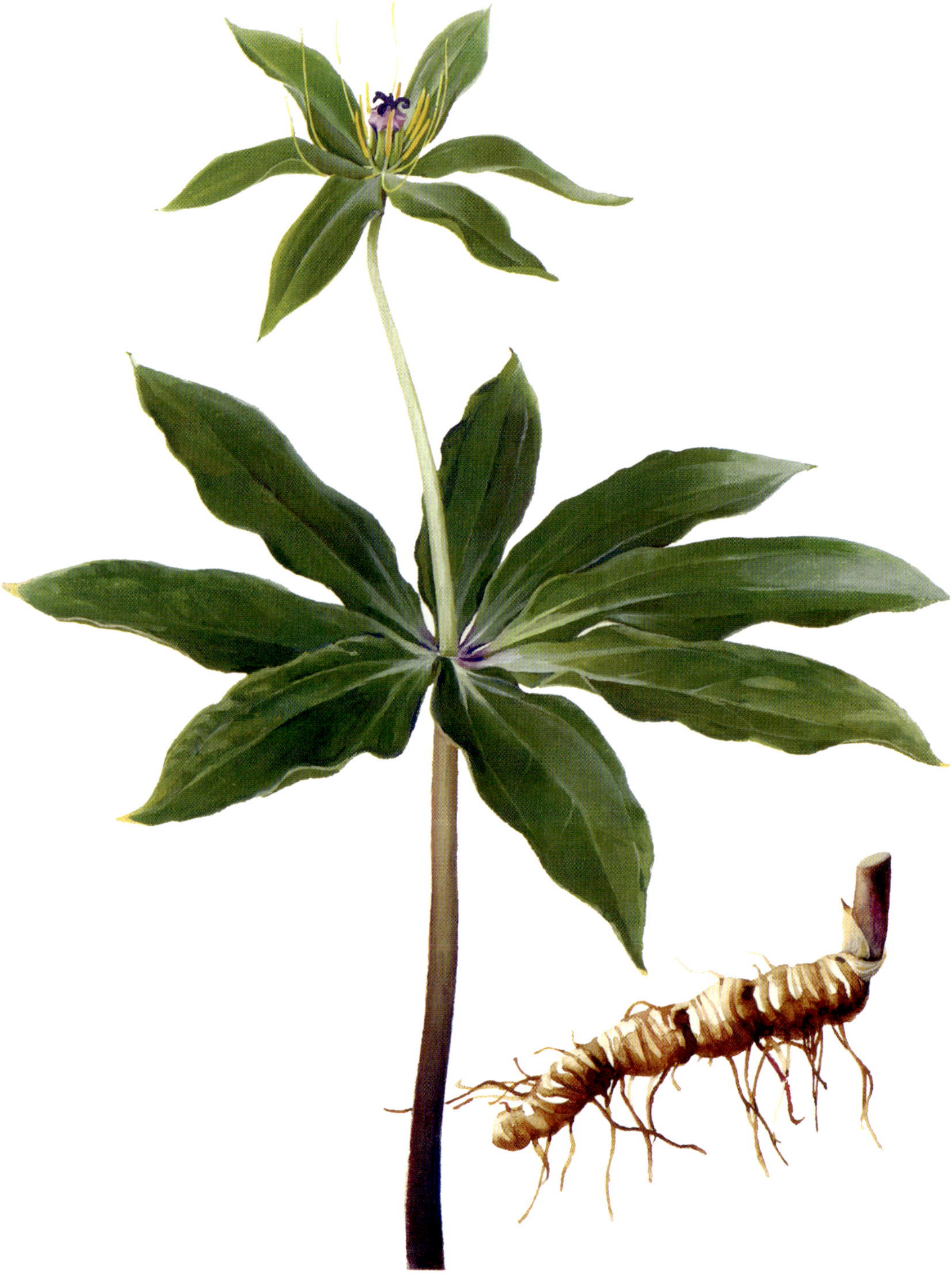

Fig. 11.105. ***Paris polyphylla*** Sm. — This plant contains pariden, peristynin, alkaloids, and the steroids saponin and diosgenin. It inhibits oncocytes and JTC-26 cells in vitro and in vivo inhibits sarcoma-37, sarcoma-180, and solid hepatocancer in mice and other animal tumors. It shows cytotoxic activity against leukemia-388 and leukemia-1210, and has been used to treat encephaloma and cancers of the nasopharynsx, esophagus, and stomach. (Hsu, et al, 1986; Minyi, 1992; Lee, 1999)

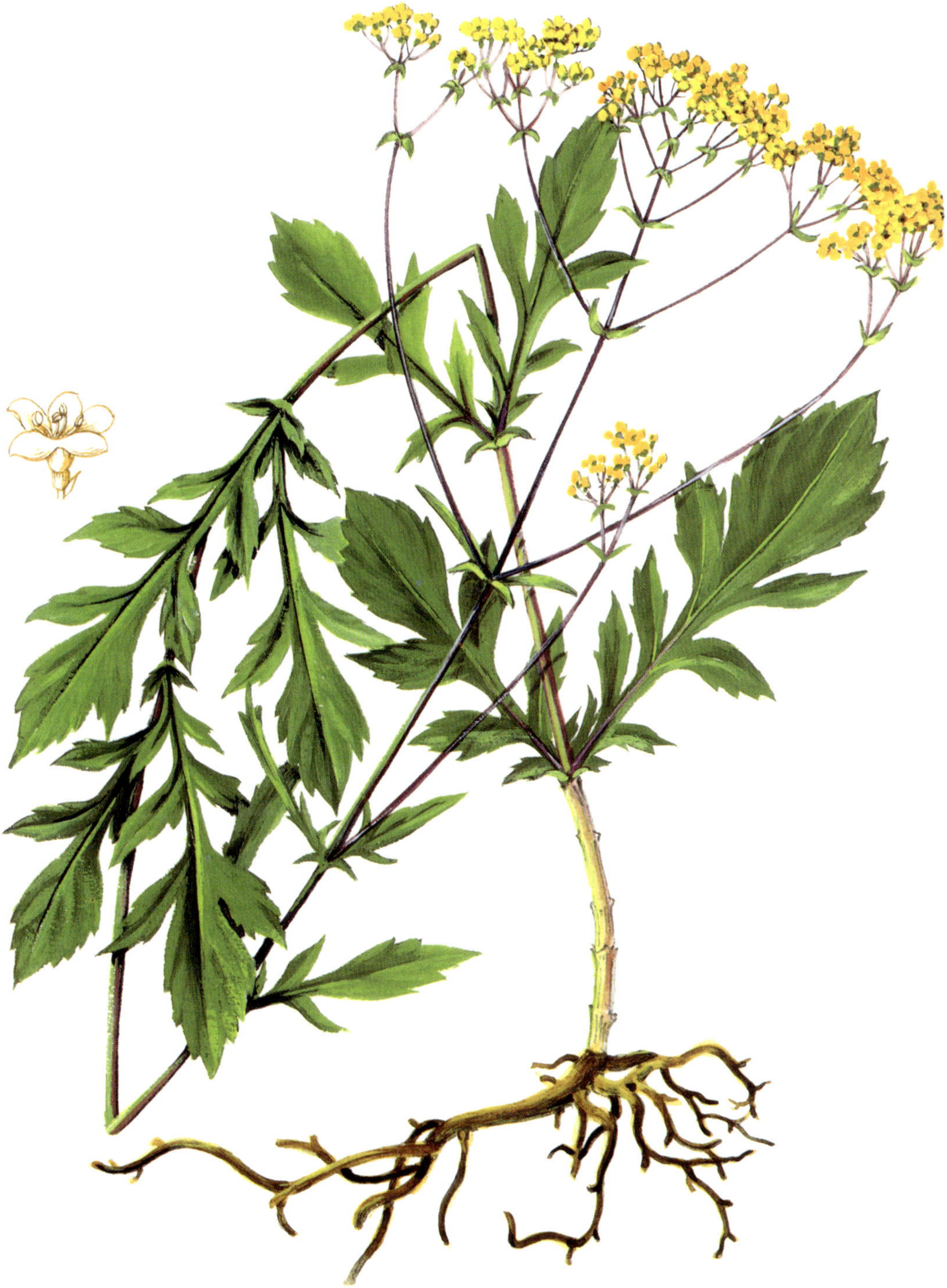

Fig. 11.106. ***Patrinia scabiosaefolia*** Fisch. — This plant contains patrinene, isopatrinene, isopentanoic acid, oleanolic acid, hederagenin, β-sitosterol-β-D-glucoside, saponins, such as patrinosides and scabiosides, sapogenin, alkaloid, and tannin. It inhibits JTC-26 cells and cancer cells of the human cervix and has been used to treat cancers of the esophagus, intestine, appendix, bladder, uterus, cervix, rectum, and skin. (Chang & But, 1986; Hsu, et al, 1986; Minyi, 1992; Lee, 1999)

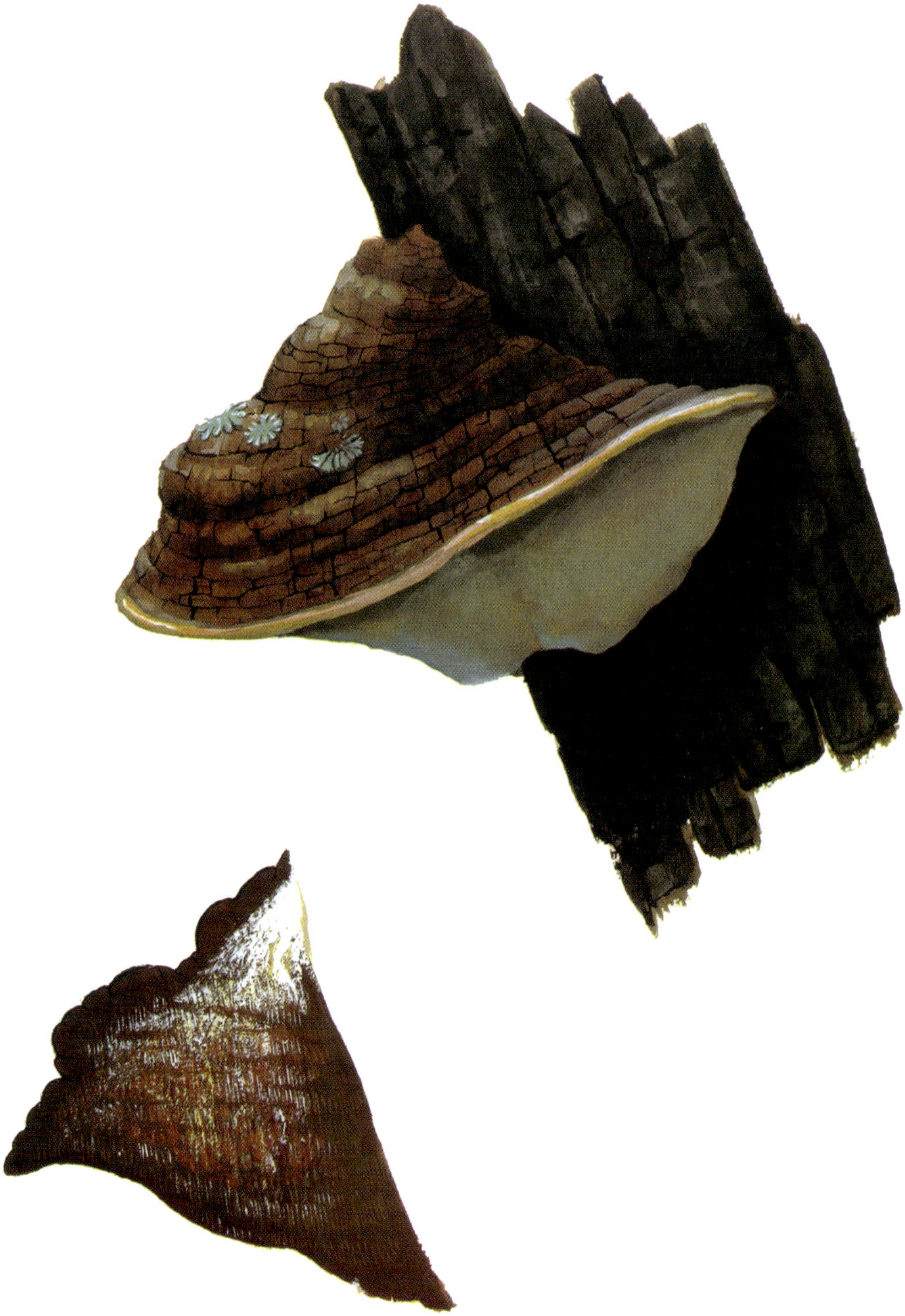

Fig. 11.107. ***Phellinus igniarius*** (Linn. ex Fr.) Quél. — This fungus grows on trees and contains polysaccharides that have antimutagenic activities and inhibit sarcoma-180 and Ehrlich's carcinoma in laboratory mice. It is also used in Siberia as a tea to prevent cancer. (Ying, et al, 1987; Halstead – unpublished data)

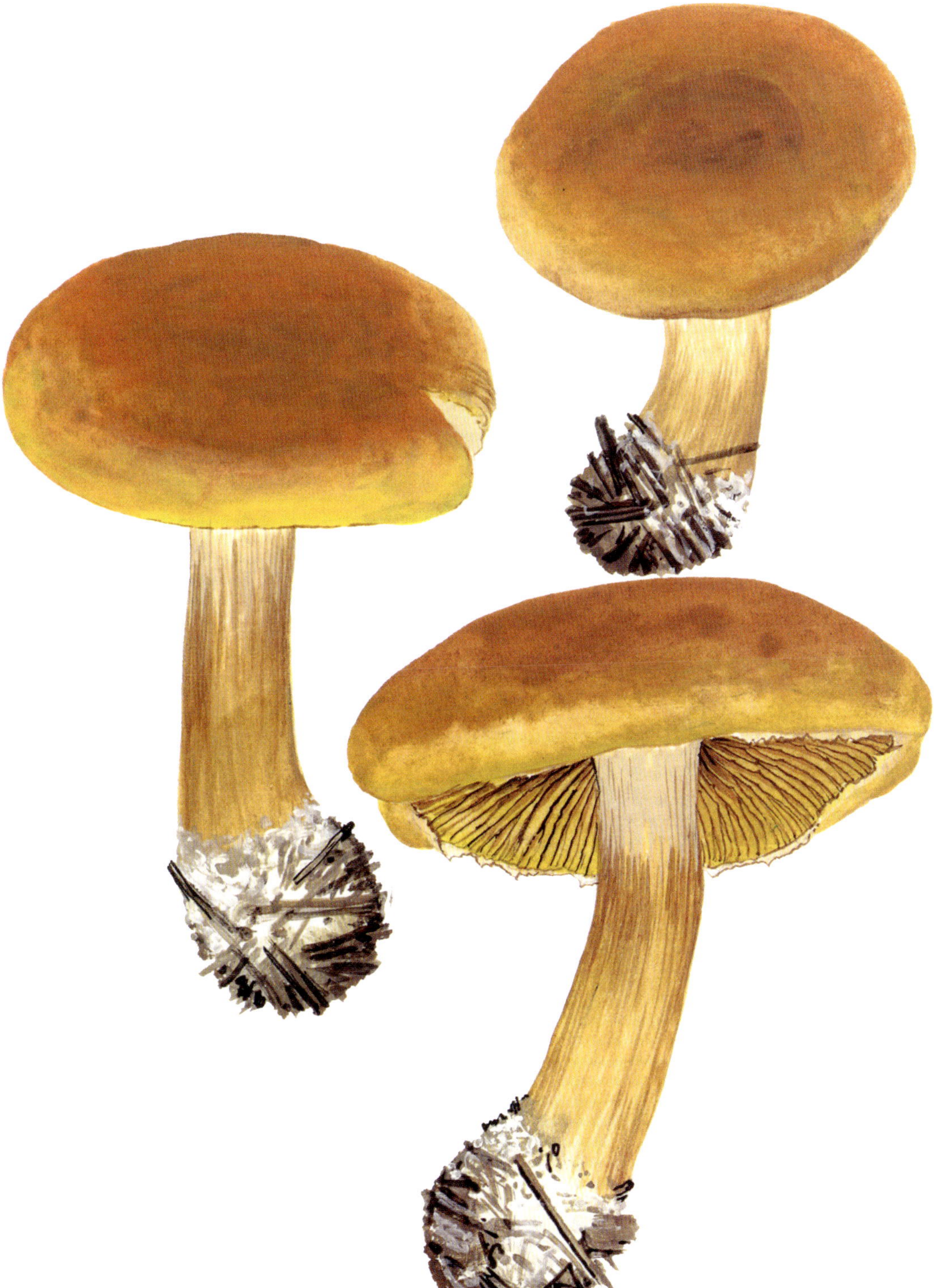

Fig. 11.108. ***Pholiota lubrica*** (Fr.) Sing. — This fungus contains polysaccharides that inhibit sarcoma-180 and Ehrlich's carcinoma (Ying, et al, 1987).

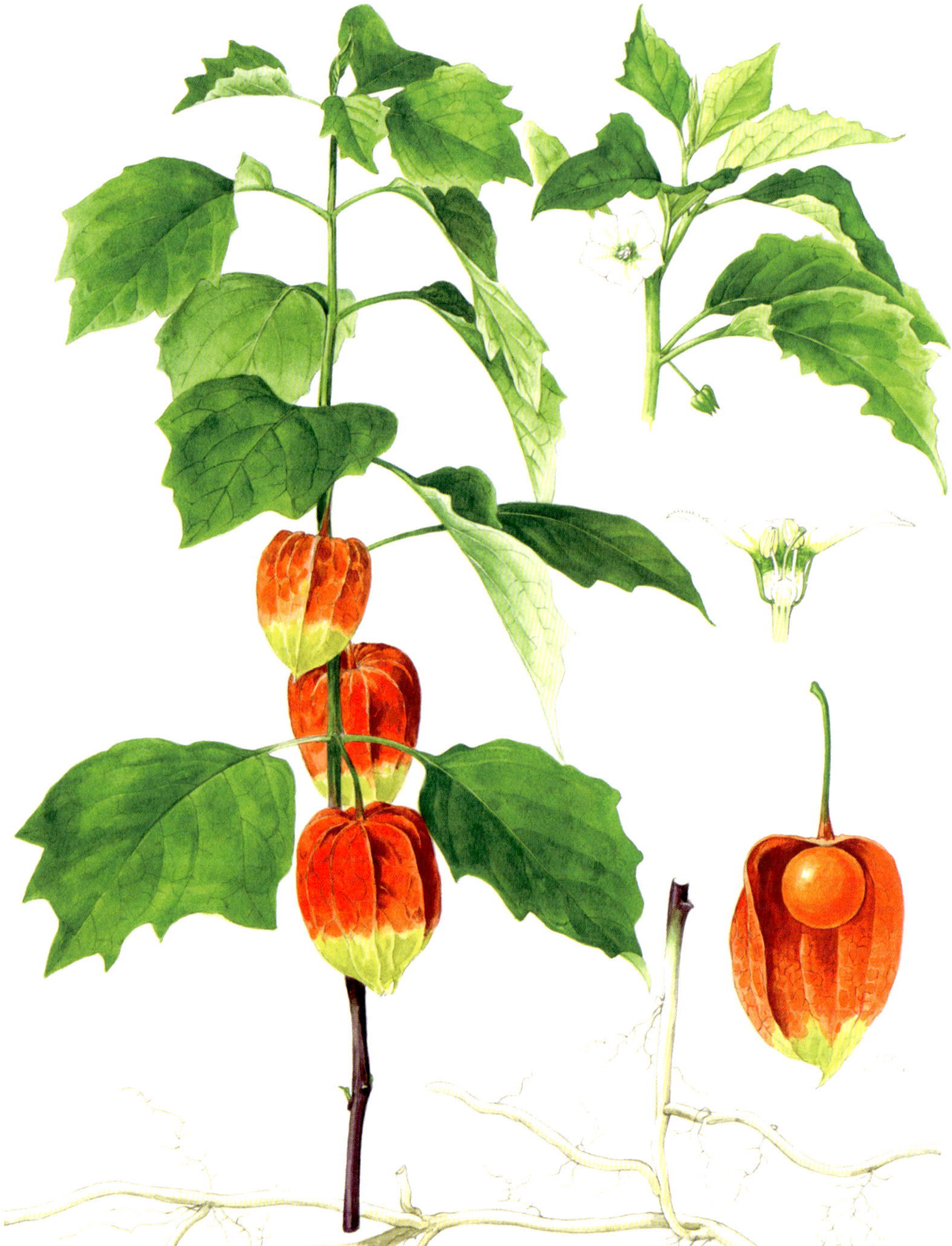


Fig. 11.109. ***Physalis alkekengi*** Linn. **var.** ***franchetti*** (Masters) Hort. — This plant contains physalins A, B, and C, physalien, tigloidine, 3-α-tigloyloxytropane, alkaloids, histonin, potassium nitrate, and vitamin C. It inhibits several human leukemia cell lines in vitro and has been used in the treatment of a variety of types of cancers. (Hsu, et al, 1986; Chiang, Jaw & Chen, 1991; Minyi, 1992; Huang, 1999)

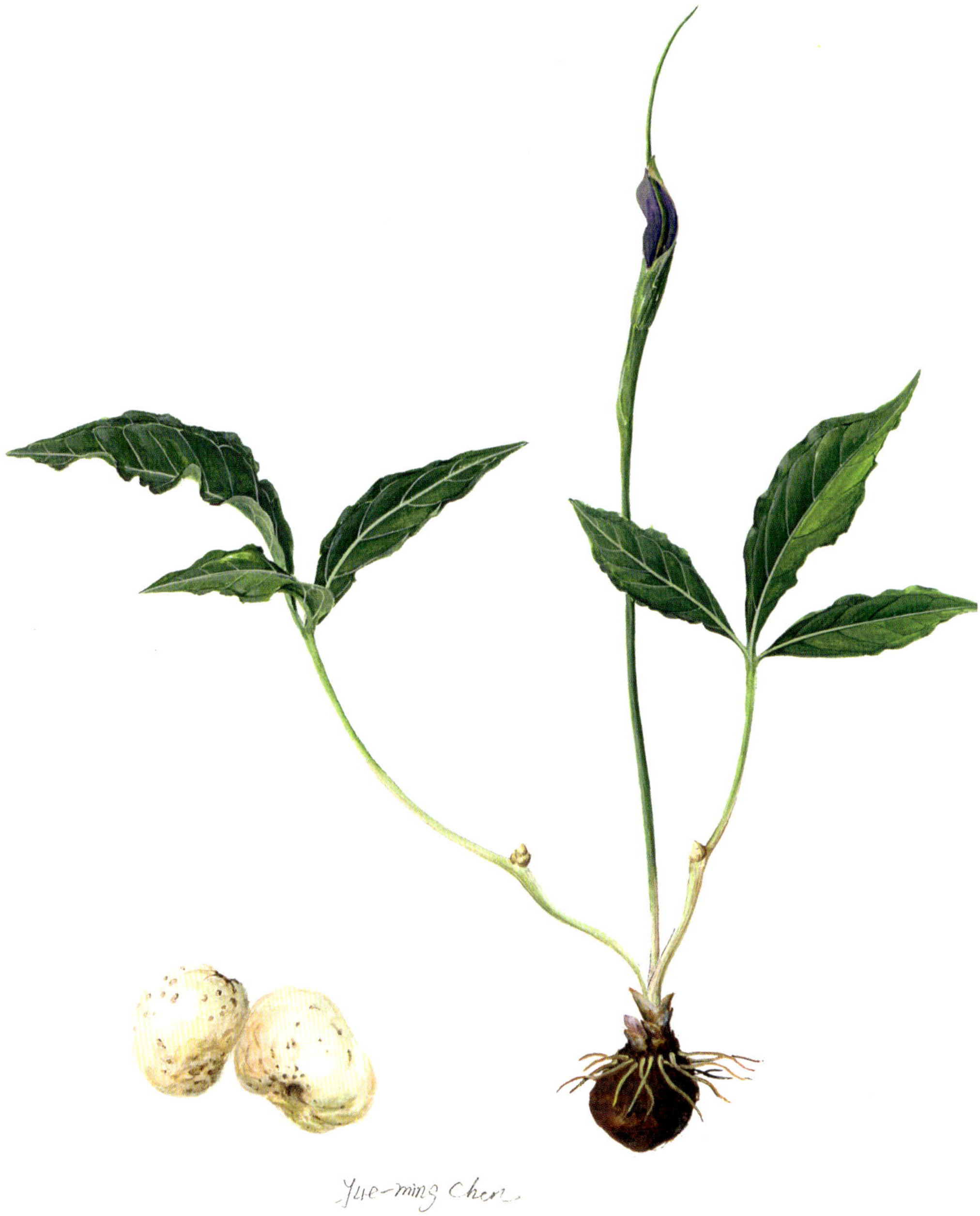


Fig. 11.110. ***Pinellia ternata*** (Thunb.) — This plant is toxic and must be used in conjunction with other herbs. It contains phenol, homogentisic acid, homogentisic acid glucoside, 3,4-dihydroxybenzaldehyde glucoside, and 3,4-dihydroxybenzaldehyde diglucoside, alkaloids, such as ephedrine and trigonelline, amino acids including arginine, aspartic acid, methionine, glutamic acid, serine, glycine, ornithine, and γ-aminobutyric acids, sugars, phytosterol, β -sitosterol, β-sitosterol glucoside, choline, palmitic acid, isoleic acid, stearic acid, octadecenoic acid, Ca-oxalate, and glucoronic acid. It inhibits liver carcinoma (HCA) in mice, JTC-26 Hela cells, sarcoma-180, cervical cancer-14, and ascitic sarcoma in rats, and has been used in the treatment of malignant lymphoma and cancers of the esophagus, stomach, heart, and cervix. (Chang & But, 1986; Hsu, et al, 1986; Minyi, .1992; Lee, 1999)

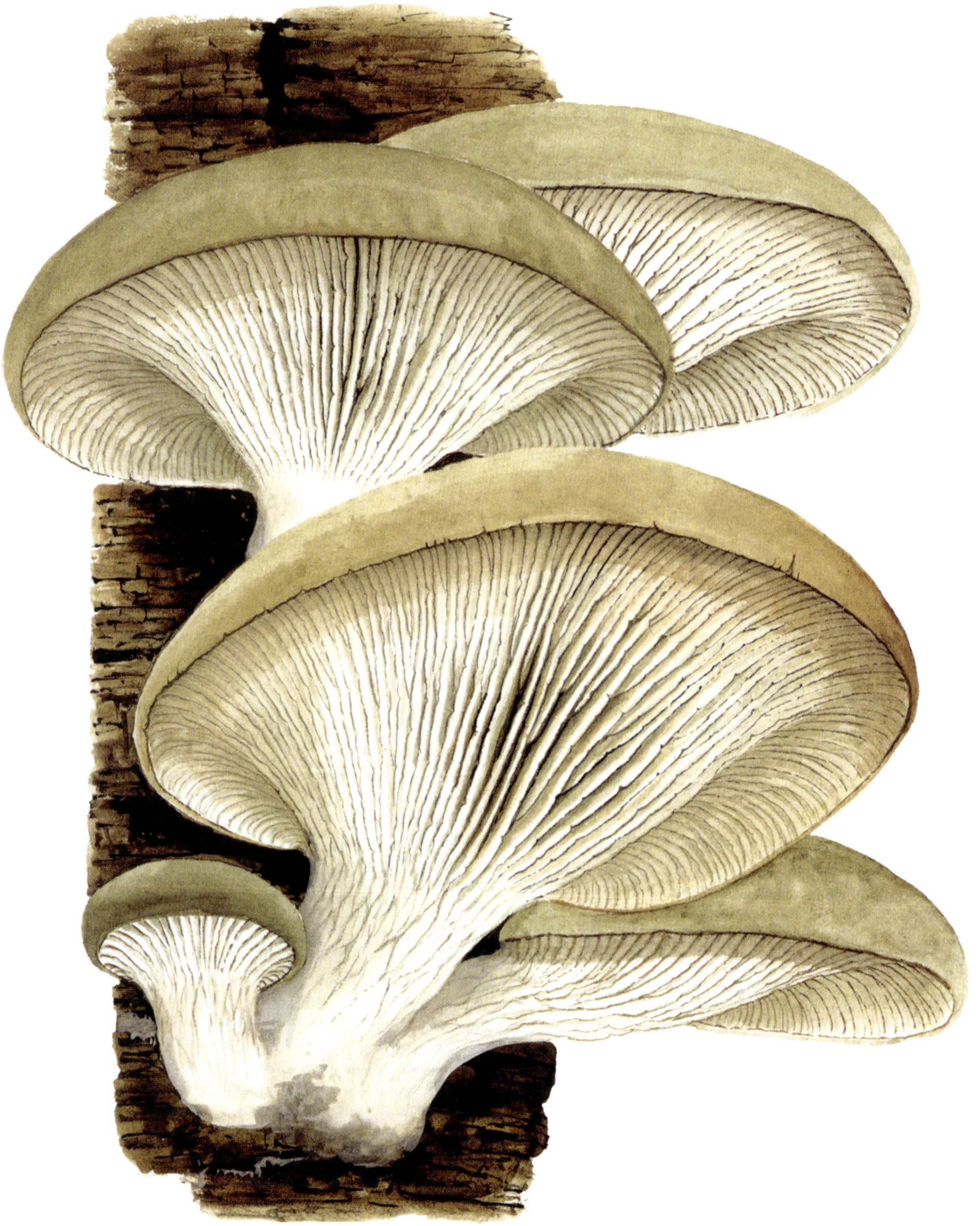

Fig. 11.111. ***Pleurotus ostreatus*** (Jacq. ex Fr.) Quél. — This fungus contains amino acids, vitamins, and polysaccharides that inhibit sarcoma-180 and Ehrlich's carcinoma in white mice (Ying, et al, 1987).

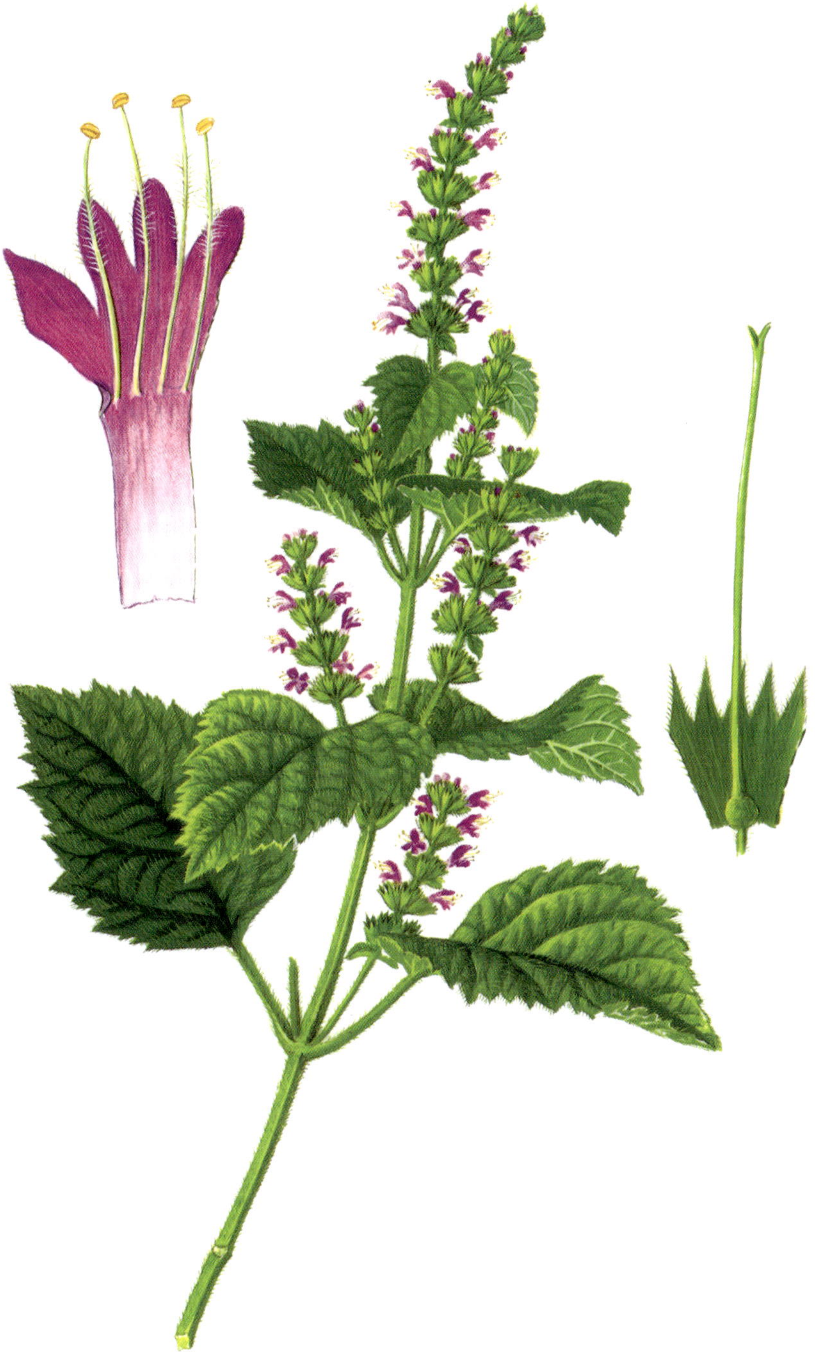

Fig. 11.112. ***Pogostemon cablin*** (Blanco) Benth. — This plant contains a large number of phytochemical constituents such as patchoulialcohol, patcholipyrideine, eugenol, cinnamic patcholipyrideine, eugenol, cinnamic aldehyde, pogostol, patchoulipyridine, epiguaipyridine, caryophylene, β-elemene, alloaromadendrene, α-patchoulene, γ-patchoulene, β-gurjunene, α-guaiene, δ-guaiene, valencene, α-gurjunene, γ-cadinene, and calamenene. It shows antimutagenic properties and has been used in China and Japan for treating cancer. (Hartwell, 1982; Hsu, et al, 1986; Miyazawa, et al, 2000; Halstead, 2002-unpublished data)

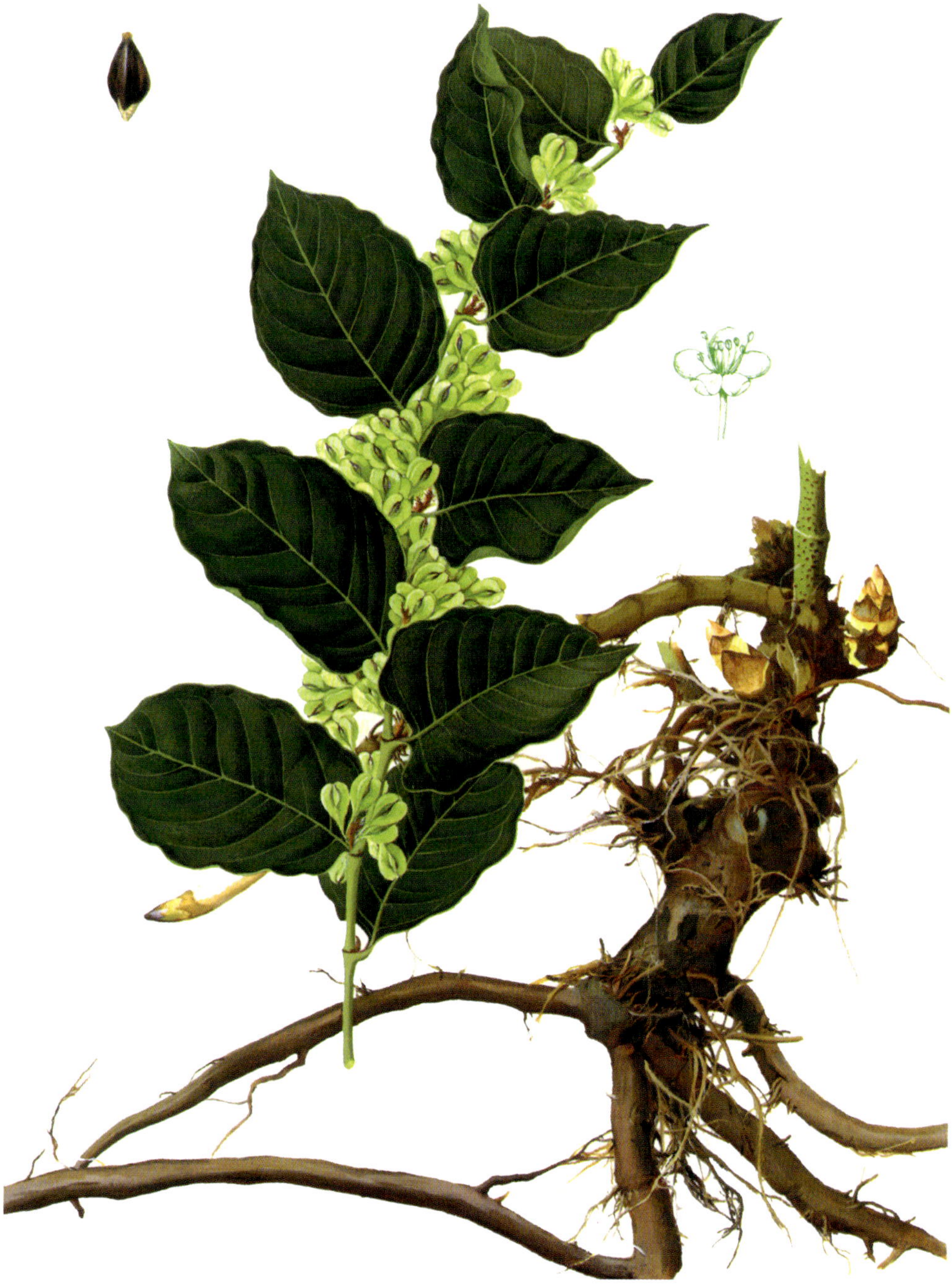

Fig. 11.113. ***Polygonum cuspidatum*** Sieb. et Zucc. — The root contains the glucosides glucofragulin, polygonin, polydatin, and polydatoside, anthraquinones emodin, emodin-monomethyl ether, and chrysophanol, the flavenoids quercitrin, isoquercitrin, reynoutrin, avicularin, rutin, and hyperin, the organic acids oxalic acid and tartaric acid, and tannins. It inhibits sarcoma-180 in mice and JTC-26 in vitro, is effective against HL-60 cell line and murine tumors such as B-16, Erlich's ascites carcinoma, HepS, and Walker's carcinoma-256, and has been used in the treatment of cancers of the stomach and intestine and for leukopenia caused by radiotherapy. (Hsu, et al, 1986; Minyi, 1992; Huang, 1999; Lee, 1999)

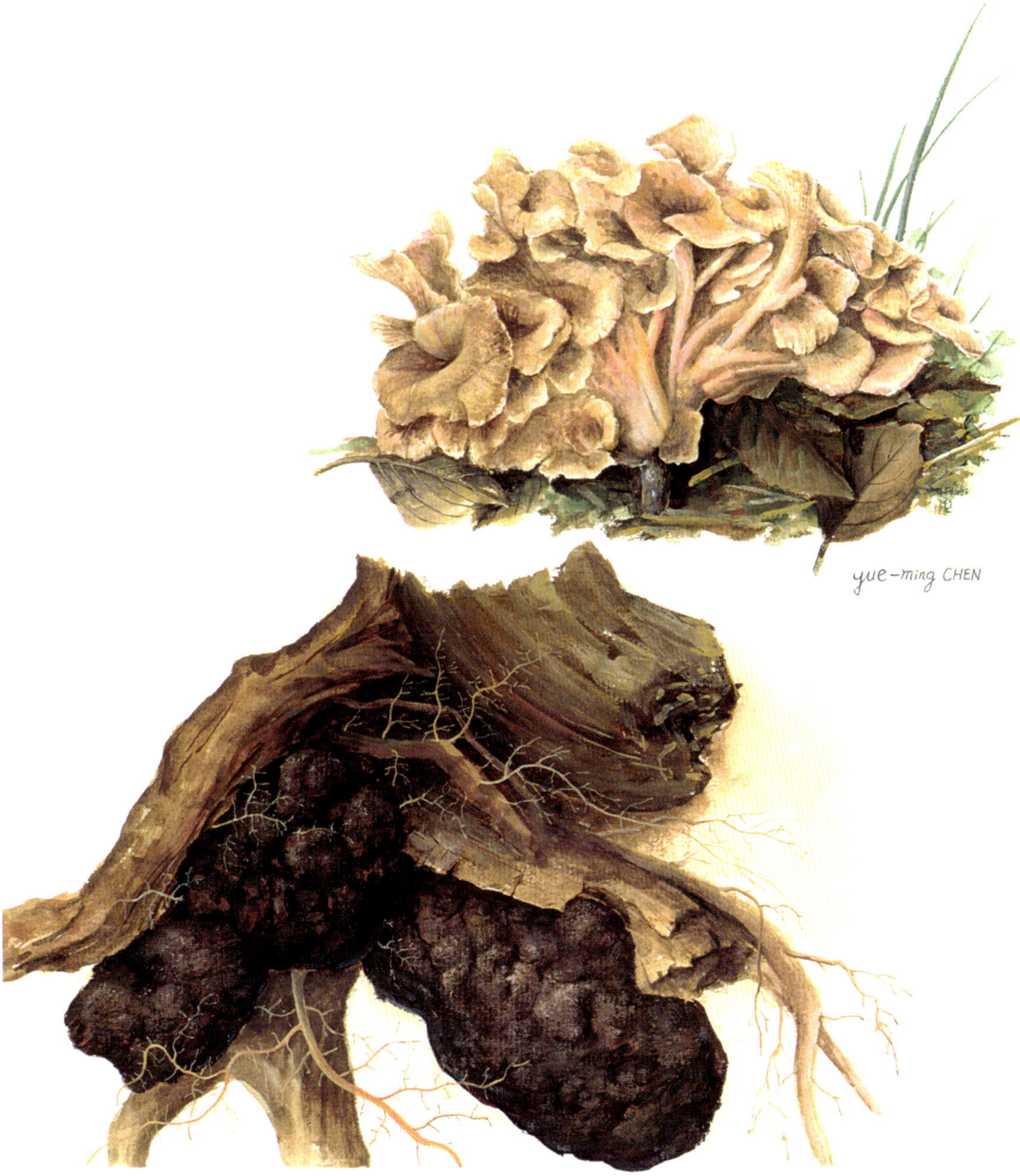


Fig. 11.114. ***Polyporus umbellatus*** (Pers.) Fries. — This is a fungus that grows on trees. It contains ergosterol, biotin and gluctan. It enhances the immune system, inhibits cancer cells in laboratory animals, and has been found useful in treating lung cancer in humans (Ying, et al, 1987).

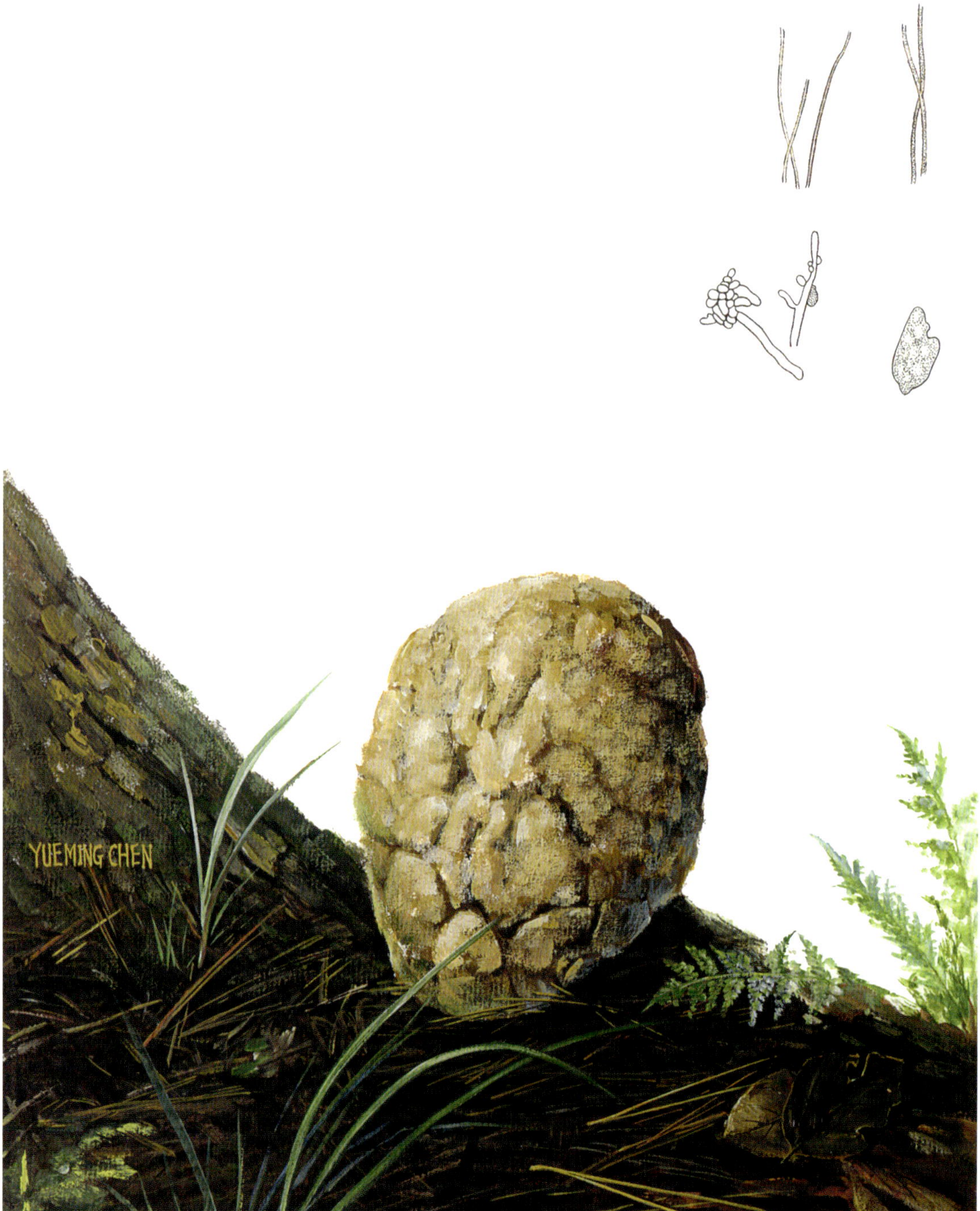


Fig. 11.115. ***Poria cocos*** (Schw.) Wolf — This plant contains ergosterol, eburicoic acid, β-pachyman, pachymic acid, tumulosic acid, 3-β-hydroxylanosta-7,9,(11),24-trien-21-oic acid, chitin, hyperin, choline, adenine, histidine, and potassium salts. It enhances the immune system, inhibits sarcoma-180 and Erlich's ascites carcinoma in mice, and has been used to treat a variety of cancers including cystocancer, uteromusculoma, and cancers of the nasopharynx, digestive tract, and breast. (Chang & But, 1986; Minyi, 1992; Lee, 1999)

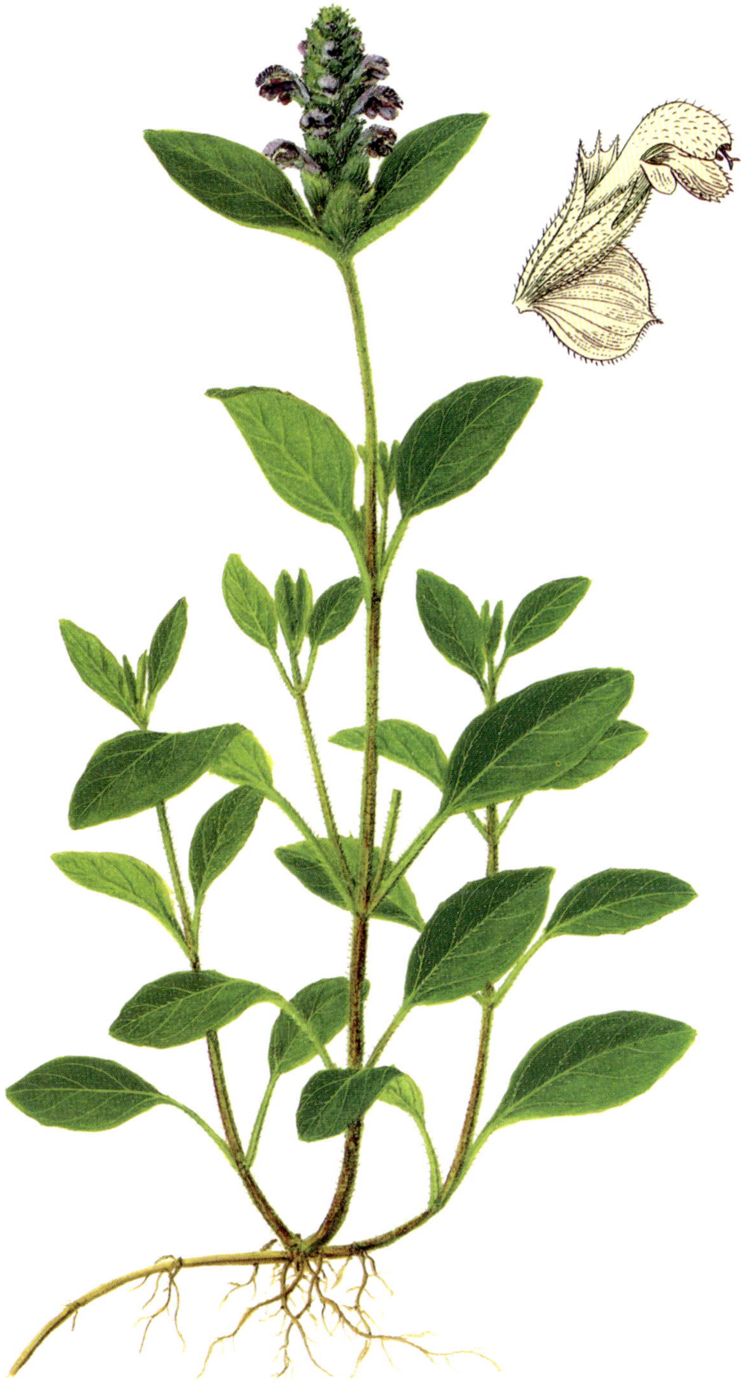

Fig. 11.116. ***Prunella vulgaris*** Linn. — This plant contains prunella oleanolic acid, ursolic acid, rutin, hyperoside, caffeic acid, vitamins $B_1$, C, and K, tannin, essential oil, alkaloids, resin, inorganic salts, delphinidin, cyanidin, d-camphor, ursolic acid, and d-fenchone. It inhibits Erlich's ascites carcinoma, sarcoma-180, and cervical cancer U-14 in mice, is effective against HL-60 cells and JTC-26, and has been used to treat a variety of cancers including lymphoma and cancers of the intracranium, thyroid, stomach, breast, and lung. (Chang & But, 1986; Hsu, et al, 1986; Lee, 1999)

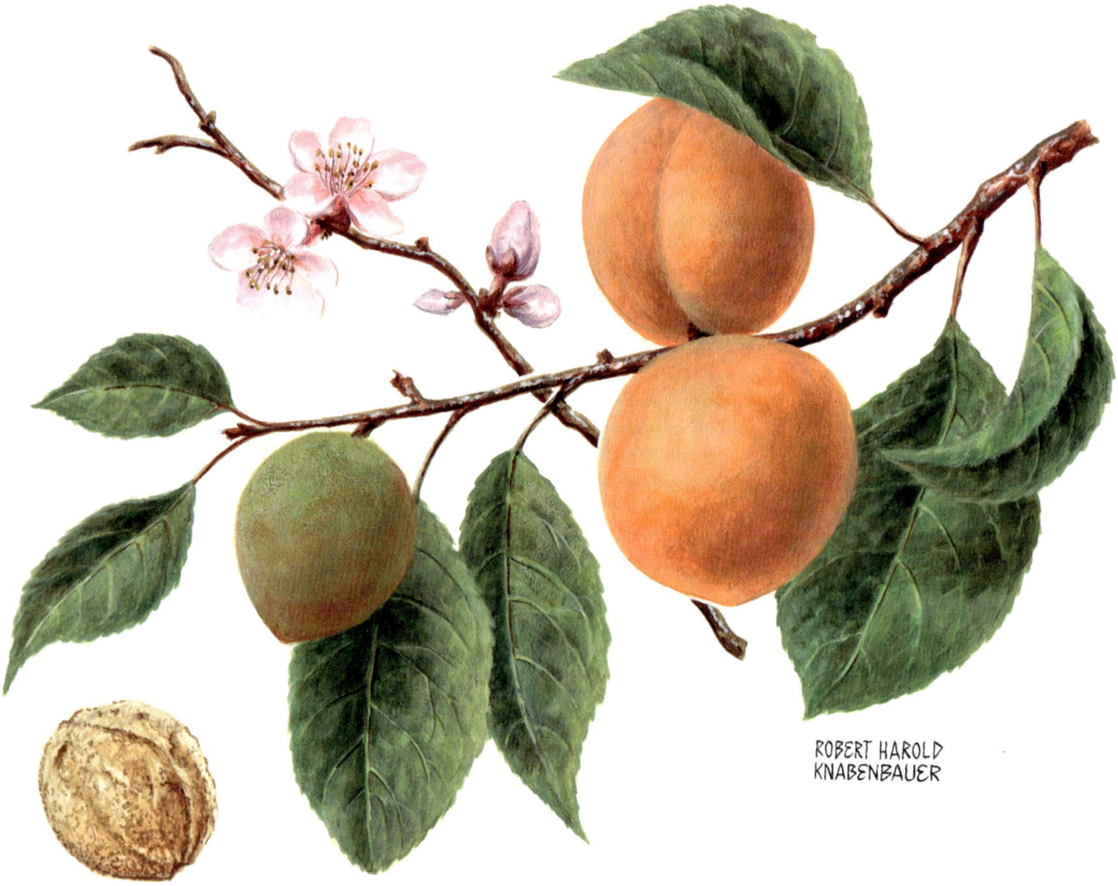


Fig. 11.117. ***Prunus armeniaca*** Linn. — The kernels contain the cyanogenic glycoside amygdalin, amygdalase, prunase, and emulsin. It has antineoplastic effects, inhibits human cervical carcinoma JTC-26 and transplanted Erlich's ascites carcinoma in mice, is effective against transplanted Walker's carcinoma-256 and transplanted Jensen sarcoma in rats, and has been used extensively throughout the world to treat cancer such as Hodgkin's disease, lymphoma, leukemia, seminoma, spindle cell sarcoma, and cancers of the esophagus, lung, heart, breast, uterus, and rectum. (Halstead, 1977; Chang & But, 1986; Lee, 1999; Halstead, 2002 - unpublished data)

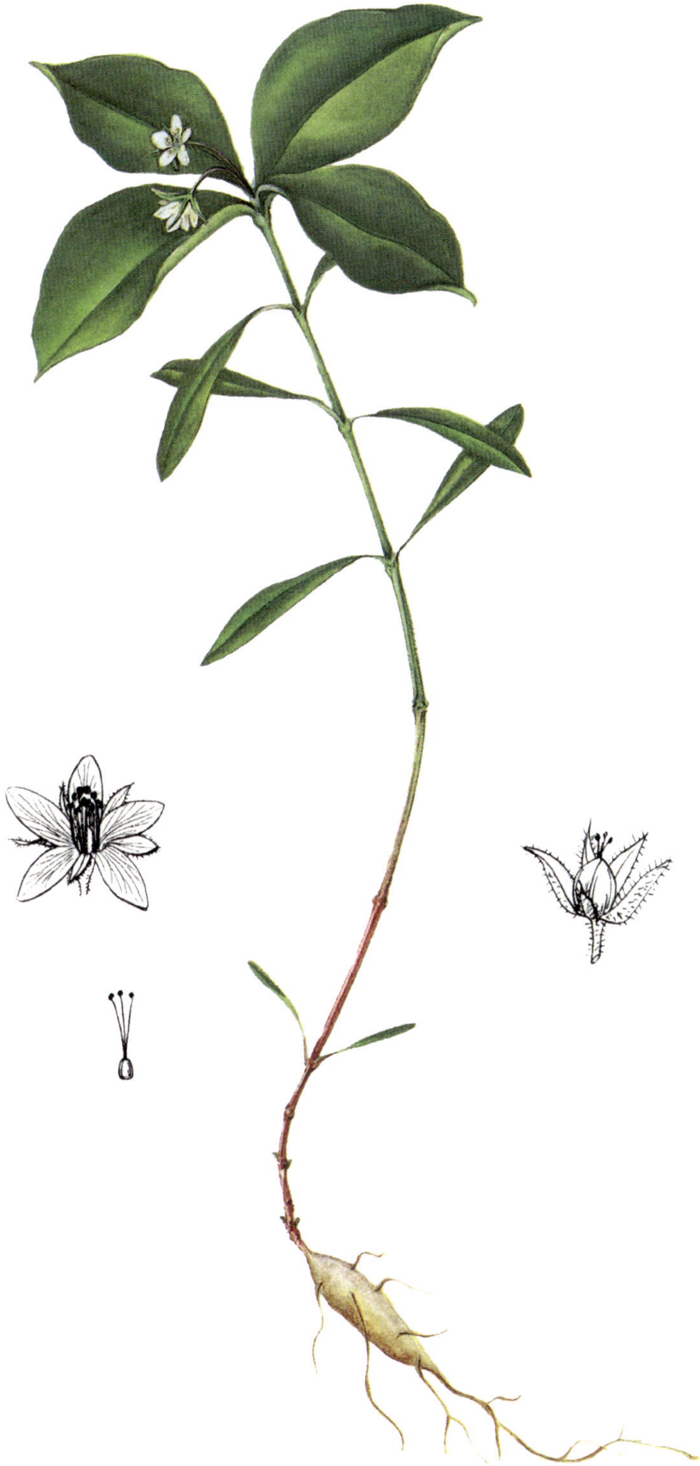

Fig. 11.118. ***Pseudostellaria heterophylla*** (Miq.) Pax ex Pax et Hoffm. — This plant contains polysaccharides that enhance the immune system and inhibit Erlich's ascites tumors in mice (Wong, et al, 1994).

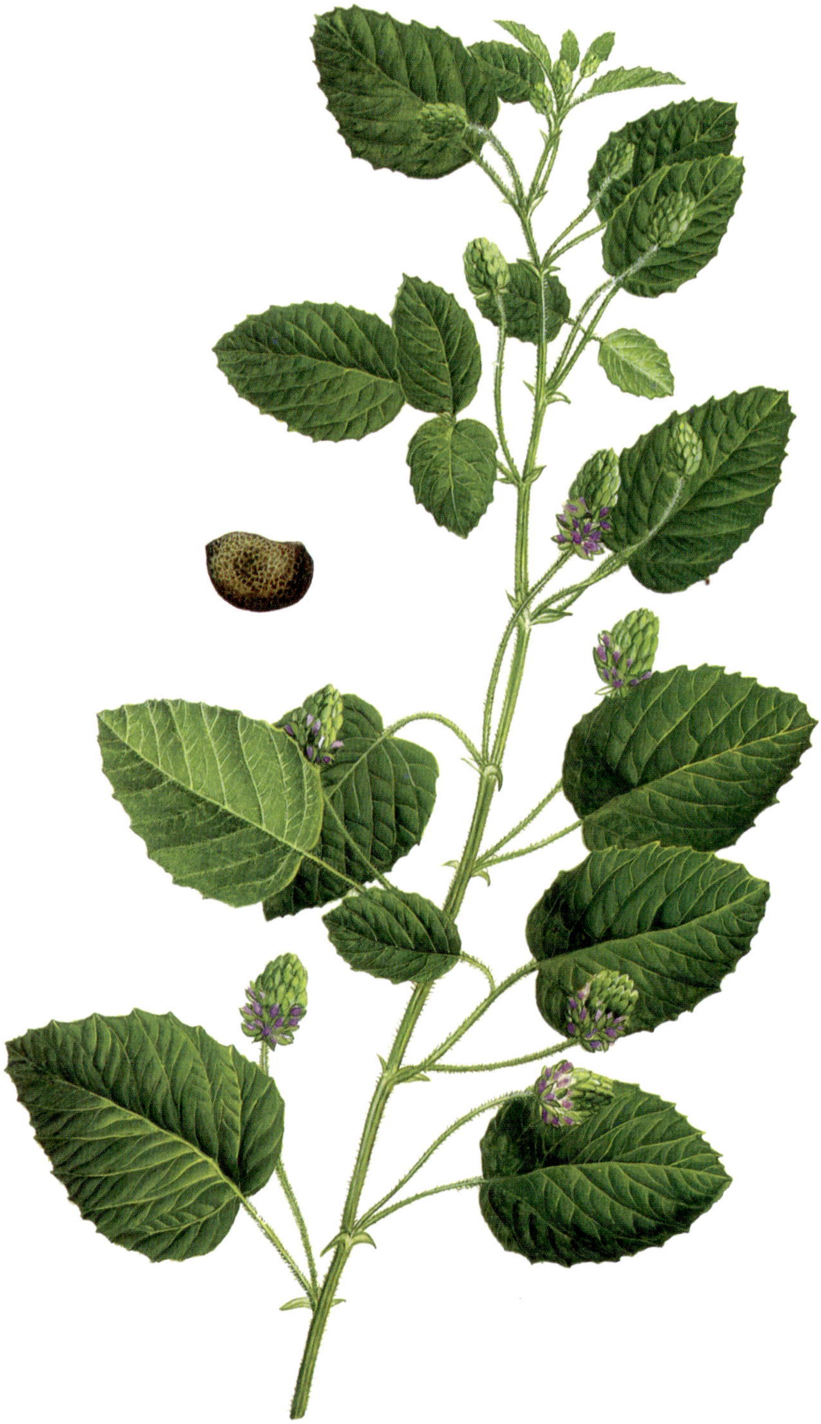

Fig. 11.119. ***Psoralea corylifolia*** Linn. — This plant contains the flavenoids corylifolin (bavachin), bavachinin, isobavachin, corylifolinin (isobavachalcone), bavachromene, neobavachalcone, coumarins, psoralen, angelicin (isoporalen), psoralidin, isopsoralidin, and corylidin, bakuchiol, raffinose, volatile oil, fixed oil, and resin. It inhibits Hela cells and sarcoma-180 in vitro and has an antineoplastic effect. (Chang & But, 1986; Hsu, et al, 1986; Latha, et al, 2000)

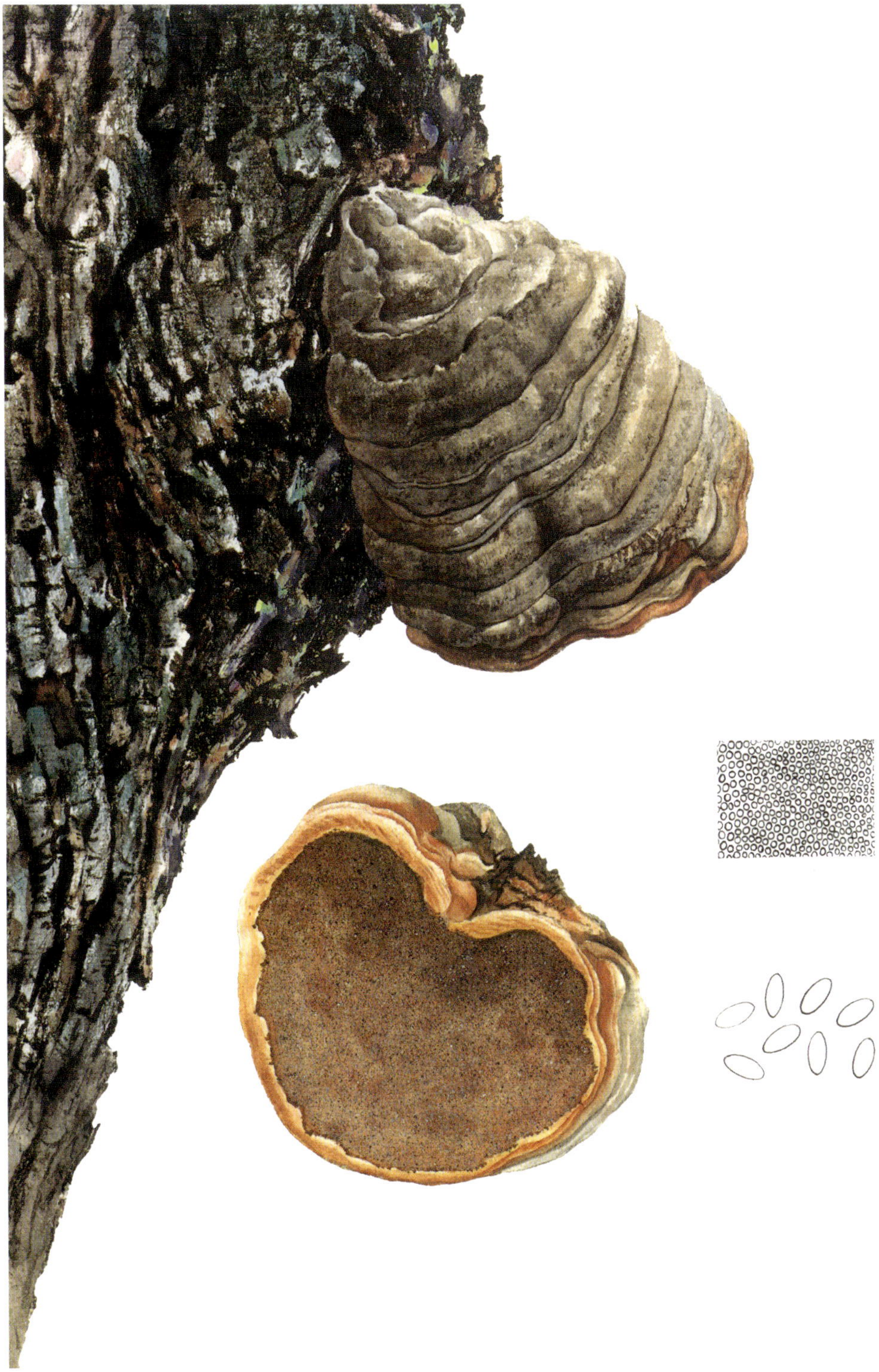

Fig. 11.120. ***Pyropolyporus fomentarius*** (Linn. ex Fr.) Teng — The sporophore of this mushroom contains polysaccharides that inhibit sarcoma-180 in mice and has been used in the treatment of cancers of the esophagus, stomach, and uterus (Ying, et al, 1987).

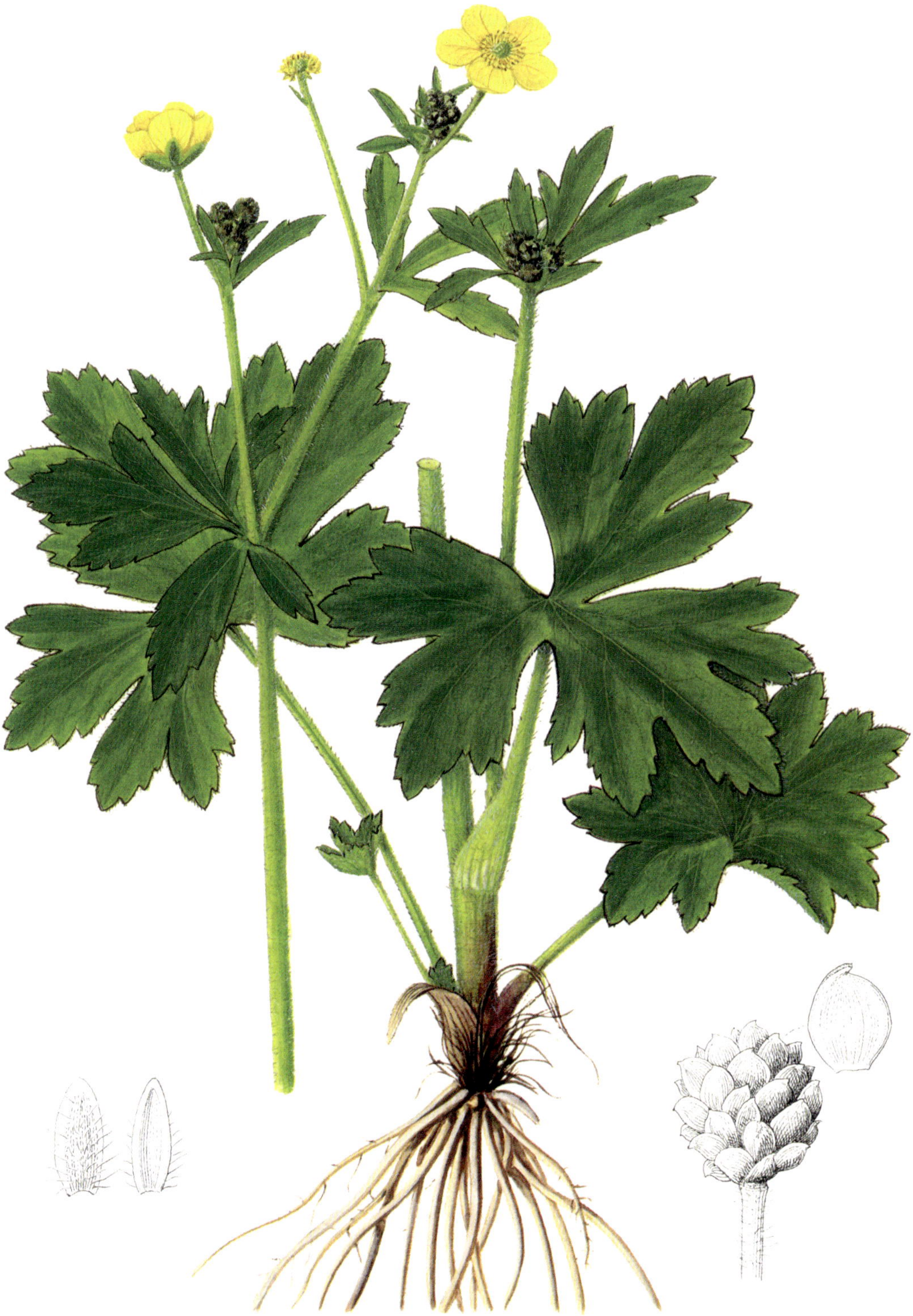

Fig. 11.121. ***Ranunculus japonicus*** Thunb. — This plant contains protoanemonin and volatile oil. It inhibits tumors and has been used to treat skin, lung, cervical, and breast cancers. (Minyi, 1992; Lee, 1999)

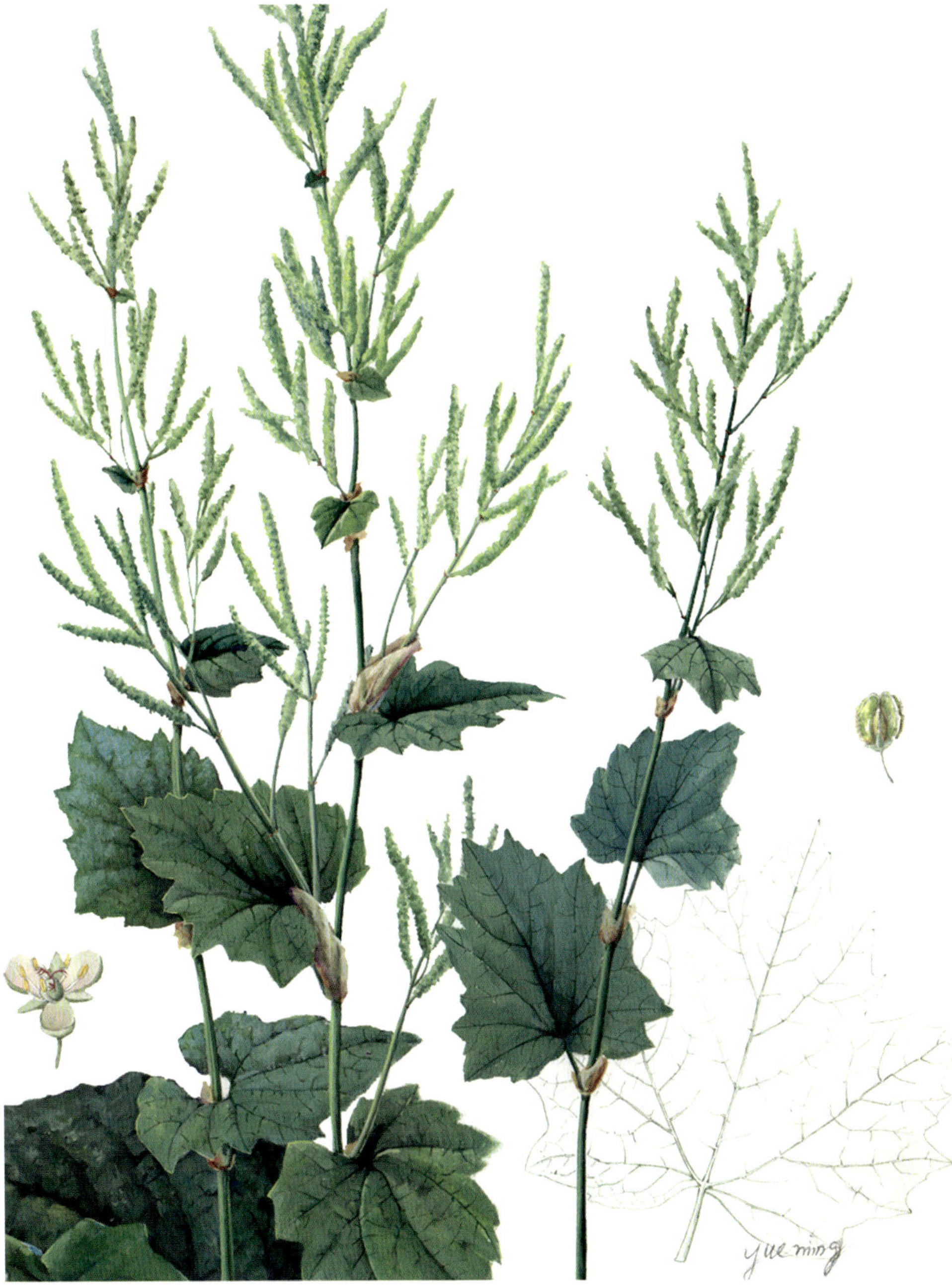


Fig. 11.122. ***Rheum officinale*** Baillon — This plant contains rhein-8-monoglucoside, physcion monoglucoside, emodin, emodin 1, citreorosein, aloe-emodin monoglucoside, aloe-emodin 8-glucoside, emodin-monoglucoside, chrysophanol, chrysophanol 1, chrysophenol monoglucoside, torachrysone, piceid, deoxyrhaponticin, 3,4',5-trihydroxy-stilbene-4'-glucoside, gallic acid, glucogallin, catechol, 4-(*p*-hydroxyphenyl)-2 butanone glucoside, sennosides A, B, and C, tannic acids, cinnamic acid, gallic acid, and catechin. It inhibits Erlich's ascites carcinoma in vitro and mice melanoma, sarcoma-37, sarcoma-180, and breast carcinoma in mice, is effective against HL-60 cells, and has been used to treat leukemia and cancers of the uterus, ovaries, and rectum. (Hsu, et al, 1986; Minyi, 1992; Huang, 1999; Lee, 1999)

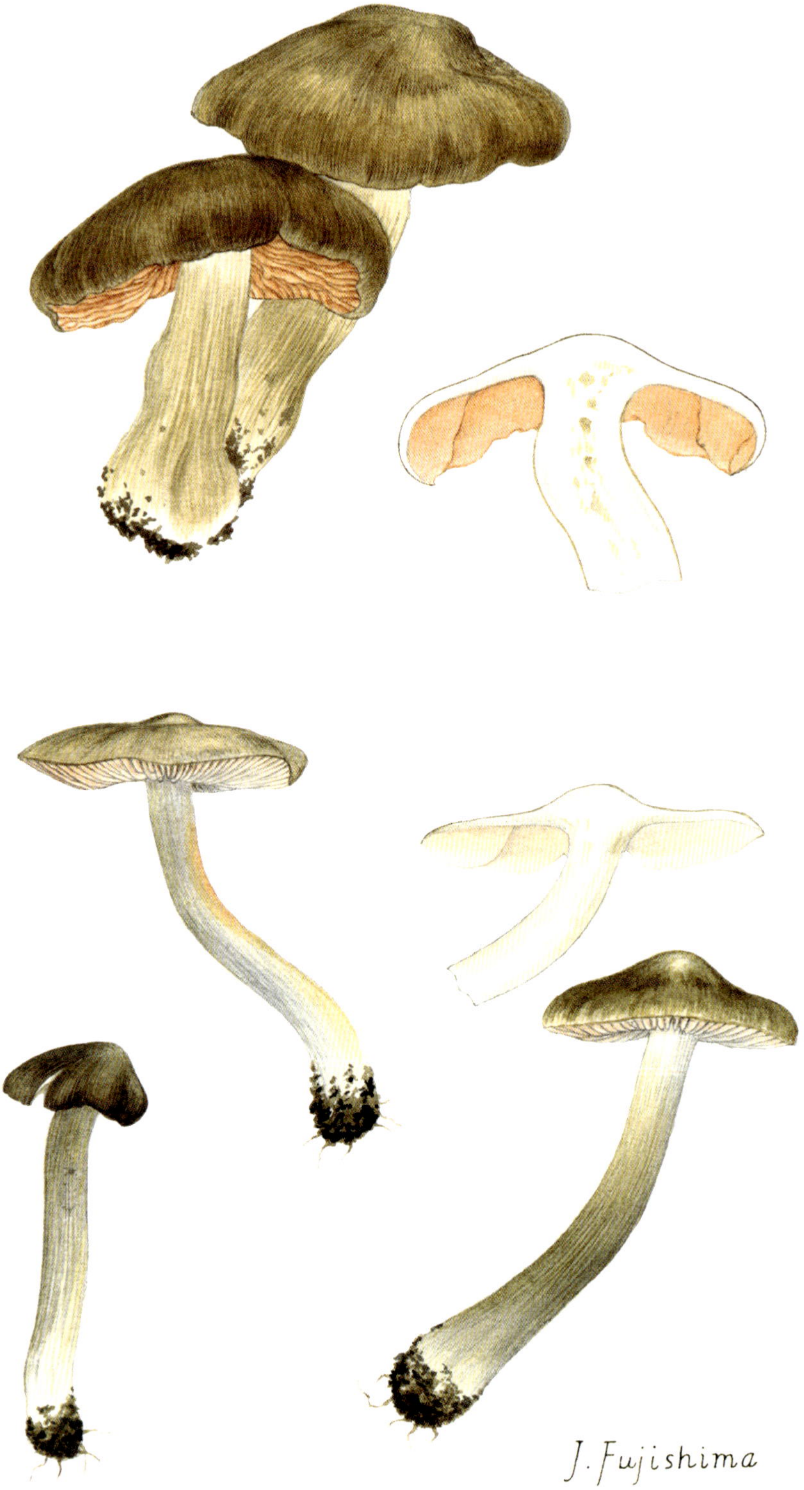


Fig. 11.123. ***Rhodophyllus clypeatus*** (Linn. ex Fr.) Quél — This mushroom contains polysaccharides that inhibit sarcoma-180 and Ehrlich's carcinoma in mice (Ying, et al, 1987).

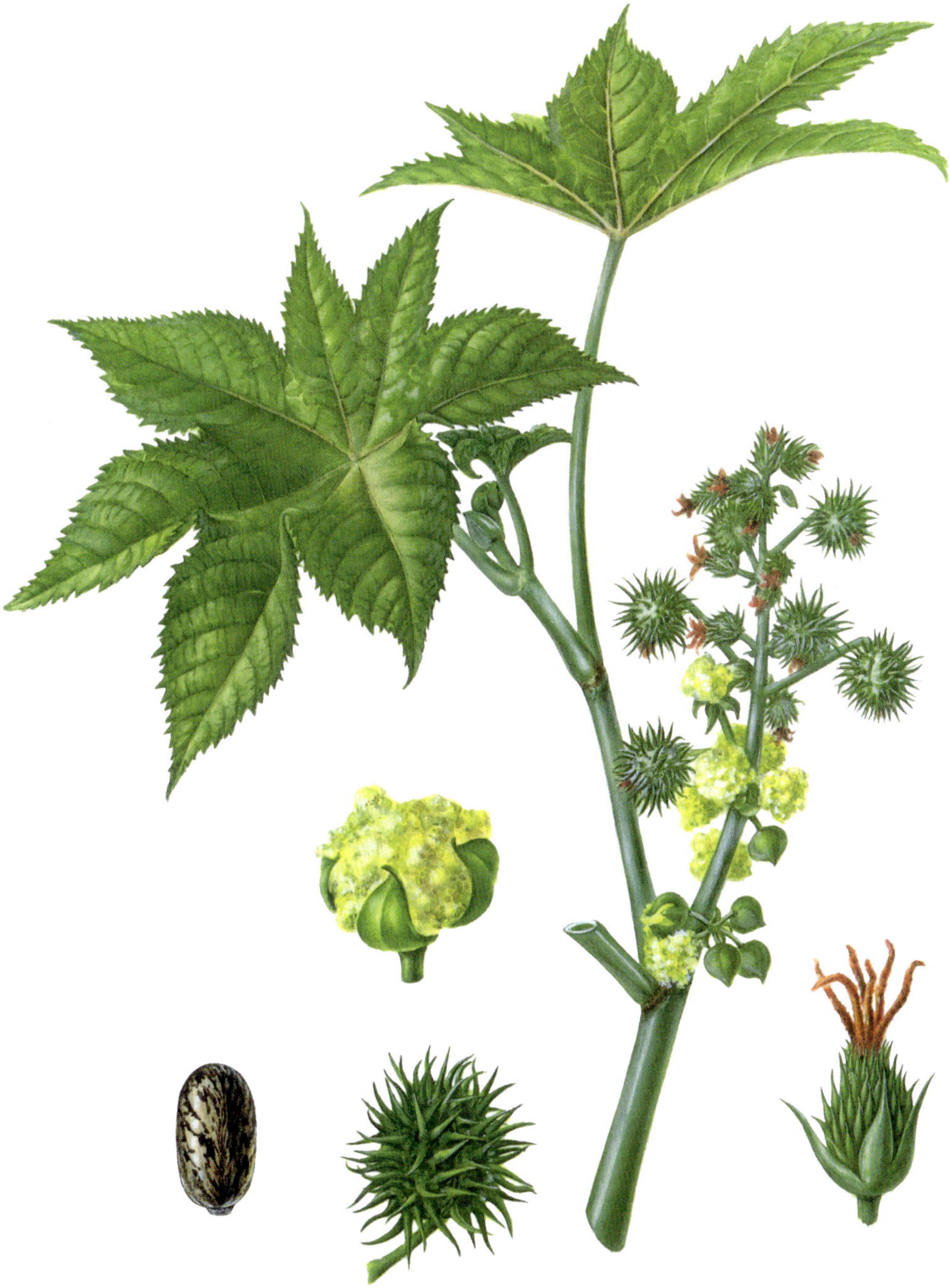

Fig. 11.124. **Ricinus communis** Linn. — This plant contains ricin, ricinine, ricinolein, glycerides of ricinoleic acid, isoricinoleic acid, oleic acid, linoleic acid, linolenic acid, sebacinic acid, stearic acid, 9,10-dihydroxystearic acid, palmitic acid, oleum, globulin, nucleoalbumin, glycoprotein, cytochrome C, lipase, and esterase. It inhibits many cancer cell strains and various animal cancer cells in vitro, is effective against transplanted animal tumors including Erlich's ascites carcinoma, sarcoma-180, cervical cancer U-14, leukemia, and ascitic hepatoma, and has been used to treat lymphosarcoma, adenocarcinoma, eryoma, colon cancer, cervical cancer, and skin cancer. (Chang & But, 1986; Hsu, et al, 1986; Minyi, 1992; Lee, 1999)

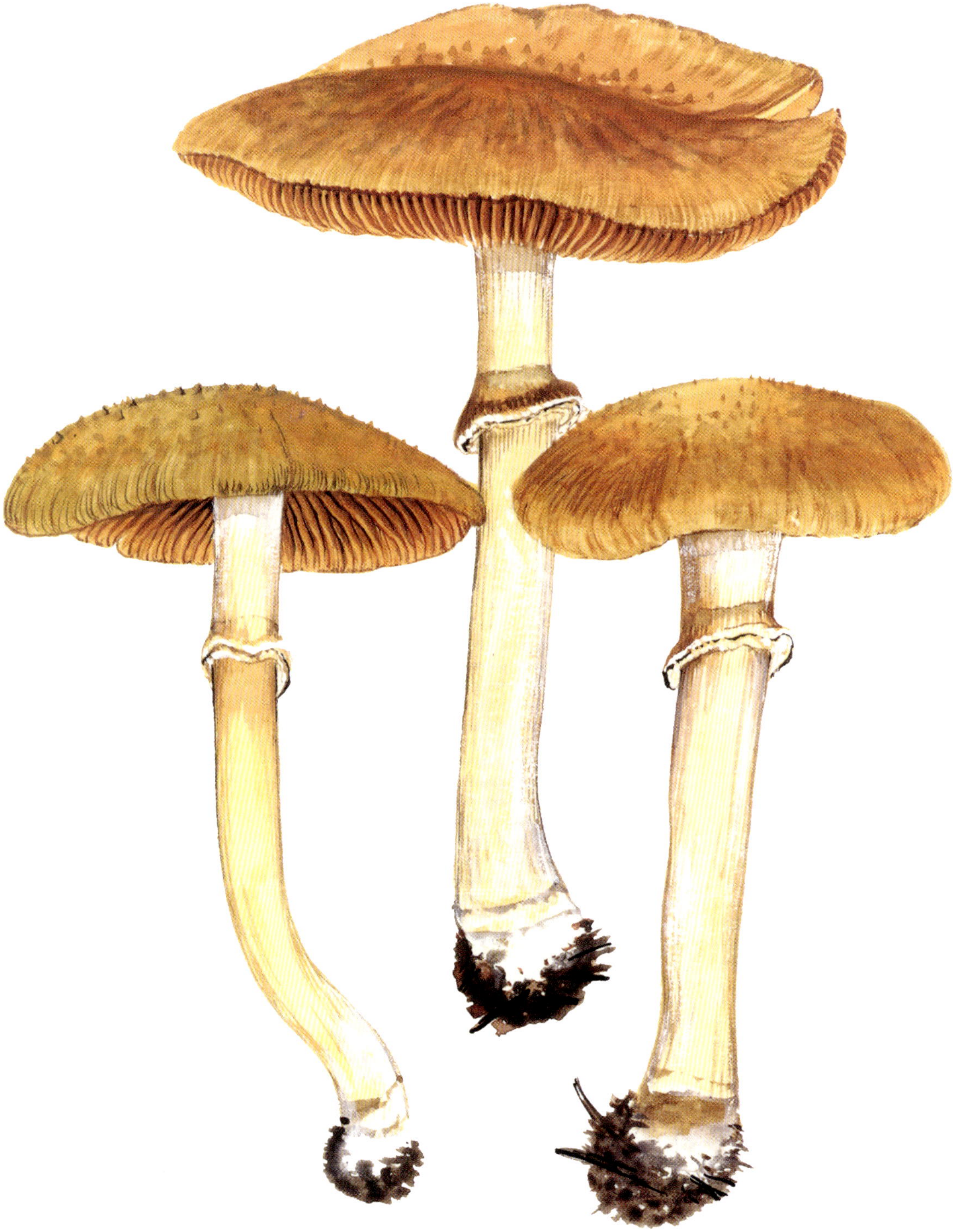

Fig. 11.125. ***Rozites caperata*** (Pers. ex Fr.) Karst. — This fungus contains polysaccharides that inhibit sacoma-180 in mice and Ehrlich's carcinoma (Ying, et al, 1987).

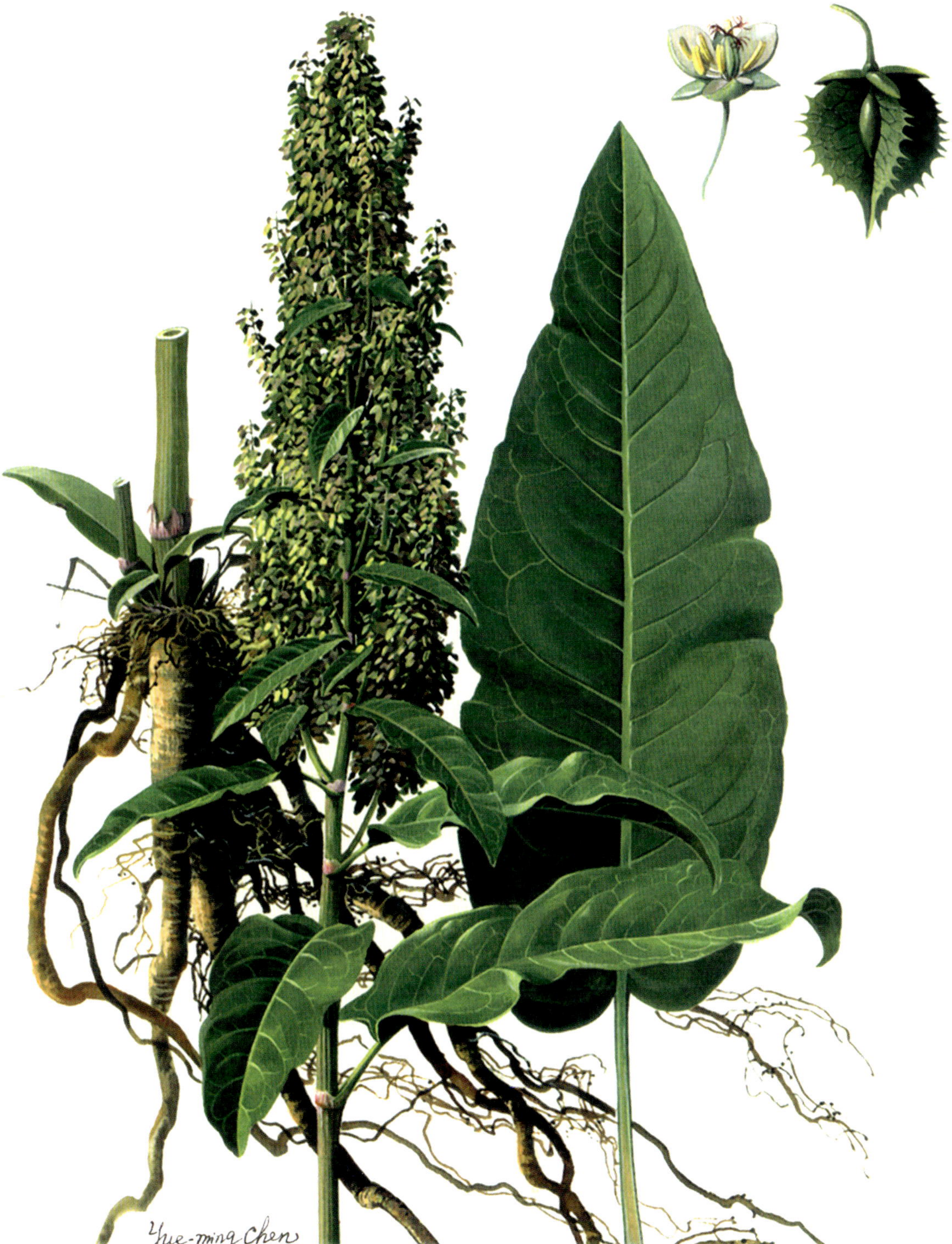


Fig. 11.126. ***Rumex japonica*** Houtt. — This plant contains emodin, which has been found to inhibit leukemia and maligniant lymphoma (Huang, 1999).

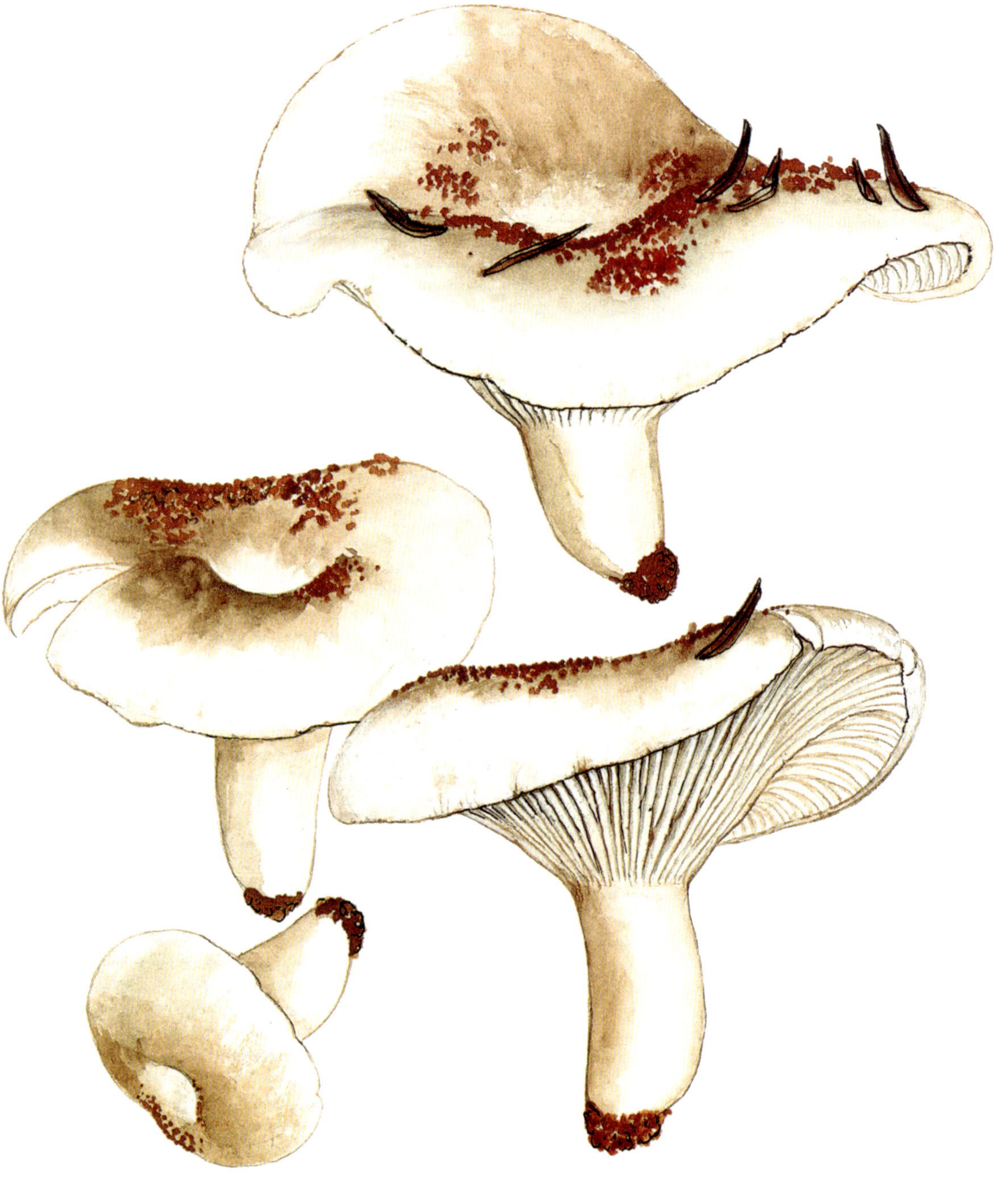

Fig. 11.127. ***Russula delica*** Fr. — This mushroom contains polysaccharides that inhibit sarcoma-180 and Ehrlich's carcinoma (Ying, et al, 1987).

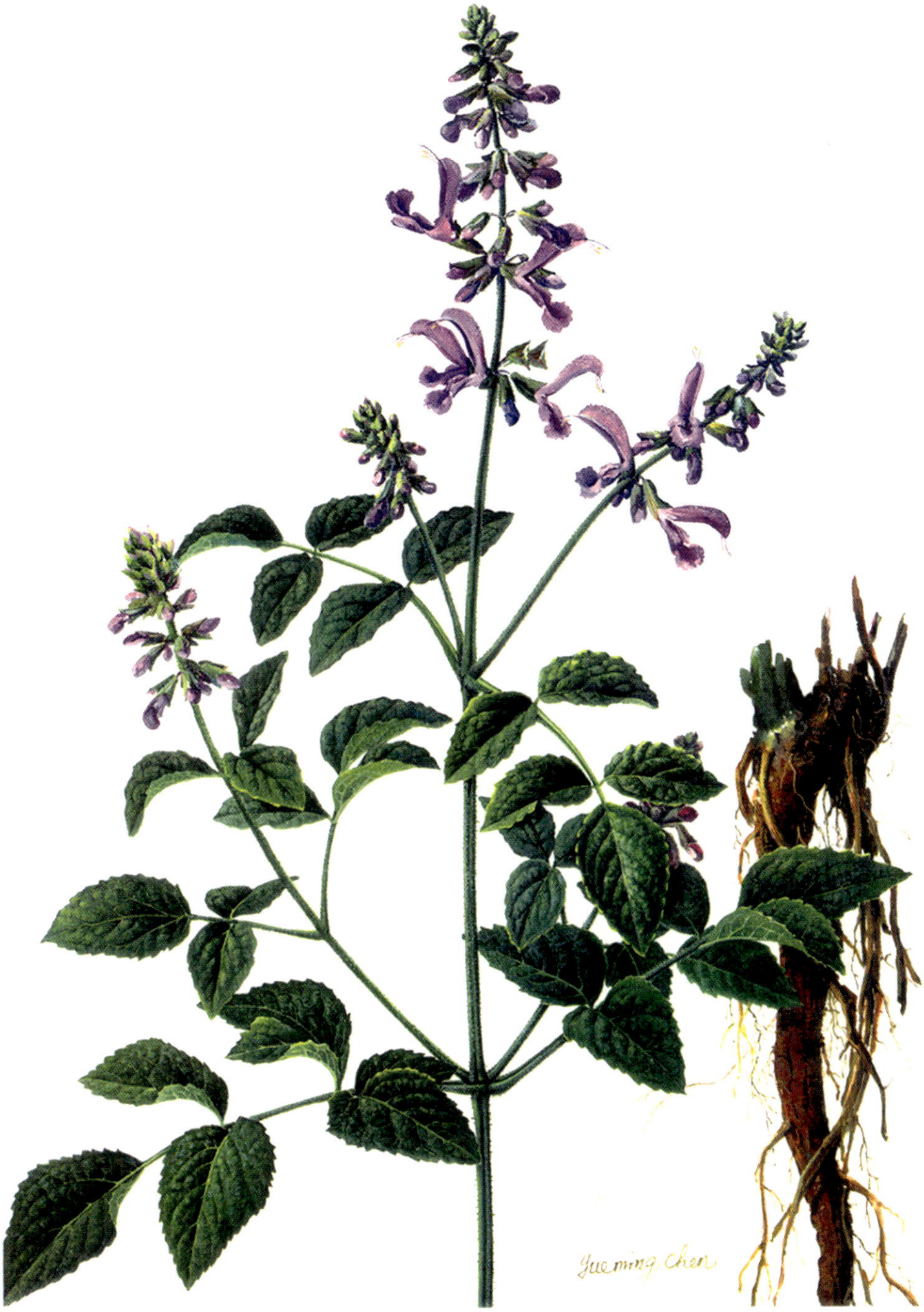


Fig. 11.128. ***Salvia miltiorrhiza*** Bge. — This plant contains tanshinones I, II$_A$, and II$_B$, isotanshinones I and II, cryptotanshinone, isocryptotanshinone, methyl tanshionate, hyroxytanshinone II$_A$, miltirone, 1-dihydrotanshinone I, salviol, protocatechuic aldehyde, protocatechuic acid, β-(3,4-dihydroxyphenyl) lactic acid, tanshinol I and II, and vitamin E and has been found to inhibit sarcoma-180 and Erlich's ascites carcinoma in laboratory mice. It has been used to treat hepatocarcinoma, hysteromyoma, pituitary chromophobe adenoma, and cancers of the esophagus, thymus gland, and abdominal cavity. (Chang & But, 1986; Minyi, 1992; Huang, 1999)

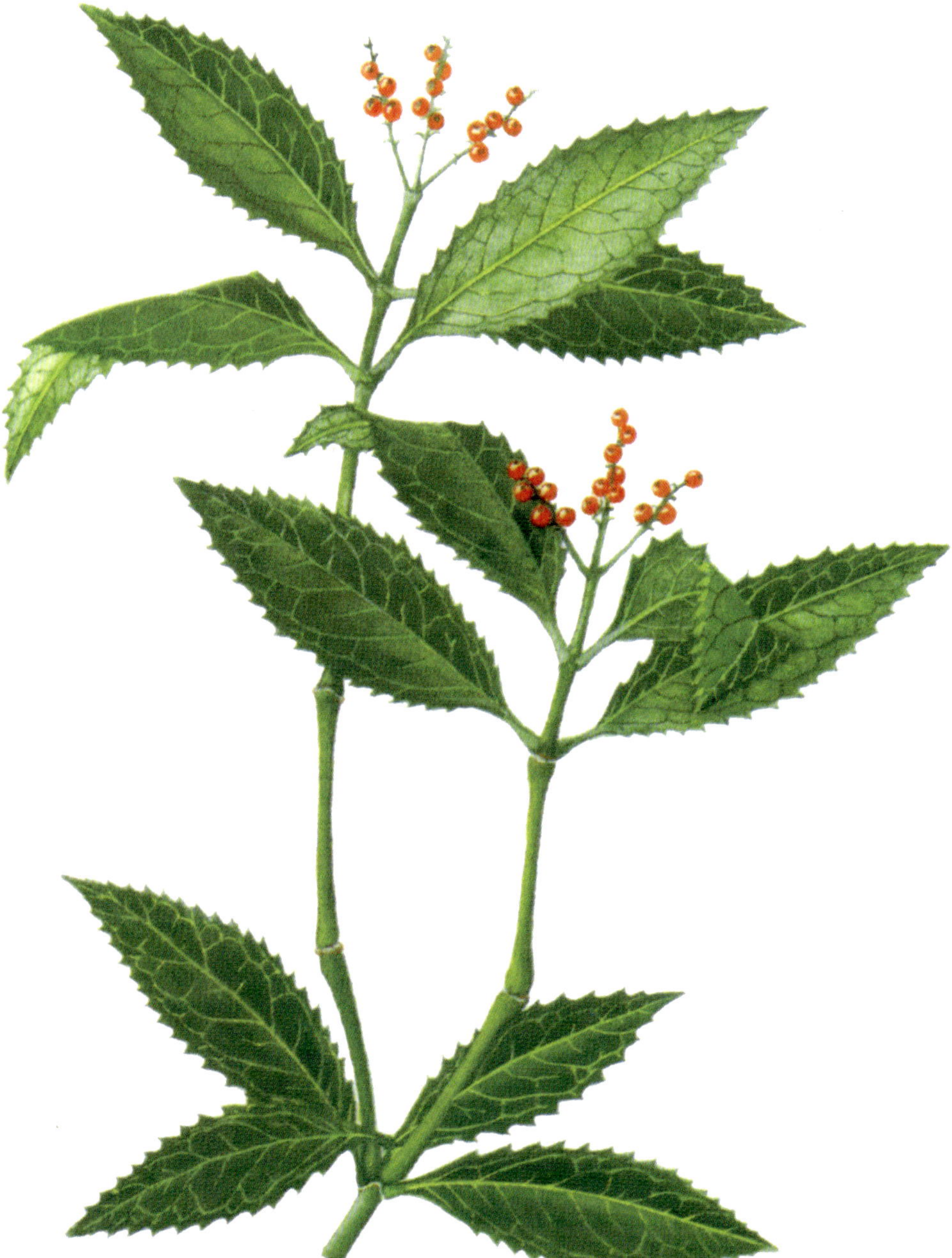

Fig. 11.129. ***Sarcandra glabra*** (Thun.) Nakei — This plant contains flavenoids, glycosides, essential oils, astilibin, isofraxidin, fumaric acid, tannic acid, succinic acid, cyanophoric glycoside, coumarins, lactones, pelargonidin-3-rhamnosyl glucoside, chloranthalactones A & D, 6,8-dimethoxy-7-hydroxycoumarin, β-sitosterol-β-D-glucoside, CI, CII, CIII, and CIV. It inhibits mouse sarcoma-180, mouse L-615, Walker's carcinoma-256, and lymphatic leukemia in vitro and tumor strains of pure bred 615 mice, $RS_{615}$, TM-755, and $CA_{615}$, and $U_{14}$, $U_{27}$, SP, and $B_{22}$, and prolongs the survival rate of mice with spontaneous leukemia ascities 771. It has been used to treat leukemia, Hodgkin's disease, and carcinomas of the thyroid, esophagus, stomach, pancreas, liver, gallbladder, urinary bladder, colon, and rectum. (Chang & But, 1986; Hsu, et al, 1986; Minyi, 1992; Huang, 1999)

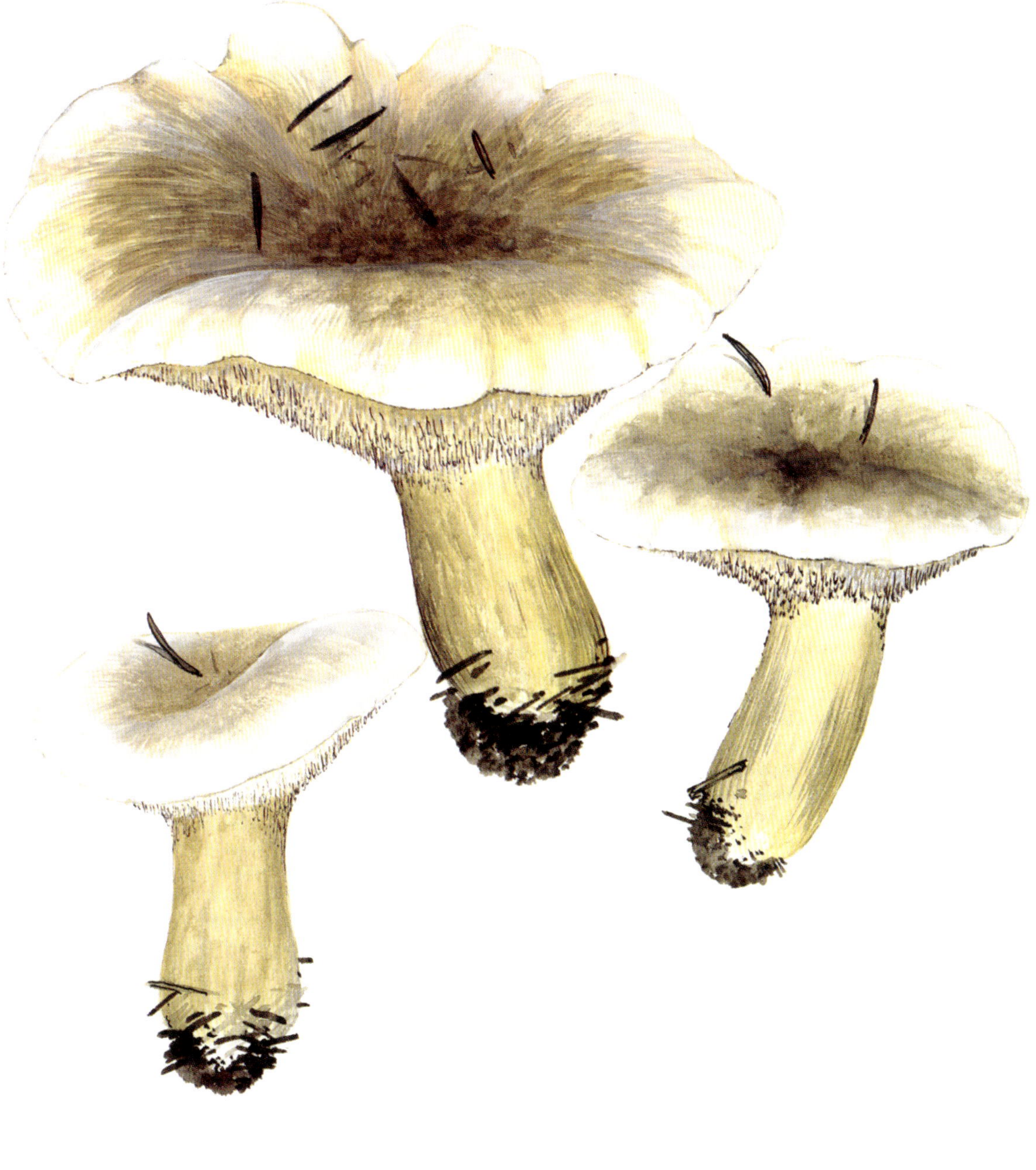

Fig. 11.130. ***Sarcodon fulgineo-albus*** (Fr.) Quél — This mushroom contains polysaccharides that have anticarcinogenic properties (Ying, et al, 1987).

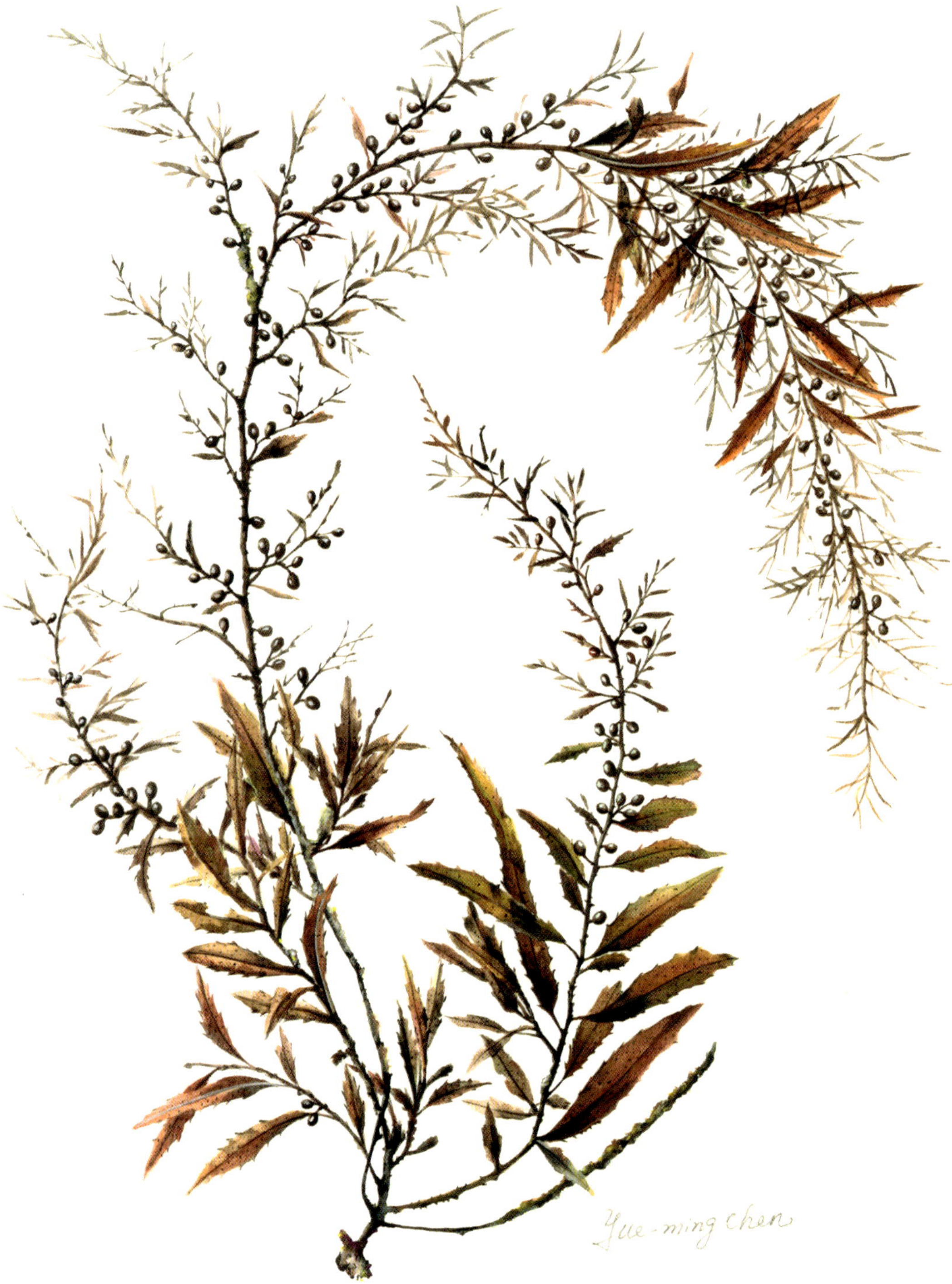


Fig. 11.131. ***Sargassum pallidum*** (Turn.) C. Ag. — This plant contains iodine, crude protein, fats, alginic acid, polypeptides, and sargassan. It inhibits uterocancer-14, sarcoma-180, HepS, and lymphoma-I of ascites type ($L_1$) and has been used to treat osteoangioma, osteoangioendothelioma, uteromusculoma, carcinoma of the parotid gland, lung cancer, and breast cancer. (Hsu, et al, 1986; Minyi, 1992; Lee, 1999)

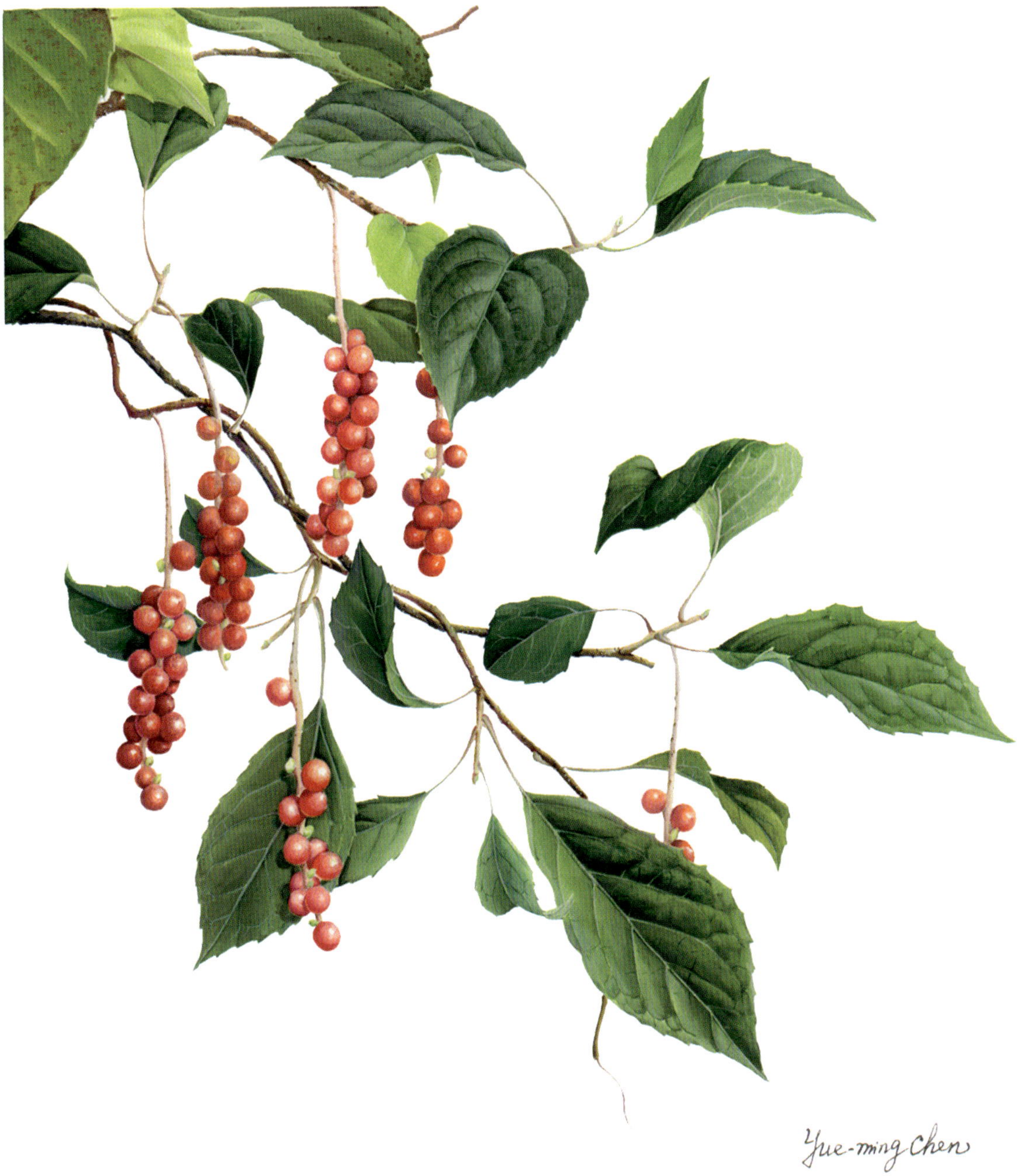


Fig. 11.132. ***Schizandra chinensis*** (Turcz.) Baill. — This plant contains several hydrocarbon derivatives such as sesquicarene, β-2-bisabolene, citral, β-chamigrene, β-chamigrenol, α-ylangene, schizandrin, γ-schizandrin, deoxyschizandrin, pseudo-schizandrin, schizandrol, gomisins A-D,F-H, and J, pregomisin, citric acid, malic acid, tartaric acid, protocatechuic acid, ascorbic acid, fumaric acid, preschisanthrin, and schisanphenol. It inhibits hepatoma ascites cells and sarcoma-180 cells and has been used to treat pulmonary carcinoma. (Hsu, et al, 1986; Huang, 1999)

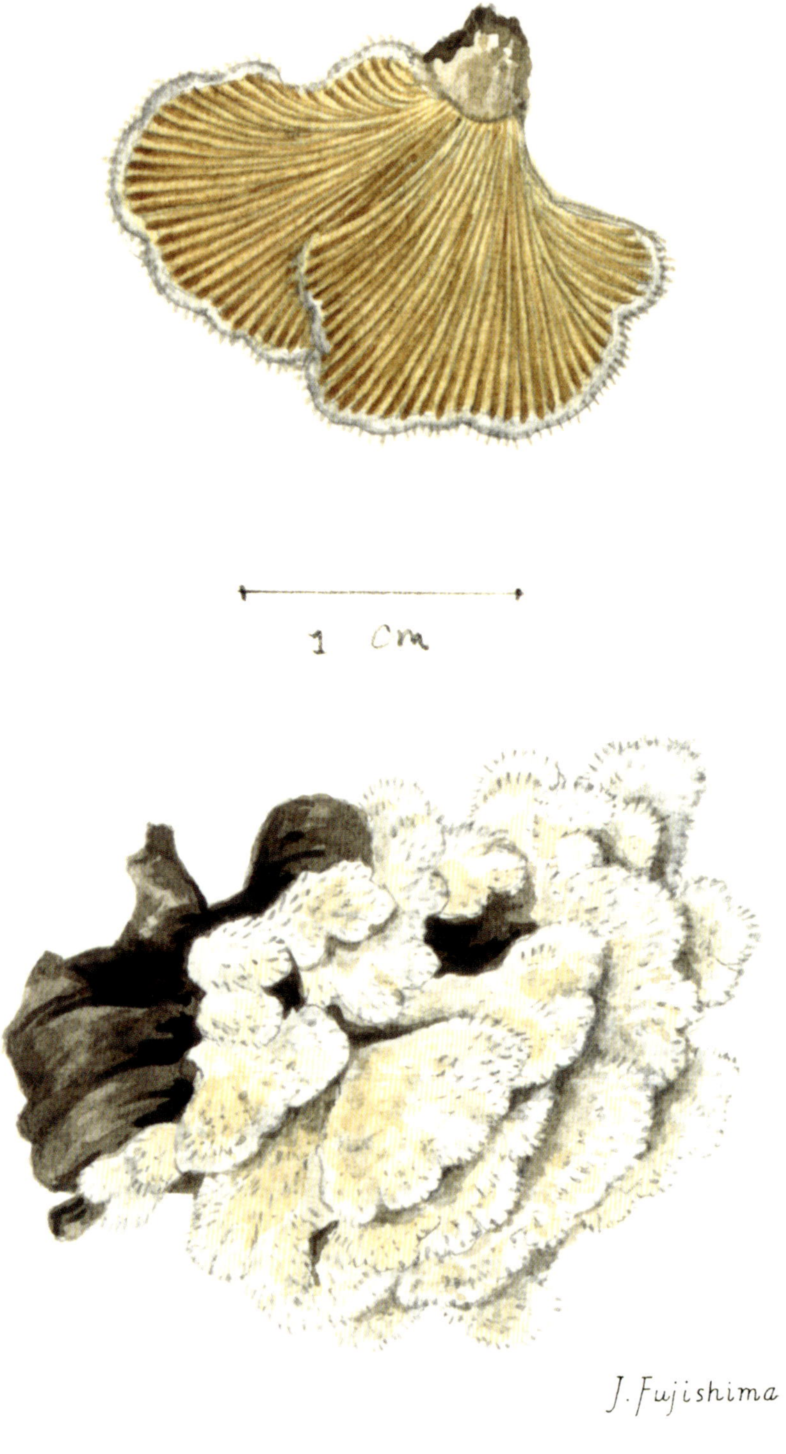


Fig. 11.133. ***Schizophyllum commune*** Fr. — This mushroom contains a polysaccharide that inhibits sarcoma-37, sarcoma-180, and Ehrlich's carcinoma in mice and Yoshida's sarcoma in rats (Ying, et al, 1987).

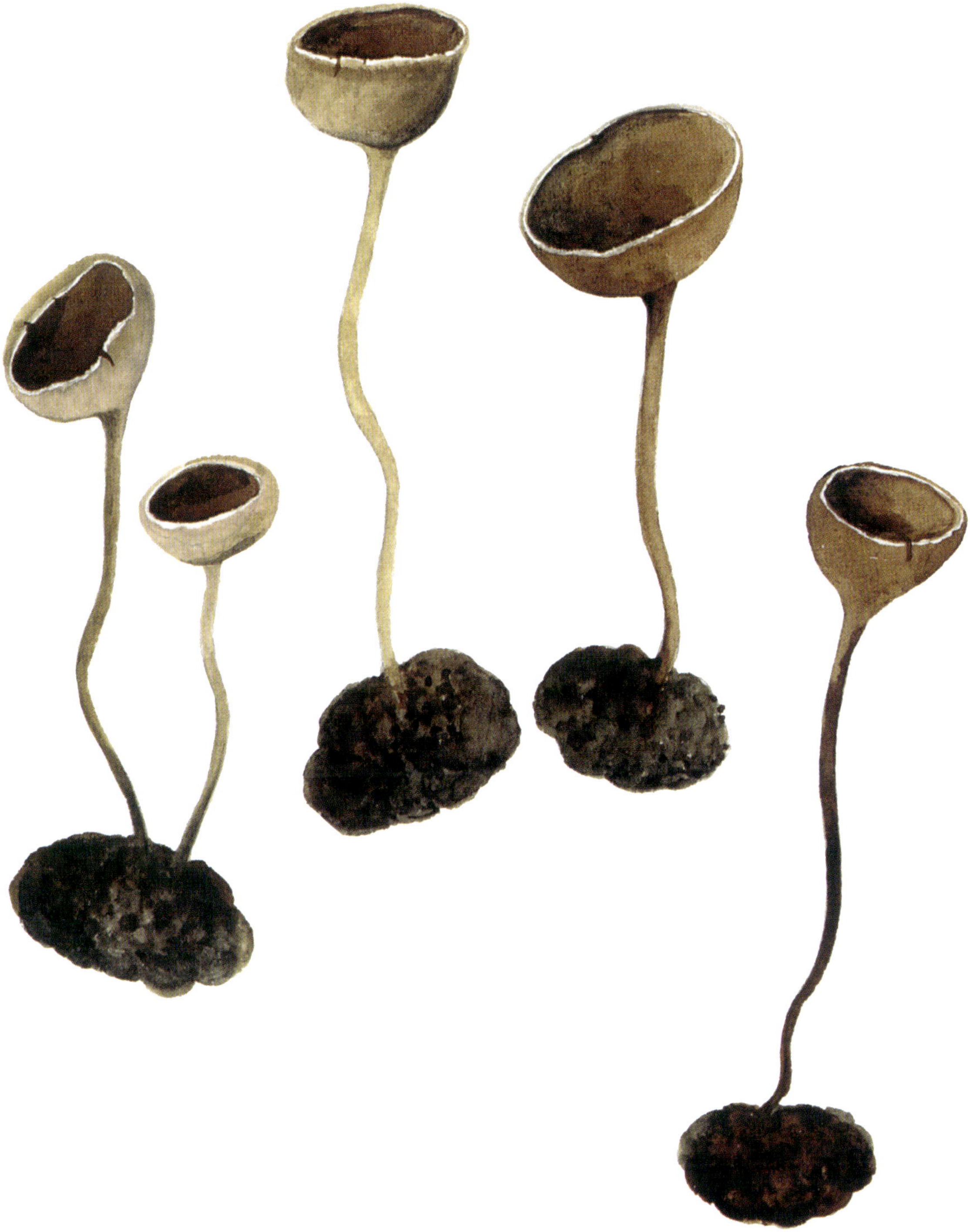

Fig. 11.134. ***Sclerotinia sclerotiorum*** (Lib.) de Bary — This mushroom contains polysaccharides that modulate the immune system and inhibit sarcoma-180 in mice and experimental pulmonary metastasis of Lewis lung carcinoma in mice. (Ying, et al, 1987; Suzuki, et al, 1991; Borchers, et al, 1999)

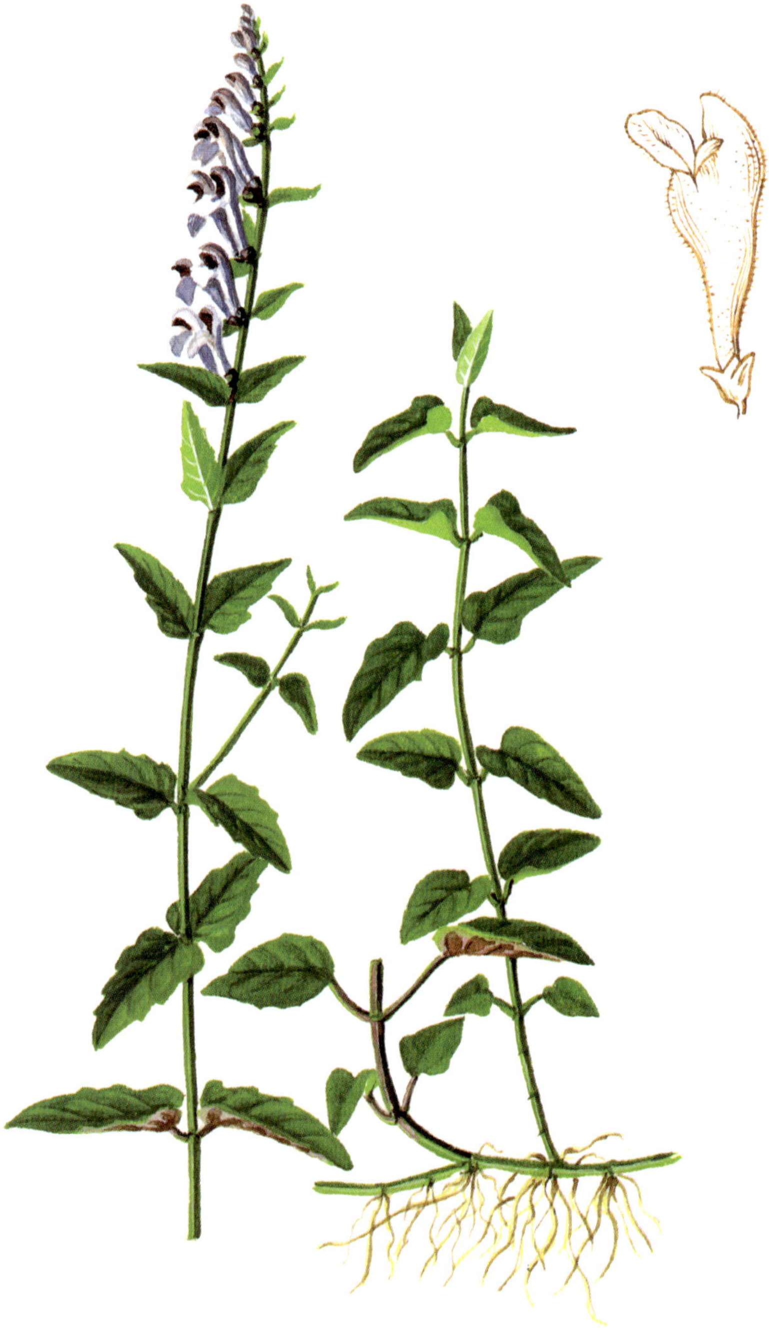

Fig. 11.135. ***Scutellaria barbata*** Don — This plant contains alkaloids, flavenoids, polysaccharides, β-sitosterol, scutellarein, scuttelarin, and carthamidin. It inhibits JTC-26 in vitro and sarcoma-180, Ehrlich's ascites carcinoma, and cerebroma-$B_{22}$ in rats; it also showed mild inhibitory effects against acute granular leukemia. It has been used to treat malignant hydatidiform mole, choriocarcinoma, chorioadenoma, fibroma of the breast, secondary pleural tumor, multiple neuroma, cancers of the nasopharynx, stomach, liver, lung, ovary, and rectum. (Siu-Cheong, 1978; Minyi, 1992; Huang, 1999; Lee, 1999)

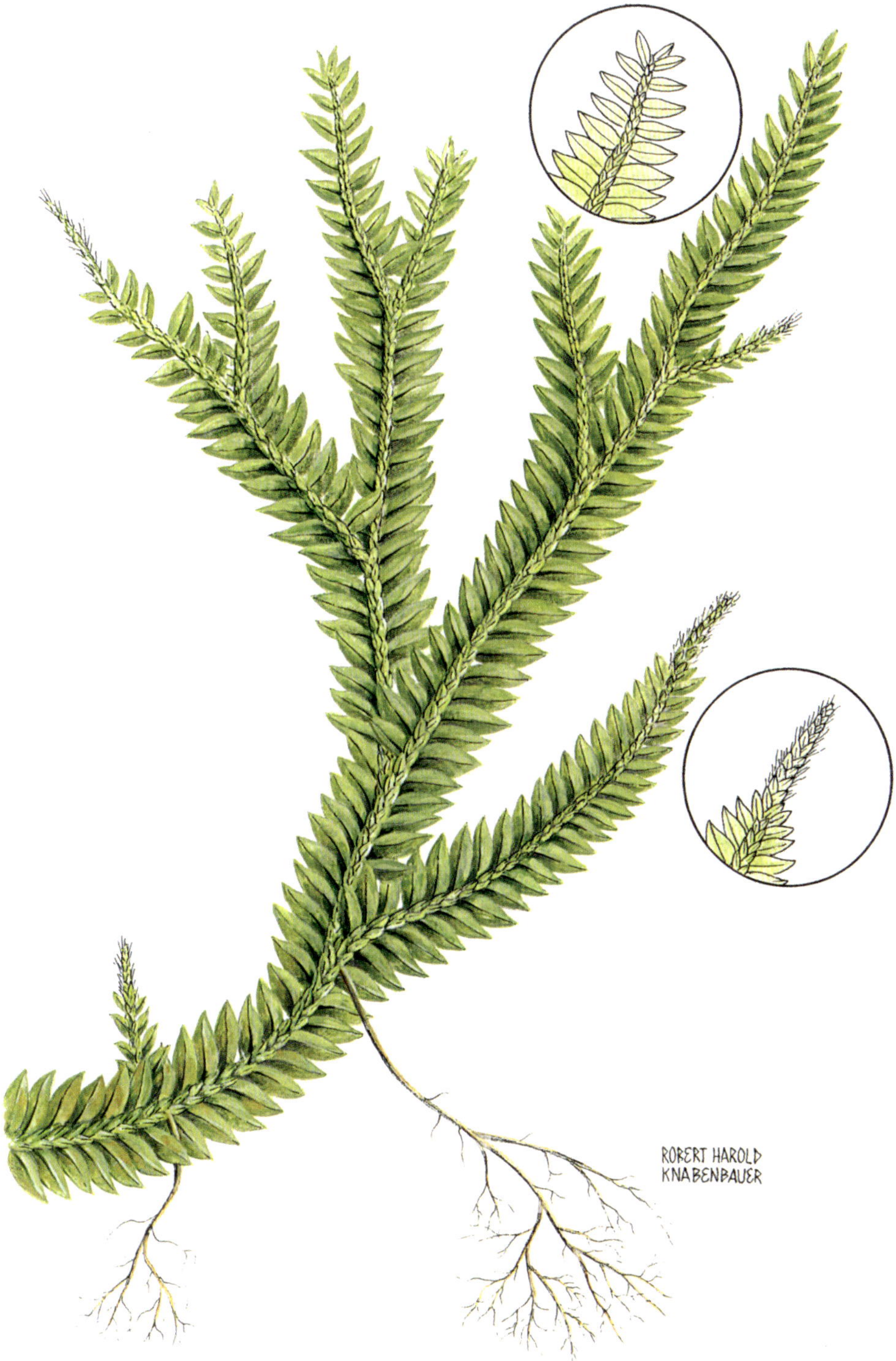


Fig. 11.136. ***Selaginella doederleinii*** Hieron. — This plant contains alkaloids, phytosterols, saponins, and shikimic acid. It has antimutagenic properties and has been used to treat chorionic epithelioma, malignant hydatid mole, and nasopharyngeal, esophageal, liver, and skin carcinomas. (Hsu, et al, 1986; Huang, 1999)

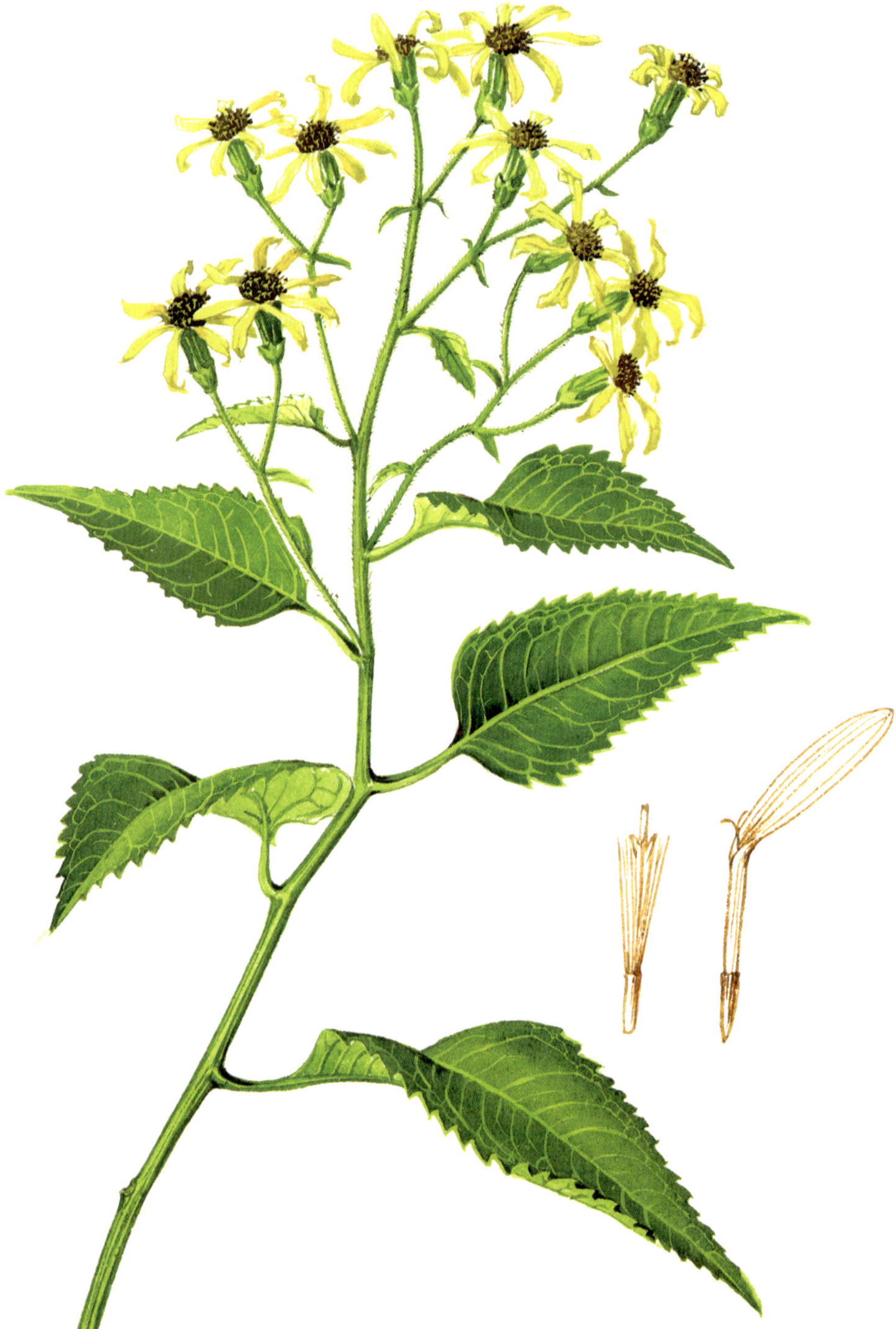

Fig. 11.137. ***Senecio scandens*** Buch.-Hamil. — This plant contains flavonxanthin, chrysanthemaxanthin, p-hydroxyphenylacetic acid, salicyclic acid, vanillic acid, pyromucic acid, hydroquinone, senecionine, seneciphylline, flavone, β-carotenoid, tannins, and alkaloids. It inhibits Walker's carcinoma-256 in rats. (Hsu, et al, 1986; Huang, 1999)

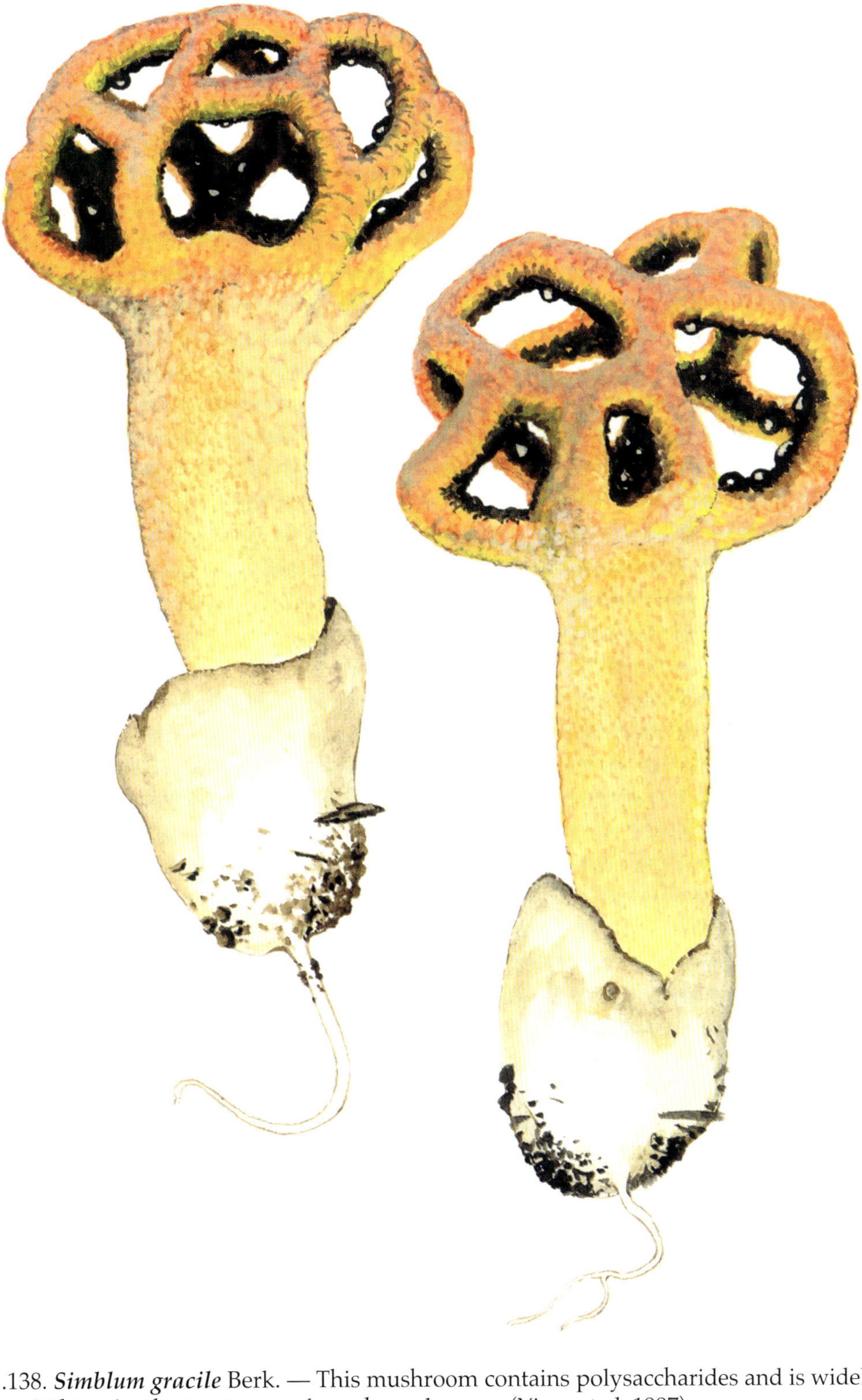

Fig. 11.138. ***Simblum gracile*** Berk. — This mushroom contains polysaccharides and is widely used in parts of China for the treatment of esophageal cancer (Ying, et al, 1987).

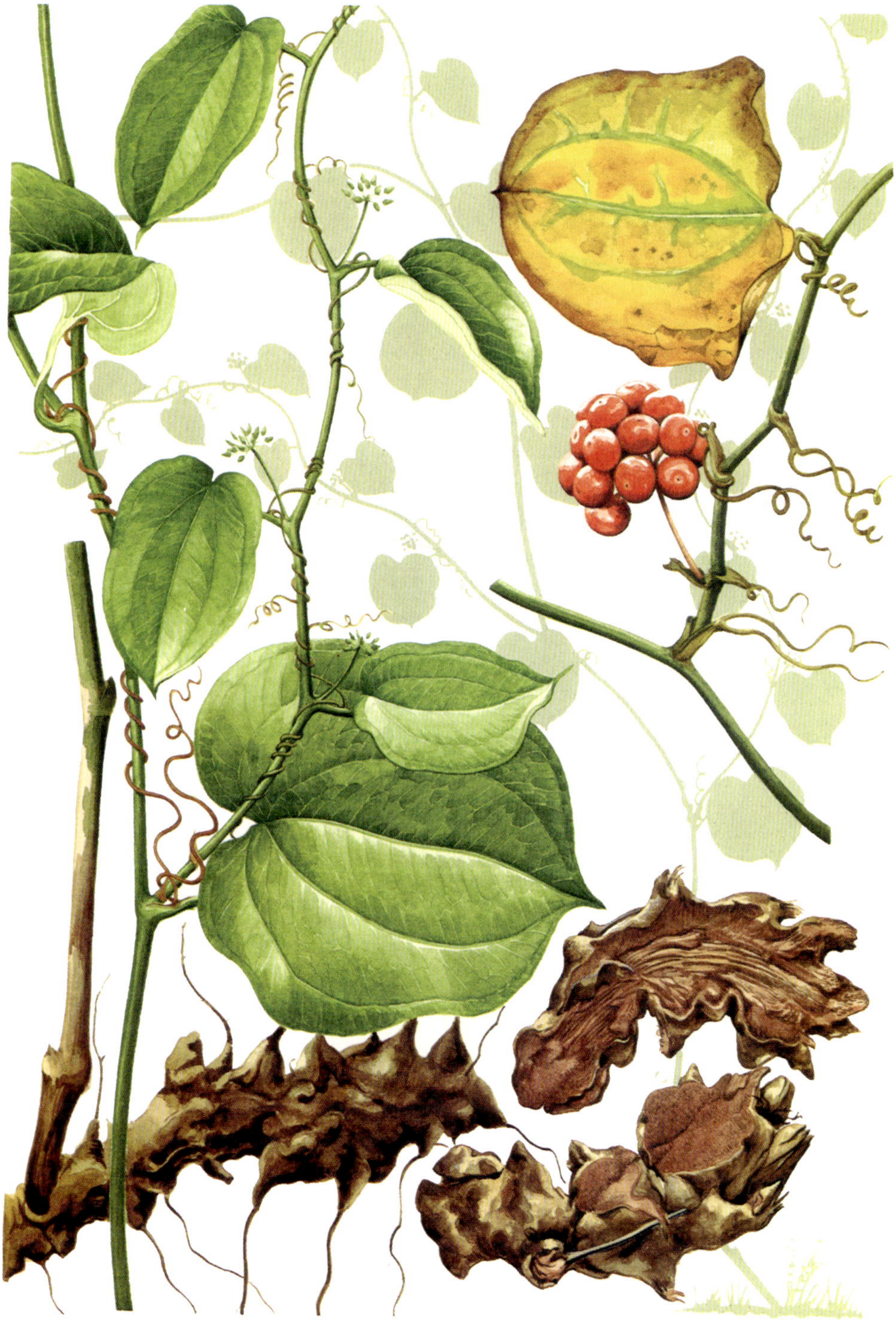

Fig. 11.139. ***Smilax china*** Linn. — This plant contains multiple steroid saponins such as smilaxsaponin A, B, and C, parillin, and smilacin. Tests reveal it is active against cancer, prolongs the life of patients with ascites sarcoma, inhibits mice sarcoma-180 and encephaloma B-22, and has been used to treat carcinomas of the nasopharynx, esophagus, stomach, intestine, heart, liver, and pancreas. (Hsu, et al, 1986; Minyi, 1992; Lee, 1999)

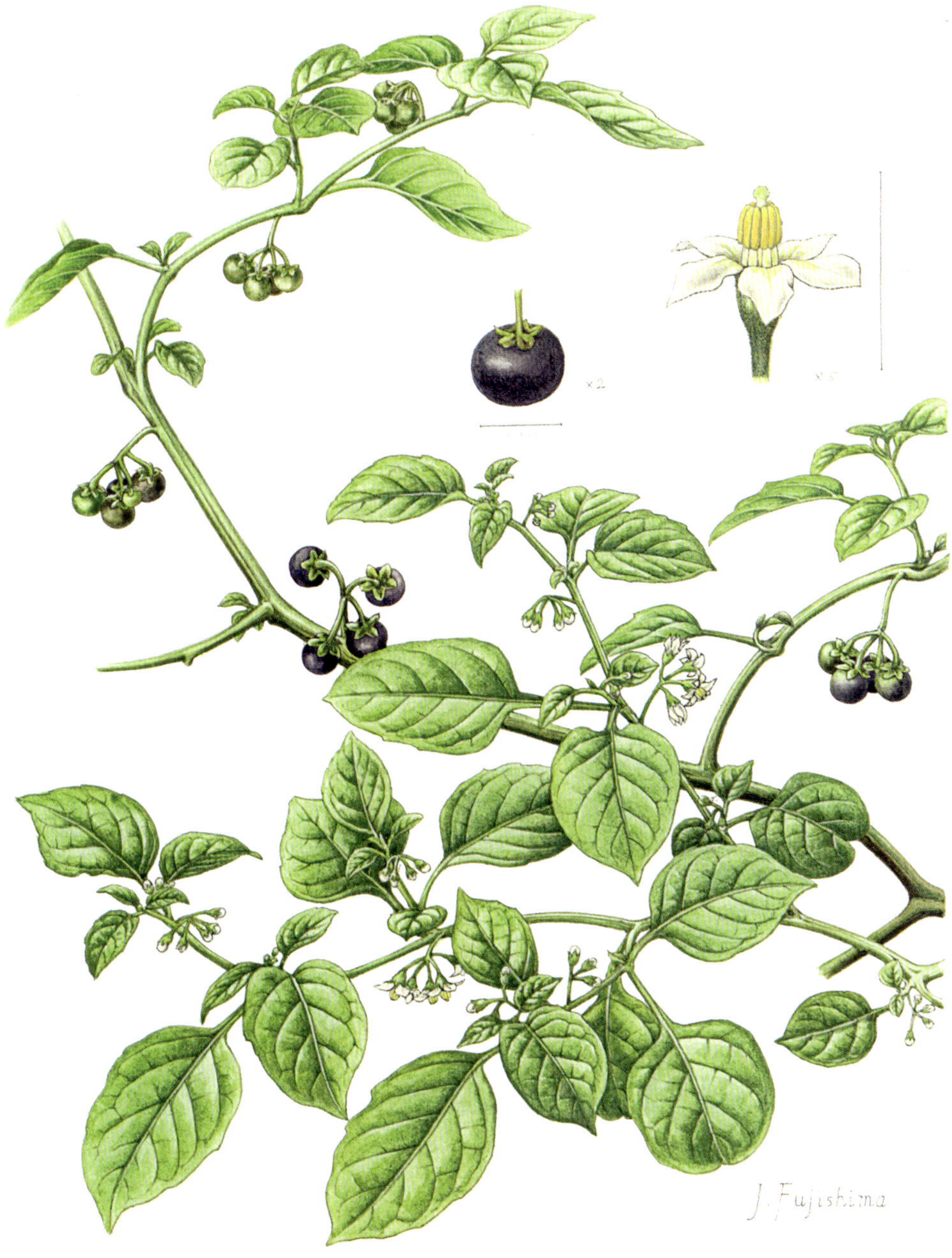


Fig. 11.140. ***Solanum nigrum*** Linn. — This plant contains the glycoalkaloids solanine, α-solanigrine, β-solanigrine (solasodamine) γ-solanigrine (solasonine), δ-solanigrine (solamargine), ε-solanigrine, and ζ-solanigrine, saponins, the genins diosgenin and tigogenin, atropine, vitamin C, and resin. It inhibits leukemia cells in vitro, Erlich's ascites carcinoma, lymphatic leukemia-615, sarcoma-37, and sarcoma-180 in rats, and stomach cancer cells in mice, has cytotoxic action against Hela cells, suppresses ascites sarcoma-180 in mice, and has been used to treat choriocarcinoma, chorioadenoma, hepatoma, leukemia, fibrosarcoma, cancerous hydrothorax, ascites, and carcinomas of the esophagus, breast, lung, liver, urinary bladder, ovary, and cervix. (Chang & But, 1986; Minyi, 1992; Huang, 1999; Lee, 1999)

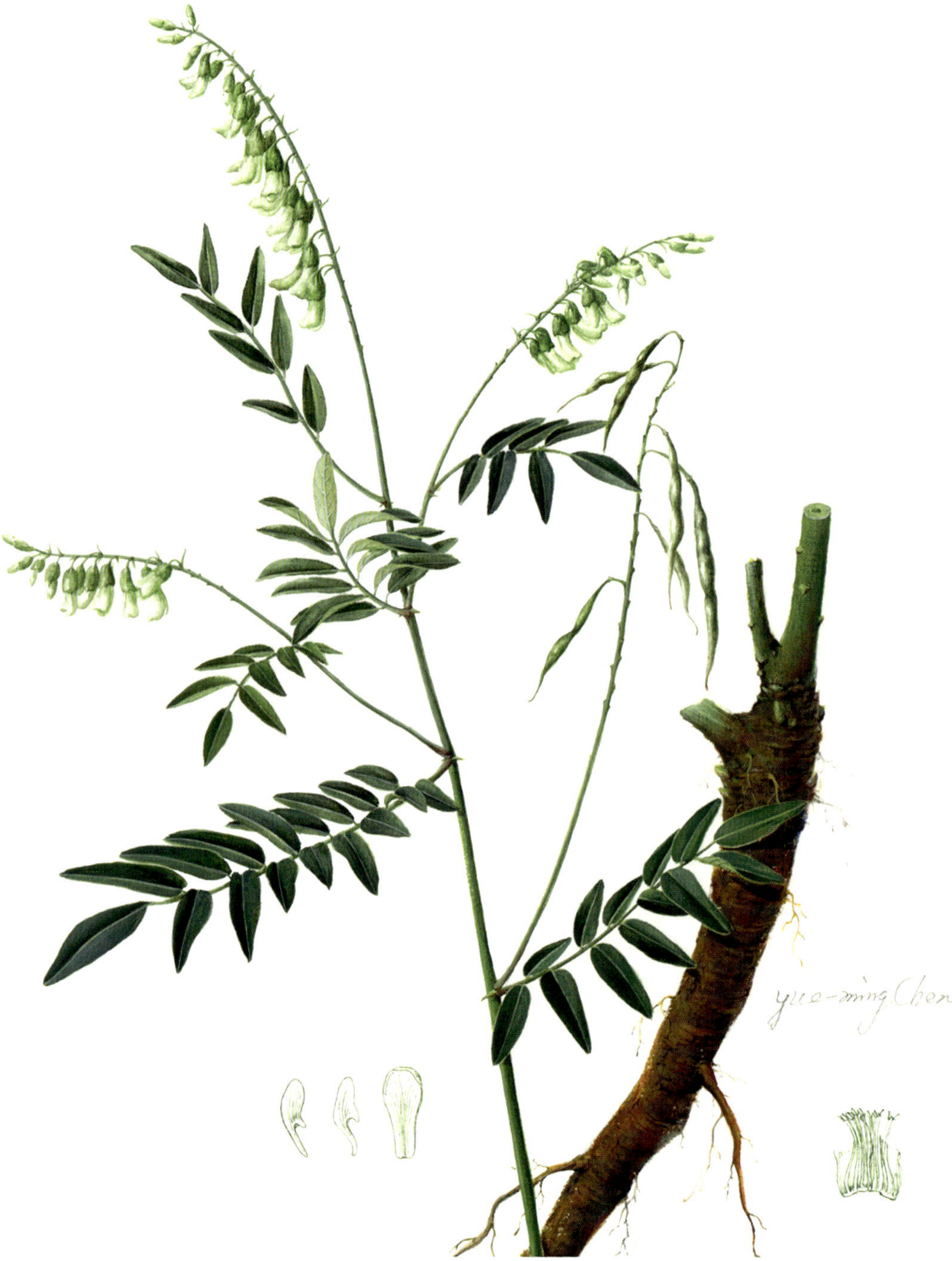


Fig. 11.141. ***Sophora flavescens*** Ait. — This plant contains the alkaloids matrine, oxymatrine, isomatrine, sophocarpine, cytisine, methylcytisine, anagyrine, baptifoline, trifolirhizin, norkurarinone, kuraridin, dehydromatrine, and sophoranol (hydroxymatrine). It has an inhibitory action against sarcoma-37 and sarcoma-180 in mice, cervical cancer-14 in rats, transplanted tumors in animals, and human stomach cancers, and prolongs the life span of mice with Erlich's ascites carcinoma. It has been used to treat cyst cancers, malignant lymphoma, cancers of the esophagus, intestine, bladder, cervix, and colon. (Chang & But, 1986; Minyi, 1992; Huang, 1999; Lee, 1999)

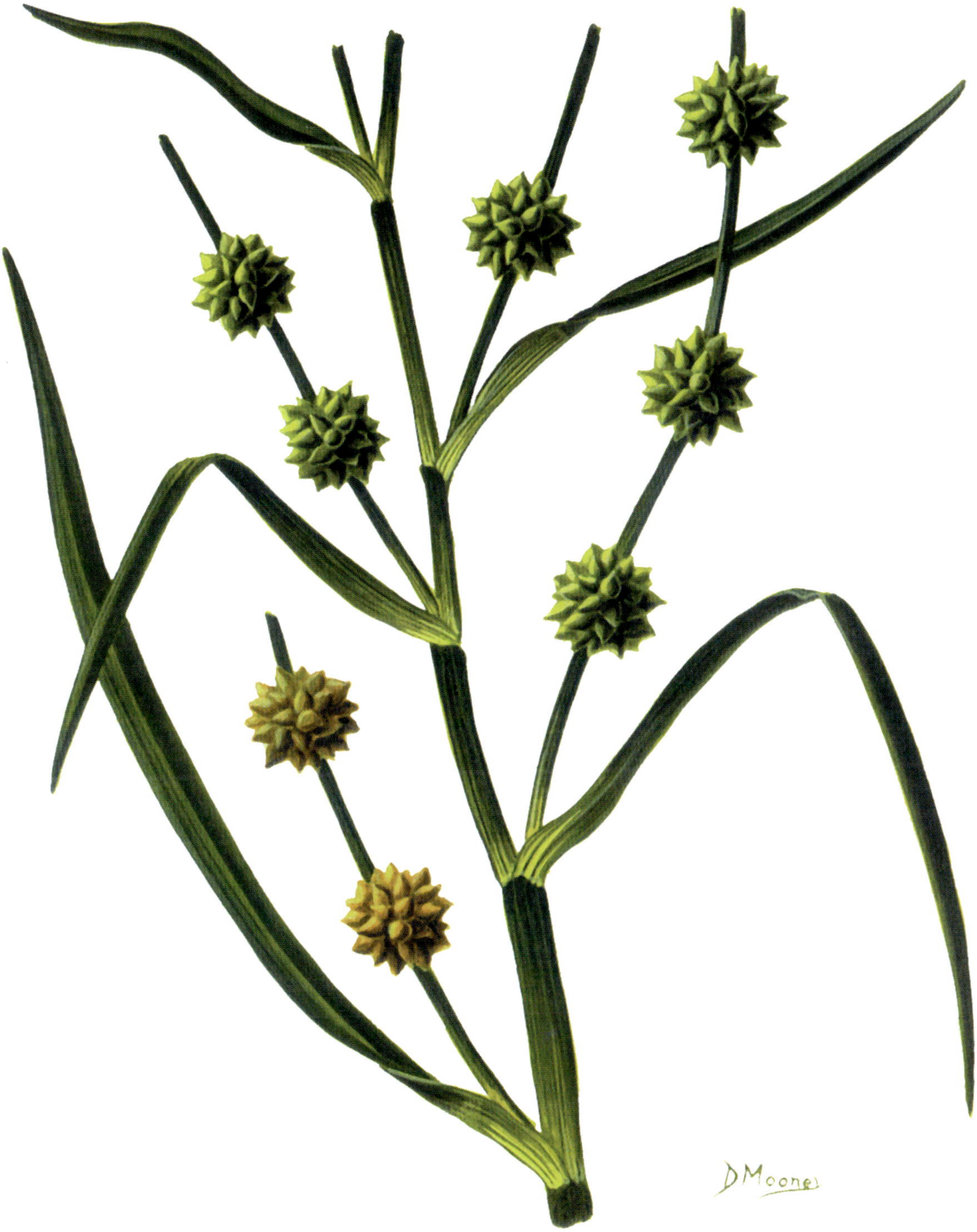


Fig. 11.142. ***Sparganium stoloniferum*** Buch.-Hamil. — This plant contains coixol, coixenolide, amino acids, and volatile oils. It inhibits tumor growth in vitro and sarcoma-180 in mice and has been used to treat thyroid adenoma and cancers of the abdominal cavity, uterus, cervix, ovary, and liver. (Minyi, 1992; Lee, 1999)

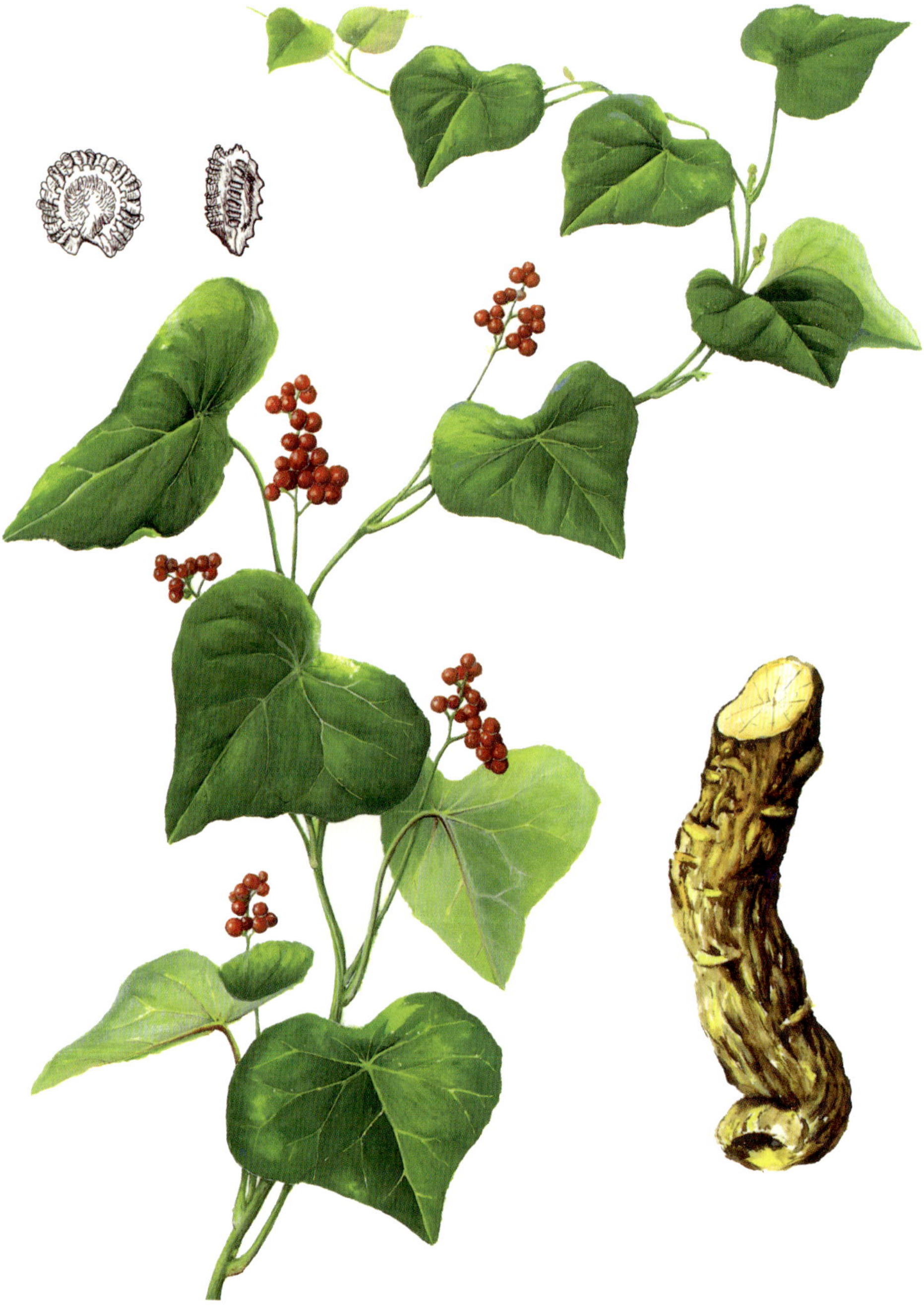

Fig. 11.143. ***Stephania tetrandra*** S. Moore — This plant contains tetrandrine, dimethyltetrandrine, fangchinoline, hanfangchin A, B, and C, cyclanoline, phenols, flavenoid glycosides, organic acids, and essential oils. It has cytotoxic activity against KB cells, Hela cells, and Hela $S_3$ cells, inhibits Erlich's ascites carcinoma, sarcoma-180, liver carcinoma BEL-7402, BEL-7405, and SMMC-7721 cells in vitro, and in vivo inhibits EAC, HepA tumors, liver carcinoma, sarcoma-45, and Walker's carcinoma-256. It also has selective anticancer properties especially against drug resistant cancer cells and has been used to treat leukemia and cancers of the nasopharynx, esophagus, heart, lung, liver, and rectum. (Chang & But, 1986; Hsu, et al, 1986; Minyi, 1992; Huang, 1999)

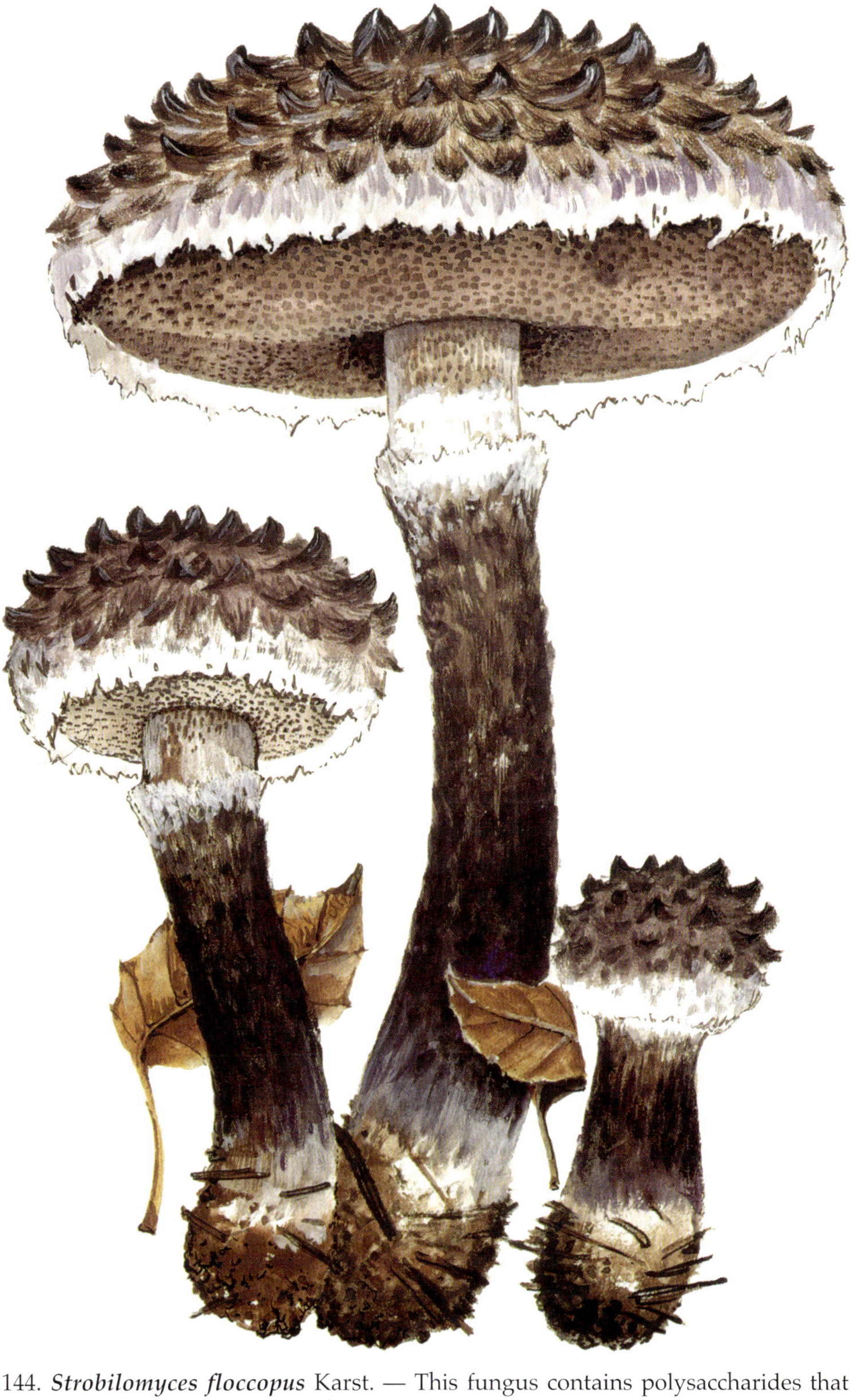

Fig. 11.144. ***Strobilomyces floccopus*** Karst. — This fungus contains polysaccharides that inhibit Ehrlich's ascites tumor in mice and Yoshida's sarcoma in rats (Ying, et al, 1987).

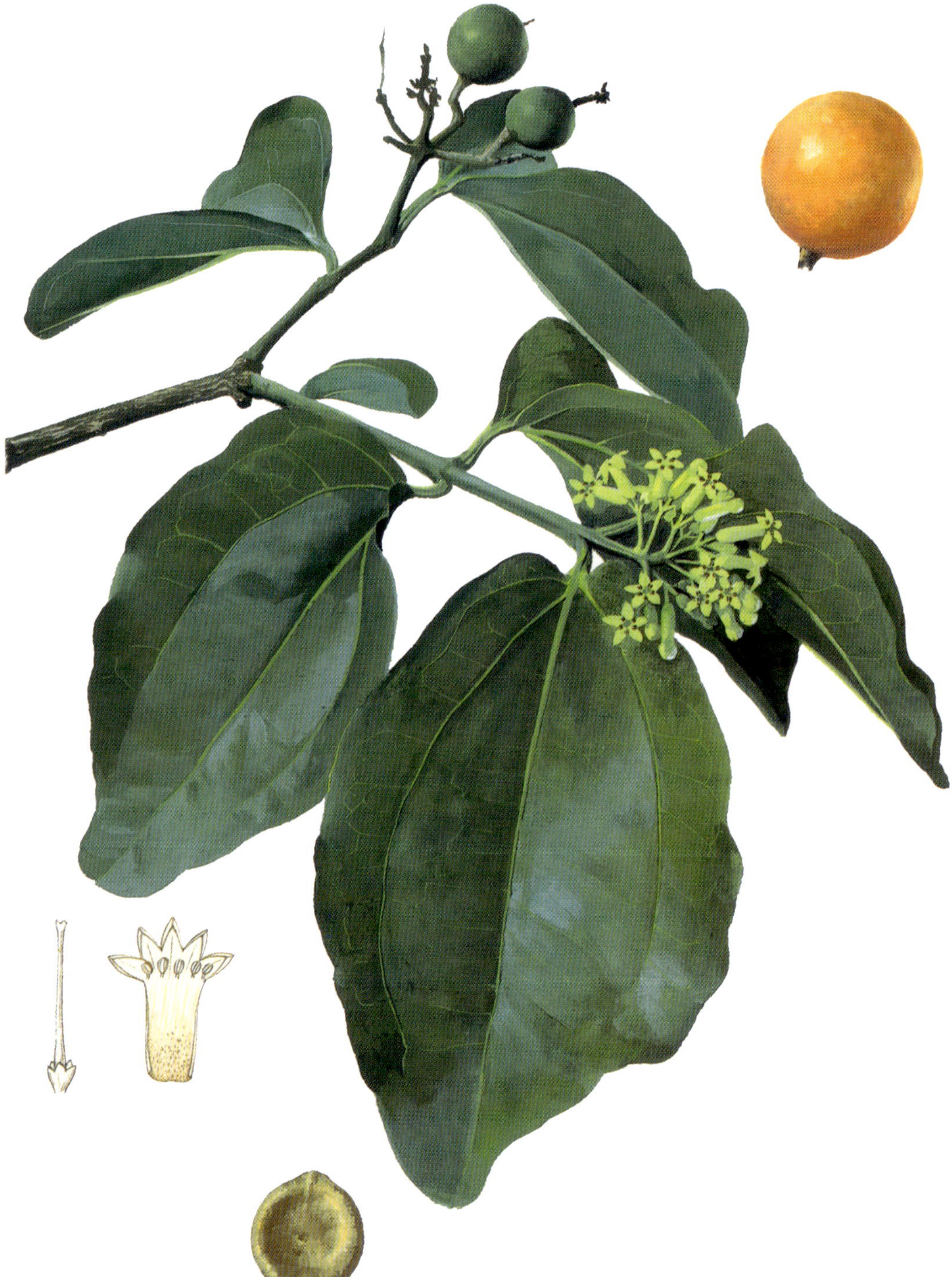

Fig. 11.145. ***Strychnos nux-vomica*** Linn. — This plant contains the alkaloids strychnine, brucine, α-colubrine, β-colubrine, tetrahydrostrychnine, brucidine, tetrahydrobrucine, vomicine, strychinicine, pseudostrychinine, and the monoterpenoid loganine. It inhibits sarcoma-180 and leukemia cells in laboratory animals and has been used to treat leukemia, skin cancer, and cancers of the brain, nasopharynx, esophagus, stomach, breast, cervix, and anus. (Hsu, et al, 1986; Minyi, 1992)

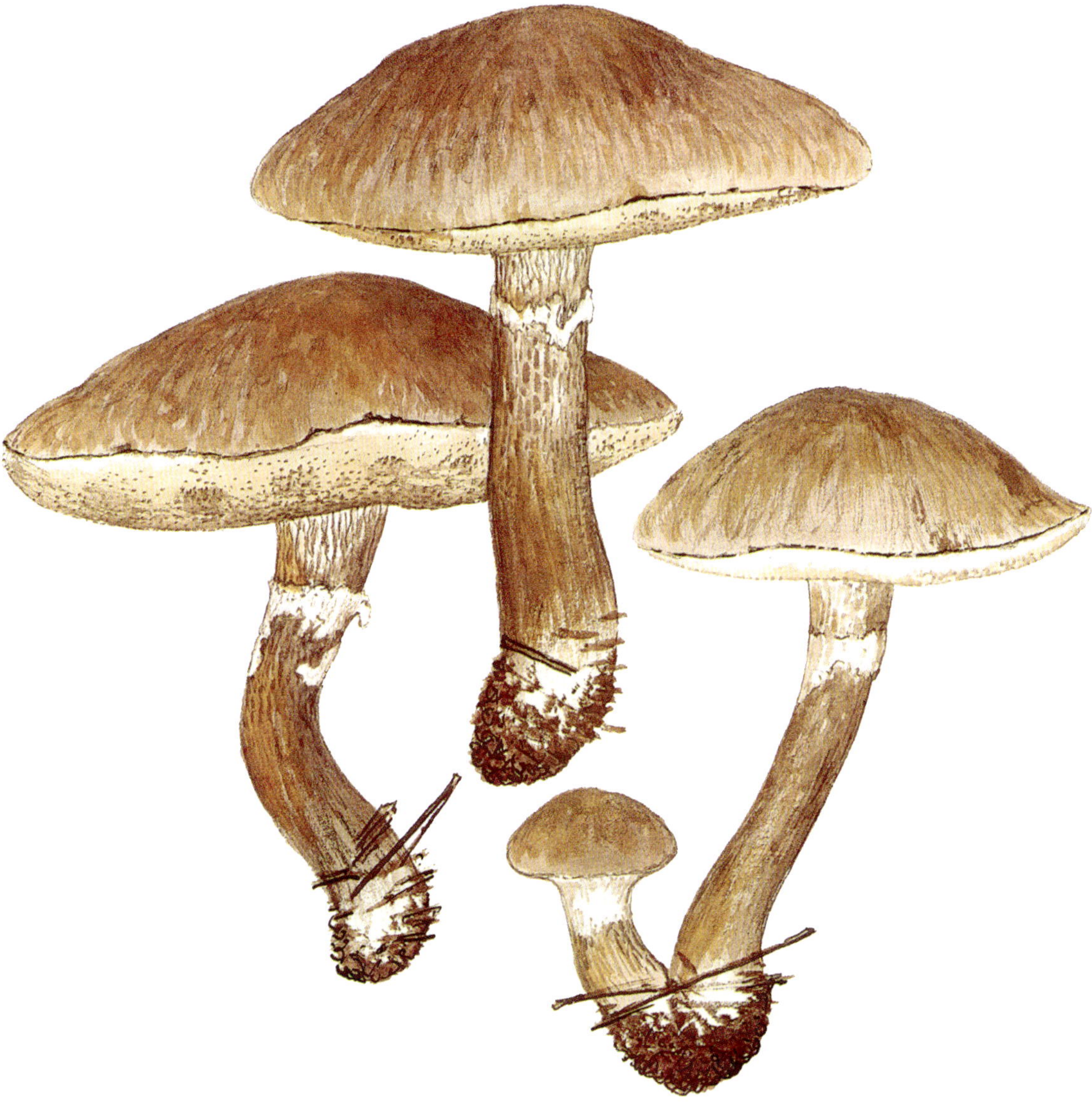

Fig. 11.146. ***Suillus aeruginascens*** (Secr.) Snell — This fungus contains polysaccharides that inhibit sarcoma-180 and Ehrlich's carcinoma (Ying, et al, 1987).

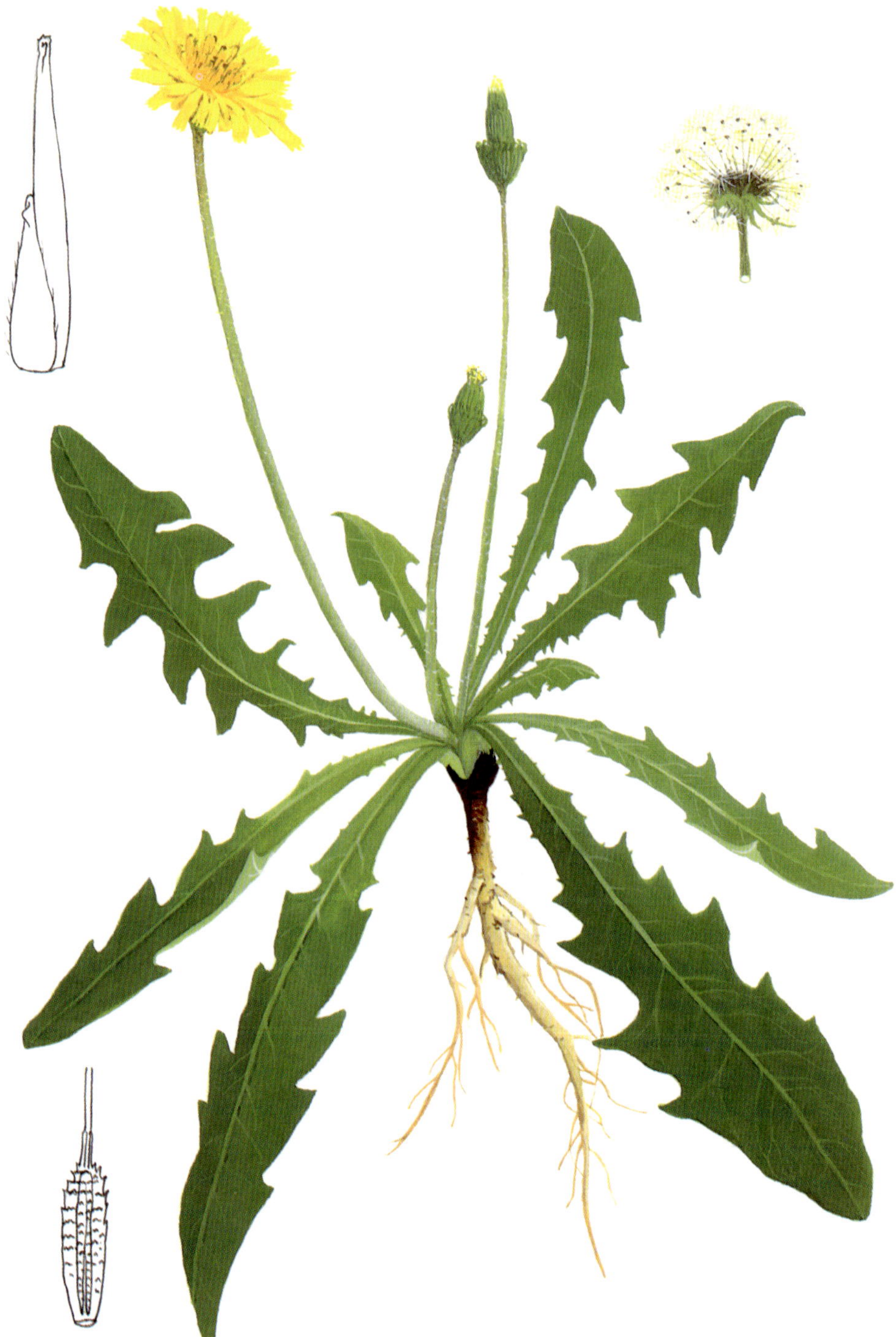

Fig. 11.147. ***Taraxacum mongolicum*** Hand.-Mazz. — This plant contains taraxasterol, choline, inulin, pectin, taraxacin, taraxarol, asparagin, and polysaccharides. It inhibits mouse sarcoma-180, Erlich's ascites carcinoma, transplanted human pulmonary cancers, is effective against mice ascites cancer, enhances the immune system, and has been used to treat angioma, leukemia, and nasopharyngeal, gingival, hard palate, breast, stomach, and cervical cancers. (Hsu, et al, 1986; Minyi, 1992; Lee, 1999)

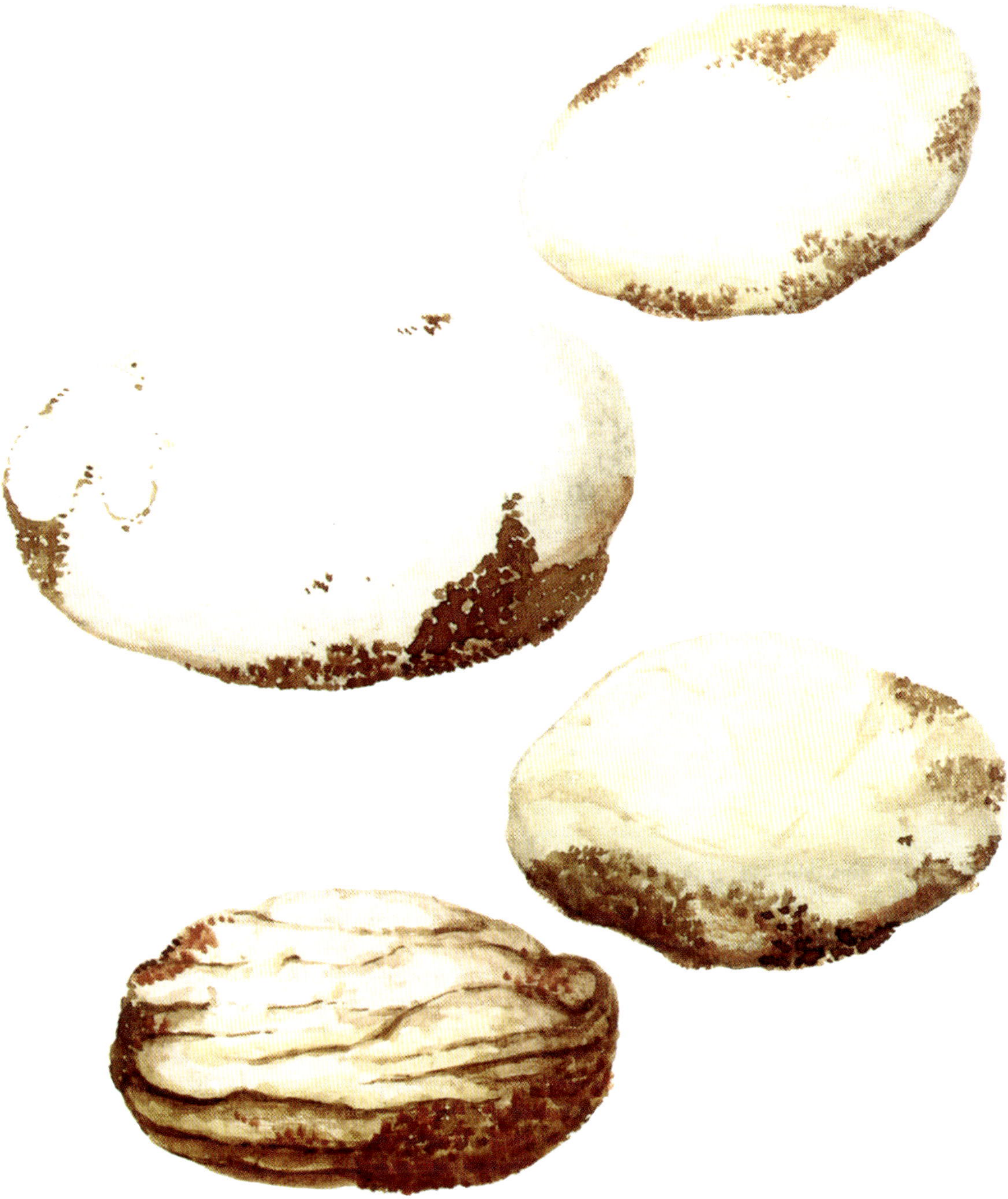

Fig. 11.148. ***Terfezia leonis*** Tul. — This fungus contains polysaccharides that inhibit tumors of the ear and anal cancers (Ying, et al, 1987).

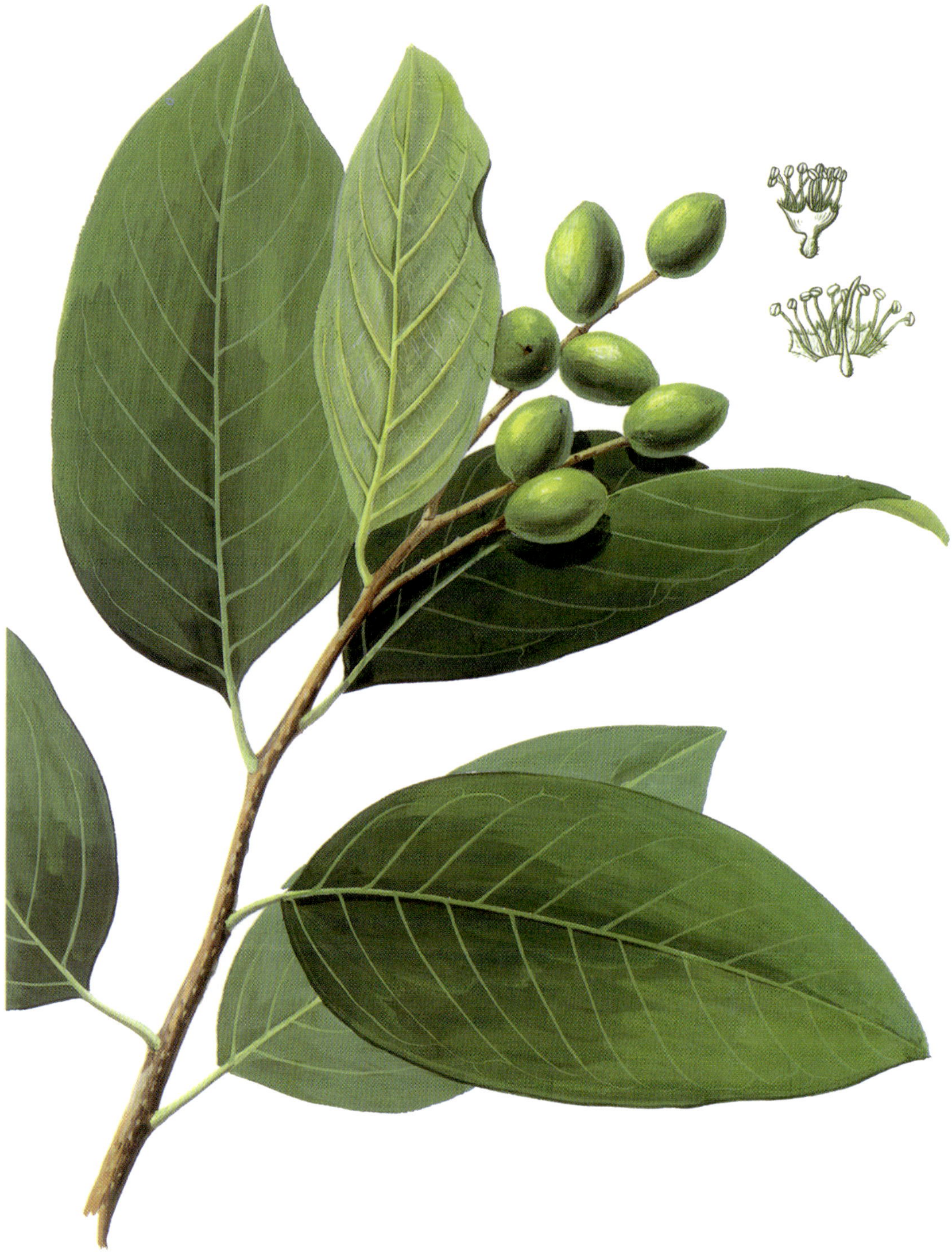

Fig. 11.149. ***Terminalia chebula*** Retz. — This plant contains chebulin, chebulinic acid, chebulagic acid, ellagic acid, gallic acid, luteoic acid, shikimic acid, quinic acid, tannins, fructose, animo acids, and sennoside A. It inhibits JTC-26 cells, fusocellular sarcoma, mouse Erlich's ascites carcinoma, and sarcoma-180 in mice, and has been used to treat esophageal, stomach, and cervical cancer. (Hsu, et al, 1986; Minyi, 1992; Lee, 1999)

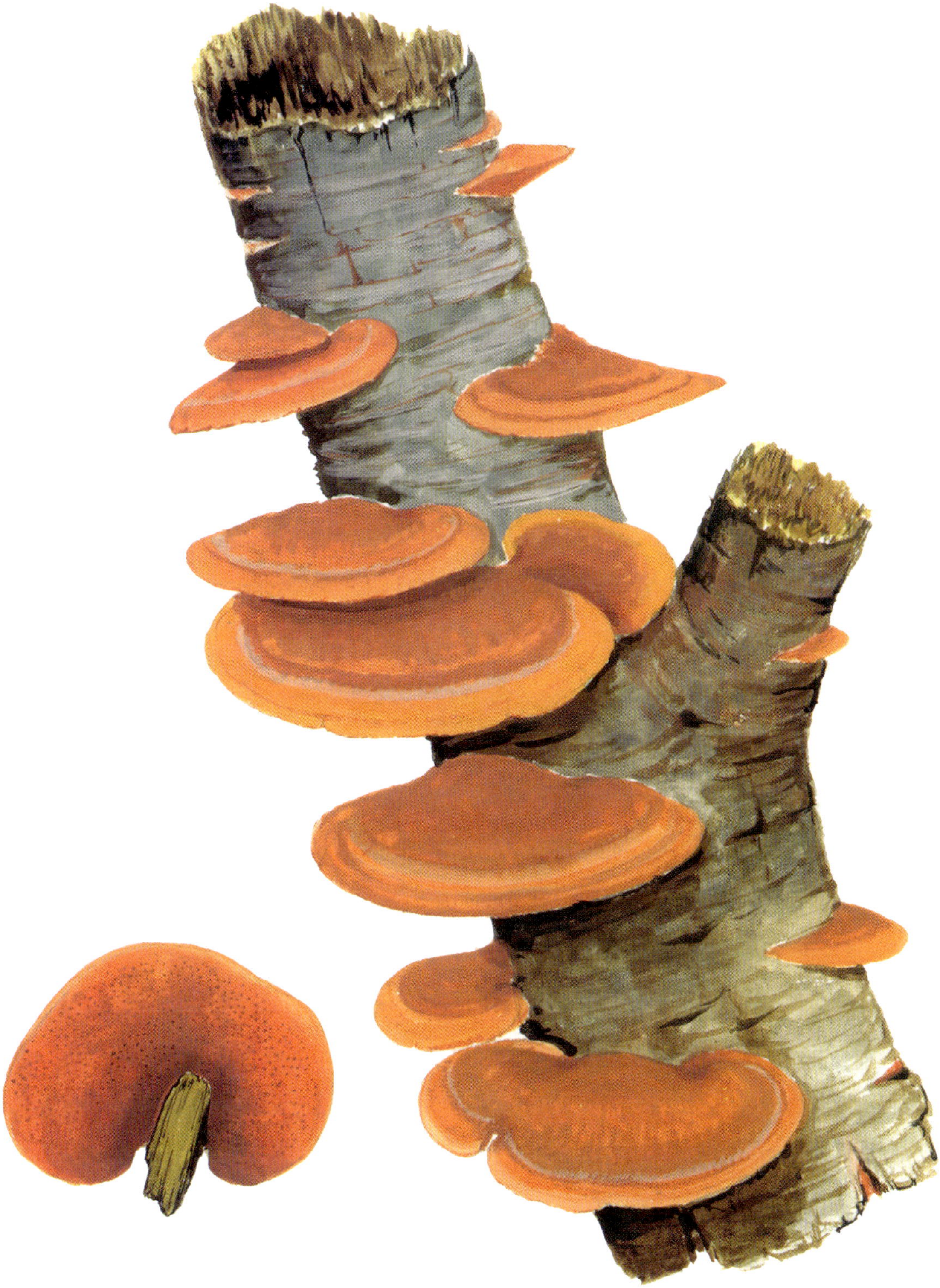

Fig. 11.150. ***Trametes cinnabarina*** (Jacq.) Fr. — This fungus contains polysaccharides that inhibit sarcoma-180 (Ying, et al, 1987).

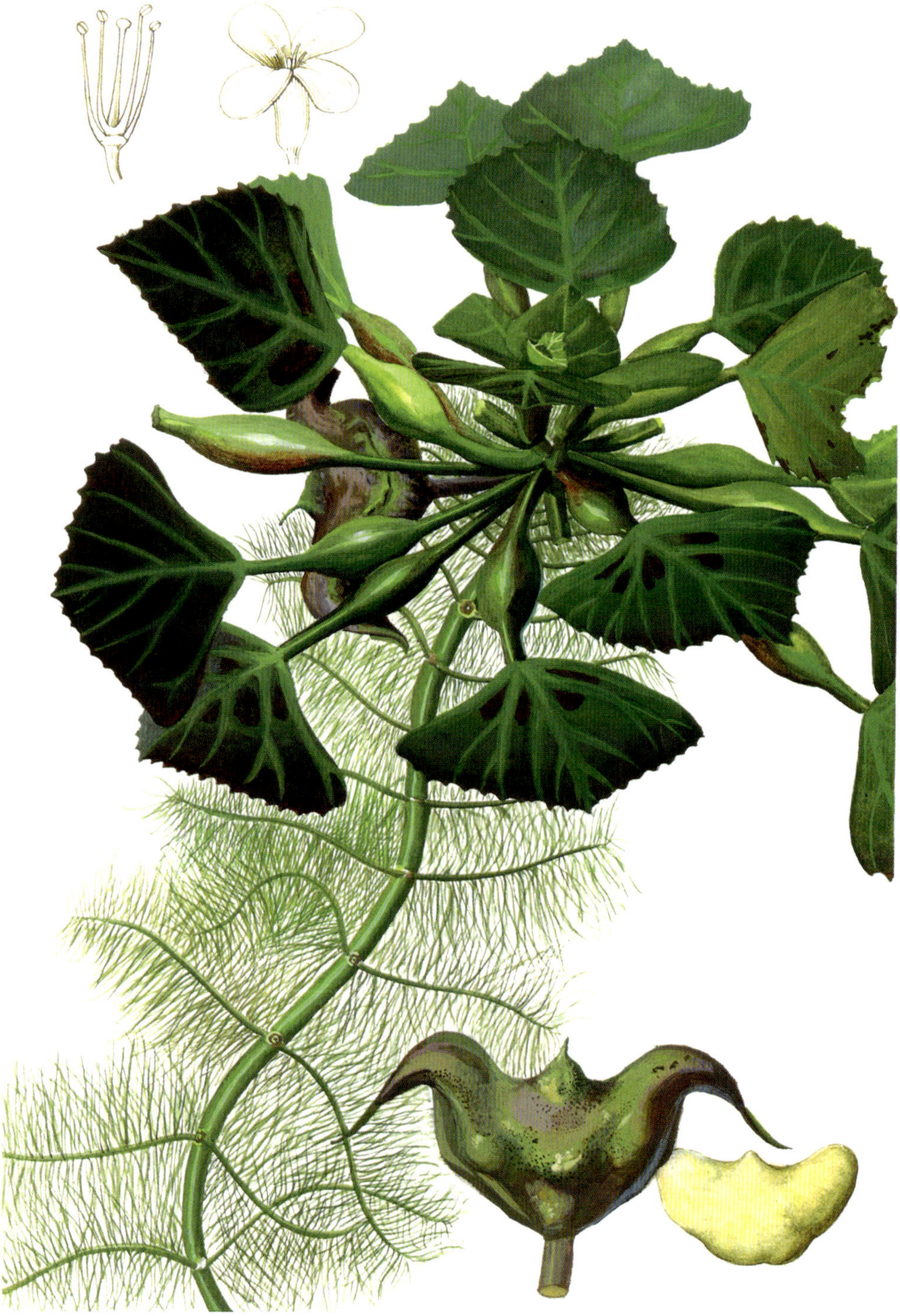

Fig. 11.151. ***Trapa bispinosa*** Roxb. — This plant contains 4,6,8,(14),22-ergostatetraen-3-one, 22-dihydrostigmast-4-en-3, 6-dione, β-sitosterol, and starch. It inhibits mice sarcoma-180, resists ascites cancer and liver cancer AH-13 in mice, exhibits a carcinostatic effect on Erlich's ascites carcinoma in vivo, and has been used to treat various cancers including cancers of the esophagus, stomach, breast, uterus, and cervix. (Hsu, et al, 1986; Minyi, 1992)

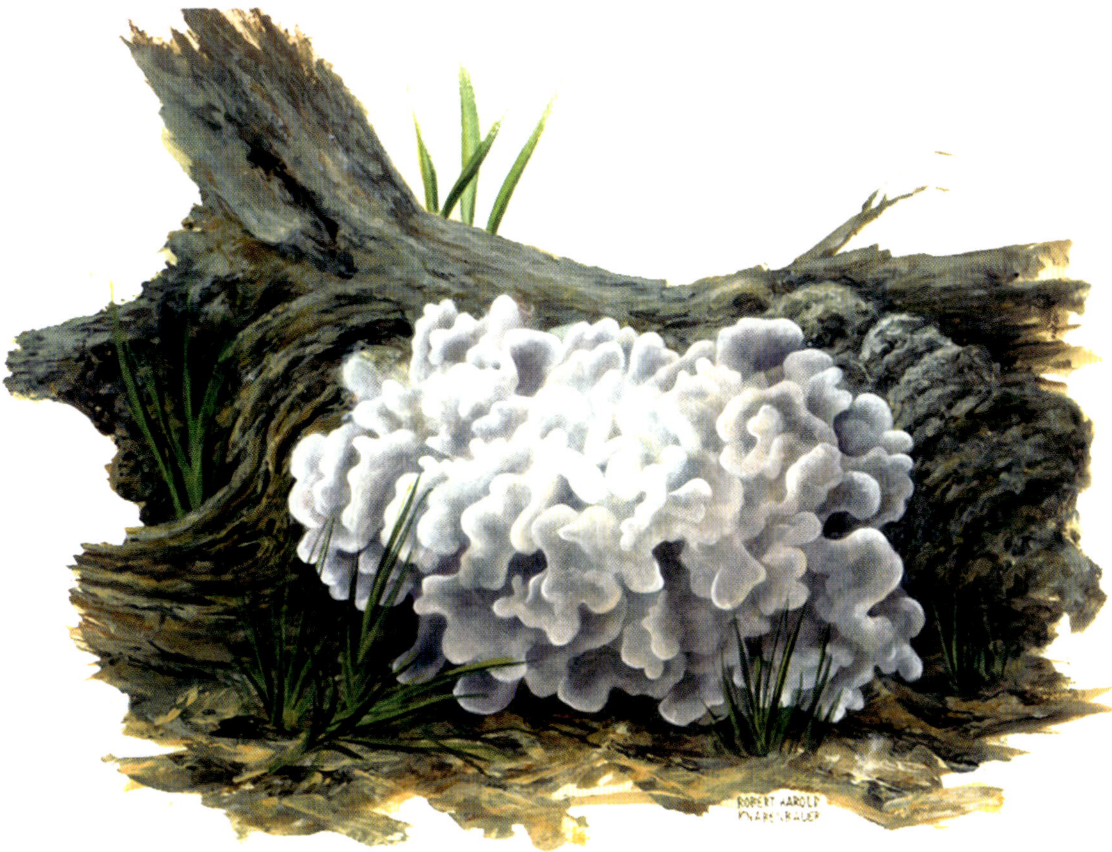

Fig. 11.152. ***Tremella fuciformis*** Berk. — This fungus contains polysaccharides, proteins, carbohydrates, inorganic salts, and vitamin B. It inhibits sarcoma-180 and Erlich's ascites carcinoma in mice, reduces the side effects from cobalt radiation, and has been used to treat hepatocarcinoma. (Hsu, et al, 1986; Minyi, 1992; Lee, 1999)

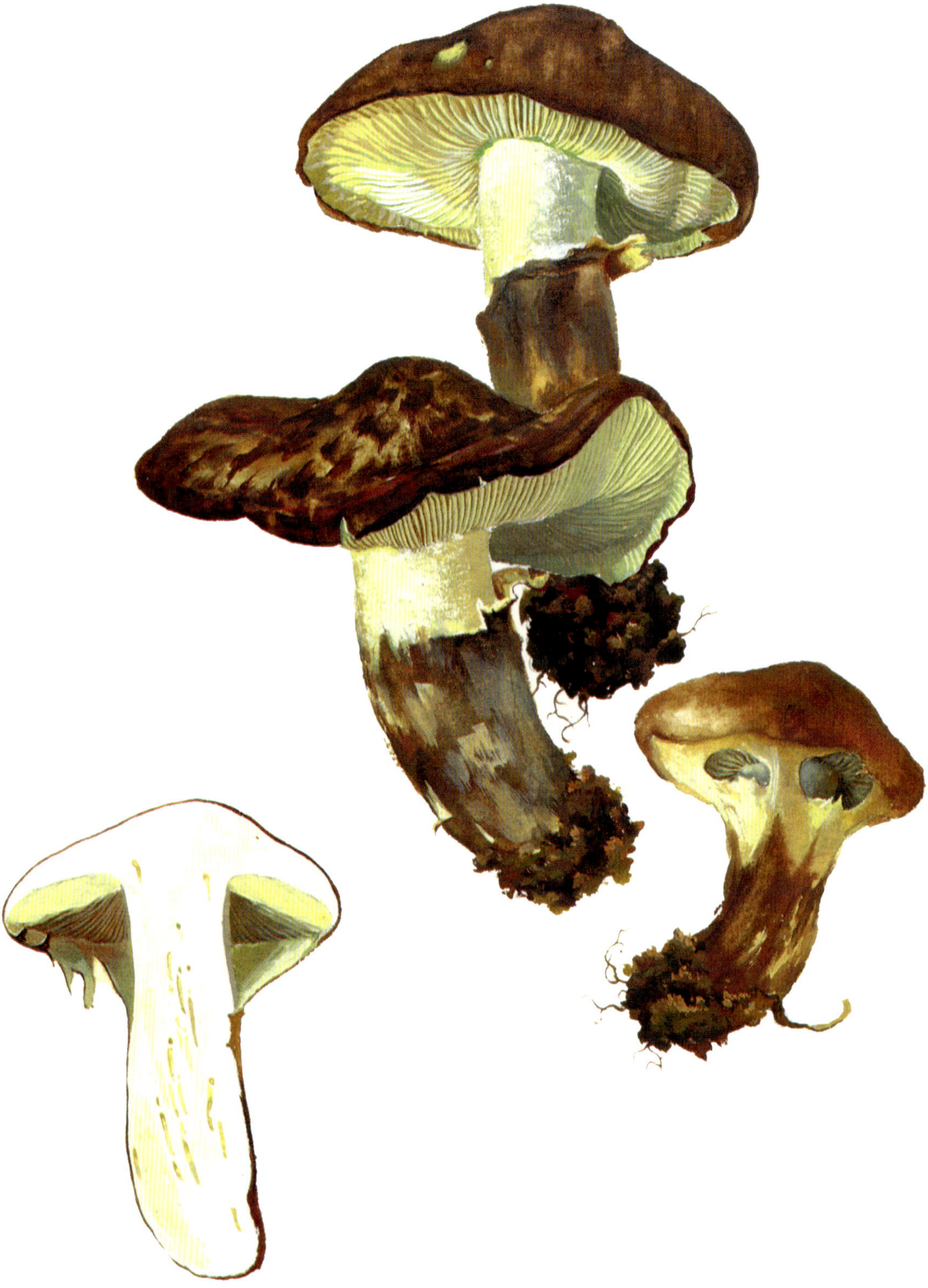

Fig. 11.153. ***Tricholoma matsutake*** (S. Ito et Imai) Sing. — This fungus contains polysaccharides that inhibit sarcoma-180 and Ehrlich's carcinoma (Ying, et al, 1987).

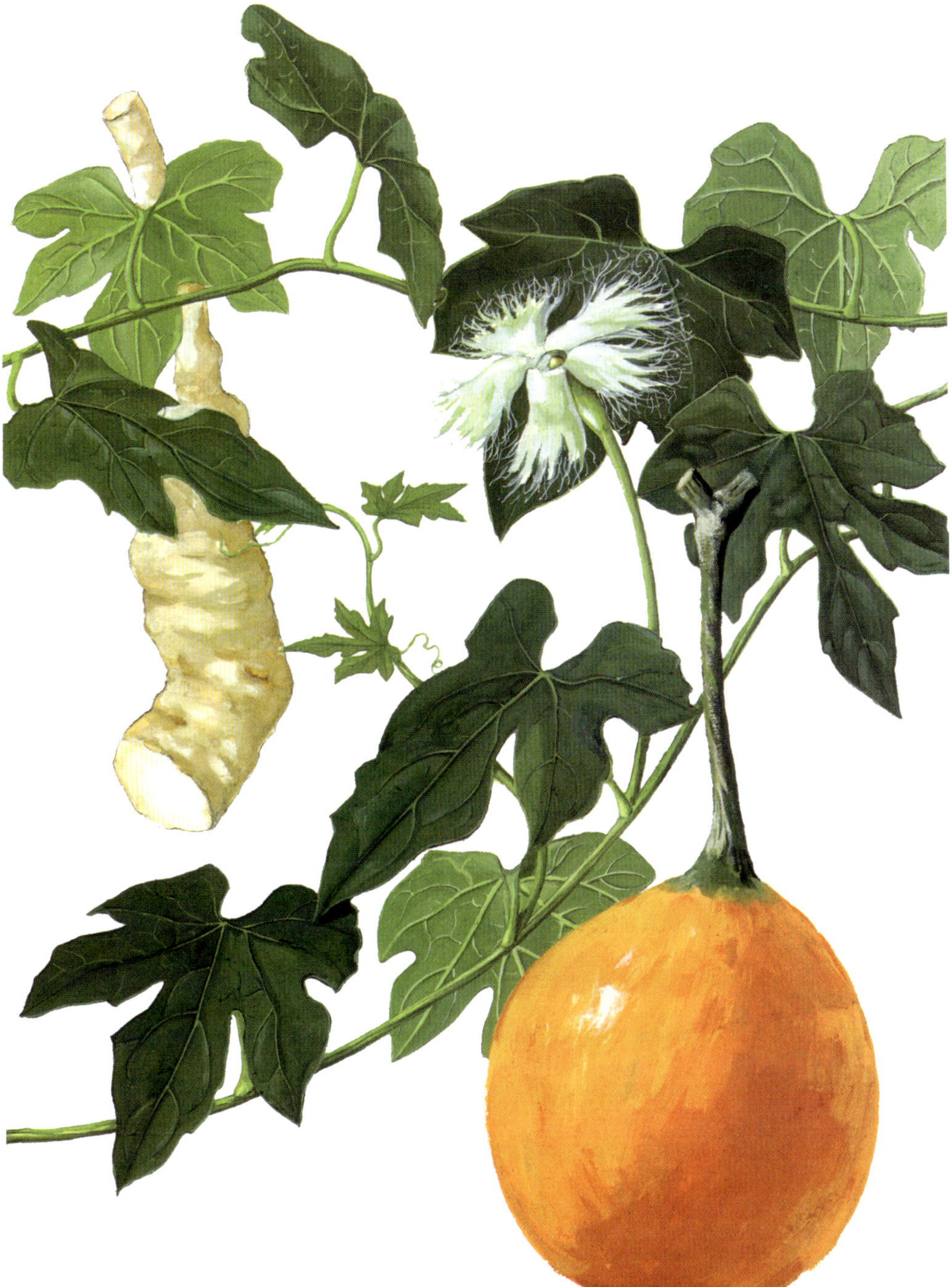

Fig. 11.154. ***Trichosanthes kirilowii*** Maxim. — It contains stigmasterol, β-sitosterol, saponin, trichosanthin, trichosanatine, curcubitacin, starch, protein, amino acids, organic acids, organic salts, resins, gums, and fatty oil. It inhibits ascites carcinoma cells, sarcoma-180, cervical cancer-14, and JTC-26 and has been used to treat chorioepithelioma, malignant hydatidiform mole, and nasopharyngeal, esophageal, stomach, and mammary cancers. (Chang & But, 1986; Hsu, et al, 1986; Huang, 1999; Lee, 1990)

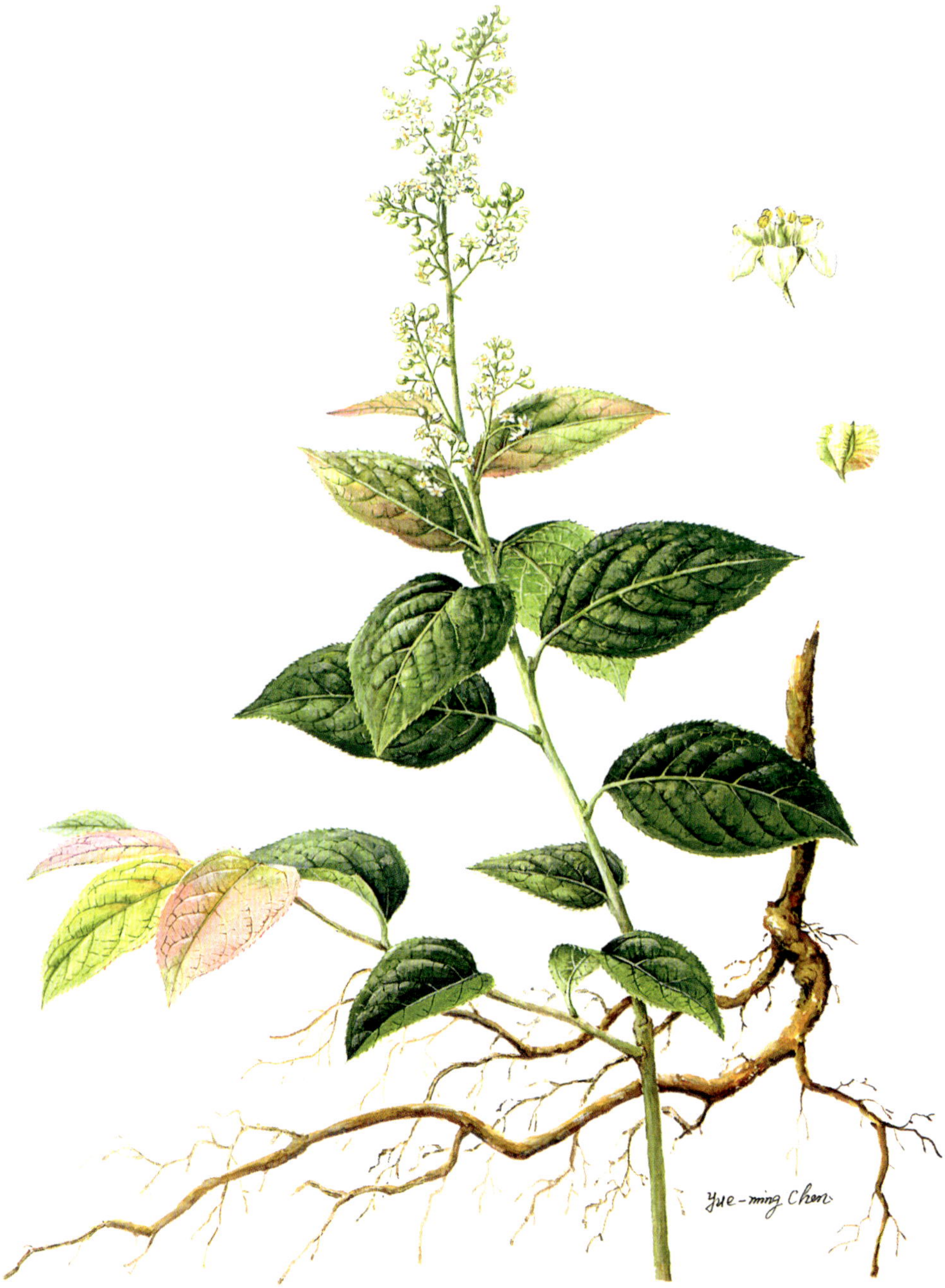


Fig. 11.155. ***Tripterygium wilfordii*** Hook. — This plant contains the alkaloids wilfordine, wilforgine, wilfortrine, wilforzine, and wilforine, the macrocyclic alkaloids celacemine, celabenzine, and celafurine, the epoxyditerpenes triptolide, tripdiolide, triptonide, triptonolide, and hypolide, tripterin (celastrol) and dulcitol, glucose and tannins. It inhibits murine cancers leukemia L-1210 and P-388, sarcoma-37, hepatoma, and Walker's carcinoma-256, prolongs the life of animals with leukemia L-615; in vitro it inhibits human nasopharyngeal cancer KB cells and cervical cancer-14, exhibits anti-tumor effects against human gastric cancer cells and mice carrying human breast tumors. It has been used in the treatment of leukemia and cancers of the esophagus, liver, and lung. (Chang & But, 1986; Minyi, 1992; Shamon, et al, 1997; Lee, 1999; Jiang, et al, 2001)

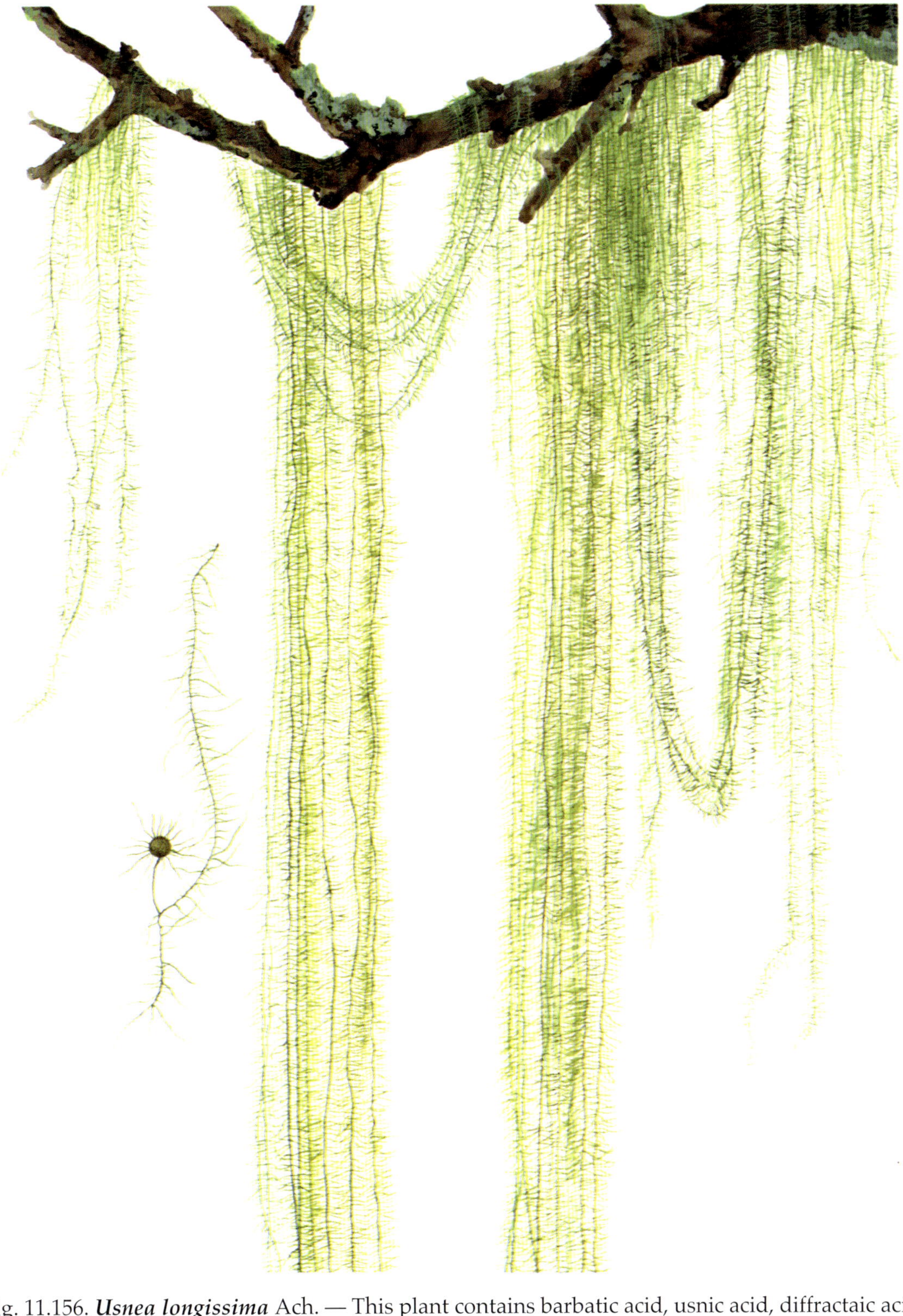

Fig. 11.156. ***Usnea longissima*** Ach. — This plant contains barbatic acid, usnic acid, diffractaic acid, ramalic acid, lichenin, and evernic acid and inhibits Erlich's ascites cells in rats (Hsu, et al, 1986).

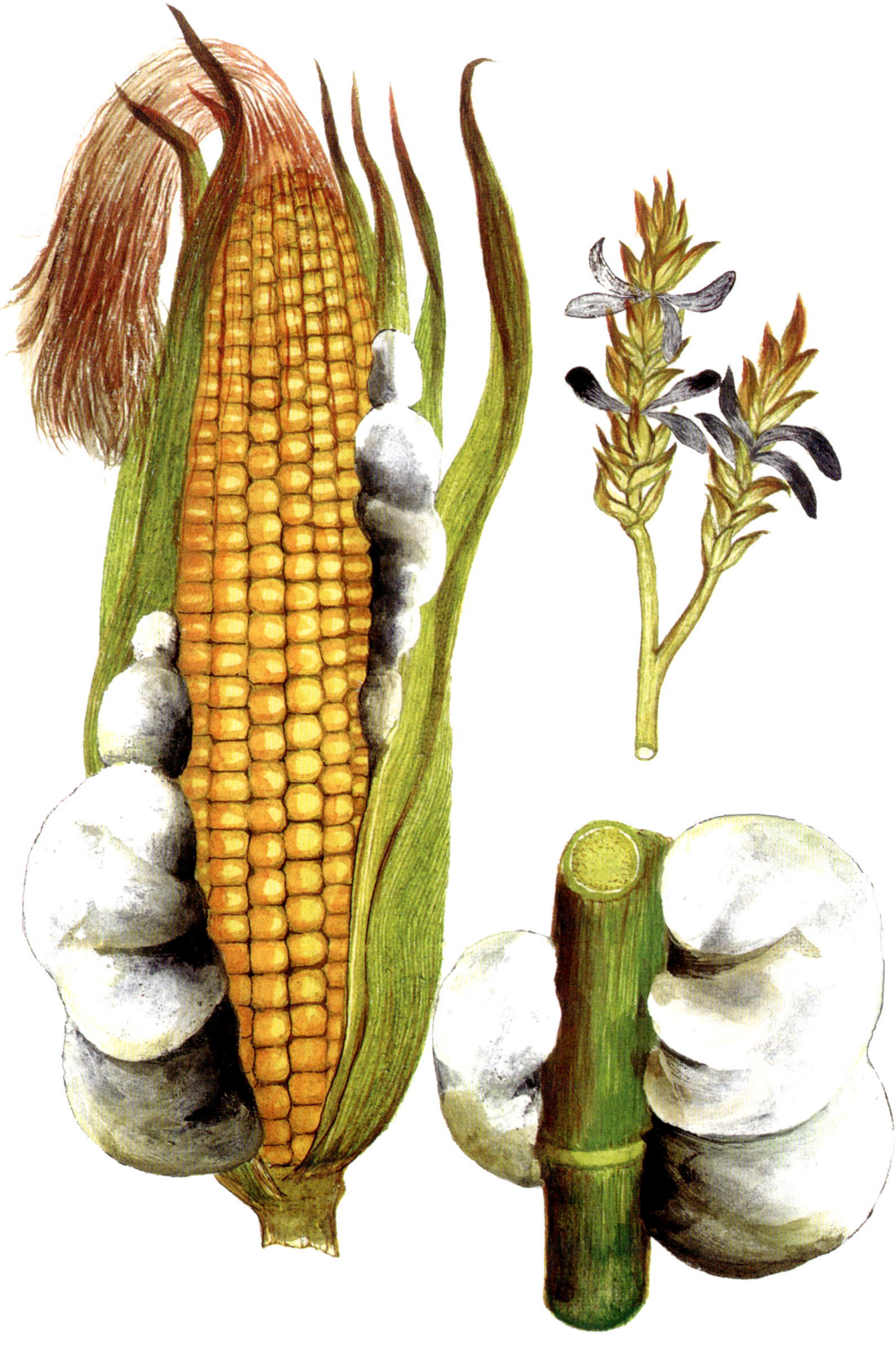

Fig. 11.157. ***Ustilago maydis*** (DC.) Corda — This fungus contains polysaccharides that inhibit sarcoma-180 in white mice (Ying, et al, 1987).

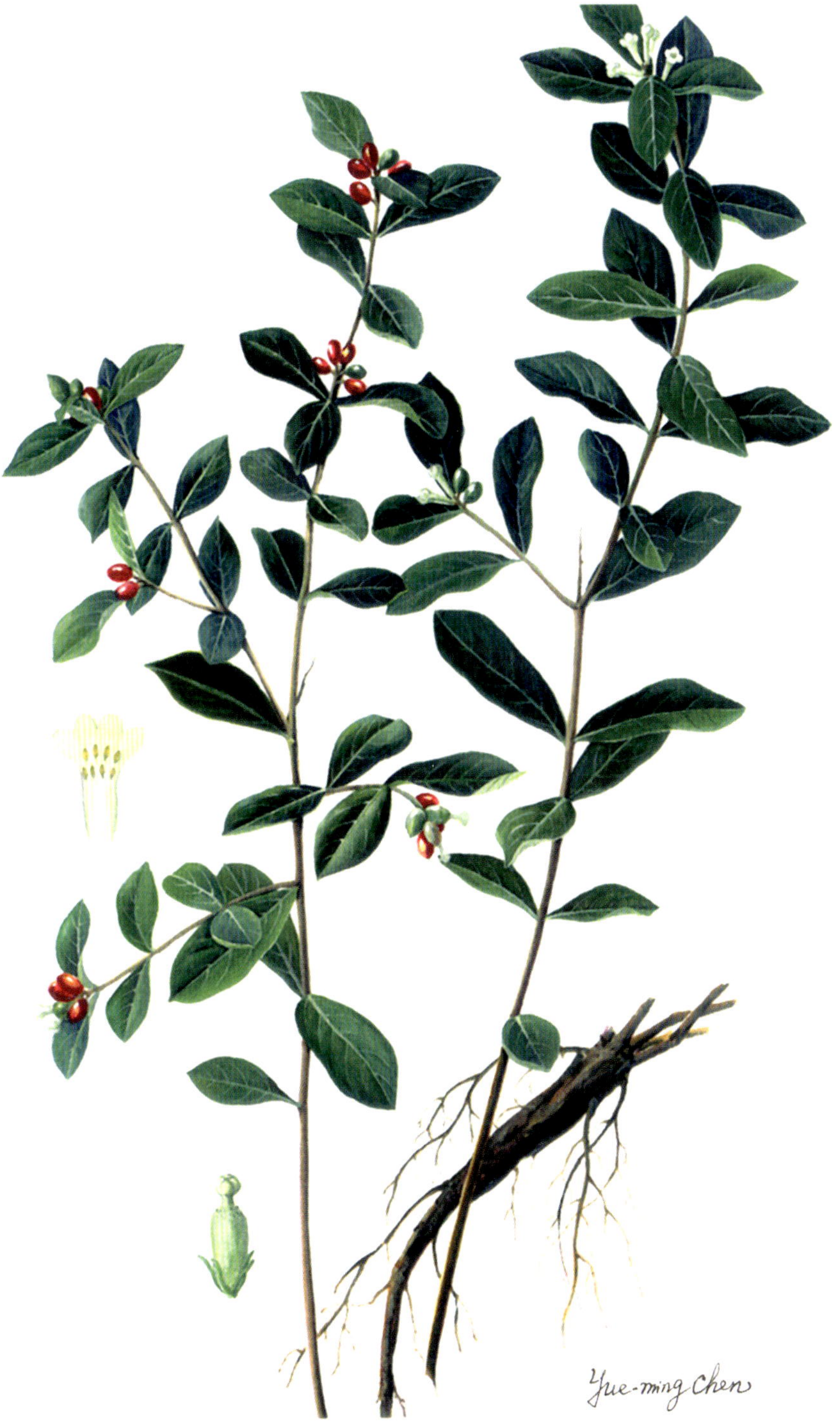


Fig. 11.158. ***Wikstroemia indica*** C. A. Meyer — This plant contains wikstroemin, daphnoretin, tricin, kaempferol-3-O-β-D-glucopyranoside, lignin, matairesinol, nortrachelogenin, and arctigenin. It inhibits lymphadenoma, cervical cancers, sarcoma-180, and Erlich's carcinoma in white mice, and has been used in the treatment of a variety of cancers including breast cancer, cervical cancer, lung cancer, liver cancer, and lymphoma. (Hsu, et al, 1986; Minyi, 1992; Lee, 1999)

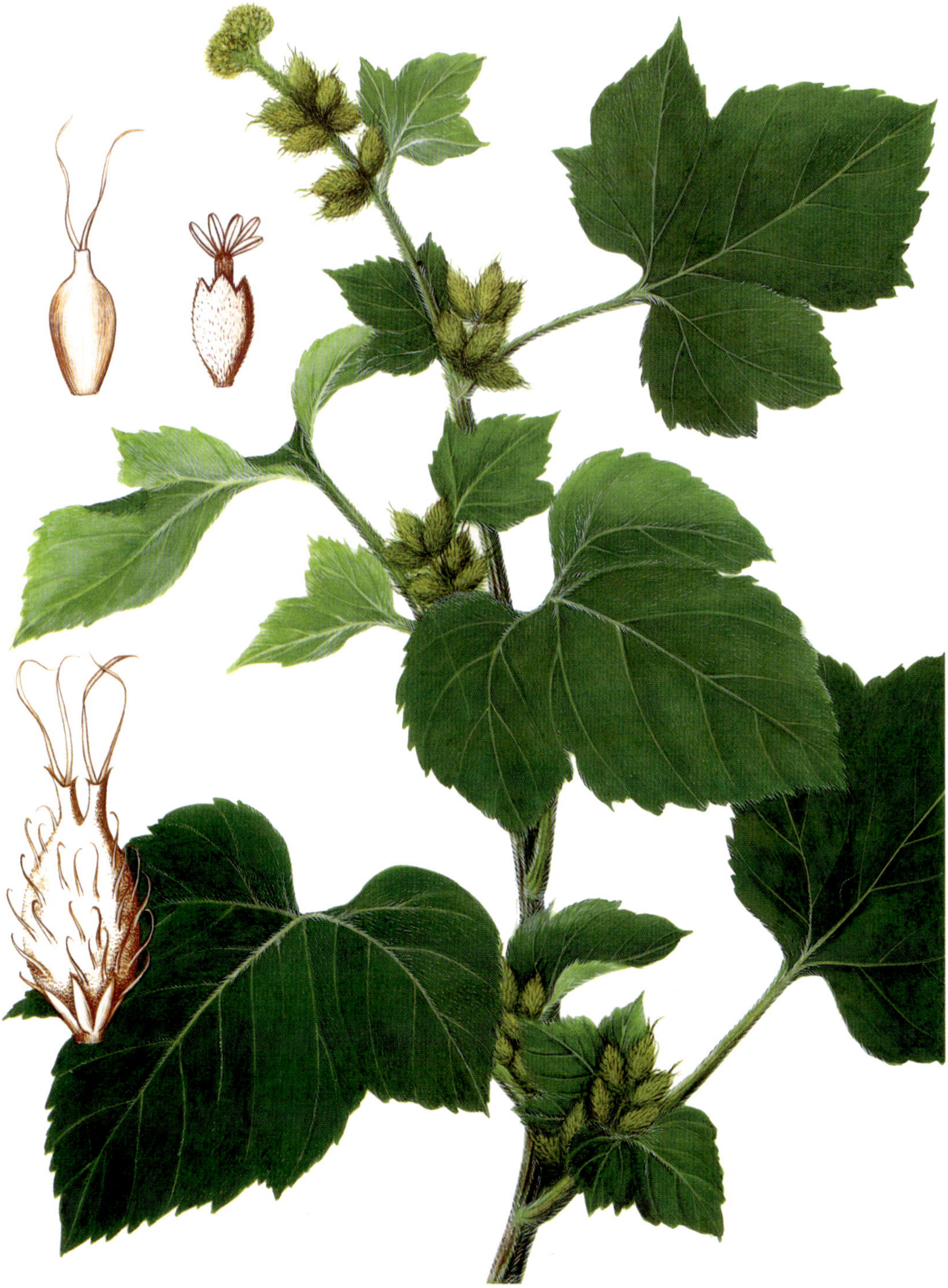

Fig. 11.159. ***Xanthium sibiricum*** Patrin. — This plant contains xanthostrumarin, β-sitosterol, xanthinol, glycosides, derivatives of chalcone, organic acids, yeasts, vitamin B, amylase, and essential oils. It inhibits sarcoma-180 in mice and JTC-26 in vivo, and can prolong the lifespan of mice with Erlich's carcinoma. It has been used in the treatment of nasopharyngeal carcinoma, thyroid adenocarcinoma, osteosarcoma, and brain tumors. (Hsu, et al, 1986; Minyi, 1992; Lee, 1999)

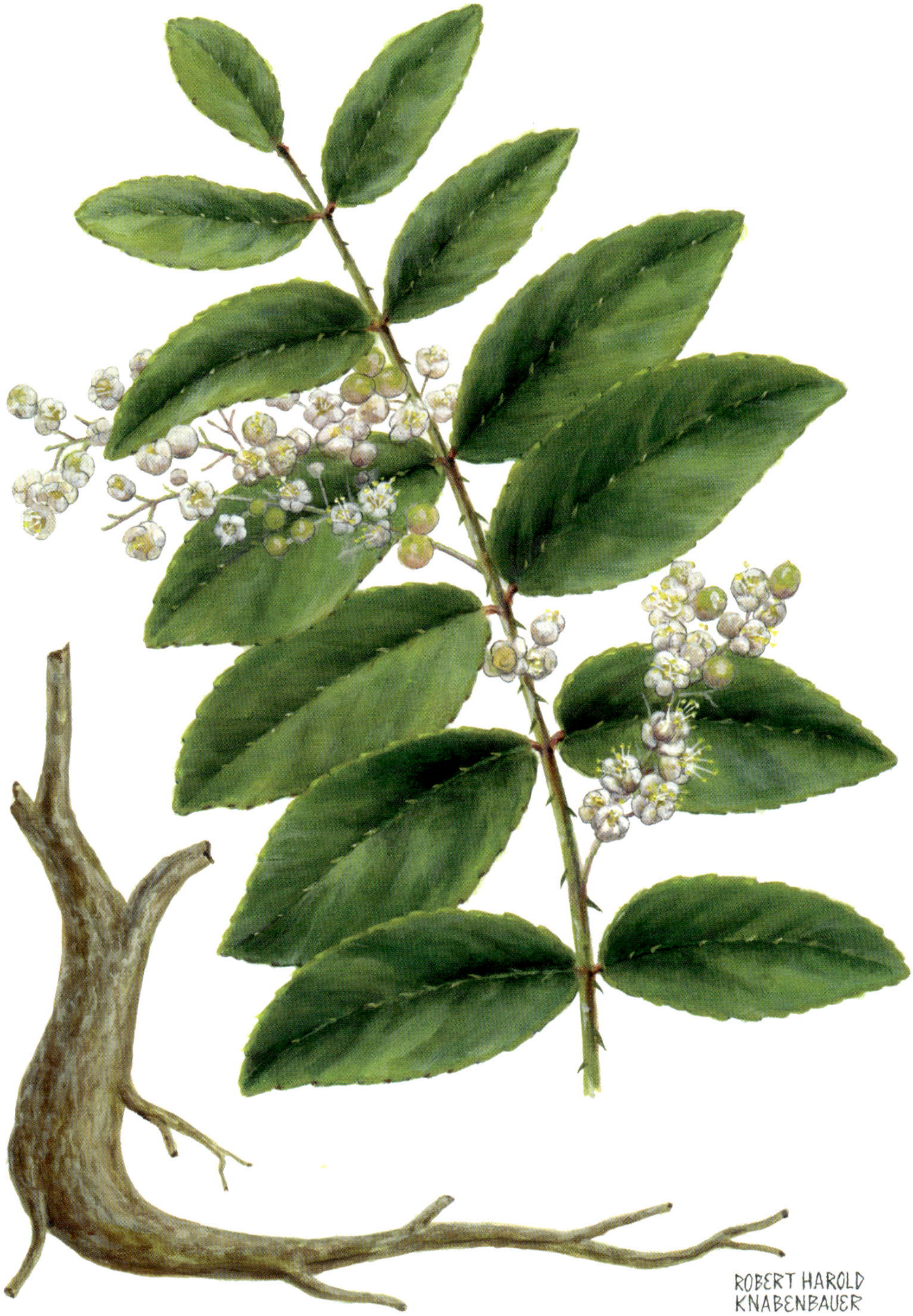


Fig. 11.160. ***Zanthoxylum nitidum*** (Roxb.) D.C. — The root contains the alkaloids nitidine, and oxynitidine, and diosmin; the leaves and nuts mainly contain volatile oils. It is effective against mouse leukemia L-1210 and P-388, lung carcinoma, Ehrlich's ascites carcinoma in rats, and sarcoma-180 in vitro and has been used to treat nasopharyngeal carcinoma. (Hsu, et al, 1986; Minyi, 1992; Huang, 1999)

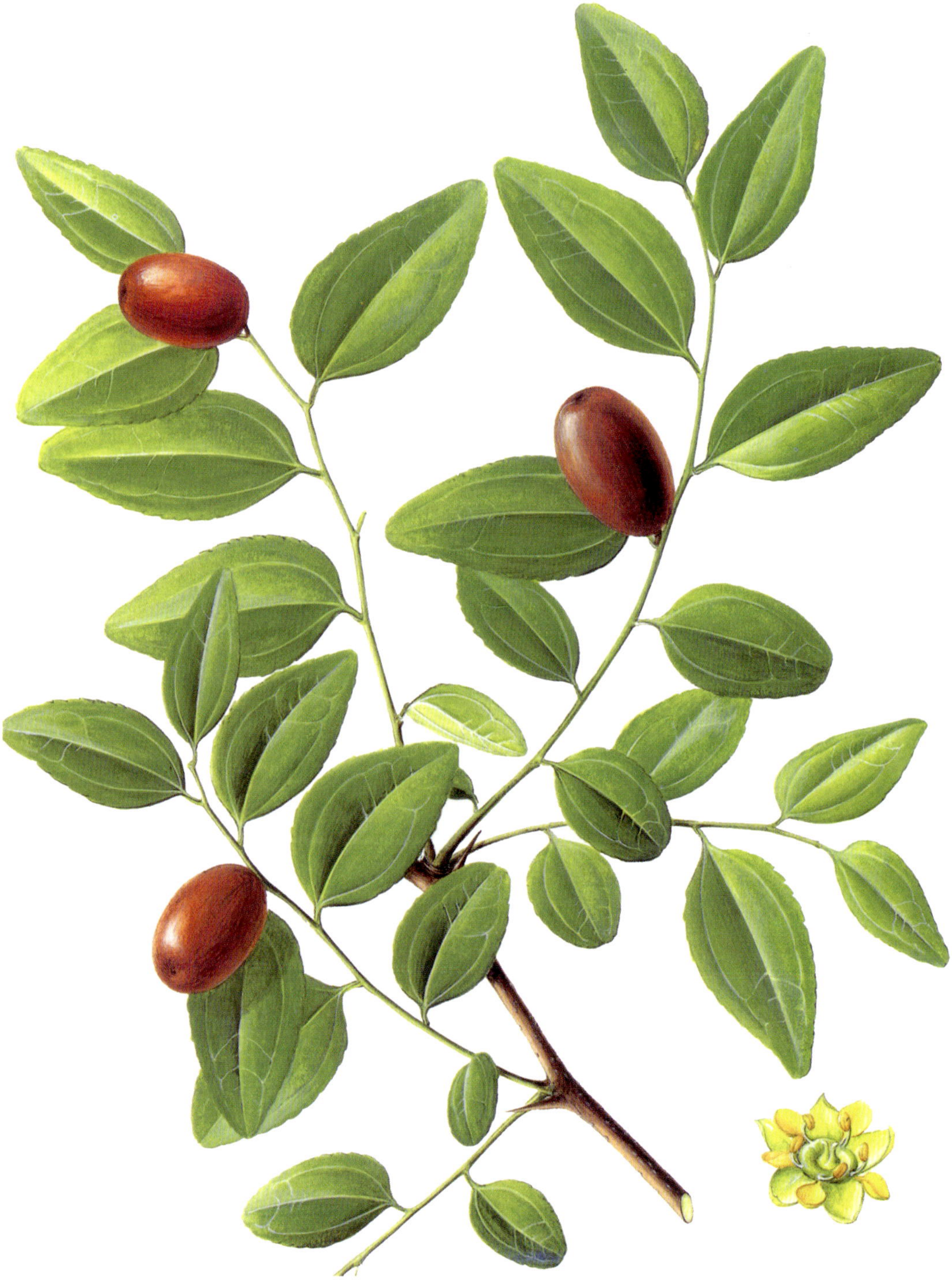

Fig. 11.161. ***Ziziphus jujuba*** Mill. — The fruit of this plant contains the saponon jujuboside, A, B, and C, the fatty acids myristic, palmitic, stearic, behenic, oleic, and linolenic acid, sitosterol, betulinic acid, betulin, crataegic acid, and cAMP. It inhibits sarcoma-180 and JTC-26 and has been used in the treatment of cervical cancer, cardiac cancer, and stomach cancer. (Hsu, et al, 1986; Minyi, 1992; Lee, 1999)

# Literature Cited


Ader, R.
1981 Psychoneuroimmunology. Academic Press, New York. 661 p.

Ader, R., Felten, D. L., and N. Cohen [Eds.]
1991 Psychoneuroimmunology. 2nd ed. Academic Press, New York. 1218 p.

Alexander, F.
1950 Psychsomatic medicine. Norton, New York. 300 p.

Ansher, S. S.
1983 Comparison of biochemical effects of BHA with those of dithiolthiones. UMI Dissertation Information Service, Michigan. 125 p.

Ansher, S. S., Dolan, P., and E. Bueding
1983 Chemoprotective effects of two dithiolthiones and of butylhydroxyanisole against carbon tetrachloride and acetaminophen toxicity. Hepatology 3(6):932-935.

Asai, K.
1980 Miracle cure. Japan Publications, Inc., Tokyo. 171 p.

Aso, H., Suzuki, F., Yamaguchi, T., et al.
1985 Induction of interferon and activation of NK cells and macrophages in mice by oral administration of Ge-132, an organic germanium compound. Microbiol. Immunol. 29(1):65-74.

Axelrod, A. E.
1971 Immune processes in vitamin deficiency states. Am. J. Clin. Nutr. 24:265-271.

Baron, S. and F. Dianzani
1977 The Interferon System: A Current Review to 1978. Univ. of Texas, Galveston. 35:1-573.

Beisel, W. R.
1975 The effects of malnutrition on immunological responses of the host: The key role of scarce amino acids. In: Western Hemisphere Nutritional Congress IV. Publ. Sci. Group, New York. pp. 313-318.
1979 Malnutrition and immune response. In: Int. Rev. Biochem. Biochemistry of Nutrition IA. [Eds.] Neuberger, A. and T.H. Jukes. Univ. Park Press, Baltimore. 27:1-19.
1980 Effects of infection on nutritional status and immunity. Fed. Proc. 39:3105-3108.

1981a Impact of infectious disease upon fat metabolism and immune functions. Cancer Res. 41:3797-3798.

1981b Iron nutrition: immunity and infection. Res. Staff Phys. pp. 37-42.

1982 Single nutrients and immunity. Am. J. Clin. Nutr. 35:417-468.

Beisel, W. R., Edelman, R., Nauss, K., et al.

1981 Single-nutrient effects on immunologicsfunctions. JAMA 245(1):53-58.

Bellanti, J. A.

1978 Immunology II. W. B. Saunders Co., Philadelphia. 813 p.

Benjamini, E. and S. Leskowitz

1991 Immunology: a short course. 2nd ed. Wiley Liss, NewYork. 459 p.

Berk, L. S., Tan, S.A., Fry, W. F., Napier, B. J., et al.

1989 Neuroendocrine and stress hormone changes during mirthful laughter. Am. J. Med. Sci. 298(6):390-396.

Berk, L. S., Tan, S. A., Napier, B. J., and W. C. Eby

1989 Eustress of mirthful laughter modifies natural killer cell activity. Clin. Res. 37(1):89.

Berk, L., Tan, S., and Fry, W.

1993 Eustress of humor associated laughter modulates specific immune system components. Annals of Behavioral Medicine 15 (Supplement): S111.

Borchers, A. T., Stern, J. S., Hackman, R. M., et al

1999 Mushrooms, tumors, and immunity. Proc. Soc. Exp. Biol. Med. 221(4):281-293.

Boyd, W.

1966 The spontaneous regression of cancer. Charles C. Thomas Publisher, Springfield. 99 p.

Brekhman, I.

1968 *Eleutherococcus*. Nauka Publishing House, Leningrad, U.S.S.R. 186 p.

1982 Personal communication to Bruce W. Halstead.

Bueding, E.

1983 Personal communication to Bruce W. Halstead.

Bueding, E., Ansher, S., and P. Dolan

1985 Anticarcinogenic and other protective effects of diothiolthiones. pp. 483-489. In: Antimutagenesis and anticarcinogenesis mechanisms. [Eds.] Shankel, D. M, Hartman, P.E., Kada, T. et al. Plenum Press, New York.

Carney, D. and K. Sikora
1990 Genes and cancer. John Wiley and Sons, New York. 348 p.

Castegnaro, M. and E. B. Sansone
1986 Chemical carcinogens. Some guidelines for handling and disposal in the laboratory. Springer-Verlag, New York. 97 p.

Chandra, R. K.
1980 Cell-mediated immunity in nutritional imbalance. Nutrition, immune response, and infectious illness. Fed. Proc. 39(13):3088-3092.
1981 Immunodeficiency in undernutrition and overnutrition. Nutrition Reviews 39(6):225-231.
1992 Effect of vitamin and trace element supplement on immune responses and infection in elderly subjects. Lancet 340:1124-1127.

Chang, H.-M. and P. P.-H. But
1986 Pharmacology and applications of Chinese materia medica. 1:1-773.
1987 Ibid 2: 775- 1320. World Scientific Publishing Co., Singapore.

Chang, J. S., Chiang, L. C., Chen, C. C., et al
2001 Antileukemic activity of *Bidens pilosula* L. var *minor* (Blume) Sherff and *Houttuynia cordata* Thunb.Am. J. Chin. Med. 29(2):303-312.

Chang, W. C., Lin Y. L., Lee, M. J., et al
1996 Inhibitory effect of crocetin on benzo(a)pyrene genotoxicity and neoplastic transformation in C3H10T1/2 cells. Anticancer Res. 16(6B):3603-3608.

Cheung, C. S. and H. E. Harrison
1983 Herbs that promote various types of immune responses. J. Am. Coll. Trad. Chinese Med. 2:21-23.

Cheung, S.-C. and N.-H. Li
1979 Chinese Medicinal Herbs of Hong Kong.

Chiang, H. C., Jaw, S. M. and P. M. Chen
1991 Inhibitory effects of physalin B and physalin F on various human leukemia cells in vitro. Anticancer Res. 12(4):1155-1162.

Ching-wei, L.
1999 General history of Chinese medicine. Peoples Medical Publishing House, Beijing. 545 p.

Chung, C. S.
1996 - 2001 Chinese color herbal drawings, 3 vols. Peoples Health Group, Beijing, China.

Cody, V., Middleton, E., and J. Harborne [Eds.]
1985 Plant flavonoids in biology and medicine. Biochemical, pharmacological, and structure-activity relationships. Alan R. Liss, New York. 558 p.

Cohen, B.I. and R.F. Raicht
1981 Plant sterols: Protective role in chemical carcinogenesis. In: Inhibition of tumor induction and development. [Eds.] M. S. Zedeck and M. Lipkin. Plenum Press, New York. 189-201.

Colburn, N. H.
1989 Chemical carcinogens. Some guidelines for handling and disposal in the laboratory. Springer-Verlag, New York. 97 p.

Cooper, G. M.
1992 Elements of human cancer. Jones and Bartlett Publishers, Boston. 354 p.

Cousins, N.
1979a Anatomy of an illness as perceived by a patient. W. W. Norton & Co., New York. 173 p.
1979b Stress. J. Am. Med. Assoc. 242:459.
1981 Human options. Berkley Books, New York. 224 p.
1983a The healing heart: antidotes to panic and helplessness. W. W. Norton & Co., New York. 288 p.
1983b Save your life. Donning Publishers, Virginia Beach. 304 p.

Culbert, M. L.
1994 Medical Armageddon. C & C Communications, San Diego, CA. Vol. 1&2:1-324; Vol. 3&4:325-707.

Culotta, E. and D. E. Koshland
1993 Emerging infections. Science 262(5142):1961.

Davis, D. L., Hoel, D., Fox, J. and A. Lopez
1990 International trends in cancer mortality in France, West Germany, Italy, Japan, England, Wales, and the USA. Lancet 336:474-481.

Davydov, M. and A. D. Krikorian
2000 *Eleutherococcus senticosus* (Rupr. & Maxim.) Maxim. (Araliaceae) as an adaptogen: a closer look. J. Ethno-Pharm. 72: 345-393.

Dubos, R.
1961 Mirage of health. Double Day, New York. 245 p.

Duke, J. A. and E. S. Ayensu
1985 Medicinal plants of China. (2 vols.) Reference Publications, Inc., Algonac, MI. 705 p.

Duke, J. and K. W. Wain
1981 Plant cancer file. Computerized by Economic Botany Laboratory, U.S. Department of Agriculture, Beltsville, MD. 278 p.

Dunbar, H. F.
1943 Psychosomatic diagnosis. Harper, New York. 741 p.

Duong, N.
1993 Medicinal Plants of Vietnam, Cambodia and Laos. Mekong Printing. SantaAna, CA. 528 p.

Engel, G. L.
1954 Selection of clinical material in psychosomatic medicine. Psychosomatic Med. 16:368-373.
1977 The need for a new medical model: a challenge for biomedicine. Science 196:129-136.

Ensminger, A. H., Ensminger, M. E., Konlande, J. E. et al
1982 Foods and nutrition encyclopedia. Pegus Press, Clovis. 1:1-1208; 2:1209-2415 p.

Everson, T. C. and W. H. Cole
1966 Spontaneous regression of cancer. W. B. Saunders Co., Philadelphia. 560 p.

Farkas, L., Gábor, M., and F. Killay [Eds.]
1974 Topics in flavonoid chemistry and biochemistry. Akadémiai Kiadó, Budapest. 286 p.

Farmer, P. B. and J. M. Walker
1985 The molecular basis of cancer. Croom Helm, London. 349 p.

Farnsworth, N. R., Akerele, O., Bingle, A. S., et al
1985 Medicinal plants in therapy. Bull. World Hlth. Org. 63(6):965-981.

Fasching, R.
1994 Tea fungus kombucha. The natural remedy and its significance in cases of cancer and other metabolic diseases. Publishing House Wilhelm Ennsthaler, Steyr, Austria. 55 p.

Fauvet, J. Roujeau, J. and R. Piet
1964 Lés Guérisons spontanées des cancers. La Revue du Practicien. 14:2177-2180.

Flavin, D. F. and A. C. Kolbe
1982 Nutritional Factors with the potential to inhabit critical pathways of tumor promotion. Proc. First Int. Symp. Modulation and Mediation of Cancer by Vitamins. Univ. Arizona Med. Center. Karger Publishing, Basel. 29 p.

Frank, G. W.
1994 Kombucha. Healthy beverage and natural remedy from the Far East. Wilhelm Ennsthaler, Steyr, Austria. 150 p.

Franks, L. M. and N. M. Teich
1991 Introduction to the cellular and molecular biology of cancer. 2nd ed. Oxford Medical Publishers, New York. 558 p.

Fundenberg, H. H., Stites, D. P., Caldwell, J. L. and J. V. Wells
1980 Basic & clinical immunology. 3rd ed. Lange Medical Publishers, Los Altos, CA. 782 p.

Gansauge, F. Ramadani, M. Pressmar, J., et al
2002 NSC-631570 (Ukrain) in the palliative treatment of pancreatic cancer. Result of a phase II trial. Lagenbecks Arch. Surg. 386(8):570-574.

Gao, Y. T., McLaughlin, J. K., Blot, W. J., et al
1994 Reduced risk of esophageal cancer associated with green tea consumption. J. Natl. Can. Inst. 86:855-858.

Garrett, L.
1994 The coming plague: newly emerging diseases in a world out of balance. Farrar, Straus and Giroux, New York. 750 p.

Geng, C.-S., Xing, S.-T., Zhou, J.-H., et al.
1989 Enhancing effect of *Lycium barbarum* polysaccharides on the interleukin-2 activity in mice. Chinese J. Pharm. Tox. 3(3):175-179.

Goldberg, B.
1993 Alternative medicine: the definitive guide. Future Medicine Publ., Puyallup, WA. 1068 p.

Gomatos, P. J., Stamatos, N. M., and R. T. Schooley
1992 Soluble CD4, immunomodulators, immunotoxins, and other approaches to anti-HIV therapy. In: AIDS. Etiology, diagnosis, treatment and prevention. 3rd ed. [Eds.] DeVita, V. T., Hellman, S., and S. A. Rosenberg. Lippincott Co., Philadelphia. pp. 406-415.

Good, R.
1981 Nutrition and immunity. J. Clin. Immu. 1(1):3-11.

Gottlieb, M. S., Wolfe, P. R. and R. Mitsuyasu
1985 Immunotherapy of the acquired immune deficiency syndrome. In: Advances in host defense mechanisms. Acquired immunodeficiency syndrome (AIDS). [Eds.] Gallin, J. L. and A. Fauci. Raven Press, New York. 5:149-170.

Graber, C. D., Goust, J. M., Glassman, A.D., et al.
1981 Immunmodulating properties of dimethylglycine in humans. J. Infect. Dis. 143(1):101-105.

Hadden, J. W. and W. E. Stewart
1981 Contemporary immunology—the lymphokines: biochemistry and biological activity. Humana Press, Cliften. 437 p.

Halliwell, B. and J. M. C. Gutteridge
1989 Free radical in biology and medicine. 2nd ed. Oxford University Press, New York. 543 p.

Halstead, B. W.
1977 Amygdalin (Laetrile) therapy. Golden Quill Publishers, Inc., Colton, CA. 7 p.

Halstead, B. W. and L. L. Hood
1980 Need for the translation of the *Pen Ts'ao Kang Mu*, the Great Herbal of China. Bull. Orient. Heal. Arts Inst. 5(7):19-43.
1984a *Eleutherococcus senticosus*. An introduction to the concept of adaptogenic medicine. Oriental Healing Arts Institute of USA, Long Beach, CA. 94 p.
1984b Natural methods to enhance immunity. Bull. Oriental Healing Arts Institute of USA 9(8):371-411.

Halstead, B. W. and T. C. Rozema
1997 The scientific basis of EDTA chelation therapy. TRC Publishing, Landrum, SC. 267 p.

Harborne, J. B. [Ed.]
1994 The flavonoids: advances in research since 1986. Chapman and Hall, London. 676 p.

Hartwell, J.
1982 Plants used against cancer. Quarterman Pubs., Lawrence, MA. 709 p.

Hayatsu, H., Arimoto, S. and T. Negishi
1988 Dietary inhibitors of mutagenesis and carcinogenesis. Mutat. Res. 202:429-446.

Higginson, J., Muir, C. S. and N. Muñoz
1992 Human cancer: epidemiology and environmental causes. Cambridge Univ. Press, Cambridge. 577 p.

Hokama, Y. and R. M. Nakamura
1982 Immunology and immunopathology basic concepts. Little Brown & Co., Boston. 528 p.

Hsu, H.-Y.
1979 Chinese herb therapy for chronic and recalcitrant diseases. Cancer. New Medico-Pharmacological Press. Taipei, Taiwan. Vol. 2:1-111.

Hsu, H.-Y., Chen, Y.-P., Shen, S., Hsu, C.-C., and H. Chang
1986 Oriental materia medica: a concise guide. Oriental Healing Arts Institute, Long Beach, CA. 932 p.

Hsu, H., Chen, Y. and M. Hong
1980 The chemical constituents of oriental herbs. Oriental Healing Arts Institute, Taiwan. 1546 p.

Hsu, H.-Y. and C.-S. Hsu
1980 Commonly used Chinese herbal formulas with illustrations. Orient. Heal. Arts Inst., Long Beach, CA. 671 p.

Huang, K. C.
1999 The pharmacology of Chinese herbs. CRC Press, Boca Raton, FL. 511 p.

Ikekawa, T., Maruyama, H., Miyano, T., et al
1985 Proflamin, a new antitumor agent: preparation, physiochemical properties and antitumor activity. Jpn J. Cancer Res. 76(2):142-148.

Iversen, O. H. [Ed.]
1988 Theories of carcinogenesis. Hemisphere Publ. Corp., New York. 327 p.
1993 New frontiers in cancer causation. Proceedings of the 2nd International Conference on Theories of Carcinogenesis. Taylor and Francis, Washington, D.C. 444 p.

Jiang, X.H., Wong, B.C., Lin, M.C., Zhu, G.H., et al
2001 Functional p53 is required for triptolide-induced apoptosis and AP-1 and nuclear factor-kappa B activation in gastric cancer cells. Oncogene 20(55):8009-8018.

Jirousek, L.
1958 Über papierchromatographische trennung von trithionen. Kurze Originalmitt. 9(45):211-212

Jirousek, L. and L. Starka
1958 Über das vorkommen von trithionen (1,2-dithiacyclopent-4-en-3-thione) in Brassicapflanzen. Naturwiss. 16(45):386-387

Katz, M., Desommier, D. D. and R. Gwadz
1982 Parasitic diseases. Springer-Verlag, New York. 264 p.

Kim, J. H., Lee, S. J., Han, Y. B., et al
1994 Isolation of isoguanosine from *Croton tiglium* and its antitumor activity. Arch. Pharm. Res. 17(2):115-118.

Kim, S. K., Ryu, S. Y., No, J., et al
2001 Cytotoxic alkaloids from *Houttuynia cordata*. Arch. Pharm. Res. 24(6):518-521.

Kojima, Y., et al
1984 Interferon inducing plants. U.S. Patent No. 4,469,685. 6 p.

Kühnau, J.
1976 The flavenoids: a class of semi-essential food components. Their role in human nutrition. Wld. Rev. Nutr. Diet. 24:117-191.

Kun, J.
1985 Carcinoma. Commercial Press, Hong Kong. 231 p.

Latha, P. G., Evans, D. A., Panikkar, K. R. and K. K. Jayavardhanan
2000 Immunomodulatory and antitumor properties of *Psoralea corylifolia* seeds. Fitoterapia 71(3):223-231.

Lee, T. H.
1999 Colour atlas of anticancer animal, plant and mineral preparations and their applications (in Chinese). Tianjin Science and Technology Translation Publishing, Corp., Tianjin, China. 352 p.

Lesser, M.
1977 Nutrition and vitamin therapy. Grove Press, New York. 240 p.

Leung, M. Y., Fung, K. P. and Y. M. Choy
1997 The isolation and characterization of an immunomodulatory and antitumor polysacchardide preparation from *Flammulina velutipes*. Immunopharmacolgy 35(3):255-263.

Levine, S. A. and P. M. Kidd
1994 Antioxidant adaptation. Its role in free radical pathology. Allergy Research Group, San Leandro, CA. 367 p.

Li, S. C.
2002 Chinese and related North American herbs. CRC Press, Boca Raton, FL. 598 p.

List, P. H. and P. C. Schmidt
1990 Phytopharmaceutical technology. CRC Press, Boca Raton, FL. 374 p.

Locke, S., Ader, R., Besedovsky, H., et al
1985 Foundations of psychoneuroimmunology. Aldine Publishing, New York. 480 p.

Lu, C. X. and B. Q. Cheng
1991 Radiosensitizing effects of *Lycium barbarum* polysaccharide for Lewis lung cancer. Zhong Xi Yi Jie He Za Zhi 11(10):611-2, 582

Luoh, H-S
1981 Frequently used Chinese medicinal materials for antineoplasms. Kwantung Science and Technical Publication Department, Kwantung, China. 248 p. (In Chinese)

MacDonald, F. and C. H. Ford
1991 Oncogenes and tumor suppressor genes. Medical Perspectives Series. [Eds.] A. P. Read and T. Brown. BIOS Scientific Publications, Oxford. 101 p.

Marshall, E.
1990 Experts clash over cancer data. Science. 250:900-902.

McBrien, D. C. H. and T. F. Slater [Eds.]
1982 Free radicals, lipid peroxidation and cancer. Academic Press, New York. 477 p.

Merck Index
1989 The Merck Index: an encyclopedia of chemicals, drugs, and biologicals. 11th ed. Merck and Co., Rahway, NJ. 1606 p.

Merigan, T. C. and R. M. Friedman
1982 Interferons. UCLA Symposium on Molecular and Cellular Biology. 25:1-81. Academic Press, New York.

Minyi, C.
1992 Anticancer Medicinal Plants. Hunan Science and Technology Publishing House. Hunan Changsba, China. 308 p.

Miyazawa, M., Okuno, Y., Nakamura, S. and H. Kosaka
2001 Antimutagenic activity of flavonoids from *Pogostemon cablin*. J. Agric. Food Chem. 48(3):642-647.

Mukhtar, H., Wang, Z. Y., Katiyar, S. K., et al
1992 Tea components: antimutagenic and anticarcinogenic effects. Prev. Med. 21: 351-360.

Mukhtar, H., Katiyar, S. K. and R. Aga-rwal
1994 Green tea and skin-anticarcinogenic effects. J. Soc. Invest. Dermat. 102(l):3-7.

Needham, J.
1980 China and the origins of immunology. Centre of Asian Studies, University of Hong Kong. 33 p.

NRC
1982 Diet, nutrition and cancer. National Academy Press, Washington, D.C. 463 p.

Oh, G. S., Pae, O. H., Oh, H., et al
2001 In vitro anti-proliferative effect of 1,2,3,4,6-penta-O-galloyl-beta-D-glucose on human hepatocellular carcinoma cell line, SK-HEP-1 cells. Cancer Lett. 174(1):17-24.

O'Regan, B. and C. Hirschberg
1993 Spontaneous remission. An annotated bibliography. Institute of Noetic Sciences, Sausalito, CA. 713 p.

Pharmacopeia Commission of the Ministry of Public Health P.R.C.
1998 Colored atlas of microscopic identification of Chinese materia medica in powdered form as specified in pharmacopeia of the People's Republic of China. Guangdong Science and Technology Press, Guangdong. 390 p.

Pizzarello, D. J. and R. L. Witcofski
1975 Basic Radiation Biology. 2nd ed. Lea and Febriger, Philadelphia. 143 p.

Plaut, S. M. and S. B. Friedman
1981 Psychosocial factors in infectious disease. In: Psychoneuroimmunology. [Ed] Alder, R. pp. 3-30. Academic Press, New York.

Porkert, M.
1979 The theoretical foundations of Chinese medicine: systems of correspondence. The MIT Press, Cambridge, MA. 368 p.

Prochaska, H. J., Santamaria, A. B. and P. Talalay
1992 Rapid detection of inducers of enzymes that protect against carcinogens. Proc. Natl. Acad. Sci. 89:2394-2398.

Reid, D. R.
1987 Chinese herbal medicine. C. F. W. Publications, Ltd., Hong Kong. 174 p.

Roitt, I. M.
1994 Essential Immunology. 8th ed. Blackwell Sci. Publ., Oxford. 448 p.

Roitt, I. M., Brostoff, J. and D. Male
1993 Immunology. 3rd ed. Mosby-Year Book, London. 381 p.

Ruddon, R. W.
1987 Cancer biology. Oxford Univ. Press, New York. 530 p.

Sakamoto, S., Yoshino, H., Shirahata, Y, et al
1992 Pharmacotherapeutic effects of kuei-chih-fu-ling-wan (keishi-bukuryo-gan) on human uterine myomas. Am. J. Chin. Med. 20(3-4):313-317.

Sarma, R. H. and M. H. Sarma
1988 DNA double helix and the chemistry of cancer. Adenine Press, New York. 254 p.

Sartippour, M. R., Liu, C., Shao, Z. M., et al
2001 *Livistona* extract inhibits angiogenesis and cancer growth. Oncol. Rep. 8(6):1355-1357.

Schindler, L. W.
1988 Understanding the immune system. Nat. Inst. Htlth. Publ. No. 88-529:1-36. U.S. Dept. Health and Human Services.

Searle, C. E.
1984 Chemical carcinogens. 2nd ed. ACS Monograph 182. American Chemical Society, Washington, D.C. 1:1-642, 2:643-137.

Selye, H.
1946 The general adaptation syndrome and the diseases of adaptation. J. Clin. Endocrinol. 6:117-230.
1973 The evolution of the stress concept. Amer. Scient. 61:692-699.

Shamon, L. A., Pezzuto, J.M., Graves, J.M., et al
1997 Evaluation of the mutagenic, cytotoxic, and antitumor pontential of triptolide, a highly oxygenated diterpene isolated from *Tripterygium wilfordii*. Cancer Lett. 112(1):113-117.

Sikora, K. Evan, G. and J. V. Watson
1991 The cancer cell. Brit. Med. Bull. 47(1):1-250p.

Silverstein, A. M.
1989 A history of immunology. Academic Press, New York. 422 p.

Siu- Cheong, C.
1978 Chinese medicinal herbs of Hong Kong. 5 vols. Hong Kong.

Song, J. Y., Yang, H. O., Pyo, S. N., et al
2002 Immunomodulatory activity of protein-bound polysaccharide extracted from *Chelidonium majus*. Arc. Pharm. Res. 25(2):158-164.

Spitz, M.R. and G.R. Newell
1992 Recommendations for cancer prevention. The University of Texas. Anderson Cancer Center. Mosby Year Book, St. Louis. 225 p.

Stites, D. P., Stobo, J. B. and J. V. Wells
1987 Basic and clinical immunology. 6th ed. Appleton and Lange, Los Altos, CA. 734 p.

Sun, A., Chia, J.-S., Wang, W.-B. and C.-P. Chiang
2004 Immunomodulating effects of "Tien-Hsien Liquid" on peripheral blood mononuclear cells and T-lymphocytes from patients with recurrent aphthous ulcerations. Am. J. of Chinese Med. 32(2):221-224.
2005 "Tien Hsien Liquid" can modulate antigen-stimulated cytokine production by T-cells from patients with recurrent aphthous ulcerations. Am. J. of Chinese Med. 33:559-571.

Sun, A., Chia, J.-S., Chiang, C.-P., Hsuen, S.-P., Du, J.-L. and W.-B. Wang
2005 The Chinese herbal medicine Tien-Hsien Liquid inhibits cell growth and induces apoptosis in a wide variety of human cancer cells. J. of Alternative and Comp. Med. 11(2):245-256.

Suzuki, I., Sakurai, T., Hasimoto, K., et al
1991 Inhibition of experimental pulmonary metastasis of Lewis lung carcinoma by orally administered beta-glucan in mice. Chem. Pharm. Bull. (Tokyo) 39(6):1606-1608.

Taylor-Papadimitriou, J [Ed.]
1985 Interferons. Their impact in biology and medicine. Oxford University Press, New York. 148 p.

Torrence, P. F.
1985 Biological response modifiers. New approaches to disease intervention. Academic Press, New York. 397 p.

Troll, W.
1980 Blocking of tumor promotion by protease inhibitors. In: Cancer: achievements, challenges and prospects for the 1980's. [Eds.] Burchenal, J. H. and H. F. Oettgen, New York. 1:549-555.

Tsung, P.-k.
1987 Anticancer and immunostimulating polysaccharides. Orient. Heal. Arts Intern. Bull. 12(1):1-10.
1989 Immune system and Chinese herbs. Institute of Chinese Herbs, Irvine, CA. 205 p.

Tsung, P.-k. and H.-y. Hsu
1986 Immunology and Chinese herbal medicine. Orient. Heal. Arts Inst., Long Beach, CA. 22 p.

Wagner, H. and A. Proksch
1985 Immunostimulatory drugs of fungi and higher plants. [English Translation] Econ. Med. Plant. Res. 1:113-153.

Wakeman, B. H.
1980 Adjuvants and immune regulation by lymphoid cells. In: Immunostimulation. [Eds.] Chedid, L., Miescher, P. A. and H. J. Mueller-Eberhard. Springer Verlag, New York. pp. 5-33.

Wallnöfer, H. and A. von Rottauscher
1965 Chinese folk medicine. Crown Publishing Co. 184 p.

Wang, C.-K.
2001 The cancer terminator. Live stories of 100 cancer sufferers. Chow Hoi Tong Cultural Enterprise, Hong Kong. 356 p.

Waring, M. J. and B. Ponder [Eds.]
1987 Biology of carcinogenesis. Cancer biology and medicine series. MTP Press, Norwell, MA. 229 p.

Wattenberg, L. W. and J. Loub
1978 Inhibition of polycyclic hydrocarbon-induced neoplasia by naturally occurring indoles. Cancer Res. 38:1410-1413.

Wattenberg, L. W., Coccia, J. B. and K. T. L. Lam
1979 Inhibitory effects of phenolic compounds on benzo(a)pyrene-induced neoplasia. Canc. Res. 40:2820-2823.

Waxman, J. and K. Sikora
1989 The molecular biology of cancer. Blackwell Scientific Publications, Oxford, England. 160 p.

WHO
1983 Traditional Medicine and Health Care Coverage. [Eds. R.H. Bannerman, J. and Ch'en W-C.] World Health Organization, Geneva. 342 p.

Wiart, C.
2000 Medicinal plants of Southeast Asia. Pelanduk Publictions, Selangor Darul Ehsan, Malaysia. 199 p.

Wijesekera, R. O. B.
1991 The medicinal plant industry. CRC Press, Boca Raton, FL. 269 p.

Wong, C. K., Leung, K. N., Fung, K. P. and Y. M. Choy
1994 The immunostimulating activities of anti-tumor polysaccharides from *Pseudostellaria heterophylla*. Int. J. Immunopharmacol. 16(4):271-277.

Wong, K. C. and L.-T. Wu
1977 Chinese medicine series 7. History of Chinese Medicine. Southern Materials Center, People's Republic of China. 906 p.

Wu, Y.
1993 Scavenging action of green tea extracts on singlet oxygen and prevention effect on lipid peroxidation. Chung Kuo I Hsueh Ko Hsueh Yuan Hsueh Pao. 15:354-359.

Xie, Z. and X. Huang
1984 Dictionary of traditional Chinese medicine. Commercial Press, Hong Kong. 428 p.

Yang, C. H.
1981 Chinese herbal medicine for anti-neoplasms. People's Public Health Publication Press, Peking. 348 p. (in Chinese)

Yeo-ruenn, L.
1994 A new compendium of materia medica. Pharmaceutical botany and Chinese medicinal plants. Science Press, Beijing. 292 p.

Ying, J., Mao, X., Ma, Q., Zong, Y. and H. Wen
1987 Icones of medicinal fungi from China. Science Press, Beijing, China. 575 p.

Yu, T. X., Ma, R. D. and L. J. Yu
2001 Structure-activity relationship of tubeimosides in anti-inflammatory, antitumor, and antitumor promoting effects. Acta. Pharmacol. Sin. 22(5):463-468.

Zhan, H., Liu, C.-G. and J.-H. Zhou
1989 Protective effects of *Lycium barbarum* polysaccharide against physical stress and $CCl_4$-induced tissue lipid metabolism changes in rats and mice. Chinese J. Pharm. Toxicol. 3(3):163-167.

Zhang, Y., Talalay, P., Cho, C.-G., et al
1992 A major inducer of anticarcinogenic protective enzymes from broccoli: isolation and elucidation of structure. Proc. Natl. Acad. Sci. 89:2399-2403.

Zhang, Y., Kensler, T. W., Cho, C.-G., et al
1994 Anticarcinogenic activities of sulforaphane and structurally related synthetic norbornyl isothiocyanates. Proc. Natl. Acad. Sci. 91:3147-3150.

Zhicen, L., et al
1987 Colour atlas of Chinese traditional drugs (Vol. 1). Science Press, Beijing. 300 p.

## Appendix One

# About The Authors

## Bruce W. Halstead, M.D.

**Birthplace:**

San Francisco, California. March 28, 1920

**Married:**

Joy Arloa Mallory, January 2, 1943
Divorced 1988.
Terri Lee Holcomb, June 25, 1988

**Children:**

Linda Glynn, May 30, 1944
Sandra Lee, September 30, 1947
David Bruce, March 16. 1951
Lawrence Douglas, November 2. 1952
Claudia Joy, December 3, 1960
Shari Lyu, April 19, 1962 (adopted)

**PRESENT POSITIONS:**

Director, International Biotoxicological Center, World Life Research Institute, Colton, CA, 92324

**ACADEMIC RECORD:**

1941 A.A. San Francisco City College - Biology
1943 B.A. University of California, Berkeley - Zoology
1948 M.D. Loma Linda University School of Medicine, Loma Linda, CA
1983 B.S. Academy of Natural Therapies, Gold Coast, North Queensland, Australia - Naturopathy & Traditional Medicine

**MILITARY RECORD:**

U.S. Army (PFC), Enlisted Reserve Corps, Army Specialized Training Program - 4 August 1942 to 18 August 1946.
U.S. Public Health Service (Asst. Surgeon) - 21 July 1947 to 20 July 1952.
U.S. Navy (Commander), Medical Corps, USNR - 1 January 1957 to 11 July 1971.
U.S. Marine Corps (Medical Officer), 4th Force Reconnaissance Co., Force Troops, FMF, U.S. Marine Corps, San Bernardino, CA - 14 September 1959 to 11 July 1971.
U.S. Navy (Commander), USNR-Retired 12 July 1971.
Consultant in Global Medicine, U.S. Navy Medical School, National Naval Medical Center, Department of the Navy, 1968.
Lecturer, Marine Biotoxicology and Soviet Medicine, School of Aerospace Medicine, U.S. Air Force, Brooks Air Force Base, Texas - 1967 to 1972.

**PROFESSIONAL EXPERIENCE:**

1935-44 Research Assistant - Department of Icthyology, California Academy of Sciences, Golden Gate Park, San Francisco, CA.
1943-44 Instructor - Department of Biology, Pacific Union College, Angwin, CA.
1944-47 Student in Medicine - Loma Linda University, Loma Linda, CA.
1947-48 Intern - Marine Hospital, U.S. Public Health Service, San Francisco, CA. (Asst. Surgeon)
1948-58 Chairman - Natural Products Section (Biotoxicology) and Assistant Director, School of Tropical and Preventive Medicine, Loma Linda University, Loma Linda, CA.
1948-58 Associate Professor - Department of Preventive Medicine, School of Medicine, Loma Linda University, Loma Linda, CA.
1950-51 Instructor - Icthyology, La Sierra College, CA. (while still on staff at L.L.U.).
1957-58 Instructor - Tropical Medicine, Division of Preventive Medicine, U.S. Naval Medical School, Bethesda, MD.
1959-present Director - World Life Research Institute, Colton, CA.
1964 Instructor - Ichthyology, Department of Biology, Walla Walla College Marine Biological Station, Anacortes, WA. (Summer)
1964-66 Research Associate - Laboratory of Neurological Research, School of Medicine, Dr. F. Russell, Loma Linda University, Los Angeles County General Hospital, Los Angeles, CA.
1967-73 Visiting Faculty - Preventive Medicine, Marine Biotoxicology and Soviet Medicine "Global Medicine Course", School of Aerospace Medicine, Department of the Air Force.
1968 Visiting Lecturer - Marine Biology, Department of Biology, Pacific Union College, Angwin, CA.
1968 Visiting Lecturer - Marine Biotoxicology Department of Epidemiology, School of Health, Loma Linda University, Loma Linda, CA.
1968 Visiting Lecturer - Marine Biotoxicology and Drugs from the Sea, Department of Pharmacy, School of Medicine, University of California, Berkeley, CA.
1968 Visiting Lecturer - Marine Biotoxicology, Department of Neurophysiology, School of Medicine, University of Southern California, Los Angeles, CA.
1969 Visiting Lecturer - Drugs from the Sea, Institute of Biologically Active Substances, Academy of Sciences of the U.S.S.R., Far Eastern Branch, Vladivostok, U.S.S.R.
1969 Visiting Lecturer - Marine Biotoxicology, School of Pharmacy, Oregon State University, Corvalis, OR.
1970 Visiting Lecturer - Drugs from the Sea, Department of Biological Sciences, University of Mississippi, Oxford, MS.
1970 Visiting Lecturer - Poisonous Marine Organisms, Royal Society of Arts and Sciences of Port Louis, Mauritius.
1972 Visiting Lecturer - "Dangerous Marine Animals — Emergencies in the Marine Environment", Department of Continuing Education in Health Sciences, School of Medicine, University of California, Los Angeles, CA.
1972 Visiting Lecturer - Poisonous Marine Organisms, Department of Environmental Toxicology, University of California, Davis, CA.
1972 Visiting Lecturer - "Global Pollution", Mississippi Junior Science Humanities Symposium, University of Mississippi, Oxford, MS.
1973 Adjunct Professor - Drugs from the Sea, Department of Pharmocognosy, School of Pharmacy, University of Mississippi, Oxford, MS.
1973 Visiting Lecturer – "Global Pollution", Department of Biological Sciences, Christian Brother's College, Memphis, TN.

1973 Lecturer – "Dangerous Marine Animals and Marine Pollution", Jean-Michel Cousteau's Project Ocean Search, Pepperdine University, Santa Monica, CA.

1973 Visiting Lecturer - Marine Biotoxicology, Department of Allied Health Professionals, Albert B. Chandler Medical Center, University of Kentucky, Lexington, KY.

1973 Lecturer – "Ocean Resources", Television Panel with Jean-Michel Cousteau, Encuentro, Tele Visa, Mexico City, Mexico.

1974 Instructor - "Diving Medicine Course", School of Medicine, University of Hawaii, Kona, HI.

1974 Visiting Lecturer - Marine Biotoxicology, Department of Allied Health Professionals, Albert B. Chandler Medical Center, University of Kentucky, Lexington, KY.

1974 Medical Officer - Expedition to Wuvulu Island, New Guinea, Jean-Michel Cousteau's Project Ocean Search, Pepperdine University, Santa Monica, CA. (August)

1974 Lecturer – "Unusual and Underutilized Drug Information Resources", Drug Information Association (Sponsored by the U.S. Food and Drug Administration and the National Library of Medicine), Williamsburg, VA.

1974 Lecturer – "Dangerous Marine Animals and Marine Pollution", Jean-Michel Cousteau's Project Ocean Search, Pepperdine University, Santa Monica, CA.

1975 External Thesis Examiner (Ph.D.) – "Toxins of the Crab, *Lophozozymus pictor*", by Yeh F. Teh, University of Singapore, Singapore.

1975 Lecturer – "Dangerous Marine Animals", Advanced Course on the Medicine and Physiology of Sport SCUBA Diving, Medical Seminars, Grand Cayman, West Indies.

1975 Lecturer – "Global Pollution", Tahoe 2,000 Mountain Lakes of the World, Lake Tahoe Environmental Education Consortium, The Cousteau Society, Lake Tahoe, NV. (November)

1976 Lecturer – "Marine Pollution", Southern California Coastal Water Research Project, Los Angeles, CA.

1977 Instructor - Expedition to Arno River, Marshall Islands, and Truk Islands, International Society of Aquatic Medicine. (August)

1978 Instructor - International Society of Aquatic Medicine, Roatan, Honduras. (January)

1978 Instructor – "Venomous Marine Animals — An In-Depth Review", Undersea Medical Society, Bonaire, Dutch Antilles. (February)

1978 Lecturer - Expedition to New Guinea - Western Islands Educational Expedition, New Guinea, Jean-Michel Cousteau Institute, University of Southern California, Los Angeles, CA. (August)

1978 Lecturer – "Current Status of Marine Biotoxicology — An Overview", Congresso Latinamericano de Toxicologia Analitica y Experimental, Carcass, Venezuela. (October)

1979 Lecturer – "Chelation Therapy in the Prevention and Treatment of Cardiovascular Disease", International Academy of Preventive Medicine, Dallas, TX. (March)

1979 Lecturer – "The Use of the Cyanogenic Glycoside Amygdalin in the Treatment of Cancer", XIV Pacific Science Congress, Khabarovsk, U.S.S.R. (August - September)

1979 Lecturer – "Adaptogenic Herbal Therapy", The Foundation for Preventive Medicine, City, MO. (October)

1979 Lecturer – "Digestive Enzymes and Absorption, N, N-Dimethylgylcine as a Metabolic Enhancer", Council on Nutrition of the American Chiropractic Association, Glendale, CA. (October)

1979 Lecturer – "Free Radical Pathology in Cancer", Fairfield Medical Centre, Montego Bay, Jamaica. (October)

1979 Lecturer – "Metabolic Therapy: An Overview", The Third International Doctor's Workshop on Amygdalin, Metabolic Therapy, and Cancer, Washington, D.C. (October)

1979 Lecturer – "Dangerous Marine Animals", International Society of Aquatic Medicine, Red Sea, Israel. (October-November)
1980 Lecturer – "Environmental Pollution as It Relates to Human Health", Systemic Nutritional Products, Acapulco, Mexico. (March)
1980 Lecturer – "Dangerous Marine Animals", Medical Seminars, San Salvador, Bahamas. (October)
1980 Lecturer – "Dangerous Marine Animals", Northwest Academy of Preventive Medicine, Maui, HI. (November)
1980 Lecturer – "Marine Biotoxicology", Department of Pharmacology, School of Medicine, University of California, Los Angeles, CA. (November)
1980 Lecturer – "Environmental Toxins as Contributors to Chronic and Degenerative Disease", The Preventive Dental Research Foundation, Los Angeles, CA. (March)
1980 Lecturer – "Poisonous and Venomous Animals of the Sea", International Society of Aquatic Medicine, San Salvador, Bahamas. (May)
1980 Panel Member – "Conventional vs. Alternative Treatments of Cancer: Are They Both Worthless?", Academy of Orthomolecular Psychiatry, San Francisco, CA. (May)
1980 Lecturer – "Dangerous Marine Animals and Marine Pollution", Expedition to Virgin Gorda, British Virgin Islands, Jean-Michel Cousteau Institute, University of Southern California, Los Angeles, CA. (July)
1980 Lecturer – "Molecular Logic in the Approach to the Treatment of Chronic Degenerative Disease", World Health Expo, Anaheim, CA. (August)
1980 Lecturer – "Chiropractic Principles", Parker Chiropractic Research Foundation, Dallas, TX. (September)
1980 Lecturer – "Chronic Degenerative Diseases and the Newer Nutritional Approaches", Council on Nutrition of the American Chiropractic Association, Lombard, IL. (September)
1981 Lecturer – "Consumer Medicine", School of Health, Loma Linda University, Loma Linda, CA. (February)
1981 Lecturer – "Current Use of Natural Therapeutics in the Treatment of Chronic Degenerative Disease", The National Naturopathic Convention, San Francisco, CA. (February)
1981 Lecturer – "Scientific Basis of EDTA Chelation Therapy for Hardening of the Arteries", Preventive Medical Seminar, Houston, TX. (March)
1981 Lecturer – "Controversial Medicine: Laetrile, DMSO, Gerovital, Chelation Therapy, Herbal Medicine, et cetra", Pacific Union College, Angwin, CA. (April)
1981 Lecturer – "DMSO, Laetrile, and EDTA, the Biochemistry Perspective", Northwest Academy of Preventive Medicine, Seattle, WA. (April)
1981 Lecturer – "Dangerous Marine Animals and Marine Pollution", Expedition to Virgin Gorda, West Indies, Jean-Michel Cousteau Institute, University of Southern California, Los Angeles, CA. (July)
1981 Lecturer – "Dangerous Marine Animals and Marine Pollution", Expedition to Maupiti, French Polynesia, Jean-Michel Cousteau Institute, University of Southern California, Los Angeles, CA. (August)
1981 Lecturer – "Dangerous Marine Animals", Westminster Hospital, Westminster, CA. (September)
1981 Lecturer – "Dangerous Marine Animals", Northwest Academy of Preventive Medicine, Kauai, HI. (November)
1982 Lecturer – "Consumer Medicine", School of Health, Loma Linda University, Loma Linda, CA. (February)
1982 Lecturer – "Whose Responsibility for Individual Health — FDA or Private Practitioner?", Alumni Association, School of Health, Loma Linda University, Loma Linda, CA. (March)

1982 Lecturer – "Dangerous Marine Animals", Medical Seminars, San Salvador, Bahamas. (October)
1982 Lecturer – "Immune Augmentation: Combatting Chronic Degenerative Diseases by Augmenting the Immune System Through Proper Nutrition", Midwest Academy of Traditional Medicine, Kansas City, MO. (October)
1982 Lecturer – "Hazardous Marine Life: Injuries and Treatment", The Foundation for Advanced Education In the Sciences, Inc., National Institutes of Health, Bethesda, MD. (November)
1982 Project Coordinator - Shark Anticancer Research, Frank Scott Enterprises, Aptos, CA.
1983 Lecturer – "Dangerous Marine Animals", California Academy of Sciences, Golden Gate Park, San Francisco, CA. (February)
1983 Lecturer – "Dangerous Marine Creatures: Things That Bite, Sting, and Poison", California Academy of Sciences, Golden Gate Park, San Francisco, CA. (February)
1983 Lecturer – "Environmental Pollution and Its Relationship to Chronic Degenerative Disease", Northwest Academy of Preventive Medicine, Maui, HI. (February)
1983 Lecturer – "Traditional Medicine", University of Redlands Science Associates, Redlands, CA. (February)
1983 Lecturer – "Chelation as an Alternative to Bypass Surgery", American Nutrition Society, Redondo Beach, CA. (March)
1983 Lecturer – "Immunotherapy and Degenerative Disease", American Biologics - Mexico, S.A. Research Hospital, Tijuana, Mexico. (April)
1983 Delegation Leader - Japan and the People's Republic of China, People-To-People International, Spokane, WA. (Project Canceled)
1983 Lecturer - Immunomodulating herbs, Morishita Conference on Natural Medicine, Tokyo, Japan. (November)
1984 Lecturer – "Dangerous Marine Animals and Marine Pollution", Guam Memorial Health Plan, Guam. (May)
1984 Lecturer – "Miscellaneous Seafood Toxins", American Chemical Society, Washington, D.C. (September)
1985 Lecturer – "Dangerous Marine Animals and Marine Pollution", Cousteau Society Inc., Project Ocean Search, Drake's Anchorage, Virgin Gorda, British Virgin Islands. (August)
1985 Lecturer – "The Present Role of Oriental Medicine in the U.S.A.", IV$^{th}$ International Congress on Oriental Medicine, Kyoto, Japan. (October) (Paper presented in absentia)
1985 Lecturer – "Ocean Pollution", Los Angeles Oceanic Society, Los Angeles, CA.
1985 Lecturer – "Immune Deficiency Disorders and Pollution", Anguilla, West Indies.
1986 Lecturer – "Natural Methods to Enhance Immunity", Oriental Healing Arts Institute, Long Beach, CA. (November)
1986 Reviewer – "Biologically Active Substances from Marine Organisms", by Dr. L. Beress. A proposal submitted to Kernforschungsanlage Julich Gesellschaft mit Beschrankter Haftung. Julich, West Germany. (November)
1986 Lecturer – "Immune Deficiency Disorders and Their Treatment", International Academy of Preventive Medicine, Denver, CO.
1986 External Thesis Examiner (Ph.D.) – "A Systematic Review of Venomous and Poisonous Marine Fishes of India", by S.S. Kora. Berhampur University, Berhampur, Orissa, India. (December)
1987 Witness - Re: Proposed Tire Burning Plant, Rialto City Council, Rialto, CA. (February)
1987 Lecturer – "Dangerous Marine Animals", New England Aquarium, Boston, MA. (October)
1988 Lecturer – "Secondary Immune Deficiency Disorders and the Use of Chinese Traditional Herbs in AIDS", Oriental Healing Arts Institute, Long Beach, CA. (April)

1988 Lecturer - "Dangerous Marine Animals", Southern California Marine Aquarium Society, (September)

1988 Lecturer – "The Use of Adaptogenic Nutritionals as Immunomodulators", Institute of Chinese Materia Medica, China Academy of Traditional Medicine, Beijing, P. R. China. (September)

1988 Lecturer – "The Use of Adaptogenic Nutritionals in the Treatment of Radiation Sickness", Institute of Medicinal Plant Development, Chinese Academy of Medical Sciences, WHO Collaborating Centre for Traditional Medicine, Beijing, P. R. China. (September)

1988 Lecturer – "The Use of Adaptogenic Nutritionals in the Treatment of Radiation Sickness", Chinese Academy of Military Medical Sciences, Beijing, P. R. China. (September)

1988 Lecturer – "Marine Biotechnology", Centro de Investigacion Cientifica y Educacion Superior de Ensenada, Ensenada, Baja California, Mexico. (November)

1988 Lecturer – "Marine Biotechnology", School of Medicine, Xochicalco University, Ensenada, Baja California, Mexico. (November)

1989 Lecturer – "Nutritional Therapy", Nature's Sunshine, Melbourne, FL. (February)

1989 Lecturer – "Nutritional Therapy", Nature's Sunshine, Atlanta, GA. (February)

1989 Lecturer – "Drugs From the Sea", Universidad Autonoma de Baja California, Ensenada, Baja California, Mexico. (April)

1989 Lecturer – "Herbal Products", Leadership meeting, Nature's Sunshine, Provo, UT. (April)

1989 Lecturer – "Poisonous Marine Animals and Their Military Significance"; "An Introduction to the Concept of Adaptogenic Nutritional Therapy for Radiation Sickness"; and "A Polythiolthione Substance Derived from Cruciferous Plants Having Antiradiation, Anticancer, and Liver Protective Properties — A PrEliminary Discussion", Institute of Radiation Medicine, Beijing, P. R. of China. (May)

1989 Lecturer – "The Use of Chinese Adaptogenic Plants in Nutrition", Institute of Medicinal Plant Development, Chinese Academy of Medical Sciences, Beijing, P.R. China. (May)

1989 Lecturer – "Marine Drugs", Joint Meeting of the Shangdong Institute of Marine Materia Medica, Institute of Marine Medicine and Food, Ocean University of Qingdao, and Editorial Department - Chinese Journal of Marine Drugs, Qingdao, P. R. China. (May)

1989 Lecturer – "Poisonous Marine Organisms and Their Military Significance", Naval Medical Research Institute, Shanghai, P. R. China. (May)

1989 Lecturer – "Taller Sorbe el Potencial de los Recursos Naturales y Acuaticos para la Produccion de Farmacos", University of Baja California, Ensenada, Baja California, Mexico. (August)

1989 Lecturer – "Nutritional Immunomodulation and Cancer Therapy", 2nd International Symp. on The Entire View on Cancer and AIDS, International Institute for Research on Metabolic Diseases and Cancer, Limassol, Cyprus. (September)

1989 Lecturer – "Angiochemistry and EDTA", American Board of Chelation Therapy Workshop, San Francisco, CA. (November)

1990 Lecturer – "Immunomodulation", 18th World Congress of Natural Medicines, Ministry of Public Health, Havana, Cuba. (April 27-29).

1990 Meeting - Deputy Prime Minister of Jamaica on Economic Development. Kingston, Jamaica. (July 10-13)

1990 Lecturer – "Alternative Medicine", School of Medicine, University of Guadalajara, Guadalajara, Mexico. (July)

1990 Lecturer – "Oriental Traditional Herbs for the Treatment of AIDS", 6th International Congress of Oriental Medicine. Tokyo, Japan. (October)

1990 Lecturer – "Free Radical Pathology and Its Immune Implications", Anaheim, CA. (November)

1991 Lecturer – "Poisonous and Venomous Marine Animal Injuries and Their Treatment", Grand Rounds Faculty Medical Lecture, Loma Linda University School of Medicine, Loma Linda, CA. (April)

1991 Lecturer – "Lipids - Their Structure, Function, and Immune Implications" (Presented in absentia by C.L. Foster), Memphis, TN. (May)

**HONORARY POSITIONS:**

1962 Member, Board of Directors, American Association of Fish and Game Biologists.

1962-70 Member, Board of Advisors, National Association of Underwater Instructors.

1967 Co-Chairman, Biology Committee (Drugs From the Sea), Marine Technology Society.

1968-present Member, Great Barrier Reef Committee of Australia, Brisbane, Australia.

1971 Member, Advisory Council, Lifebound, Ltd., Arvada, CO.

1971 Member, Board of Directors, Resources Recovery, Inc., Long Beach, CA.

1971 Member, Scientific Advisory Board, Environmental Defense Fund.

1972 Member, Water and Waste Task Force, Comprehensive Health Planning Association, Riverside, San Diego and Imperial Counties, CA.

1973 Member, Honorary Board of Directors, Environmental Education Group.

1973 Member, Scientific Advisory Board, Island Resources Foundation, St. Thomas, U.S. Virgin Islands.

1974 Vice President, International Association of Environmental Medicine and Biology, Paris.

1975 Member, Advisory Board, International Society of Aquatic Medicine.

1975 Member, Board of Directors, American Academy of Medical Preventics.

1980-85 Member, Board of Governors, National Health Federation.

1980 Member, International Board of Scientific and Nutritional Advisors, American International Hospital, Zion, IL.

1980 Senior Research Fellow, Island Resources Foundation, St. Thomas, U.S. Virgin Islands.

1980-81 President, American Academy of Medical Preventics, Los Angeles, CA.

1982-83 Board Chairman, Academy of Medical Preventics, Los Angeles, CA.

1984 Member, Board of Advisors, Oriental Healing Arts International University, Long Beach, CA.

1984 Member, Scientific Advisory Board, World Health Research Center, Pompano Beach, FL.

1985-present Member, Board of Directors, International Congress of Oriental Medicine, Kyoto, Japan.

1985 Honorary Advisor to the Academy of Natural Therapies, Gold Coast, North Queensland, Australia.

1989 Honorary Advisor to the Institute of Radiation Medicine, Chinese Academy of Military Medical Sciences, Beijing, P. R. China.

**CONSULTANT:**

1955 Consultant - Air Force Survival Problems, George Washington University, Wright-Patterson Air Force Base, OH. (U.S. Air Force Contract No. AF 18 [66]-1190)

1956-58 Editorial Consultant - Poisonous Marine Animals, *Journal of the American Medical Association*, Chicago, IL.

1958 Consultant - Japanese Minamata Disease, National Institute of Neurological Diseases and Blindness, U.S. Public Health Service, Washington, D.C.

1959-present Editorial Consultant - *Excerpta Medica*, International Abstracting Service, Amsterdam, Holland.

1962-67 Consultant - New Drug Development, Pitman-Mooree Co., Dow Chemical Co., Indiaheim, CA.
1964 Consultant - Oceanography, Marine Technology Group, North American Aviation, Inc., Miami, FL.
1965 Consultant - Special Study Section on Biotoxicology and Natural Products, Research Grants Review Branch, Division of Research Grants, National Institutes of Health, Bethesda, MD.
1966-present Editorial Consultant - *Clinical Toxicology*, Marcel Dekker, New York.
1967 Consultant - Toxic Marine Organisms, Battelle Memorial Research Institute, Columbus, OH.
1968 Consultant - Biotoxicology, Global Medicine Program, School of Aerospace Medicine, U.S. Air Force, Brooks A.F.B., TX.
1968 Consultant - Global Medicine, U.S. Naval Medical School, National Naval Medical Center, Department of the Navy, Bethseda, MD.
1968 Consultant - Marine Intoxicants, Informal Committee, World Health Organization of the United Nations, Geneva, Switzerland.
1969 Consultant - Joint IMCO, FAO, UNESCO, WMO Group of Experts on the Scientific Aspects of Marine Pollution, Food and Agriculture Organization of the United Nations, London, England.
1969 Consultant - Marine Aquaculture, Aquarium Systems, Inc., Wickliffe, OH.
1969 Consultant - Marine Chemistry, Institute of Biologically Active Substances, Far Eastern Branch, Siberian Department, The Academy of Sciences of the U.S.S.R., Vladivostok, U.S.S.R.
1969 Consultant - Ocean Research Laboratory, Westinghouse Research Laboratories, Westinghouse Electric Corp., San Diego, CA.
1969-70 Consultant - Marine Intoxications, Caribbean Fisheries Development Project, Food and Agriculture Organization of the United Nations, Rome, Italy.
1970 Consultant - Committee on Man's Underwater Activities, Marine Technology Society, Washington, D.C.
1970 Consultant - Fishery Development Project, Food and Agriculture Organization of the United Nations, Mauritius, Indian Ocean.
1970 Consultant - Joint IMCO, FAO, UNESCO, WMO, WHO, IAEA, UN Group of Experts on the Scientific Aspects of Marine Pollution, World Health Organization of the United Nations, Paris, France.
1970 Consultant (Rapporteur) - Section on Effects of Pollutants on Quality of Marine Products, Marine Pollution Conference, Food and Agriculture Organization of the United Nations, Rome, Italy.
1970 Consultant - Tempo-Ambon, Indonesian Oceanographic Project, General Electric Company, Ambon, Indonesia.
1971 Consultant - Biotoxicology, Global Medicine Program, School of Aerospace Medicine, U.S. Air Force, Brooks Air Force Base, TX.
1971 Consultant - Expert Advisory Panel on Food Additives, World Health Organization of the United Nations, Geneva, Switzerland.
1971 Participant - Fourth Annual Blimp Whalewatch Operation, American Cetacean Society, San Pedro, CA.
1971 Consultant - Joint IMCO, FAO, UNESCO, WMO, WHO, IAEA, UN Group of Experts on the Scientific Aspects of Marine Pollution, World Health Organization of the United Nations, Rome, Italy.
1971 Consultant - Science Advisory Board, Environmental Defense Fund, Washington, D.C.

1971 World Health Organization Consultant, Inter-Governmental Working Group on Marine Pollution, Second Session, United Nations Conference on the Human Environment, Ottawa, Canada. (November).

1972 Consultant - Task Force on Water and Waste Problems, Comprehensive Health Planning Association of Riverside County, Riverside, CA.

1973 Consultant - Ecotoxicology Working Group, Scientific Committee on Problems of the Environment (SCOPE), International Council on Scientific Unions (ICSU), Paris, France.

1973 Editorial Consultant - *Diving World*, Colton, CA.

1973 Consultant - Environmental Problems, Santa Monica Island, William L. Bates Organization, Los Angeles, CA.

1973 Consultant - International Committee, First World Congress of Medicine and Biology of the Environment, Association Internationale de Medicine et Biologiede l'Environment, Paris, France.

1975 Consultant - Resources and Land Committee, California State Legislature, Sacramento, CA.

1978 Consultant - Conference on Paralytic Shellfish Poisoning, World Health Organization of the United Nations, West Berlin, F.R. Germany. (December)

1980-87 Consultant - Expert Advisory Panel on Food Hygiene, World Health Organization of the United Nations, Geneva, Switzerland.

1982-83 Consultant - Nutritional Products, World Institute of Health, Grand Cayman, British West Indies.

1983 Consultant - EDTA Study, American International Hospital, Zion, IL.

1983 Consultant - Hyperbaric Oxygen, Frenco Laboratories, Dallas, TX.

1983 Consultant - Nutritional Products, Farady Laboratories, Hillside, NJ.

1983 Consultant - Nutritional Products, I'm Living Proof International, Inc., Houston, TX.

1986-87 Consultant - Nutritional Products, Sun Chlorella California, Inc., Torrance, CA.

1991 Report: "The toxicological Effects to Human Beings Resulting From Potentially Hazardous Wastes - Fertilizers, Herbicides, Fungicides, and Insecticides", Ron Barto Ground Water Consultants, Big Bear Lake, California. (June)

1992 Consultant - Preproposal Review on "The relationship between toxicity, unpalatability, antibiosis, and antifouling in marine resources from Indonesia", Board on Science and Technology for International Development (BOSTID), National Research Council, United States Academy of Science, Washington, D.C. (February)

1996 Consultant - Ocean Pollution, The State of Koror, Republic of Palau. (January)

**LEGISLATIVE AND COURT APPEARANCES (Expert Witness):**

1964 An R & D program in natural products as they relate to international economic development and our national security. Presented to: President's Commission on Marine Science, Engineering, and Resources, Washington, D.C.

1969 Ocean resources and marine biomedicine. Presented to: Hearings before the Subcommittee on Oceanography of the Committee on Merchant Marine and Fisheries, U.S. House of Representatives, Congressman Jerry L. Pettis, Washington, D.C.

1969 Recommendations to the President's Commission on Marine Science, Engineering, and Resources for the establishment of National Institute of Marine Medicine and Pharmacology. Presented to: Hearings before the Subcommittee on Oceanography of the Committee on Merchant Marine and Fisheries, U.S. House of Representatives, Congressman Alton Lennon, Washington, D.C.

1970 Use of marine biodynamic substances. Presented to: Republican Task Force on Earth Resources and Population, U.S. House of Representatives, Congressman George Bush, Washington, D.C.

1975 Speaker - "Marine Pollution." Governor E. Brown and California State Legislature with Jacques Cousteau, Sacramento, California.

1975 United States of America vs. Military Supply Agency. Re: Smuggling art carvings out of Rhodesia, Federal Grand Jury, Los Angeles, California.

1975 States Postal Department vs. Posten. Re: Mail fraud in the use of Siberian ginseng, Eleutherococcus senticosus, Administrative Law Proceedings, Los Angeles, California.

1975 Louisiana State Board of Medical Examiners vs. Evers. Re: Use of chelation therapy, Board of Medical Examiners, New Orleans, Louisiana.

1975 Royal Commissions into Exploratory and Production Drilling for Petroleum in the Area of the Great Barrier Reef vs. Great Barrier Reef Committee. Re: Marine Pollution, Brisbane, Australia.

1976 United States Food and Drug Administration vs. Evers. Re: Use of chelation therapy, U.S. Federal Court, New Orleans Louisiana.

1976 Scientific Board and Advisory Panel on Internal Medicine of the California Medical Association vs American Academy of Medical Preventics. Re: Scientific basis of chelation therapy, Hearing of the Board of the California Medical Association, Los Angeles, California.

1976 Phillips vs Alsleben. Re: Use of chelation therapy, Superior Court, Santa Ana, California.

1977 California Board of Medical Quality Assurance vs Hackethal. Re: Medical incompetence, Superior Court, San Bernardino, California.

1977 Speaker - "Amygdalin and Laetrile." California State Senate Committee on Health and Welfare (Senate Bill 245), Sacramento, California.

1977 United States of America vs Bradford, *et al*. Re: Conspiracy to smuggle Laetrile, U.S. Federal Court, San Diego, California.

1977 Banning of Laetrile from interstate commerce by FDA. Presented to: Subcommittee on Health and Scientific Research, Committee on Human Resources, U.S. Senate, Senator Ted Kennedy, Washington, D.C.

1977 U.S. Food and Drug Administration vs. Evers. Re: Use of Laetrile, U.S. Federal Court, Atlanta, Georgia.

1977 Glen L. Rutherford vs. United States of America. Re: Use of Laetrile, U.S. Federal Court, Oklahoma City, Oklahoma.

1978 Scott vs. McDonald. Re: Use of Laetrile, Superior Court, Atlanta, Georgia.

1978 Speaker - "Laetrile and Freedom of Choice." Idaho State Legislature Health Committee, Boise, Idaho.

1978 Speaker - "Laetrile and Freedom of Choice." Massachusetts State Legislature Health Committee, Boston, Massachusetts.

1978 Bolinger vs Medicare. Re: Payment for the treatment of atherosclerosis in chelation therapy, Riverside, California.

1978 Sanchez vs Roston. Re: Medical malpractice, Superior Court, Santa Ana, California.

1978 New York, Saratoga County Department of Social Services vs John Fofbaeur, *et al*. Re: Use of Laetrile, Superior Court, Saratoga Springs, New York.

1979 People vs Couture. Re: Use of oxygen colonics, Superior Court, Santa Ana, California.

1979 Speaker - "Amygdalin and Laetrile." California State Senate Committee on Health and Welfare (Senate Bill 1101), Senator W. Campbell, Sacramento, California.

1979 People of the Commonwealth of Massachusetts vs Gerald and Diane Green. Re: Custody of a minor and the use of metabolic therapy (Laetrile), Superior Court, Plymouth, Massachusetts.

1979 Speaker - "Freedom of Choice in Alternate Forms of Medical Care." California State Assembly Health Committee, Huntington Beach, California.

1979 United States of America vs Food Science Laboratories Inc. Re: Vitamin B15, U.S. Federal Court, Chicago, Illinois.

1980 United States Securities Exchange Commission vs Bioptics. Re: Operations of the Bioptics Corporation, Los Angeles, California.

1980 State of California vs Athena Products, Ltd. Re: Misbranding of labels on vitamin-mineral nutrients, Superior Court, Los Angeles, California.

1980 R.W. Bradford, Committee for Freedom of Choice in Cancer Therapy, American Biologics, M.L. Culbert, and Bruce W. Halstead, M.D. for His Cancer Patients vs National Cancer Institute, Mayo Clinic, United States Department of Health Education, and Welfare, Public Health Service, National Institutes of Health, United States Food and Drug Administration, and the United States of America. Re: Injunction to stop the testing of amygdalin in the treatment of cancer on human beings, U.S. Federal Court, San Diego, California.

1980 Conservatorship of the Estate and Person of Ariya Dahmma Thera, Superior Court, Indio, California.

1980 Glen L. Rutherford, *et al* vs United States of America, *et al* (United States Food and Drug Administration, United States Customs). Re: The legality of Laetrile, U.S. Federal Court, Oklahoma City, Oklahoma.

1981 United States Postal Service vs Dunmore Corporation. Re: Human requirements for zinc, Administrative Law Proceedings, Washington, D.C.

1981 United States Postal Service vs Athena Products, Ltd. Re: Misbranding of labels on vitamin-mineral nutrients, Administrative Law Proceedings, Atlanta, Georgia.

1981 Michaelis *et al* vs Califano, *et al*. Re: Unconstitutional search and seizure, Superior Court, Columbus, Ohio.

1981 Williams vs Donato. Re: Vitamin A poisoning, Superior Court, Whittier, California.

1981 Hammons vs Harper. Re: Cancer therapy, Superior Court, Los Angeles, California.

1981 Eastwood vs Lincoln National Life Insurance Company. Re: Payment for the treatment of cancer with Laetrile, Superior Court, San Francisco, California.

1981 Reagan vs United States of America. Re: Metallic poisoning, U.S. Federal District Court, Las Vegas, Nevada.

1981 Smith vs Ann Bhuket, M.D. Re: Chelation therapy, Superior Court, Dallas, Texas.

1982 Fitzpatrick vs Frent, D.O. Re: Chelation therapy and Wilson's Disease, Superior Court, Detroit, Michigan.

1982 French vs California Goat Dairymen's Association, *et al*. Re: Lead poisoning from goat's milk, Superior Court, Riverside, California.

1982 Sullivan, *et al* vs Henry, *et al*. Re: Laetrile toxicity, U.S. Federal District Court, Atlanta, Georgia.

1982 Board of Medical Quality Assurance of the State of Californiavs John C. Luly, D.C. Re: Colon therapy, Superior Court,San Diego, California. (Consultant Only).

1983 Bresee vs Harper, M.D. Re: Cancer therapy, Superior Court, Los Angeles, California.

1983 Furnire vs Hamdan, M.D. Re: Cirrhosis of the liver resulting from hypervitaminosis A, Superior Court, Princeton, New Jersey.

1983 People of the State of California vs World Institute of Health, *et al*. Re: Efficacy of Gerovital ($GH_3$), California State Hearing Before Attorney General's Office, San Diego, California.

1983 Phillip E. Hoke vs Life Insurance Company of America, *et al*. Re: Fish poisoning, Superior Court, Santa Barbara, California.

1983 U.S. Postal Service vs Nutritional research. Re: Glucomannan nutritional product, Superior Court, Newport Beach, California.

1984 State of Idaho vs Cyrus E. Maxfield. Re: Colon therapy, Superior Court, Boise, Idaho.

1985 Elmore vs Word, *et al.* Re: Medical malpractice, Columbia, South Carolina.
1985 Federal Trade Commission vs Arthur Furman, M.D. Re: Use of hair analysis in diagnosis of disease, U.S. Federal Court, Washington, D.C.
1985 Silva vs Bluepoint, *et al.* Re: Paralytic shellfish poisoning, Superior Court, San Francisco, California.
1989 Ruffalo vs Medical Board. Re: Use of Chelation Therapy, Fair Hearing Medical Board, New York, New York.
1989 Cavigliano vs Teledyne Aeronautics. Re: PCB poisoning, Superior Court, San Diego, California.
1989 Boling vs The Sunrider Corporation. Re: Review of constituents contained in herbal preparations, Arizona.
1989 Vopel vs Vons Grocery Co. Re: Poisoning by ENDRIN contaminated sugar, Superior Court, El Cahon, California.
1990 Fox vs Montalbano. Re: Recurring exposure of spouse to AIDS virus due to delay in testing husband for blood transfusion related AIDS, San Diego, California.
1990 Tomarchio vs Pueblo International. Re: Ciguatera poisoning from injesting shark meat, Superior Court, Ft. Lauderdale, Florida.
1990 Vickie Blake vs General Electric. Re: LEXAN intoxication, Federal Court, Pheonix City, Alabama.
1990 Kisiel vs Mark's Fish and Pets. Re: Lionfish sting, Superior Court, Burbank, California.
1990 Tessa Cason vs The Bren Company. Re: Natural Gas Poisoning, Superior Court, San Diego, California.
1991 Bertha O. Gonzales vs. Denny's Restaurant. Re: Shellfish intoxication, Superior Court, Ventura, California. (Case dismissed out of court).
1991 Reed vs. Bank of Hemet. Re: Toxicological evaluation of Joedna Reed, Superior Court, Los Angeles, California.
1996 Workmen's Comp. vs. Lola Biro. Re: Chlorine Poisoning, Superior Court, Santa Ana, California.

**HONORS:**

President of the Senior Class, School of Medicine, Loma Linda University, Loma Linda, CA, 1946-47.
Listed as one of the 12 Outstanding Young Men in California by the California Junior Chamber of Commerce, 1955.
Distinguished Achievement Award, Men of Achievement, Cambridge, England, 1956.
Carlos Lamar Award, in Recognition of Achievement and Research in Chelation Therapy. American Academy of Medical Preventics, 28 September 1975.
Humanitarian Award, Cancer Control Society, 14th Annual Cancer Convention, Los Angeles, CA, 5 July 1986.
Presented the Bronze Medal of the Academy in Appreciation for Lecture on Treatment of Radiation Sickness with Adaptogenic Chinese Herbs, Academy of Military Medical Sciences, Beijing, P. R. China, 13 September 1988.
Reconocimiento, for lecture on "The potential use of natural resources (terrestrial and aquatic) for the development of new pharmacuetical products in Mexico." University of Baja California, Ensenada, Baja California, Mexico, 23 August 1989.

Listed In: American Men in Science
Aquatic Biologists of the World
Dictionary of International Biography
Leaders in American Science

Personalities of the West and Midwest
Pioneers In Diving
Who's Who in America
Who's Who in Frontier Science and Technology
Who's Who in the West
World's Who's Who in Science

**MEMBERSHIPS IN SCIENTIFIC SOCIETIES (Past and Present):**

Academia Nacional de Medicina de Buenos Aires
Academy of Natural Therapies - Fellow
American Academy of Clinical Toxicology
American Academy of Medical Preventics - Charter Fellow
American Association for the Advancement of Science - Fellow
American Institute of Biological Sciences
American Institute of Chemists - Fellow
American Institute of Fishery Research Biologists - Fellow
American Naturopathic Medical Association
American Microscopical Society
American Ordnance Association
American Society of Ichthyologists and Herpetologists
American Society of Limnology and Oceanography
American Society of Pharmacognosy
American Society of Tropical Medicine and Hygiene
Association for Tropical Biology
California Academy of Sciences - Fellow
Confederacion International Asociaciones de Medicinas Alternatives Naturales
The Cousteau Society
The Explorers Club, New York
Great Barrier Reef Committee of Australia
Hollywood Academy of Medicine
International Academy of Preventive Medicine
International Kirlian Research Association
International Society on Toxicology - Founding Fellow
International Underwater Explorers Society - Honorary Life Member
Island Resources Foundation
Marine Technology Society
National Geographic Society
Northwest Academy of Preventive Medicine - Fellow
Oceanic Society
New York Academy of Sciences - Fellow
Royal Society of Arts and Sciences of Mauritius
Royal Society of Tropical Medicine and Hygiene (London, England)
Royal Society of Health (England) - Fellow
Royal Society Zoological Society of New South Wales
San Francisco Aquarium Society
Sigma Xi
Society of Environmental Toxicology
Society for Experimental Biology and Medicine
Society of Systematic Zoology

Undersea Medical Society, Inc.
Washington Academy of Sciences
Western Society of Naturalists
Wilderness Medical Society - Founding Member

**FOREIGN TRAVEL:**

AFRICA: Angola, Egypt, Ethiopia, Kenya, Libya, Morocco, South Africa, Somalia, Tanzania, Uganda, Zimbabwe.
ASIA: Afghanistan, Burma, Cambodia, Cyprus, Hong Kong, India Indonesia, Israel, Japan, Laos, Lebanon, Macao, Malta, Nepal, Pakistan, Pescadores Islands, People's Republic of China, Phillipines, Rhodes, Ryukyu Islands, Saudi Arabia, Siberia (U.S.S.R.), South Korea, Syria, Taiwan, Thailand, Turkey, Vietnam.
EUROPE: Austria, Azore Islands, Belgium, Bulgaria, Czechoslovakia, Denmark, England, Estonia, Finland, France, Germany, Greece, Holland, Hungary, Iceland, Ireland, Italy, Latvia, Lichtenstein, Monaco, Norway, Poland, Portugal, Romania, Scotland, Spain, Sweden, Switzerland, U.S.S.R., Wales.
CARIBBEAN: Antigua, Aruba, Bahamas, Barbados, Bonaire, British Virgin Islands, Cayman Islands, Cuba, Curacao, Granada, Haiti, Jamaica, Martinique, Netherlands Antilles, Puerto Rico, Saba, Saint Lucia, Saint Vincent, Tobago, Trinidad, U.S. Virgin Islands.
NORTH AMERICA: Baja California, Canada, Greenland, Mexico, United States (most of the U.S. including Alaska and Hawaii).
CENTRAL AMERICA: Costa Rica, El Salvador, Guatemala, Honduras, Nicaragua, Panama, San Benitos Island.
SOUTH AMERICA: Argentina, Bolivia, Brazil, Colombia, Ecuador, Peru, Uruguay, Venezuela.
OCEANIA: Australia, Canton Island, Caroline Islands, Cocos Islands, Eniwetok, Fiji Islands, French Polynesia, Galapagos Islands, Guam, Hermit Islands, Johnston, Kwajalein, Line Islands, Mariana Islands, Marshall Islands, Midway, New Caledonia, New Guinea, New Hebrides Islands, New Zealand, Ninigo Islands, Palawu, Papua, Palmyra, Phoenix Islands, Ponapay, Samoa (U.S.), Saipan, Solomon Islands, Tiniane, Tonga Islands, Truck, Wake, West Samoa, Wuvulu, Yap.
INDIAN OCEAN: Madagascar, Mauritius, Reunion.

**PUBLICATIONS:**

**1938**

(1) Clark, H.W. and B.W. Halstead
*Decapterus scombrinus* (Valenciennes) in Monterey Bay. Copeia (4):205.

**1949**

(2) Halstead, B.W.
Octopus bites in human beings. Leafl. Malac. 1(5):17-22.
(3) Halstead, B.W.
Problems concerning medical ichthyology and future plans of the Department of Ichthyology and Herpetology. School of Tropical and Preventive Medicine, College of Medical Evangelists, Loma Linda, CA. 16 p. (Limited distribution)
(4) Halstead, B.W. and R. Ryckman
Injurious effects from contacts with millipedes. Med. Arts Sci. 3(1):16-18, 1 fig.

**1950**

(5) Halstead, B.W.
The capture of a wattled eel-pout, *Lycodes palearis*, from Fidalgo Island, Washington, and the distributional record of this species. Copeia (4):317.

(6) Halstead, B.W.
The levitical laws and disease transmission by animals. 7 p. (Limited distribution)

(7) Halstead, B.W.
Mosaic law substantiated. Rev. Herald 127(3):13.

(8) Halstead, B.W. and F.R. Modglin
A preliminary report on the venom apparatus of the batray, *Holorhinus californicus*. Copeia (3):165-175, 6 figs.

**1951**

(9) Halstead, B.W.
Ichthyotoxism - a neglected medical problem! Med. Arts Sci. 5(4):115-121, 8 figs.

(10) Halstead, B.W.
Injurious effects from the sting of the scorpionfish, *Scorpaena guttata*. California Med. 74:395-396, 1 pl.

(11) Halstead, B.W.
Poisonous fish - a medical-military problem. Office of Naval Research, Research Reservists, Department of the Navy, Washington, D.C., NAVEXOS P-510:10-16, 8 figs.

(12) Halstead, B.W.
The role of CME in basic medial research. The Journal 22(5):18-19.

**1952**

(13) Halstead, B.W.
Concerning fish poisoning on Saipan. (Limited distribution)

(14) Halstead, B.W.
Concerning fish poisoning on Midway Islands. (Limited distribution)

(15) Halstead, B.W.
Poisonous fish. J. Am. Med. Assoc. 149 (16):1513.

(16) Halstead, B.W. and N.C. Bunker
Poisonous fishes of Saipan. 53p. (Limited distribution)

(17) Halstead, B.W. and N.C. Bunker
Stingray attacks and their treatment. Am. J. Trop. Med. Hyg. 2(1):115-128, 12 figs.

(18) Halstead, B.W. and N.C. Bunker
The venom apparatus of the ratfish, Hydrolagus colliei. Copeia (3):128-138, 1 pl., 4 figs.

(19) Ryckman, R.E. and B.W. Halstead
Report of a case of human nasal myiasis by the greenbottle fly, *Phaenicia sericata*, in San Bernardino County, California. Am. J. Trop. Med. Hyg. 1(4):711-712.

**1953**

(20) Halstead, B.W.
On the results of feeding poisonous puffer fish to nontoxic California marine fishes. (Limited distribution)

(21) Halstead, B.W.
The orthopedic arthrometer for the precise measurement of angles in systematic ichthyology. Copeia (4):241.

(22) Halstead, B.W.
Poisonous fishes and fish poisoning. In: Research Reviews. NAVEXOS P-510, Department of the Navy, Washington, D.C. pp. 23-25.
(23) Halstead, B.W.
Some general considerations of the problem of poisonous fish and ichthyosarcotoxism. Copeia (1):31-33.
(24) Halstead, B.W.
The effect of the commercial canning process upon puffer poison. California Fish Game 39(2):219-228, 1 fig.
(25) Halstead, B.W., Kuninobu, L.S., and H.G. Hebard
Catfish stings and the venom apparatus of the Mexican catfish, *Galeichthys felis* (Linneaus). Trans. Am. Microsc. Soc. 72(4):297-314, 6 figs.
(26) Goe, D.R. and B.W. Halstead
A preliminary report of the toxicity of the gulf puffer, *Sphoeroides annulatus*. California Fish Game 39(2):229-232, 1 fig.
(27) Holloway, J.E., Bunker, N.C., and B.W. Halstead
The venom of *Urobatis halleri* (Cooper), the round stingray. California Fish Game 39(1):77-82, 1 fig.
(28) Ocampo, R.R., Halstead, B.W., and F.R. Modglin
The microscopic anatomy of the caudal appendage of the spotted eagleray, *Aetobatus narinari* (Euphrasen), with reference to the venom apparatus. Anat. Rec. 115(1):87-99, 3 pls.

**1954**

(29) Halstead, B.W.
A note regarding the toxicity of the fishes of the skipjack family, Katsuwonidae. California Fish Game 40(1):61-63.
(30) Halstead, B.W.
Regarding clinical characteristics of fish poisoning. (Limited distribution).
(31) Halstead, B.W. and N.C. Bunker
A survey of the poisonous fishes of Johnston Island. Zoologica 39(2):61-77, 1 fig.
(32) Halstead, B.W. and N.C. Bunker
A survey of the poisonous fishes of the Phoenix Islands. Copeia (1):1-11, 5 figs.
(33) Halstead, B.W. and R.C. Habekost
Experiments on the toxicity of *Pseudosuberites pseudos* Dickinson. l p. (Limited distribution)
(34) Halstead, B.W. and W.M. Lively, Jr.
Poisonous fishes and ichthyosarcotoxism. U.S. Arm. Forces Med. J. 5(2):157-175, 13 figs.
(35) Halstead, B.W. and R.D. Macomber
Moray eel injection records. ll p. (Unpublished)
(36) Halstead, B.W. and R.J. Ralls
Results of dialyzing some fish poisons. Science 119(3083):160-161.
(37) Halstead, B.W. and R.L. Schall
Poisonous fishes of La Plata Island. 7 p. (Unpublished)
(38) Halstead, B.W., and R.L. Smith
Presence of an axillary venom gland in the Oriental catfish, *Plotosus lineatus*. Copeia (2):153-154.
(39) Berry, S.S. and B.W. Halstead
Octopus bites - a second report. Leafl. Malac. 1(11):59-65, 1 fig.

**1955**

(40) Halstead, B.W., Chitwood, M.J., and F.R. Modglin
The anatomy of the venom apparatus of the zebrafish, *Pterois volitans* (Linneaus). Anat. Rec. 122(3):317-333, 3 pls., 16 figs.

(41) Halstead, B.W., Chitwood, M.J., and F.R. Modglin
The venom apparatus of the California scorpionfish, *Scorpaena guttata* Girard. Trans. Am. Microsc. Soc. 74(2):145-158, 15 figs.

(42) Halstead, B.W., Ocampo, R.R., and F.R. Modglin
A study on the comparative anatomy of the venom apparatus of certain North American stingrays. J. Morphol. 97(1):1-21, 4 pls., 20 figs.

(43) Halstead, B.W. and D.W. Schall
Poisonous fishes of Palau. (Limited distribution)

(44) Halstead, B.W. and D.W. Schall
Poisonous fishes of Tahiti. (Limited distribution)

(45) Halstead, B.W. and D.W. Schall
Poisonous fishes of the Gulf of California. (Limited distribution)

(46) Halstead, B.W. and D.W. Schall
Poisonous fishes of the Marshall Islands. 5 p. (Limited distribution)

(47) Halstead, B.W. and D.W. Schall
A report on the poisonous fishes captured during the Woodrow G. Krieger expedition to the Galapagos Islands. In: Essays in the Natural Sciences in Honor of Captain Allan Hancock. University of Southern California Press, Los Angeles. Pp. 147-172, 2 pls.

(48) Dawson, E.Y., Alleem, A.A., and B.W. Halstead
Marine algae from Palmyra Island with special reference to the feeding habits and toxicology of reef fishes. Allan Hancock Found. Publs. (17):1-39, 12 figs.

(49) Goe, D.R. and B.W. Halstead
A case of fish poisoning from Caranx ignobilis Forskal from Palmyra Island, with comments on the sensitivity of the mouse injection technique for the screening of toxic fishes. Copeia (3):238-240.

(50) Habekost, R.C., Fraser, I.M., and B.W. Halstead
Observations on toxic marine algae. J. WA. Acad. Sci. 45(4):101-103.

(51) Ralls, R.J., and B.W. Halstead
Moray eel poisoning and a preliminary report on the action of the toxin. Am. J. Trop. Med. Hyg. 4(1):136-140.

(52) Whitley, G.P. and B.W. Halstead
An annotated bibliography of the poisonous and venomous fishes of Australia. Rec. Aust. Mus. 23(5):211-227.

**1956**

(53) Halstead, B.W.
Animal phyla known to contain poisonous marine animals. In: E.E. Buckley and N. Porges [Eds.], Venoms. American Association for the Advancement of Science, Washington, D.C. pp. 9-27.

(54) Halstead, B.W.
Current status of research on Pacific poisonous fishes and ichthyosarcotoxism. In: E.E. Buckley and N. Porges [Eds.], Venoms. American Association for the Advancement of Science, Washington, D.C. pp. 29-32.

(55) Halstead, B.W.
Poisonous fishes and their relationship to marine food resources in the Pacific area. Proc. 8th Pac. Sci. Congr. 3:321-330.
(56) Halstead, B.W.
Toxic marine organisms. In: Handbook of Biological Data. National Research Council, WADC Tech. Rept. 56-273. pp. 424-426. (ASTIA No. AD-110501).
(57) Halstead, B.W.
Venomous mollusks. Rep. Am. Malac. Un. 23:1.
(58) Halstead, B.W., Chitwood, M.J., and F.R. Modglin
Stonefish stings and the venom apparatus of *Synanceja horrida* (Linnaeus). Trans. Am. Microsc. Soc. 75(4):381-397, 12 figs.
(59) Halstead, B.W. and D.W. Schall
A report on the poisonous fishes captured during the Woodrow G. Krieger expedition to Cocos Island. Pac. Sci. 10(1):103-109, 1 fig.
(60) Halstead, B.W. and C. Teel
Regarding venom apparatus in *Muraena helena*. (Limited distribution).

**1957**

(61) Halstead, B.W.
Dorland's Illustrated Medical Dictionary (Contributor). 23rd/ ed. W.B. Saunders Co., Philadelphia. 1598 p.
(62) Halstead, B.W.
Jellyfish stings and their medical management. U.S. Arm. Forces Med. J. 8(11):1587-1602, 11 figs.
(63) Halstead, B.W.
Mysterious outbreaks of fish poisoning. Experimental Diving Unit, U.S. Naval Medical School, Washington, D.C. 8 p. (Limited distribution).
(64) Halstead, B.W.
Preventative medicine manual on sea snakes. U.S. Naval Medical School Graduate Training Course for Medical Officers, Bethesda, MD. 12 p. (Limited distribution).
(65) Halstead, B.W.
The public health significance of the recent outbreaks of poisoning by marine organisms in Japan. U.S. Naval Medical School, National Naval Medical Center, Bethesda, MD. 11 p. (Limited distribution).
(66) Halstead, B.W.
Unexploited ocean resources. Med. Arts Sci. 11(2):72-75.
(67) Halstead, B.W.
Wealth of the seas. 5 p. (Limited distribution).
(68) Halstead, B.W.
Weever stings and their medical management. U.S. Arm. Forces Med. J. 8(10):1441-1451, 8 figs.
(69) Halstead, B.W., Kawabata, T., and T.F. Judefind
The public health significance of the recent outbreaks of poisoning by marine organisms in Japan. In: Proceeding of the 9th/ Science Congress. Pacific Association, Bangkok. 11 p. (Limited distribution).
(70) Halstead, B.W. and M.H. McLaughlin
Fish poisoning. Life Health 72(7):10-11, 32.
(71) Halstead, B.W., Modglin, F.R., and G.D. Kuhn
On the morphology of the hairs of the rare deep sea fish, *Mirapinna esau*. Annl. Mag. Nat. Hist., Series 12, 10:767-768.

(72) Halstead, B.W. and F.E. Russell
Animal toxins, Part 3: Marine organisms. In: W.S. Spector [Ed.], Handbook of Biological Data. W. B. Saunders and Co., Philadelphia. 7 p.

(73) Kawabata, T., Halstead, B.W., and T.F. Judefind
A report of a series of recent outbreaks of unusual cephlopod and fish intoxications in Japan. Am. J. Trop. Med. Hyg. 6(5):935-939.

(74) Schantz, E.J., Halstead, B.W., McFarren, E.F., Bond, R.M., and W.B. Page
Conference on shellfish toxicology. U.S. Public Health Service, Special Publications. 126 p., 5 figs. (Limited distribution).

**1958**

(75) Halstead, B.W.
Beware!! The zebrafish. All Pets (Sept.):27-32, illust.

(76) Halstead, B.W.
Class Diplopoda (millipedes). In: J. DeCoursey, [Ed.], Medical Entomology. U.S. Naval Medical School, National Naval Medical Center, Bethesda, MD. Pp. 22-23.

(77) Halstead, B.W.
The deadly fugu - mysterious fish of ancient Japanese emperors. 7 p. (Unpublished).

(78) Halstead, B.W.
Global medicine and CME. CME Alumni J. 29(5):10-13.

(79) Halstead, B.W.
Jellyfish stings and their medical management. S. Afr. Practnr. 3(3):43-48, 11 figs.

(80) Halstead, B.W.
Poisonous and venomous marine organisms. In: D.W. Wright, Medical Zoology. (Unpublished). 106 p.

(81) Halstead, B.W.
Poisonous fishes. Pub. Health Rep. 73(4):302-312, 11 figs.

(82) Halstead, B.W.
Poisonous fish-like vertebrates. [Appendix B]. U.S. Naval Medical School, National Naval Medical Center, Bethesda, MD. 39 p.

(83) Halstead, B.W.
The relationship of traumogenous fishes to man. AIBS Symposium. 16 p. (Limited distribution).

(84) Halstead, B.W.
Results of an investigation on a series of outbreaks in Japan caused by the eating of marine organisms. Natl. Inst. Health Consultantship, 1-22 September 1958. 4 p. (Limited distribution).

(85) Halstead, B.W.
Skin disorders most frequently encountered by the fishing industry. 2 p. (Limited distribution).

(86) Halstead, B.W.
Venomous fishes. U.S. Naval Medical School Graduate Training Course for Medical Officers, Bethesda, MD. 39 p. (Limited distribution).

(87) Halstead, B.W. and R.F. Modglin
Weeverfish stings and the venom apparatus of weevers (*Trachinus*). Z. Tropenmed. Parasit. 9(2):129-146, 12 figs.

(88) Halstead, B.W. and D.W. Schall
A report on the poisonous fishes of the Line Islands. Acta. Trop. 15(3):193-233.

(89) Courville, D.A., Halstead, B.W., and D.W. Hessel
Marine biotoxins: Isolation and properties. Chem Rev. 58(2):235-248.

**1959**

(90) Halstead, B.W.
Dangerous Marine Animals. Cornell Maritime Press, Cambridge. 146 p., 88 figs.

(91) Halstead, B.W.
Environmental hazards. In: U.S. Navy Diving Manual, Part 1, NAVSHIPS 250-538. U.S. Department of the Navy, Washington, D.C. Pp. 158-175.

(92) Halstead, B.W. and W.M. Lively, Jr.
Poisonous fishes and ichthyosarcotoxism. PACAF Command Surgeon's Newsletter 1(1):1-5.

**1960**

(93) Hessel, D.W., Halstead, B.W., and N.H. Peckham
Marine biotoxins. I. Ciguatera poison: Some biological and chemical aspects. Annl. NY Acad. Sci. 90(3):788-797, 4 figs.

**1961**

(94) Halstead, B.W.
Candiru - the human parasitic catfish of the Amazon. 9 p. (Unpublished).

(95) Halstead, B.W.
Marine biotoxins - a wealth of new drugs for the future. 9 p. (Unpublished).

(96) Halstead, B.W.
Sting rays. J. Am. Med. Assoc. 175(6):541.

(97) Halstead, B.W.
Venomous fishes. In: P. Gray, [Ed.], The Encyclopedia of the biological sciences. Reinhold Publishing Corp., New York. pp. 1049-1051.

**1962**

(98) Halstead, B.W.
Biotoxins, allergies, and other disorders. In: G. Borgstrom, [Ed.], Fish as Food, Vol. 2: Nutrition, Sanitation, and Utilization. Academic Press, New York. pp. 521-540.

**1963**

(99) Halstead, B.W.
First aid treatment of shark bites - general comments. In: P.W. Gilbert, [Ed.], Sharks and Survival. D.C. Health and Co., Boston. pp. 495-496.

(100) Halstead, B.W.
Quest for new drugs. J. Am. Pharm. Assoc. N53(3):129-130, illust.

(101) Halstead, B.W., Hessel, D.W., and J. Suchy
An investigation of ciguatera poison. Final Report, Army Chemical Corps., Grant No. DA-CML-18-108-61-g-19, June 1961 - Sept. 1962. 9 p. (Limited distribution).

(102) Halstead, B.W. and L.R. Mitchell
A review of the venomous fishes of the Pacific area. In: H.L. Keegan and W.V. MacFarlane, [Ed.], Venomous and Poisonous Animals and Noxious Plants of the Pacific Area. Pergamon Press, New York. pp. 173-202, 16 figs.

**1964**

(103) Halstead, B.W.
Fish poisoning - their diagnosis, pharmacology, and treatment. Clin. Pharmacol. Ther. 5(5):615-627.

(104) Halstead, B.W.
An R&D program in natural products as they relate to international economic development and our national security. Ocean Engineering. N. Am. Aviat. 8(1):100-114.

(105) Halstead, B.W., Carscallen, L.J., and F.E. Russell
Animal toxins, Part 3: Marine organisms. In: P.L. Altmanard and D.S. Ditter, [Eds.], Biology Data Book. Federal American Society of Experimental Biology, Washington, D.C. pp. 336-344.

(106) O'Neal, P.L., Halstead, B.W., and L.D. Howard, Jr.
Injury to human tissues from sea urchin spines. California Med. 101:199-202.

**1965**

(107) Halstead, B.W.
Dorland's Illustrated Medical Dictionary (Contributor). 24th ed. W.B. Saunders Co., Philadelphia. 1724 p.

(108) Halstead, B.W.
In memorium - Yevgeniy N. Pavlovskiy (1884-1965). Toxicon 3:169-170.

(109) Halstead, B.W.
Poisonous and Venomous Marine Animals of the World. U.S. Government Printing Office, Washington, D.C. Vol I, 994 p., illust.

**1966**

(110) Halstead, B.W.
Aspectos medicos de los animales marinos venenosos. Acad. Nac. Med. Buenos Aires 44(2). 1 p.

(111) Halstead, B.W.
Field report on the epidemiology of biotoxications from eating the livers of polar bears and other arctic mammals. (Limited distribution)

(112) Halstead, B.W.
Venomous marine animals of Brazil. Mem. Inst. Butanan 33(1):1-26.

**1967**

(113) Halstead, B.W.
Medical ichthyology - the unknown science. Presented to: The Marine Technology Society, Washington, D.C. 11p. (Limited distribution)

(114) Halstead, B.W.
National goals in biomedical oceanography and recommendations for achieving these goals. Presented to: Marine Technology Society, Washington, D.C. 11 p. (Limited distribution)

(115) Halstead, B.W.
Need for a national institute of marine medicine and pharmacology. Presented to: Marine Technology Society, Washington, D.C. 20 p. (Limited distribution)

(116) Halstead, B.W.
Poisonous and Venomous Marine Animals of the World. U.S. Government Printing Office, Washington, D.C. Vol. 2, 1070 p., illust.

(117) Halstead, B.W. and A.E. Dalgleish
The venom apparatus of the European stargazer, *Uranoscopus scaber* Linnaeus. In: F.E. Russell and P.R. Saunders, [Eds.], Animal Toxins. Pergamon Press, New York. pp. 177-186, 10 figs.

(118) Halstead, B.W.
Marine biotoxins, new foods, and drugs from the sea. Presented to: Marine Technology Society, University of Rhode Island. 10p. (Limited distribution).

**1968**

(119) Halstead, B.W.
Marine biological hazards. J. Ocean Technol. 2(3):46-49.

(120) Halstead, B.W.
Marine biotoxins and marine food resources. 11 p. (Unpublished)

(121) Halstead, B.W.
Marine biotoxins, new foods, and drugs from the sea. In: Drugs From the Sea. Transactions of the Drugs From the Sea Symposium, University of Rhode Island, 27-29 August 1967. Marine Technology Society, Washington, D.C. pp. 229-239.

(122) Halstead, B.W.
Marine biotoxins, world food supply, and the need for an international surveillance program. Presented to: Consultants on the Problems of Toxicants in Marine Food Products, World Health Organization, Geneva, 18-22 Nov. 1968. 6 p. (Limited distribution)

(123) Halstead, B.W.
New drugs from the sea - the state of the art. Presented to: Oceanography as an Investment, 2nd/ Annual Conference, 2-4 December 1968. 12 p.

(124) Halstead, B.W.
Powerful poisons in marine organisms - a factor in using foods from the sea. Maritime 2:5-6,10.

(125) Halstead, B.W.
The significance of marine biotoxins to marine protein concentrates and food from the sea. Presented to: Seminar on Ichthyosarcotoxism, South Pacific Commission, French Polynesia, 16-22 August 1968. 21 p. (Limited distribution)

(126) Der Marderosian, A.H., Youngken, H.W., Jr., and B.W. Halstead
An outline for a new course in marine pharmacognosy. Am. J. Pharm. Educ. 32:219-245, 3 figs.

(127) Rice, R.D. and B.W. Halstead
Report of fatal cone shell sting by *Conus geographus* Linnaeus. Toxicon 5:223-224.

**1969**

(128) Halstead, B.W.
Dangerous marine animals. Text for proposed book by Doug Falkner. 9 p. (Unpublished).

(129) Halstead, B.W.
Dangerous marine animals. Unit 16-B. Supplement to Naval Medical School Kinescope Film No. HA-PMB-722. U.S. Naval Medical School, National Naval Medical Center, Bethesda, MD. 14 p.

(130) Halstead, B.W.
Hazardous marine life. In: J.J. Meyers, C.H. Holm and R.F. McAllister, [Eds.], Handbook of Ocean and Underwater Engineering. McGraw-Hill Book Co., New York. Pp. 10/23-10/44.

(131) Halstead, B.W.
Marine biodynamic chemicals - a neglected resource. Congressional Record, 2 October 1969. pp. E8090-E8092.

(132) Halstead, B.W.
Marine biotoxins: A new source of medicinals. Lloydia 32(4):484-488.
(133) Halstead, B.W.
Ocean resources and marine biomedicine. Congressional Record, 3 June 1969. 115(91):E4568-E4570.
(134) Halstead, B.W.
The sea—source of life-giving substances. 13 p. (Limited distribution)
(135) Halstead, B.W.
The significance of marine biotoxins to marine protein concentrates and food from the sea. Restricted communication to President's Commission on Marine Science, Engineering and Resources for preparation of: Our Nation and the Sea. U.S. Government Printing Office, Washington, D.C. 21 p.
(136) Halstead, B.W.
Statement regarding the recommendation for the establishment of a National Institute of Marine Medicine and Pharmacology. In: Hearing before the subcommittee on merchant marine fisheries. House of Representatives. U.S. Government Printing Office, Washington, D.C. (No. 91-5). pp. 465-486.
(137) Halstead, B.W.
Toxicology of marine animals. In: F.E. Firth, [Ed.], Encyclopedia of Marine Resources. Van Nostrand Reinhold Co., New York. pp. 675-687, 13 figs.
(138) Rathjen, W.E. and B.W. Halstead
Report on two fatalities due to sting-rays. Toxicon 6:301-302.

**1970**

(139) Halstead, B.W.
Dangerous marine animals. [In Russian]; Hydrometerological Publishers, Leningrad, U.S.S.R. 160 p., illust.
(140) Halstead, B.W.
Investigations on fish poisoning. Caribbean Fishery Development Project (Phase 2), Food and Agriculture Organization of the United States (FI: SF/CAR. Reg. 189). 16 p.
(141) Halstead, B.W.
Pharmacological testing of blue-green algae for constituents having therapeutic value. In: Water Pollution Control Research Series. U.S. Government Printing Office, Washington, D.C. (No. 5501-0123) 13 p.
(142) Halstead, B.W.
Poisonous and Venomous Marine Animals of the World. U.S. Government Printing Office, Washington, D.C. Vol. 3, 1006 p., illust.
(143) Halstead, B.W.
Recommendations to the President's commission on marine science, engineering, and resources for a national program in marine biomedicine. In: H.W. Youngken, Jr., [Ed.], Food-Drugs From the Sea. Marine Technology Society, Washington, D.C. pp. 11-21.
(144) Halstead, B.W.
Toxicity of marine organisms caused by pollutants. Presented to: FAO Technical Conference on Marine Pollution and Its Effect on Living Resources and Fishing, 9-18 December 1970. Food and Agriculture Organization of the United Nations, FIR: MP/70/R-6 (WM/ A8087). 21 p.
(145) Halstead, B.W. and D.D. Danielson
Death from the depths. Oceans 3(6):14-25, illust.

(146) Halstead, B.W.
Human fatality due to ingestion of the crab *Demania* sp. in the Philippines. Clin. Toxicol. 3(4):609-611.

(147) Bagnis, R., Berglund, F., Elias, P.S., Van Esch, G.J., Halstead, B.W., and K. Kojima.
Problems of toxicants in marine food products. 1. Marine biotoxins. Bull. WHO 42:69-88. (Written by B.W.H.)

(148) Cooke, T.S. and B.W. Halstead
Report of stingings by coelenterate *Rhizophysa eysenhardti* Gegenbaur in California waters. Clin. Toxicol. 3(4):589-595, 5 figs.

(149) Levy, S., Masry, D., and B.W. Halstead
Report of stingings by the sea anemone *Triactis producta* Kluzinger from Red Sea. Clin. Toxicol. 3(4):637-643, 4 figs.

(150) Mote, G.E., Halstead, B.W., and Y. Hashimoto
Occurrence of toxic crabs in the Palau Islands. Clin. Toxicol. 3(4):597-607, 3 figs.

**1971**

(151) Halstead, B.W.
Cancer & other abnormalities in fish. In: Water Pollution, Fish Disease, & Human Health. Hearing before the Subcommittee on Fisheries & Wildlife Conservation of the Committee on Merchant Marine Fisheries, House of Representatives, 91st/ Congress, Ser. No. 91-42. U.S. Government Printing Office, Washington, D.C. pp. 351-409 (355-363, 404-405).

(152) Halstead, B.W.
Drugs from the sea. This is Japan (18):45-46.

(153) Halstead, B.W.
Marine pollution and human health. California Med. 115(6):61-62.

(154) Halstead, B.W.
Pollution problems relating to oil drilling on the Great Barrier Reef. Presented to: The Australian Royal Commission's Hearings on Oil Drilling on the Great Barrier Reef, Brisbane, 21-22 June 1971. (Unpublished, but included in the official proceedings of the hearings)

(155) Halstead, B.W.
The sting of the sea. Emerg. Med. 3(7):64-79.

(156) Halstead, B.W.
Toxicological aspects of marine pollution. Presented to: GESAMP, Report No. 3, Rome, 22-27 February 1971. 15 p.

(157) Halstead, B.W.
Venomous coelenterates: hydroids, jellyfishes, corals,and sea anemones. In: W. Bucherl, E. Buckley, and V. Deulofeu, [Eds.], Venomous Animals and Their Venoms. Academic Press, New York. 3:395-417,10 figs.

(158) Halstead, B.W.
Venomous echinoderms and annelids: Starfishes, sea urchins, sea cucumbers, and segmented worms. In: W. Bucherl, E. Buckley, and V. Deulofeu, [Eds.], Venomous Animals and Their Venoms. Academic Press, New York. 3:419-441, 10 figs.

(159) Halstead, B.W.
Venomous fishes. In: W. Bucherl, E. Buckley, and V. Deulofeu, [Eds.], Venomous Animals and Their Venoms. Academic Press, New York. 2:587-626, 22 figs.

(160) Halstead, B.W., and L. Halstead Baldwin
Mistress of mankind. Skin Diver 20(3):14-17.

(161) Halstead, B.W., and K.J. Beukema
Proposal for the establishment of a natural products institute for the economic development of underdeveloped countries. Presented to: Marine Technology Society, Washington, D.C. 21 p. (Limited distribution)

(162) Halstead, B.W., Engen, P.C., and D.D. Danielson
Morphology of the venom organs of the rabbitfishes (family Teuthidae). In: A. de Vies and E. Kochva, [Eds.], Toxins of Animal and Plant Origin. Tel-Avis University. 1:121-157, 29 figs.

(163) Cooke, T.S. and B.W. Halstead
Errata to: Report of stingings by the coelenterate, *Rhizophysa eysenhardti* Gegenbaur, in California waters (Clin. Toxicol. 3(4):589-595). Clin. Toxicol. 4(2):302.

(164) Hansen, P.A. and B.W. Halstead
The venomous sea anemone *Actinodendron plumosum* Haddon of South Vietnam. Micronesia 7(1/2):123-136, 5 figs.

**1972**

(165) Halstead, B.W.
Final report: Monograph on poisonous plants of the world. National Library of Medicine, National Institutes of Health, Grant No. 5 (RO1-LM-00072-05). 15 p. (Limited distribution)

(166) Halstead, B.W.
A golden guide to environmental organizations. Golden Press, New York. 63 p.

(167) Halstead, B.W.
Pharmaceuticals from the sea. New Scient. 56(823):564-567.

(168) Halstead, B.W.
Toxicity of marine organisms caused by pollutants. In: M. Ruivo, [Ed.], Marine Pollution and Sea Life. Fishing News (Books) Ltd., London. pp. 584-594.

(169) Halstead, B.W.
A working paper on the surveillance of biotoxins in marine food products. Presented to: GESAMP, Geneva. 31 p. (Limited distribution)

(170) Halstead, B.W. and L. Halstead Baldwin
Mares envenendados? [In Spanish]; Salud Mundial (May):16-21.

(171) Halstead, B.W. and L. Halstead Baldwin
O mar - sinais de perigo para o homem. [In Portuguese]; A Saude Do Mundo (May):16-21.

(172) Halstead, B.W., and L. Halstead Baldwin
The sea - danger signals for man. [In Russian]; Zdrovie Mira (May):16-21.

(173) Halstead, B.W., Danielson, D.D., Baldwin, W.J., and P.C. Engen
Morphology of the venom apparatus of the leatherback fish *Scomberoides sanctipetri* (Cuvier). Toxicon 10:249-258, 5 figs.

(174) Halstead, B.W. and L. Halstead Baldwin
Die meere - Gefahrensignale fur den menschen. [In German]; Weltgesundheit (May):16-21.

(175) Halstead, B.W. and L. Halstead Baldwin
Le danger qui viet de la mer. [In French]; Sante du Monde (May):16-21.

(176) Halstead, B.W. and L. Halstead Baldwin
The sea, danger signals for man. World Health (May):16-21.

(177) Roche, E.T. and B.W. Halstead
The venom apparatus of California rockfishes (family Scorpaenidae). California Department of Natural Resources, Division of Fish and Game, Fish Bulletin 156. 49 p., 45 figs.

**1973**

(178) Halstead, B.W.
Aquatic resources. Diving World 1(4):189-191.

(179) Halstead, B.W.
Concept of toxicity indicator profiles. Presented to: GESAMP as a World Health Organization Consultant. 4 p. (Limited distribution)

(180) Halstead, B.W.
Death from the sea. Life Health 88(5):18-20, 7 figs.

(181) Halstead, B.W.
Marine pollution and the pharmaceutical scientist. Am. J. Pharm. Educ. 37:267-275.

(182) Halstead, B.W.
Portuguese man-of-war stings. In: H.F. Conn, [Ed.], Current Therapy. W. B. Saunders, Co., Philadelphia. pp. 870.

(183) Halstead, B.W.
Sea of death. 30 p. (Limited distribution)

(184) Halstead, B.W., and K.W. Cox
A fatal case of poisoning by the red spotted crab *Carpilius maculatus* (Linnaeus) in Mauritius. Proc. Roy. Soc. Arts Sci. Mauritius 4(2):27-30, 1 pl.

(185) Halstead, B.W., and K.W. Cox
An investigation on fish poisoning in Mauritius. Proc. Roy. Soc. Arts Sci. Mauritius 4(2)1-26, 4 pls.

**1974**

(186) Halstead, B.W.
Chelation Therapy. Life and Health Medical Group, Loma Linda, CA. 10 p.

(187) Halstead, B.W.
Chelation Therapy. World Life Research Institute, Colton. 7 p. (Limited distribution)

(188) Halstead, B.W.
Dorland's Illustrated Medical Dictionary (Consultant). 25th ed. W. B. Saunders Co., Philadelphia. 1748 p.

(189) Halstead, B.W.
Marine biotoxicology. In: F. Coulston, [Ed.], Global Aspects of Chemistry, Toxicology and Technology as Applied to the Environment: Environmental Quality and Safety. Academic Press, New York. 3:212-239.

(190) Halstead, B.W.
Marine biotoxins - an important group of environmental poisons. Presented to: First World Congress on Environmental Medicine and Biology, UNESCO, Paris, 1-5 July 1974. 19 p. (Limited distribution)

(191) Halstead, B.W.
Portuguese man-of-war stings. In: H.F. Conn, [Ed.], Current Therapy. W. B. Saunders Co., Philadelphia. pp. 867.

**1975**

(192) Halstead, B.W.
Poisonous animals and plants. In: Encyclopedia Britannica, 15th ed. 14:606-616, 6 pls.

(193) Halstead, B.W.
Chelation Therapy. Life Force, Inc., San Bernardino, CA. 14 p.

(194) Halstead, B.W.
Chelation Therapy. Life and Health Medical Group, Loma Linda, CA. 11 p. (Revised)

(195) Halstead, B.W.
A dying sea. Presented to: California State Legislature - Resources and Land Committee, State Capitol, Sacramento, 10 March 1975. 13 p. (Limited distribution)

(196) Halstead, B.W.
Poisonous and venomous marine animals. In: The Ocean World of Jacques Cousteau. Danbury Press, New York. 20:54-71.

(197) Halstead, B.W., and H.W. Harper
Evaluation of EDTA chelation therapy in coronary occlusive disease - clinical protocol. 14 p. (Unpublished)

(198) Halstead, B.W. and B.L. Landa
Tropical Fish. Golden Press, New York. 160 p., illust.

(199) Halstead, B.W.
Toxic Fish and Mollusks. Information Bulletin No. 12. Air Training Command. Environmental Information Division. Maxwell Air Force, Alabama. (Info. Used in this bulletin is Dr. Halstead's three-volume work on *Poisonous and Venemous Marine Animals of the World*).

**1976**

(200) Halstead, B.W.
Biotoxins: The poisons of life. In: 1977 Yearbook of Science and the Future. Encyclopedia Britannica, Inc., Chicago. pp. 220-233.

(201) Halstead, B.W.
Chelation Therapy. Life and Health Medical Group, Redlands, CA. 14 p.

(202) Halstead, B.W.
Dangerous sea creatures (Consultant). In: T.A. Dozier, Wild, Wild World of Animals. Time Life Films, New York. 128 p., illust.

(203) Halstead, B.W.
Hazardous marine life. In: R. Strauss, [Ed.], Diving Medicine. Grune and Stratton, New York. pp. 227-256, 9 figs.

(204) Halstead, B.W.
Health maintenance program - general information circular. Life and Health Medical Group, Redlands, CA. 5 p.

(205) Halstead, B.W.
Hyperbaric oxygen therapy. Life and Health Medical Group, Redlands, CA. 10 p.

(206) Halstead, B.W.
Hyperbaric Oxygen Therapy. Golden Quill Publishers, Inc., Colton, CA. 26 p., 2 figs. (Revised)

(207) Halstead, B.W.
Shellfish emotionalism. Clin. Toxicol. 9(1):1-2.

(208) Halstead, B.W.
Use of chelating agents in heavy metal poisoning. Presented to: Proceeding of the 1st International Symposium on Industrial Wastes and Environment, Caracas, Venezuela, 14-19 November 1976. 35 p. (Limited distribution)

(209) Scharffenberg, R.S., Scharffenberg, M.D., and B.W. Halstead
EDTA chelation literature. Author index, 81 p. Subject index, 57 p. American Academy of Medical Preventics, North Hollywood, CA.

(210) Halstead, B.W.
Edible and Hazardous Marine Life. Air Training Command. Environmental Information Division. Maxwell Air Force Base, Alabama. (Advice and photos support by B.W. Halstead).

**1977**

(211) Halstead, B.W.
Amygdalin fact sheet. 11 p. (Unpublished)

(212) Halstead, B.W.
Amygdalin (Laetrile) routine - clinical protocol. 4 p. (Unpublished)

(213) Halstead, B.W.
Amygdalin (Laetrile) Therapy. Choice Publications, Inc., Los Altos. 47 p.

(214) Halstead, B.W.
Biochemical basis of EDTA - chelation therapy. Presented to: Health Care Horizons Seminar, American International Hospital, Zion. 72 p.

(215) Halstead, B.W.
Biotoxins from the oceans of the world as a source of new pharmaceutical agents. Drug Information Bulletin, College of Pharmacy, University of Cincinnati. (Abstract only)

(216) Halstead, B.W.
Chelation therapy explained by Life-Health group. Redlands Facts, Area News, Peoples Column, January. 1 p.

(217) Halstead, B.W.
Portuguese man-of-war (jellyfish) stings. In: H.F. Conn,[Ed.], Current Therapy. W. B. Saunders Co., Philadelphia. pp. 925.

**1978**

(218) Halstead, B.W.
Amygdalin (Laetrile) Therapy. Golden Quill Publishers, Inc., Colton, CA. 47 p. (Revised)

(219) Halstead, B.W.
Bioecological aspects: Ecological biogenesis of paralytic shellfish poisoning, Preliminary Report. Presented to: World Health Organization Paralytic Shellfish Poisoning Conference, West Berlin, 5-8 December 1978. 5 p. (Limited distribution)

(220) Halstead, B.W.
Dangerous marine animals. In: Handbook of Zoo and Aquarium Keepers - The Prevention of Keeper's Accidents by Animals. [In Japanese]; Japan Zoo Aquarium Association. pp. 67-84.

(221) Halstead, B.W.
Dangerous Marine Animals. Cornell Maritime Press, Centreville. 208 p., 16 pls., 110 figs. (Revised)

(222) Halstead, B.W.
Gerovital (Procaine) Therapy. Golden Quill Publishers, Inc., Colton, CA. 9 p.

(223) Halstead, B.W.
Gerovital (Procaine) Therapy. Golden Quill Publishers, Inc., Colton. 19 p. (Revised)

(224) Halstead, B.W.
Hyperbaric oxygen therapy. J. No. W. Acad. Prev. Med. 2(1):10-13.

(225) Halstead, B.W.
Life-giving substances from the sea - an untapped biomedical resource. In: Proposal to the People's Republic of China for a joint Chinese-American Helicopter Conquest of Oomolangma Feng (Mt. Everest). William Hall Group, March 1978. 20 p. (Limited distribution)

(226) Halstead, B.W.
Metabolic Cancer Therapy. Golden Quill Publishers, Inc., Colton, CA. 19 p.

(227) Halstead, B.W.
Poisonous and Venomous Marine Animals of the World. The Darwin Press, Inc., Princeton. Rev. ed., 1043 p., illust.

(228) Halstead, B.W.
Portuguese man-of-war (jellyfish) stings. In: H.F. Conn, [Ed.], Current Therapy. W. B. Saunders Co., Philadelphia. pp. 881.

(229) Halstead, B.W.
Procurement of crude pharmaceutical products. Presented to: Undersea Medical Society Symposium on New Drugs From the Sea. 11 p. (Limited distribution)

(230) Halstead, B.W.
Toxicological aspects and detection of the toxin(s). Presented to: World Health Organization Paralytic Shellfish Poisoning Conference, West Berlin, 5-8 December 1978. 1 p. (Limited distribution)

(231) Halstead, B.W.
Toxicological aspects of marine pollution. Eff. Water. Treatment J. 11(12):671-673.

(232) Halstead, B.W.
World Life Research Institute Brochure. World Life Research Institute, Colton. 12 p.

(233) Halstead, B.W., Engen, P.C., and A.T. Tu
The venom and venom apparatus of the sea snake *Lapemis hardwicki* Gray. Zool. J. Linnean Soc. 63(4):371-396, 17 figs.

(234) McCabe, M.J., Hammon, W.M., Halstead, B.W., and T.H. Newton
A fatal brain injury caused by a needlefish. Neuroradiology 15:137-139, 3 figs.

**1979**

(235) Halstead, B.W.
America's health fraud. The Mature Am.:10-11.

(236) Halstead, B.W.
Chelation therapy. Rev. ed. Golden Quill Pub., Colton, CA. 22 p.

(237) Halstead, B.W.
Chelation therapy notebook. Public Scrutiny (7):7,9.

(238) Halstead, B.W.
Contributor - Report of the World Health Organization expert consultation on paralytic shellfish poisoning, 5-8 December 1978, West Berlin, Germany. WHO, Final Report. 15 p.

(239) Halstead, B.W.
Contributor - Report of the World Health Organization expert consultation on paralytic shellfish poisoning, 5-8 December 1978, West Berlin, Germany. WHO, Preliminary Report. 15 p. [In Japanese].

(240) Halstead, B.W.
Contributor - Report of the World Health Organization expert consultation on paralytic shellfish poisoning, 5-8 December 1978, West Berlin, Germany. WHO, Final Report. 15 p. [In Japanese].

(241) Halstead, B.W.
Podiatrists alerted to beach stings. Podiatry News 17(2):1,4.

(242) Halstead, B.W.
The Scientific Basis of EDTA Chelation Therapy. Golden Quill Publishers, Inc., Colton, CA. 113 p., 15 figs.

(243) Halstead, B.W.
The toxicology of amygdalin (Laetrile). In: R. W. Bradford and M. L. Culbert, [Eds.], The Metabolic Management of Cancer. Robert W. Bradford Foundation, Los Altos, CA. pp. 63-68.

(244) Halstead, B.W.
The use of cyanogenic glycoside amygdalin in the treatment of cancer. Presented to: The 14th Pacific Science Congress, Khabarovsk, U.S.S.R., 20 August – 5 Sept. 1979. 17 p. (Limited distribution).

**1980**

(245) Halstead, B.W.
The cancer "cure". 16 p. (Limited distribution)

(246) Halstead, B.W.
Dangerous Marine Animals. 2nd ed. Cornell Maritime Press, Centreville, MD. 208 p., 16 pls., 110 figs.

(247) Halstead, B.W.
Hyperbaric Oxygen Therapy. Golden Quill Publishers, Inc., Colton, CA. 26 p., 2 figs. (Revised)

(248) Halstead, B.W.
Metabolic Cancer Therapy. Golden Quill Publishers, Inc., Colton, CA. 28 p. (Revised)

(249) Halstead, B.W.
Two routes of medicine. Chem. Sci. 8:35-36. [In Russian].

(250) Halstead, B.W., and L.L. Hood
Need for the translation of the Pen Ts'ao Kang Mu, the great herbal of China. Bull. Orient. Heal. Arts Inst. 5(7):19-43.

(251) Halstead, B.W.
*Eleutherococcus* has a tremendous future! Chemistry & Life:40.

**1981**

(252) Halstead, B.W.
Chelation Therapy. Golden Quill Publishers, Inc., Colton, CA. 29 p. (Revised)

(253) Halstead, B.W.
Current status of marine biotoxicology - an overview. Clin. Toxicol. 18(1)1-24.

(254) Halstead, B.W.
Portuguese man-of-war (jellyfish) stings. In: H.F. Conn,[Ed.], Current Therapy. W. B. Saunders Co., Philadelphia. pp. 991-992.

(255) Halstead, B.W.
Preface. In: J.M. Hoffman, The Missing Link. Professional Press Publishing Co., Valley Center. 424 p.

(256) Halstead, B.W., and S.A. Youngberg
The DMSO Handbook. Golden Quill Publishers, Inc., Colton, CA. 130 p.

**1982**

(257) Halstead, B.W.
Immune augmentation therapy. Anabolism 1(3):7-8.

(258) Halstead, B.W.
Now you can use DMSO for a healthier life. Mod. Health Rep. 14:1-8.

(259) Halstead, B.W.
Stings of the sea. Emerg. Med. 14(13):183-210.

(260) Auerbach, P.S. and B.W. Halstead
Marine hazards: Attacks and envenomations. J. Emerg. Nursing 8(3):115-122.

(261) Williams, D.R., and B.W. Halstead
Medical progress review: Chelating agents in medicine. J. Clin. Toxicol. 19(10):1081-1115.

**1983**

(262) Auerbach, P.S. and B.W. Halstead
Hazardous marine life. In: Auerbach, P. S. and E. C. Geeher, [Eds.], Management of Wilderness and Environmental Emergencies. Macmillan Publ. Co., New York. pp. 213-259.

(263) Halstead, B.W. and L.L. Hood
Amazon house call. Dolphin Log (December):12-13.

(264) Halstead, B.W. and L.L. Hood
Siberian ginseng: New hope for the hopelessly tired. Let's Live 51(12):68-71.

(265) Halstead, B.W., and L.L. Hood
Marine drugs: New hope from the sea. Aquasphere 17(2):2-7.

**1984**

(266) Halstead, B.W. and E.J. Schantz
Intoxicacion paralitica por mariscos. [In Spanish]; World Health Organization, Geneva, Switzerland. Offset Publication No. 79. 60 p.

(267) Halstead, B.W. and E.J. Schantz
L' intoxication paralytique par fruits de mer. [In French]; World Health Organization, Geneva, Switzerland. Offset Publication No. 79. 60 p.

(268) Halstead, B.W. and E.J. Schantz
Paralytic shellfish poisoning. World Health Organization, Geneva, Switzerland. Offset Publication No. 79. 60 p.

(269) Halstead, B.W. and J.G. Defares
Kleine gids voor de chelatietherapie. [In Dutch]; Centre Orthomoleculaire, Boerhaavelaan 8, Leiden, Holland. 64 p.

(270) Halstead, B.W. and L.L. Hood
Natural methods to enhance immunity. Bull. Orient. Heal. Arts Inst. 9(8):371-421.

(271) Halstead, B.W., and L.L. Hood
*Eleutherococcus senticosus* Siberian ginseng: An introduction to the concept of adaptogenic medicine. Oriental Healing Arts Institute, Long Beach, CA. 94 p.

(272) Halstead, B.W.
Miscellaneous seafood toxicants. In: E.P. Ragelis [Ed.], Seafood Toxins, American Chemical Society, Washington, D.C. pp. 37-51.

**1985**

(273) Halstead, B.W.
Coelenterate stings: Hydroids, jellyfishes, sea anemones, coral cuts, and their treatment. In: Edlich, R. F. and D. A. Spyker, [Eds.], Current Emergency Therapy, Aspen Systems Corp., Rockville. Pp. 827-834.

(274) Halstead, B.W.
Immune augmentation therapy. J. Int. Acad. Prev. Med. 9(1):5-19.

**1986**

(275) Halstead, B.W.
AIDS genetically engineered? Freedom Fighter (January):1-12.

(276) Halstead, B.W.
Our pollution is destroying us. Voice of the People, The San Bernardino Sun (Sunday, August 31):I4

(277) Halstead, B.W.
The present status of traditional oriental medicine in the U.S.A. In: Proceedings of 4th International Congress of Oriental Medicine, 19-21 October 1986, Kyoto, Japan. pp. 56-61.

**1987**

(278) Halstead, B.W.
Tire-burning plant. Voice of the People, San Bernardino Sun (Sunday, January 18):D3.

(279) Halstead, B.W.
Coelenterate (Cnidarian) stings and wounds. In: R. M. Mandojana, [Ed.], Clinics in Dermatology. 5(3):8-13.

(280) Halstead, B.W., and J.M. Vinci
Venomous fish stings (Ichthyoacanthotoxicoses). In: R. M. Mandojana, [Ed.], Clinics in Dermatology. 5(3):29-35.

(281) Halstead, B.W.
AIDS, cancer, radiation will wreck 'orthodox' medicine in U.S., lead to needed health reform. The Choice 13(2):14-15.

**1988**

(282) Halstead, B.W. and J.M. Vinci
Biology of poisonous and venomous marine animals. In: A. T. Tu [Ed.], Marine Toxins and Venoms: Handbook of Natural Toxins. Marcel Dekker, Inc., New York. 3:1-30.

(283) Halstead, B.W.
Radiation sickness, AIDS, and cancer. Quantum Med. 1(1,2):120-127.

(284) Halstead, B.W.
Poisonous and Venomous Marine Animals of the World. 2nd rev. ed. Darwin Press, Inc., Princeton. 1168 p., illust.

**1989**

(285) Halstead, B.W.
Secondary immune deficiency disorders and the use of Chinese traditional herbs in AIDS. In: B.C. Enger and E.R. Long, [Eds.], AIDS Immunity and Chinese Medicine. Oriental Healing Arts Institute, Long Beach, CA. pp. 28-34.

(286) Auerbach, P.S. and B.W. Halstead
Hazardous aquatic life. In: Auerbach, P. S. and E. C. Geehr, [Eds.], Management of Wilderness and Environmental Emergencies. 2nd ed. C.V. Mosby Co., St. Louis. pp. 933-1028.

(287) Halstead, B.W.
Introduction. In: M.L. Culbert, Aids, Hope, Hoax, and Hoopla. The Bradford Foundation, Chula Vista, CA. 9 p.

**1990**

(288) Halstead, B.W., Auerbach, P., and D. Campbell
Colour Atlas of Dangerous Marine Animals. Wolfe Medical Publishing, Ltd., London, England. 192 p.

(289) Halstead, B.W., and C.L. Foster
Drugs from the sea. Chinese J. Mar. Drugs. 9(1):1-32.

(290) Halstead, B.W.
Introduction. In: M.L. Culbert, AIDS, Hope, Hoax, and Hoopla, 1990's Updated ed. The Bradford Foundation, Chula Vista. 8 p.

**1991**

(291) Halstead, B.W.
State wastes water. Voice of the People, The San Bernardino Sun (Sunday, April 9).

(292) Halstead, B.W.
Free radical pathology and its immunological consequences: Free radical pathology. J. Adv. Med. 4(2):93-105.

(293) Halstead, B.W.
Free radical pathology and its immunological consequences: Adaptogenic nutrition. J. Adv. Med. 4(3):167-184.

**1992**

(294) Halstead, B.W. and R.L. Haddock
A fatal outbreak of poisoning from the ingestion of red seaweed *Gracilaria tsuda* in Guam - Review of the oral marine biotoxicity problem. J. Nat. Tox. 1(1): 87-115

(295) Halstead, B.W.
Dangerous Aquatic Animals of the World: A Color Atlas. Darwin Press. Princeton, NJ. 284 p.

(296) Halstead, B.W., Foster, C. L., et al.
Cuban marine algae as sources of potent antiherpetic and anticholinesterase metabolites. Nat. Tox. 1(2):39-45.

**1993**

(297) Halstead, B.W. and L.L. Hood
Poisonous and Venomous Marine Animals and Plants of Southern Asia. In: Toxin-Related Diseases. Poisons Originating From Plants, Animals, and Spoilage. [Ed.] Anthony T. Tu. Oxford & IBH Publishing Co. Pvt. Ltd., New Delhi. pp. 137-236.

**1994**

(298) Halstead, B.W.
Fish Toxins. In: Foodborne Disease Handbook, Diseases Caused By Hazardous Substances. Marcel Dekker, Inc. New York. pp 463-496.

(299) Halstead, B.W.
Other Poisonous Marine Animals. In: Foodborne Disease Handbook, Diseases Caused By Hazardous Substances. Marcel Dekker, Inc., New York. pp. 497-528.

**1995**

(300) Halstead, B.W. and P.S. Auerbach
Injuries from non-venomous aquatic animals. In: Wilderness Medicine, Management of Wilderness and Environmental Emergencies, 3rd ed. Mosby-Year Book, Inc., St. Louis, MO. pp 1303-1326.

(301) Halstead, B.W., Auerbach, P.S. and D. Campbell
Colour Atlas of Dangeous Marine Animals. (In Japanese) Wolf Medical Publishing, Ltd., London, England. 192 pgs.

(302) Halstead, B.W.
Dangerous Marine Animals. 3rd Edition. Cornell Maritime Press. Centerville, MD. 275 pgs.

**1996**

(303) Halstead, B.W.
Marine Animal Injuries. In: Conn's Current Therapy. [Ed.] R. E. Rakel. W. B. Saunders, Philadelphia. pp. 1147-1149.

**1997**

(304) Halstead, B.W. and T. C. Rozema
The Scientific Basis of EDTA Chelation Therapy. Second Edition. TRC Publishing, Landum, SC. 267 p.

**1999**

(304) Halstead, B.W.
Fossil Stony Coral Minerals and Their Nutritional Application. Health Digest Publishing Co., Cannon Beach, OR. 141 pgs.

**2000**

(306) Halstead, B.W.
Fish Toxins. In: Foodborne Disease Handbook: Volume 4: Seafood and Environmental Toxins. [Eds.] Hui, Kitts, Stanfield. Marcel Dekker, Inc., New York. pp. 23-50.

(307) Halstead, B.W.
Other Poisonous Marine Animals. In: Foodborne Disease HAndbook: Volume 4: Seafood and Environmental Toxins. [Eds.] Hui, Kitts, Stanfield. Marcel Dekker, Inc., New York. pp. 51-76.

(308) Halstead, B.W.
Marine Animal Injuries. In: Conn's Current Therapy. [Ed.] R. E. Rakel. W. B. Saunders, Philadelphia. pp. 1141-1144.

(309) Halstead, B.W. and T. C. Rozema
Marine Animal Injuries. In: Advances in Medicine. [Ed.] R. F. Edlich. ABI Professional Publications. pp. 703-715.

**2001**

(310) Halstead, B.W.
The Microbial Biogenesis of Aquatic Biotoxins. Toxicological Methods.

**Works in Progress**

(311) Halstead, B.W.
Chinese Adaptogenic Nutritional Therapy for AIDS, Cancer, and Radiation Sickness. Approx. 900 pgs.

(312) Halstead, B.W.
Medicinal and Poisonous Plants of Amazonia and Adjacent Regions.

(313) Halstead, B.W. and L. C. Medrano
United States Military Survival Manual - Dangerous Animals of the Middle East Region. Darwin Press, Princeton, NJ. Approx. 250 pgs.

(312) Halstead, B.W.
Medicinal and Poisonous Plants of Amazonia and Adjacent Regions.

(314) Halstead, B.W.
Laetrile and Cancer Politics--The Cancer Holocaust.

# Terri-Lee Holcomb Halstead

**Birthplace:**

San Bernardino, California. June 17,1952 (5th generation, Holcomb, in San Bernardino County.)

**Married:**

1988 - Bruce W. Halstead, MD

**Family:**

Daughter of W.R. Holcomb and Pearl L. Pennington Holcomb
Brothers: John Stewart (Deceased)
William W. Holcomb, Attorney at Law
Robert G. Holcomb, Teacher

**PROFESSION:**

Corporate President, Bio-Defense Nutritionals, Inc., Grand Terrace, CA
Nutritional Consultant (Training received under Dr. Bruce W. Halstead)

**PRESENT POSITIONS:**

President, Bio-Defense Nutritionals, 21891 Vivienda Avenue, Grand Terrace, CA 92313
Scientific Advisory Board in Ethnobotany, World Life Research Institute, 23000 Grand Terrace, CA 92313

**PROFESSIONAL EXPERIENCE:**

| | |
|---|---|
| 1989 – Present | President - Bio-Defense Nutritionals, Inc., Grand Terrace, CA In 1989 Terri founded Bio-Defense Nutritionals. She has since been responsible for all aspects of the companies operations. |
| 1986 - 1996 | Served as Administrator and vice-president of Rancho Mediterrania Medical Clinic (a preventive health care clinic) and Loma Linda Diagnostic Health Group. She was required to spend 30-40 hours per week in this capacity. She served under the medical directorship of Dr. Bruce Halstead. |
| 1986 - 1996 | Worked as a nutritional consultant at Rancho Mediterranea Medical Clinic. This practice dealt with chronic degenerative diseases, anti-aging, virus disorders, chronic fatigue, heart disease and general preventive health practices. |
| 1985 - 1988 | Research Assistant - World Life Research Institute, Colton, CA |
| 1984 | Pre-school Teacher - Temple Emmanuel, San Bernardino, CA |
| 1981 - 1983 | Administrative Director - Operation Second Chance, School of Opportunities, San Bernardino, CA |
| 1973 | Assistant Campaign Manager Holcomb Mayoral Campaign, San Bernardino, CA |
| 1972 | District Manager - Democratic Headquarters for McGovern Campaign, San Bernardino County, CA |

**EDUCATIONAL BACKGROUND:**

| | |
|---|---|
| 1970 | Graduated from San Gorgonio High School with honors. Also served on student council three years and was the student selected for a seven week exchange program the summer of 1969 to Tachikawa, Japan. |

1970 - 1971 Youth for Understanding, exchange program to West Berlin, Germany. Studied German culture, language, and their political system.

1971 Began undergraduate studies University of California, Santa Barbara – Political Science major.

Fall of 1972 – Fall of 1973 Political Science field work. Youth Director for George McGovern's campaign in San: Bernardino, California. Assistant campaign manager Holcomb Mayoral Campaign, San Bernardino, California.

1973 - 1977 Continued studies at the University of California, Santa Barbara (changed major to liberal studies). Completed junior year with a total of 113 credits. Began study and practice of Yoga. Also began the studies of herbal medicine, nutrition, and oriental medicine.

1981 - 1982 San Bernardino Valley College. Completed early childhood education teaching credential program.

1985 World Life Research Institute, studying ethnobotany, biochemistry, plant physiology, immunology, nutrition, oriental medicine, and several alternative clinical therapies -chelation therapy, hyperbaric oxygen therapy, among others.

1986 - 1988 San Bernardino Valley College. Pre-med course work in Biology, Chemistry, Microbiology, and Environmental Biology.

**LECTURES & PROFESSIONAL EXPERIENCE ABROAD:**

1988 Participant – Ethnobotanical Conference, Mexico City, Mexico (Feb.)

1988 Participant – 3rd International Congress of Oriental Medicine, Soeul, Korea (Sept.)

1988 Lecturer – Institute of Medicinal Plant Development, Chinese Academy of Medical Sciences, Beijing, P.R. China. (Sept.)

1989 Seminar – Institute of -Radiation Medicine, Beijing, P. R. China. (May)

1989 Lecturer – Institute of Medicinal Plant Development, Chinese Academy of Medical Sciences, Beijing, P.R. China. (May)

1989 Conference with Dr. Yan Sun, Cancer Institute, Chinese Academy of Medical Sciences, Beijing, P.R. China. (May)

1989 Seminar – Joint meeting of the Shangdong Institute of Marine Materia Medica, Institute of Marine Medicine and Food, Ocean University of Qingdao, and Editorial Department, Chinese Journal of Marine Drugs, Qingdao, P.R. China. (May)

1989 Special Guest – Lao-Shan Monastery, Quingdao, P.R. China. (May)

1989 Guest Lecturer – Naval Medical Research Institute and Hospital, Shanghai, P.R. China (May)

1989 Special Guest – Hin-wing Yeong, Director, Chinese Medicinal Material Research Center, Chinese University of Hong Kong, Hong Kong. (June)

1989 Conference with Brion Research Institute, Taiwan, P.R. China. (June)

1989 Participant – 2nd Intl. Symp. on The Entire View on Cancer and AIDS, International Inst. for Research on Metabolic Diseases and Cancer, Limassol, Cyprus. (Sept.)

1989 Participant – Expedition to Athens, Pathmos, Crete, Spetsies, and Rhodes, Greece. (October)

1989 Guest Lecturer – "Potential of Medicinal Products from the Ocean", University of Baja California, Ensenada, Mexico. (November)

1990 Guest Lecturer – 18th World Congress of Natural Medicines, Ministry of Public Health, Havana, Cuba. (April)

1990 Lecturer – University of Guadalajara, Guadalajara, Mexico. (July)

1990 Special Guest – Assistant Prime Minister, Jamaica. (July)

**PUBLICATIONS:**

Phillips, M. A. and T.L. Holcomb
1987 Chelation therapy: An alternate to bypass surgery.

Foster, C.L. Holcomb, T.L. and M.A. Phillips
1989 Chelation therapy: An alternate to bypass surgery. The Hemmitt News.

## Appendix Two

# About the Artist Robert "Bob" H. Knabenbauer

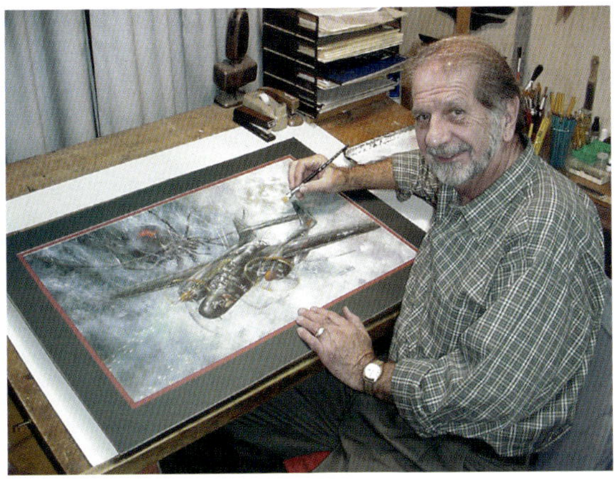

Born in Appleton, Wisconsin on March 26, 1940, Bob's family moved to Los Angeles, California when he was just three years old. From a tender age of seven, Bob knew his calling was to become an artist. After graduating from St. John Vienney High School in Los Angeles, he enrolled simultaneously in the intensive commercial art curriculum at the Los Angeles Trade Technical College and evening Adult Education classes in technical illustration. His goal was to create space illustrations, which at the time was a rare skill since the space program had not yet begun.

Bob's work experience has taken him from aviation and space to the scientific and medical fields.

- AUTONETICS, a division of North American Aviation
  Anaheim, California
  1959-1960 Technical illustration
- AEROSPACE CORPORATION
  El Segundo, California
  1960-1971 Space and industrial artist working with security clearance; received certificate of appreciation for working on the Mercury Project, the first U.S. manned flight into space; promoted to position as industrial illustrator and model maker at the San Bernardino operations facility requiring TOP SECRET clearance, lasting from mid-1960 to mid-1971.
- LOMA LINDA UNIVERSITY MEDICAL CENTER
  Loma Linda, California
  1971 - Present Chief artist and medical illustrator, working with doctors and staff doing textbook and journal artwork. This opportunity lead to numerous publication recognitions and personal experiences in surgery, with autopsies, and court cases.

Among Bob's achievements are his winnings of first place in the 1974 Association of Medical Illustrator's Convention competition showing Chelation Function (used on cover of one of Dr. Bruce Halstead's books), and second place for 3-D Modeling (in plastic) of the insect Triatoma infestans, or the kissing bug, as well as numerous awards for fine art and technical illustration.

His continued education has included years of night classes in scientific illustration and model making, industrial design and illustration, technical art, rendering techniques, fine art, forensic reconstruction, etc.

Bob first met Dr. Bruce Halstead of the World Life Research Institute while working for Aerospace Corporation in 1966 and has been illustrating his books ever since. When asked about their working relationship, Bob was quick to remark, "I first consider Bruce one of my best friends and I've learned much about biological and plant subjects from him."

Bob lives in Loma Linda, California with his wife, Sandi. He has one son, John, and one daughter, Cindy, from a prior marriage. Bob's children have given him four wonderful grandchildren and, along with Sandi's family, they enjoy a total of eleven grandchildren. Bob's hobbies include painting aviation and nautical subjects in historic settings, mostly WWII and sunken ships. He also builds and details 1/72 WWI aircraft models and wooden sailing ships, repairs damaged ceramic and pottery pieces, and enjoys wood carving.

# Index

# Other Books by Bruce W. Halstead, M.D.

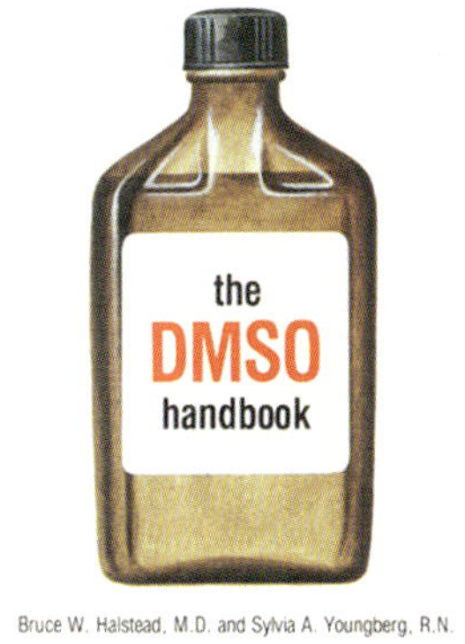


***The DMSO Handbook: A Complete Guide to the History and Use of DMSO***
by B. W. Halstead and S. A. Youngberg
Publ. by Golden Quill Publishers, Inc.
©1981

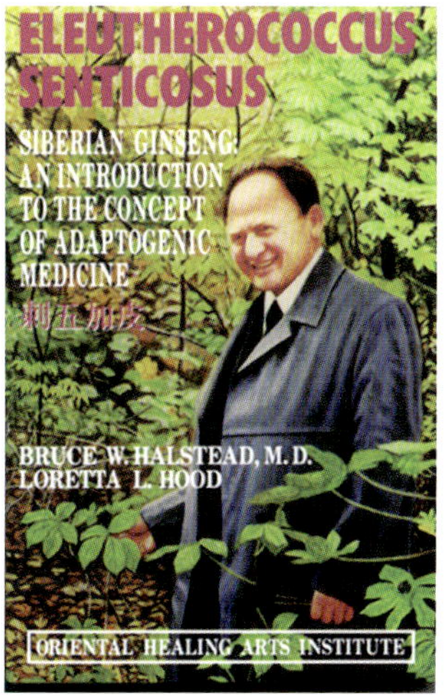


***Eleutherococcus senticossus, Siberian Ginseng: An Introduction to the Concept of Adaptogenic Medicine***
by B. W. Halstead and L. L. Hood
Publ. by Oriental Healing Arts Institute, Long Beach, CA
©1984

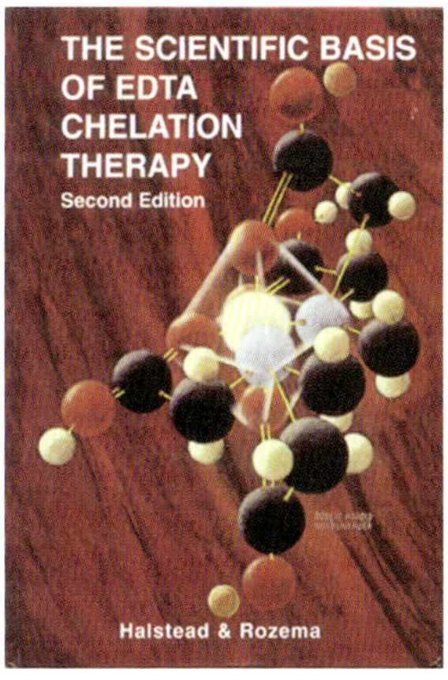


***The Scientific Basis of EDTA Chelation Therapy*, 2nd Ed.**
by B. W. Halstead and T. C. Rozema
Publ. by TRC Publishing, Landrum, SC
©1997

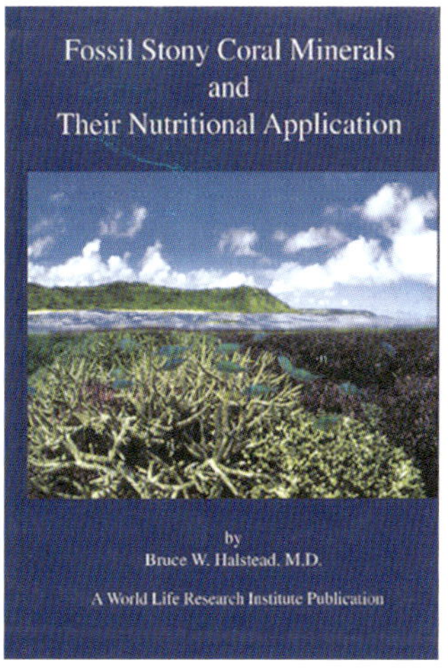


***Fossil Stony Coral Minerals and Their Nutritional Application***
by B. W. Halstead
Publ. by Health Digest Publishing Co., Cannon Beach, OR
©1999

***Dangerous Aquatic Animals of the World: A Color Atlas***
by B. W. Halstead
Publ. by The Darwin Press, Inc., Princeton, NJ
©1992

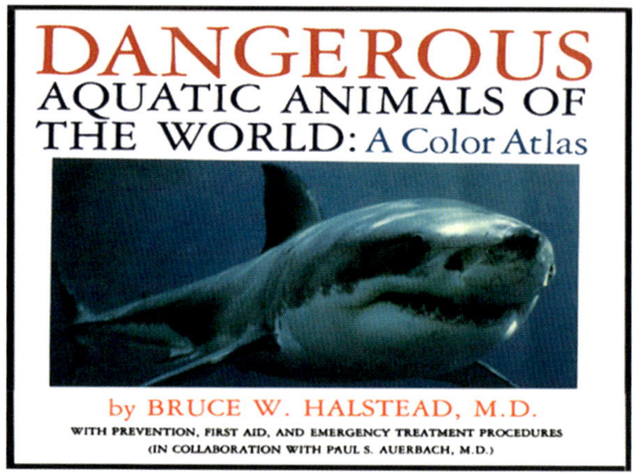


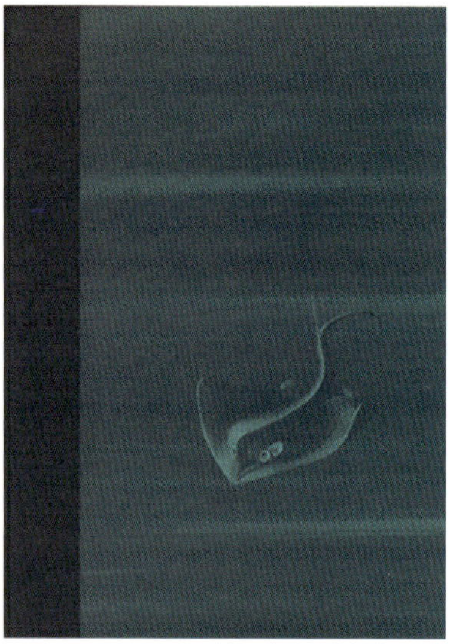

***Poisonous and Venomous Marine Animals of the World (Vol. I - III)***
by B. W. Halstead
Publ. by U.S. Govt. Printing Office
©1965

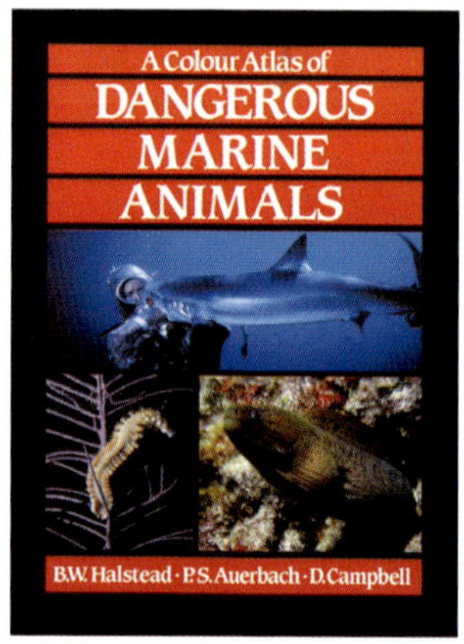


***A Colour Atlas of Dangerous Marine Animals***
by B. W. Halstead, P. S. Auerbach, D. R. Campbell
Publ. by Wolfe Medical Publications Ltd, London
©1990

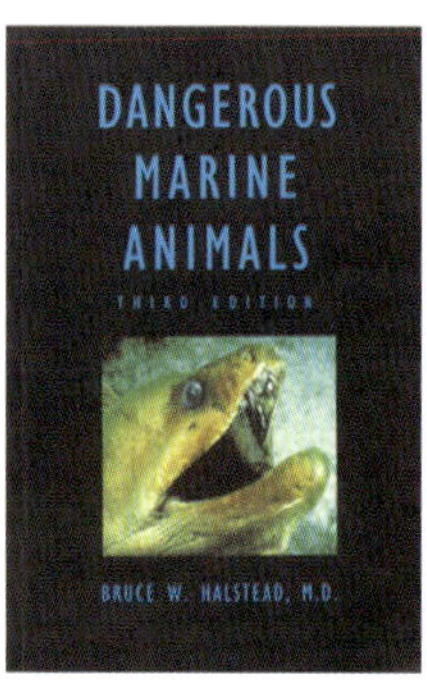


***Dangerous Marine Animals, 3rd Ed.***
by B. W. Halstead
Publ. by Cornell Maritime Press, Centreville, MD
©1995

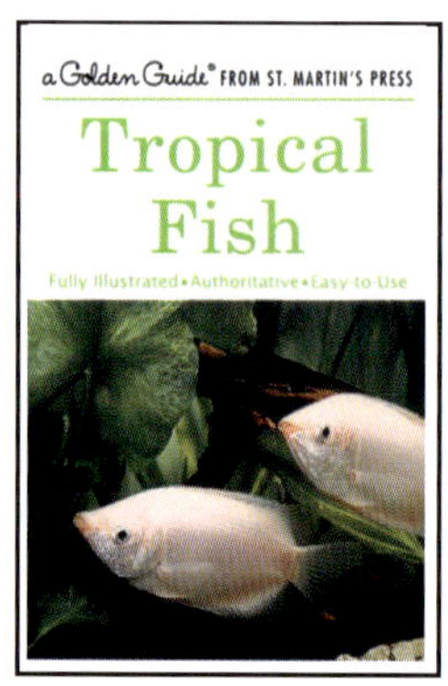


***Tropical Fish: A Guide For Setting Up and Maintaining An Aquarium for Tropical Fish and Other Animals***
by B. W. Halstead and B. L. Landa
Publ. by St. Martin's Press
©2001